# **FREE** Study Skills Videos/DVD Offer

Dear Customer,

Thank you for your purchase from Mometrix! We consider it an honor and a privilege that you have purchased our product and we want to ensure your satisfaction.

As part of our ongoing effort to meet the needs of test takers, we have developed a set of Study Skills Videos that we would like to give you for FREE. These videos cover our *best practices* for getting ready for your exam, from how to use our study materials to how to best prepare for the day of the test.

All that we ask is that you email us with feedback that would describe your experience so far with our product. Good, bad, or indifferent, we want to know what you think!

To get your FREE Study Skills Videos, you can use the **QR code** below, or send us an **email** at studyvideos@mometrix.com with *FREE VIDEOS* in the subject line and the following information in the body of the email:

- The name of the product you purchased.
- Your product rating on a scale of 1-5, with 5 being the highest rating.
- Your feedback. It can be long, short, or anything in between. We just want to know your impressions and experience so far with our product. (Good feedback might include how our study material met your needs and ways we might be able to make it even better. You could highlight features that you found helpful or features that you think we should add.)

If you have any questions or concerns, please don't hesitate to contact me directly.

Thanks again!

Sincerely,

Jay Willis
Vice President
jay.willis@mometrix.com
1-800-673-8175

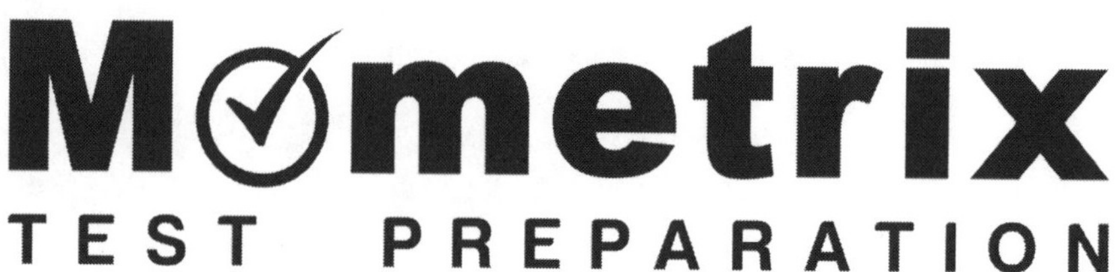

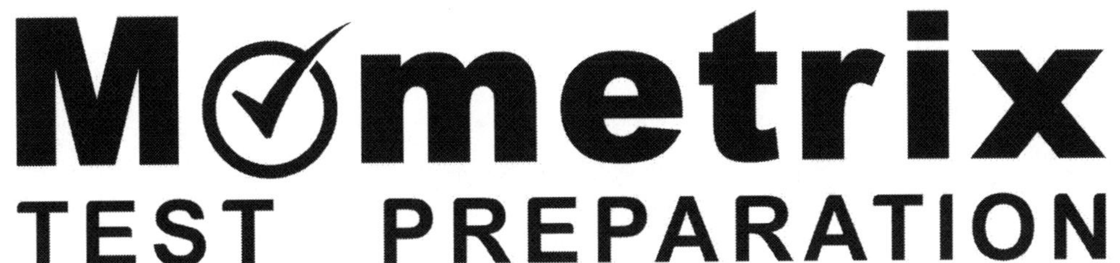


# CEN

## Study Guide 2023-2024

### CEN Exam Secrets Review Book

**Full-Length Practice Test**

**Step-by-Step Video Tutorials**

## 4th Edition

Written and edited by the Mometrix Nursing Certification Test Team

Printed in the United States of America

This paper meets the requirements of ANSI/NISO Z39.48-1992 (Permanence of Paper).



Paperback
ISBN 13: 978-1-5167-2212-9
ISBN 10: 1-5167-2212-4

# Dear Future Exam Success Story

First of all, **THANK YOU** for purchasing Mometrix study materials!

Second, congratulations! You are one of the few determined test-takers who are committed to doing whatever it takes to excel on your exam. **You have come to the right place.** We developed these study materials with one goal in mind: to deliver you the information you need in a format that's concise and easy to use.

In addition to optimizing your guide for the content of the test, we've outlined our recommended steps for breaking down the preparation process into small, attainable goals so you can make sure you stay on track.

We've also analyzed the entire test-taking process, identifying the most common pitfalls and showing how you can overcome them and be ready for any curveball the test throws you.

Standardized testing is one of the biggest obstacles on your road to success, which only increases the importance of doing well in the high-pressure, high-stakes environment of test day. Your results on this test could have a significant impact on your future, and this guide provides the information and practical advice to help you achieve your full potential on test day.

**Your success is our success**

**We would love to hear from you!** If you would like to share the story of your exam success or if you have any questions or comments in regard to our products, please contact us at **800-673-8175** or **support@mometrix.com**.

Thanks again for your business and we wish you continued success!

Sincerely,
The Mometrix Test Preparation Team

**Need more help? Check out our flashcards at:**
**http://mometrixflashcards.com/CEN**

# TABLE OF CONTENTS

# Introduction

**Thank you for purchasing this resource!** You have made the choice to prepare yourself for a test that could have a huge impact on your future, and this guide is designed to help you be fully ready for test day. Obviously, it's important to have a solid understanding of the test material, but you also need to be prepared for the unique environment and stressors of the test, so that you can perform to the best of your abilities.

For this purpose, the first section that appears in this guide is the **Secret Keys**. We've devoted countless hours to meticulously researching what works and what doesn't, and we've boiled down our findings to the five most impactful steps you can take to improve your performance on the test. We start at the beginning with study planning and move through the preparation process, all the way to the testing strategies that will help you get the most out of what you know when you're finally sitting in front of the test.

We recommend that you start preparing for your test as far in advance as possible. However, if you've bought this guide as a last-minute study resource and only have a few days before your test, we recommend that you skip over the first two Secret Keys since they address a long-term study plan.

If you struggle with **test anxiety**, we strongly encourage you to check out our recommendations for how you can overcome it. Test anxiety is a formidable foe, but it can be beaten, and we want to make sure you have the tools you need to defeat it.

# Secret Key #1 – Plan Big, Study Small

There's a lot riding on your performance. If you want to ace this test, you're going to need to keep your skills sharp and the material fresh in your mind. You need a plan that lets you review everything you need to know while still fitting in your schedule. We'll break this strategy down into three categories.

## Information Organization

Start with the information you already have: the official test outline. From this, you can make a complete list of all the concepts you need to cover before the test. Organize these concepts into groups that can be studied together, and create a list of any related vocabulary you need to learn so you can brush up on any difficult terms. You'll want to keep this vocabulary list handy once you actually start studying since you may need to add to it along the way.

## Time Management

Once you have your set of study concepts, decide how to spread them out over the time you have left before the test. Break your study plan into small, clear goals so you have a manageable task for each day and know exactly what you're doing. Then just focus on one small step at a time. When you manage your time this way, you don't need to spend hours at a time studying. Studying a small block of content for a short period each day helps you retain information better and avoid stressing over how much you have left to do. You can relax knowing that you have a plan to cover everything in time. In order for this strategy to be effective though, you have to start studying early and stick to your schedule. Avoid the exhaustion and futility that comes from last-minute cramming!

## Study Environment

The environment you study in has a big impact on your learning. Studying in a coffee shop, while probably more enjoyable, is not likely to be as fruitful as studying in a quiet room. It's important to keep distractions to a minimum. You're only planning to study for a short block of time, so make the most of it. Don't pause to check your phone or get up to find a snack. It's also important to **avoid multitasking**. Research has consistently shown that multitasking will make your studying dramatically less effective. Your study area should also be comfortable and well-lit so you don't have the distraction of straining your eyes or sitting on an uncomfortable chair.

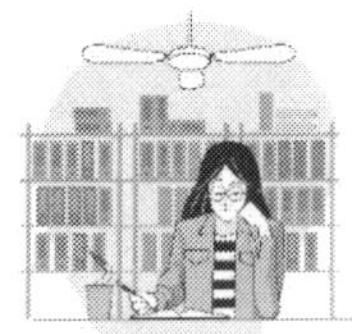

The time of day you study is also important. You want to be rested and alert. Don't wait until just before bedtime. Study when you'll be most likely to comprehend and remember. Even better, if you know what time of day your test will be, set that time aside for study. That way your brain will be used to working on that subject at that specific time and you'll have a better chance of recalling information.

Finally, it can be helpful to team up with others who are studying for the same test. Your actual studying should be done in as isolated an environment as possible, but the work of organizing the information and setting up the study plan can be divided up. In between study sessions, you can discuss with your teammates the concepts that you're all studying and quiz each other on the details. Just be sure that your teammates are as serious about the test as you are. If you find that your study time is being replaced with social time, you might need to find a new team.

# Secret Key #2 – Make Your Studying Count

You're devoting a lot of time and effort to preparing for this test, so you want to be absolutely certain it will pay off. This means doing more than just reading the content and hoping you can remember it on test day. It's important to make every minute of study count. There are two main areas you can focus on to make your studying count.

## Retention

It doesn't matter how much time you study if you can't remember the material. You need to make sure you are retaining the concepts. To check your retention of the information you're learning, try recalling it at later times with minimal prompting. Try carrying around flashcards and glance at one or two from time to time or ask a friend who's also studying for the test to quiz you.

To enhance your retention, look for ways to put the information into practice so that you can apply it rather than simply recalling it. If you're using the information in practical ways, it will be much easier to remember. Similarly, it helps to solidify a concept in your mind if you're not only reading it to yourself but also explaining it to someone else. Ask a friend to let you teach them about a concept you're a little shaky on (or speak aloud to an imaginary audience if necessary). As you try to summarize, define, give examples, and answer your friend's questions, you'll understand the concepts better and they will stay with you longer. Finally, step back for a big picture view and ask yourself how each piece of information fits with the whole subject. When you link the different concepts together and see them working together as a whole, it's easier to remember the individual components.

Finally, practice showing your work on any multi-step problems, even if you're just studying. Writing out each step you take to solve a problem will help solidify the process in your mind, and you'll be more likely to remember it during the test.

## Modality

*Modality* simply refers to the means or method by which you study. Choosing a study modality that fits your own individual learning style is crucial. No two people learn best in exactly the same way, so it's important to know your strengths and use them to your advantage.

For example, if you learn best by visualization, focus on visualizing a concept in your mind and draw an image or a diagram. Try color-coding your notes, illustrating them, or creating symbols that will trigger your mind to recall a learned concept. If you learn best by hearing or discussing information, find a study partner who learns the same way or read aloud to yourself. Think about how to put the information in your own words. Imagine that you are giving a lecture on the topic and record yourself so you can listen to it later.

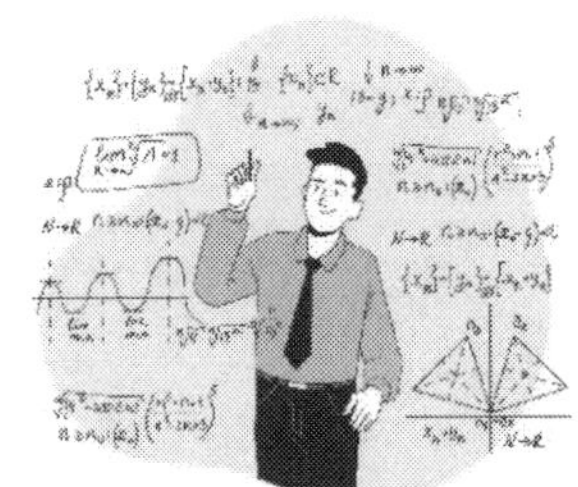

For any learning style, flashcards can be helpful. Organize the information so you can take advantage of spare moments to review. Underline key words or phrases. Use different colors for different categories. Mnemonic devices (such as creating a short list in which every item starts with the same letter) can also help with retention. Find what works best for you and use it to store the information in your mind most effectively and easily.

# Secret Key #3 – Practice the Right Way

Your success on test day depends not only on how many hours you put into preparing, but also on whether you prepared the right way. It's good to check along the way to see if your studying is paying off. One of the most effective ways to do this is by taking practice tests to evaluate your progress. Practice tests are useful because they show exactly where you need to improve. Every time you take a practice test, pay special attention to these three groups of questions:

- The questions you got wrong
- The questions you had to guess on, even if you guessed right
- The questions you found difficult or slow to work through

This will show you exactly what your weak areas are, and where you need to devote more study time. Ask yourself why each of these questions gave you trouble. Was it because you didn't understand the material? Was it because you didn't remember the vocabulary? Do you need more repetitions on this type of question to build speed and confidence? Dig into those questions and figure out how you can strengthen your weak areas as you go back to review the material.

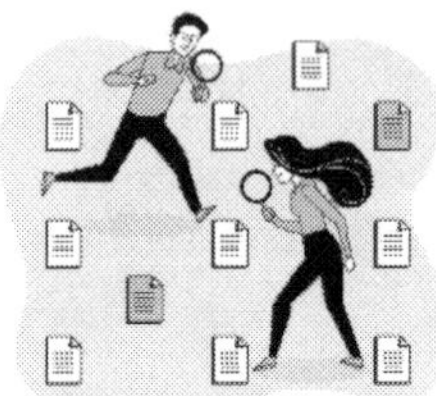

Additionally, many practice tests have a section explaining the answer choices. It can be tempting to read the explanation and think that you now have a good understanding of the concept. However, an explanation likely only covers part of the question's broader context. Even if the explanation makes perfect sense, **go back and investigate** every concept related to the question until you're positive you have a thorough understanding.

As you go along, keep in mind that the practice test is just that: practice. Memorizing these questions and answers will not be very helpful on the actual test because it is unlikely to have any of the same exact questions. If you only know the right answers to the sample questions, you won't be prepared for the real thing. **Study the concepts** until you understand them fully, and then you'll be able to answer any question that shows up on the test.

It's important to wait on the practice tests until you're ready. If you take a test on your first day of study, you may be overwhelmed by the amount of material covered and how much you need to learn. Work up to it gradually.

On test day, you'll need to be prepared for answering questions, managing your time, and using the test-taking strategies you've learned. It's a lot to balance, like a mental marathon that will have a big impact on your future. Like training for a marathon, you'll need to start slowly and work your way up. When test day arrives, you'll be ready.

Start with the strategies you've read in the first two Secret Keys—plan your course and study in the way that works best for you. If you have time, consider using multiple study resources to get different approaches to the same concepts. It can be helpful to see difficult concepts from more than one angle. Then find a good source for practice tests. Many times, the test website will suggest potential study resources or provide sample tests.

# Practice Test Strategy

If you're able to find at least three practice tests, we recommend this strategy:

## Untimed and Open-Book Practice

Take the first test with no time constraints and with your notes and study guide handy. Take your time and focus on applying the strategies you've learned.

## Timed and Open-Book Practice

Take the second practice test open-book as well, but set a timer and practice pacing yourself to finish in time.

## Timed and Closed-Book Practice

Take any other practice tests as if it were test day. Set a timer and put away your study materials. Sit at a table or desk in a quiet room, imagine yourself at the testing center, and answer questions as quickly and accurately as possible.

Keep repeating timed and closed-book tests on a regular basis until you run out of practice tests or it's time for the actual test. Your mind will be ready for the schedule and stress of test day, and you'll be able to focus on recalling the material you've learned.

# Secret Key #4 – Pace Yourself

Once you're fully prepared for the material on the test, your biggest challenge on test day will be managing your time. Just knowing that the clock is ticking can make you panic even if you have plenty of time left. Work on pacing yourself so you can build confidence against the time constraints of the exam. Pacing is a difficult skill to master, especially in a high-pressure environment, so **practice is vital**.

Set time expectations for your pace based on how much time is available. For example, if a section has 60 questions and the time limit is 30 minutes, you know you have to average 30 seconds or less per question in order to answer them all. Although 30 seconds is the hard limit, set 25 seconds per question as your goal, so you reserve extra time to spend on harder questions. When you budget extra time for the harder questions, you no longer have any reason to stress when those questions take longer to answer.

Don't let this time expectation distract you from working through the test at a calm, steady pace, but keep it in mind so you don't spend too much time on any one question. Recognize that taking extra time on one question you don't understand may keep you from answering two that you do understand later in the test. If your time limit for a question is up and you're still not sure of the answer, mark it and move on, and come back to it later if the time and the test format allow. If the testing format doesn't allow you to return to earlier questions, just make an educated guess; then put it out of your mind and move on.

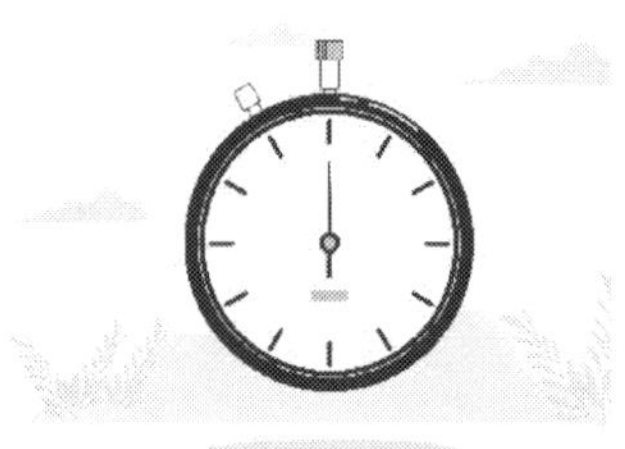

On the easier questions, be careful not to rush. It may seem wise to hurry through them so you have more time for the challenging ones, but it's not worth missing one if you know the concept and just didn't take the time to read the question fully. Work efficiently but make sure you understand the question and have looked at all of the answer choices, since more than one may seem right at first.

Even if you're paying attention to the time, you may find yourself a little behind at some point. You should speed up to get back on track, but do so wisely. Don't panic; just take a few seconds less on each question until you're caught up. Don't guess without thinking, but do look through the answer choices and eliminate any you know are wrong. If you can get down to two choices, it is often worthwhile to guess from those. Once you've chosen an answer, move on and don't dwell on any that you skipped or had to hurry through. If a question was taking too long, chances are it was one of the harder ones, so you weren't as likely to get it right anyway.

On the other hand, if you find yourself getting ahead of schedule, it may be beneficial to slow down a little. The more quickly you work, the more likely you are to make a careless mistake that will affect your score. You've budgeted time for each question, so don't be afraid to spend that time. Practice an efficient but careful pace to get the most out of the time you have.

# Secret Key #5 – Have a Plan for Guessing

When you're taking the test, you may find yourself stuck on a question. Some of the answer choices seem better than others, but you don't see the one answer choice that is obviously correct. What do you do?

The scenario described above is very common, yet most test takers have not effectively prepared for it. Developing and practicing a plan for guessing may be one of the single most effective uses of your time as you get ready for the exam.

In developing your plan for guessing, there are three questions to address:

- When should you start the guessing process?
- How should you narrow down the choices?
- Which answer should you choose?

## When to Start the Guessing Process

Unless your plan for guessing is to select C every time (which, despite its merits, is not what we recommend), you need to leave yourself enough time to apply your answer elimination strategies. Since you have a limited amount of time for each question, that means that if you're going to give yourself the best shot at guessing correctly, you have to decide quickly whether or not you will guess.

Of course, the best-case scenario is that you don't have to guess at all, so first, see if you can answer the question based on your knowledge of the subject and basic reasoning skills. Focus on the key words in the question and try to jog your memory of related topics. Give yourself a chance to bring the knowledge to mind, but once you realize that you don't have (or you can't access) the knowledge you need to answer the question, it's time to start the guessing process.

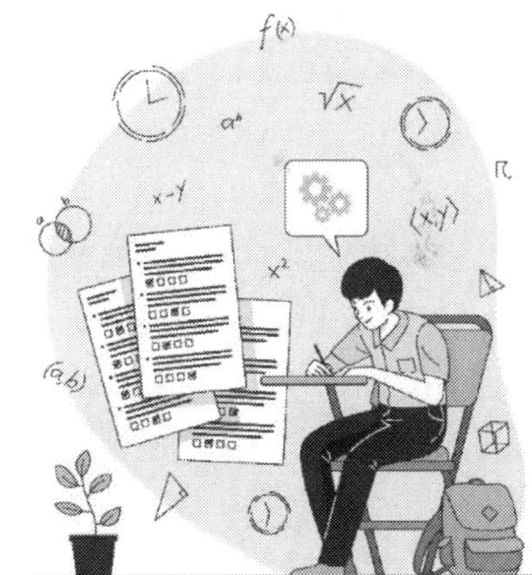

It's almost always better to start the guessing process too early than too late. It only takes a few seconds to remember something and answer the question from knowledge. Carefully eliminating wrong answer choices takes longer. Plus, going through the process of eliminating answer choices can actually help jog your memory.

**Summary**: Start the guessing process as soon as you decide that you can't answer the question based on your knowledge.

## How to Narrow Down the Choices

The next chapter in this book (**Test-Taking Strategies**) includes a wide range of strategies for how to approach questions and how to look for answer choices to eliminate. You will definitely want to read those carefully, practice them, and figure out which ones work best for you. Here though, we're going to address a mindset rather than a particular strategy.

Your odds of guessing an answer correctly depend on how many options you are choosing from.

| Number of options left | 5 | 4 | 3 | 2 | 1 |
|---|---|---|---|---|---|
| Odds of guessing correctly | 20% | 25% | 33% | 50% | 100% |

You can see from this chart just how valuable it is to be able to eliminate incorrect answers and make an educated guess, but there are two things that many test takers do that cause them to miss out on the benefits of guessing:

- Accidentally eliminating the correct answer
- Selecting an answer based on an impression

We'll look at the first one here, and the second one in the next section.

To avoid accidentally eliminating the correct answer, we recommend a thought exercise called **the $5 challenge**. In this challenge, you only eliminate an answer choice from contention if you are willing to bet $5 on it being wrong. Why $5? Five dollars is a small but not insignificant amount of money. It's an amount you could afford to lose but wouldn't want to throw away. And while losing $5 once might not hurt too much, doing it twenty times will set you back $100. In the same way, each small decision you make—eliminating a choice here, guessing on a question there—won't by itself impact your score very much, but when you put them all together, they can make a big difference. By holding each answer choice elimination decision to a higher standard, you can reduce the risk of accidentally eliminating the correct answer.

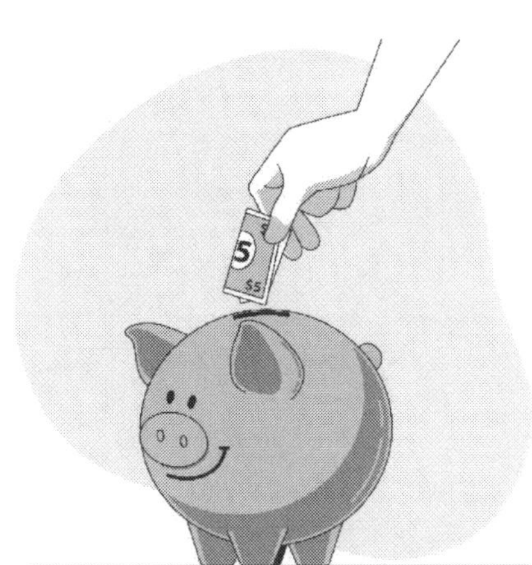

The $5 challenge can also be applied in a positive sense: If you are willing to bet $5 that an answer choice *is* correct, go ahead and mark it as correct.

**Summary**: Only eliminate an answer choice if you are willing to bet $5 that it is wrong.

## Which Answer to Choose

You're taking the test. You've run into a hard question and decided you'll have to guess. You've eliminated all the answer choices you're willing to bet $5 on. Now you have to pick an answer. Why do we even need to talk about this? Why can't you just pick whichever one you feel like when the time comes?

The answer to these questions is that if you don't come into the test with a plan, you'll rely on your impression to select an answer choice, and if you do that, you risk falling into a trap. The test writers know that everyone who takes their test will be guessing on some of the questions, so they intentionally write wrong answer choices to seem plausible. You still have to pick an answer though, and if the wrong answer choices are designed to look right, how can you ever be sure that you're not falling for their trap? The best solution we've found to this dilemma is to take the decision out of your hands entirely. Here is the process we recommend:

**Once you've eliminated any choices that you are confident (willing to bet $5) are wrong, select the first remaining choice as your answer.**

Whether you choose to select the first remaining choice, the second, or the last, the important thing is that you use some preselected standard. Using this approach guarantees that you will not be enticed into selecting an answer choice that looks right, because you are not basing your decision on how the answer choices look.

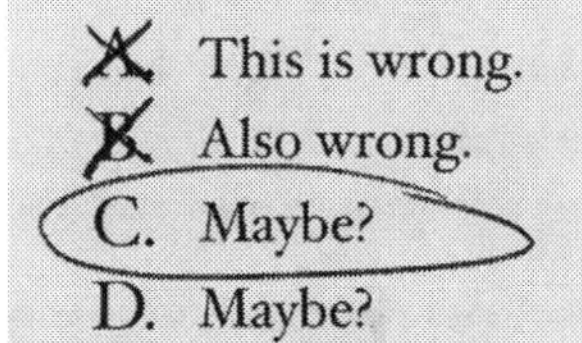


This is not meant to make you question your knowledge. Instead, it is to help you recognize the difference between your knowledge and your impressions. There's a huge difference between thinking an answer is right because of what you know, and thinking an answer is right because it looks or sounds like it should be right.

**Summary**: To ensure that your selection is appropriately random, make a predetermined selection from among all answer choices you have not eliminated.

# Test-Taking Strategies

This section contains a list of test-taking strategies that you may find helpful as you work through the test. By taking what you know and applying logical thought, you can maximize your chances of answering any question correctly!

It is very important to realize that every question is different and every person is different: no single strategy will work on every question, and no single strategy will work for every person. That's why we've included all of them here, so you can try them out and determine which ones work best for different types of questions and which ones work best for you.

## Question Strategies

### ⊘ Read Carefully

Read the question and the answer choices carefully. Don't miss the question because you misread the terms. You have plenty of time to read each question thoroughly and make sure you understand what is being asked. Yet a happy medium must be attained, so don't waste too much time. You must read carefully and efficiently.

### ⊘ Contextual Clues

Look for contextual clues. If the question includes a word you are not familiar with, look at the immediate context for some indication of what the word might mean. Contextual clues can often give you all the information you need to decipher the meaning of an unfamiliar word. Even if you can't determine the meaning, you may be able to narrow down the possibilities enough to make a solid guess at the answer to the question.

### ⊘ Prefixes

If you're having trouble with a word in the question or answer choices, try dissecting it. Take advantage of every clue that the word might include. Prefixes can be a huge help. Usually, they allow you to determine a basic meaning. *Pre-* means before, *post-* means after, *pro-* is positive, *de-* is negative. From prefixes, you can get an idea of the general meaning of the word and try to put it into context.

### ⊘ Hedge Words

Watch out for critical hedge words, such as *likely, may, can, sometimes, often, almost, mostly, usually, generally, rarely,* and *sometimes.* Question writers insert these hedge phrases to cover every possibility. Often an answer choice will be wrong simply because it leaves no room for exception. Be on guard for answer choices that have definitive words such as *exactly* and *always.*

### ⊘ Switchback Words

Stay alert for *switchbacks.* These are the words and phrases frequently used to alert you to shifts in thought. The most common switchback words are *but, although,* and *however.* Others include *nevertheless, on the other hand, even though, while, in spite of, despite,* and *regardless of.* Switchback words are important to catch because they can change the direction of the question or an answer choice.

### ⊘ Face Value

When in doubt, use common sense. Accept the situation in the problem at face value. Don't read too much into it. These problems will not require you to make wild assumptions. If you have to go beyond creativity and warp time or space in order to have an answer choice fit the question, then you should move on and consider the other answer choices. These are normal problems rooted in reality. The applicable relationship or explanation may not be readily apparent, but it is there for you to figure out. Use your common sense to interpret anything that isn't clear.

# Answer Choice Strategies

## ANSWER SELECTION

The most thorough way to pick an answer choice is to identify and eliminate wrong answers until only one is left, then confirm it is the correct answer. Sometimes an answer choice may immediately seem right, but be careful. The test writers will usually put more than one reasonable answer choice on each question, so take a second to read all of them and make sure that the other choices are not equally obvious. As long as you have time left, it is better to read every answer choice than to pick the first one that looks right without checking the others.

## ANSWER CHOICE FAMILIES

An answer choice family consists of two (in rare cases, three) answer choices that are very similar in construction and cannot all be true at the same time. If you see two answer choices that are direct opposites or parallels, one of them is usually the correct answer. For instance, if one answer choice says that quantity *x* increases and another either says that quantity *x* decreases (opposite) or says that quantity *y* increases (parallel), then those answer choices would fall into the same family. An answer choice that doesn't match the construction of the answer choice family is more likely to be incorrect. Most questions will not have answer choice families, but when they do appear, you should be prepared to recognize them.

## ELIMINATE ANSWERS

Eliminate answer choices as soon as you realize they are wrong, but make sure you consider all possibilities. If you are eliminating answer choices and realize that the last one you are left with is also wrong, don't panic. Start over and consider each choice again. There may be something you missed the first time that you will realize on the second pass.

## AVOID FACT TRAPS

Don't be distracted by an answer choice that is factually true but doesn't answer the question. You are looking for the choice that answers the question. Stay focused on what the question is asking for so you don't accidentally pick an answer that is true but incorrect. Always go back to the question and make sure the answer choice you've selected actually answers the question and is not merely a true statement.

## EXTREME STATEMENTS

In general, you should avoid answers that put forth extreme actions as standard practice or proclaim controversial ideas as established fact. An answer choice that states the "process should be used in certain situations, if..." is much more likely to be correct than one that states the "process should be discontinued completely." The first is a calm rational statement and doesn't even make a definitive, uncompromising stance, using a hedge word *if* to provide wiggle room, whereas the second choice is far more extreme.

## BENCHMARK

As you read through the answer choices and you come across one that seems to answer the question well, mentally select that answer choice. This is not your final answer, but it's the one that will help you evaluate the other answer choices. The one that you selected is your benchmark or standard for judging each of the other answer choices. Every other answer choice must be compared to your benchmark. That choice is correct until proven otherwise by another answer choice beating it. If you find a better answer, then that one becomes your new benchmark. Once you've decided that no other choice answers the question as well as your benchmark, you have your final answer.

### ✓ Predict the Answer

Before you even start looking at the answer choices, it is often best to try to predict the answer. When you come up with the answer on your own, it is easier to avoid distractions and traps because you will know exactly what to look for. The right answer choice is unlikely to be word-for-word what you came up with, but it should be a close match. Even if you are confident that you have the right answer, you should still take the time to read each option before moving on.

## General Strategies

### ✓ Tough Questions

If you are stumped on a problem or it appears too hard or too difficult, don't waste time. Move on! Remember though, if you can quickly check for obviously incorrect answer choices, your chances of guessing correctly are greatly improved. Before you completely give up, at least try to knock out a couple of possible answers. Eliminate what you can and then guess at the remaining answer choices before moving on.

### ✓ Check Your Work

Since you will probably not know every term listed and the answer to every question, it is important that you get credit for the ones that you do know. Don't miss any questions through careless mistakes. If at all possible, try to take a second to look back over your answer selection and make sure you've selected the correct answer choice and haven't made a costly careless mistake (such as marking an answer choice that you didn't mean to mark). This quick double check should more than pay for itself in caught mistakes for the time it costs.

### ✓ Pace Yourself

It's easy to be overwhelmed when you're looking at a page full of questions; your mind is confused and full of random thoughts, and the clock is ticking down faster than you would like. Calm down and maintain the pace that you have set for yourself. Especially as you get down to the last few minutes of the test, don't let the small numbers on the clock make you panic. As long as you are on track by monitoring your pace, you are guaranteed to have time for each question.

### ✓ Don't Rush

It is very easy to make errors when you are in a hurry. Maintaining a fast pace in answering questions is pointless if it makes you miss questions that you would have gotten right otherwise. Test writers like to include distracting information and wrong answers that seem right. Taking a little extra time to avoid careless mistakes can make all the difference in your test score. Find a pace that allows you to be confident in the answers that you select.

### ✓ Keep Moving

Panicking will not help you pass the test, so do your best to stay calm and keep moving. Taking deep breaths and going through the answer elimination steps you practiced can help to break through a stress barrier and keep your pace.

## Final Notes

The combination of a solid foundation of content knowledge and the confidence that comes from practicing your plan for applying that knowledge is the key to maximizing your performance on test day. As your foundation of content knowledge is built up and strengthened, you'll find that the strategies included in this chapter become more and more effective in helping you quickly sift through the distractions and traps of the test to isolate the correct answer.

Now that you're preparing to move forward into the test content chapters of this book, be sure to keep your goal in mind. As you read, think about how you will be able to apply this information on the test. If you've already seen sample questions for the test and you have an idea of the question format and style, try to come up with questions of your own that you can answer based on what you're reading. This will give you valuable practice applying your knowledge in the same ways you can expect to on test day.

**Good luck and good studying!**

# Cardiovascular Emergencies

## Cardiovascular Assessment

### Assessment of the Cardiovascular System

**Cardiovascular assessment** includes questioning the patient for any family history of death at a young age or other cardiovascular diseases. Elderly African-American males are at highest risk for cardiovascular problems. One must question the patient about edema, chest pain, dyspnea, fatigue, vertigo, syncope or other changes in consciousness, weight gain, and leg cramps or pain. If chest pain is a symptom, one must ask about the intensity, timing, location, any radiation, quality, meaning to the patient, factors that aggravate or alleviate the pain, nausea, dyspnea, diaphoresis, or any other accompanying symptoms. Physical assessment includes assessment of vital signs, heart and lung sounds, skin assessment, radial, popliteal, and pedal pulses, circulation and sensation of extremities, and auscultation of the aorta, renal, iliac, and femoral arteries for bruits. Blood should be taken for a lipid profile and electrolytes. The patient must be helped to modify risk factors such as hypertension, smoking, diabetes, obesity, hyperlipidemia, inactivity, and stress.

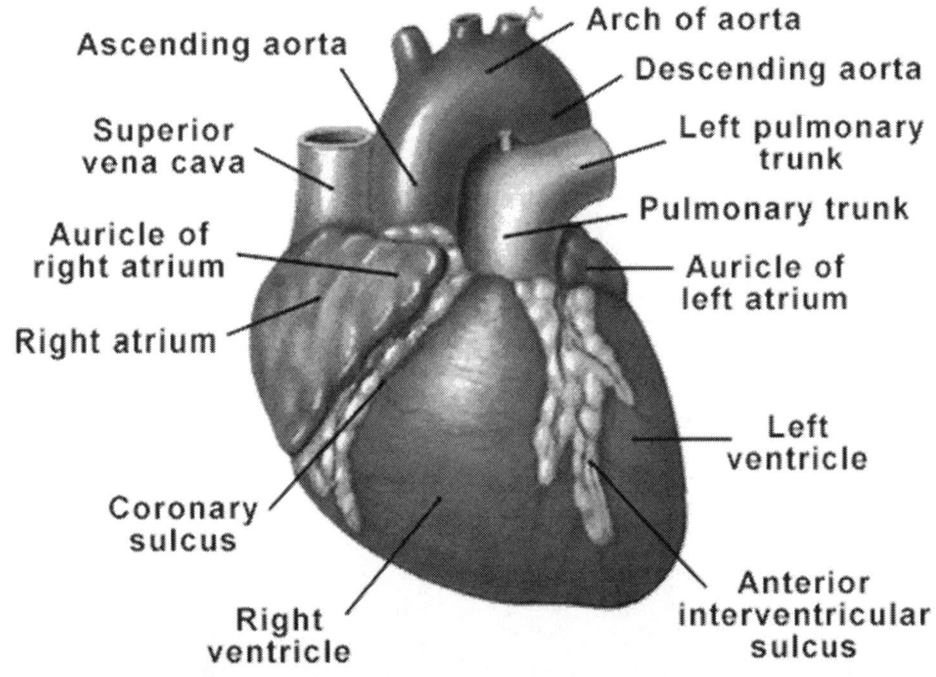


**Review Video: Cardiovascular Assessment**
Visit mometrix.com/academy and enter code: 323076

**Review Video: Circulatory System**
Visit mometrix.com/academy and enter code: 376581

**Review Video: Heart Blood Flow**
Visit mometrix.com/academy and enter code: 783139

## ASSESSMENT OF HEART SOUNDS

Auscultation of heart sounds can help to diagnose different cardiac disorders. Areas to auscultate include the aortic area, pulmonary area, Erb's point, tricuspid area, and the apical area. The **normal heart sounds** represent closing of the valves.

- The **first heart sound** (S1) "lub" is closure of the mitral and tricuspid valves (heard at apex/left ventricular area of the heart).
- The **second heart sound** (S2) "dub" is closure of the aortic and pulmonic valves (heard at the base of the heart). There may be a slight splitting of the S2.

The time between S1 and S2 is systole and the time between S2 and the next S1 is diastole. Systole and diastole should be silent although ventricular disease can cause gallops, snaps, or clicks and stenosis of the valves or failure of the valves to close can cause murmurs. Pericarditis may cause a friction rub.

Additional heart sounds:

- **Gallop rhythms**: S3 commonly occurs after S2 in children and young adults but may indicate heart failure or left ventricular failure in older adults (when heard with patient lying on left side). S4 occurs before S1, during the contracting of the atria when there is ventricular hypertrophy, found in coronary artery disease, hypertension, or aortic valve stenosis.
- **Opening snap**: Unusual high-pitched sound occurring after S2 with stenosis of mitral valve from rheumatic heart disease
- **Ejection click**: Brief high-pitched sound after S1; aortic stenosis
- **Friction rub**: Harsh, grating holosystolic sound; pericarditis
- **Murmur**: Sound caused by turbulent blood flow from stenotic or malfunctioning valves, congenital defects, or increased blood flow. Murmurs are characterized by location, timing in the cardiac cycle, intensity (rated from Grade I to Grade VI), pitch (low to high-pitched), quality (rumbling, whistling, blowing) and radiation (to the carotids, axilla, neck, shoulder, or back).

## CARDIAC MONITORING

Cardiac monitoring includes the evaluation of different intervals and segments on the electrocardiogram:

- **QT interval**: This is the complete time of ventricular depolarization and repolarization, which begins with the QRS segment and ends when the Y wave is completed. Typically, duration usually ranges from 0.36 to 0.44 seconds, but this may vary depending on the heart rate. If the heat rate is rapid, the duration is shorter and vice versa. Certain medications can prolong the QT interval, in such cases monitoring this is critical. A prolonged QT interval puts the patient at risk for R-on-T phenomenon, which can result in dangerous arrhythmias.
- **ST segment**: This is an isoelectric period when the ventricles are in a plateau phase, completely depolarized and beginning recovery and repolarization. Deflection is usually isoelectric, but may range from -0.5 to +1mm. If the ST segment is ≥0.5 mm below the baseline, it is considered depressed and may be an indication of myocardial ischemia. Depression may also indicate digitalis toxicity. If the ST segment is elevated ≥1 mm above baseline, this is an indication of myocardial injury.

## MAP

The MAP **(mean arterial pressure)** is most commonly used to evaluate perfusion as it shows pressure throughout the cardiac cycle. Systole is one-third and diastole two-thirds of the normal cardiac cycle. The MAP for a blood pressure of 120/60 is calculated as follows:

$$\text{MAP} = \frac{\text{Diastole} \times 2 + \text{Systole}}{3}$$

$$MAP = \frac{60 \times 2 + 120}{3} = \frac{240}{3} = 80$$

Normal range for mean arterial pressure is 70-100 mmHg. A MAP of greater than 60 mmHg is required to perfuse vital organs, including the heart, brain, and kidneys.

## Oxygen Saturation as it Relates to Hemodynamic Status

Hemodynamic monitoring includes monitoring **oxygen saturation** levels, which must be maintained for proper cardiac function. The central venous catheter often has an oxygen sensor at the tip to monitor oxygen saturation in the right atrium. If the catheter tip is located near the renal veins, this can cause an increase in right atrial oxygen saturation; and near the coronary sinus, a decrease.

- Increased oxygen saturation may result from left atrial to right atrial shunt, abnormal pulmonary venous return, increased delivery of oxygen or decrease in extraction of oxygen.
- Decreased oxygen saturation may be related to low cardiac output with an increase in oxygen extraction or decrease in arterial oxygen saturation with normal differences in the atrial and ventricular oxygen saturation.

## Electrocardiogram

The electrocardiogram records and shows a graphic display of the electrical activity of the heart through a number of different waveforms, complexes, and intervals:

- **P wave**: Start of electrical impulse in the sinus node and spreading through the atria, muscle depolarization
- **QRS complex**: Ventricular muscle depolarization and atrial repolarization
- **T wave**: Ventricular muscle repolarization (resting state) as cells regain negative charge
- **U wave**: Repolarization of the Purkinje fibers

A modified lead II ECG is often used to monitor basic heart rhythms and dysrhythmias:

- Typical placement of leads for 2-lead ECG is 3-5 cm inferior to the right clavicle and left lower ribcage. Typical placement for a 3-lead ECG is (RA) right arm near shoulder, (LA) $V_5$ position over 5th intercostal space, and (LL) left upper leg near groin.

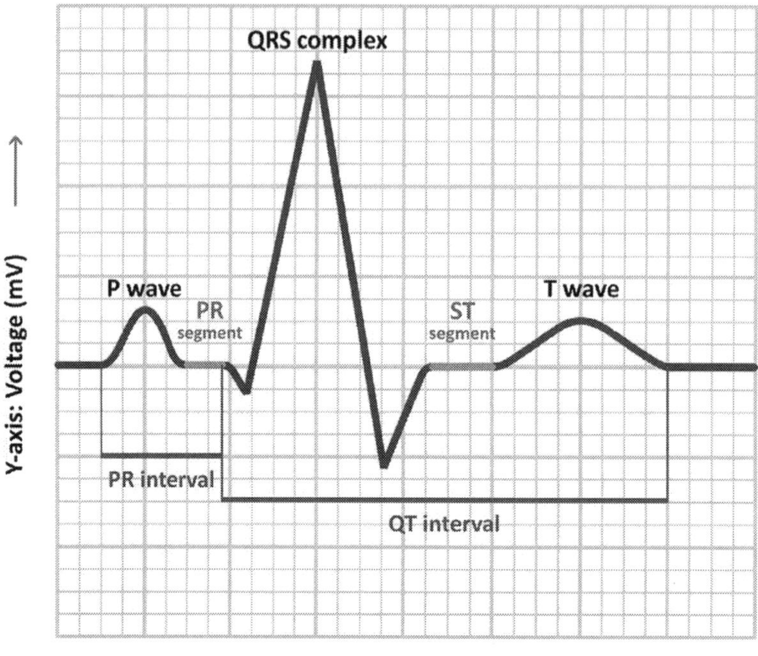


## ADMINISTRATION OF 12-LEAD ECG

The electrocardiogram provides a graphic representation of the electrical activity of the heart. It is indicated for chest pain, dyspnea, syncope, acute coronary syndrome, pulmonary embolism, and possible MI. The standard **12 lead ECG** gives a picture of electrical activity from 12 perspectives through placement of 10 body leads:

- 4 limb leads are placed distally on the wrists and ankles (but may be placed more proximally if necessary).
- Precordial leads:
    - V1: Right sternal border at 4th intercostal space
    - V2: Left sternal border at 4th intercostal space
    - V3: Midway between V2 and V4
    - V4: Left midclavicular line at 5th intercostal space
    - V5: Horizontal to V4 at left anterior axillary line
    - V6: Horizontal to V5 at left midaxillary line

In some cases, additional leads may be used:

- Right-sided leads are placed on the right in a mirror image of the left leads, usually to diagnose right ventricular infarction through ST elevation.

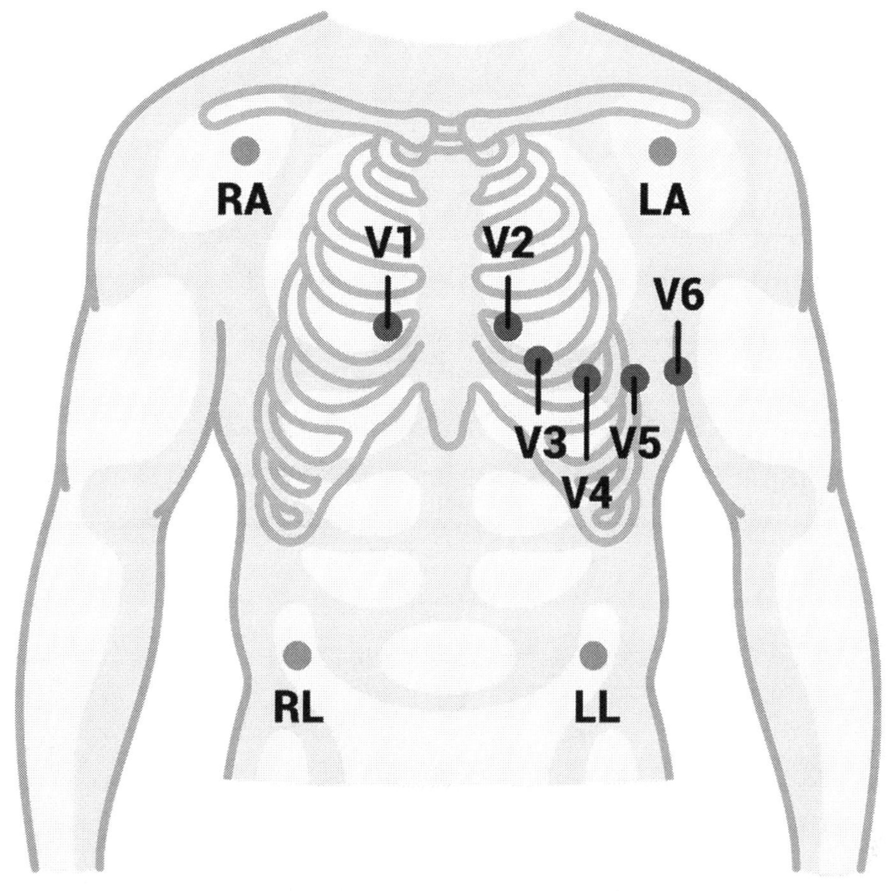


**Review Video: 12 Lead ECG**
Visit mometrix.com/academy and enter code: 962539

## Cardiac Output

Cardiac output (CO) is the amount of blood pumped through the ventricles during a specified period. Normal cardiac output is about 5 liters per minutes at rest for an adult. Under exercise or stress, this volume may multiply 3 or 4 times with concomitant changes in the heart rate (HR) and stroke volume (SV). The basic formulation for calculating cardiac output is the heart rate (HR) per minute multiplied by the stroke volume (SR), which is the amount of blood pumped through the ventricles with each contraction. The stroke volume is controlled by preload, afterload, and contractibility.

$$\text{CO}\left(\frac{\text{mL}}{\text{min}}\right) = \text{HR}\left(\frac{\text{beats}}{\text{min}}\right) \times \text{SV (mL)}$$

The heart rate is controlled by the autonomic nervous system. Normally, if the heart rate decreases, stroke volume increases to compensate. The exception to this would be cardiomyopathies, so bradycardia results in a sharp decline in cardiac output.

## Cardiac Index

Cardiac index (CI) is the cardiac output (CO) divided by the body surface area (BSA). This is essentially a measure of cardiac output tailored to the individual, based on height and weight, measured in liters/min per square meter of BSA.

- Normal value: 2.2–4.0 L/min/$m^2$

## Stroke Volume

Stroke volume (SV) is the amount of blood pumped through the left ventricle with each contraction, minus any blood remaining inside the ventricle at the end of systole.

- Normal values: 60–70 mL
- Formula:

$$\text{SV (mL)} = \text{CO}\left(\frac{\text{mL}}{\text{min}}\right) \div \text{HR}\left(\frac{\text{beats}}{\text{min}}\right)$$

## Pulmonary Vascular Resistance and Ejection Fraction

**Pulmonary vascular resistance (PVR)** is the resistance in the pulmonary arteries and arterioles against which the right ventricle has to pump during contraction. It is the mean pressure in the pulmonary vascular bed divided by blood flow. If PVR increases, SV decreases.

- Normal value: 1.2–3.0 units or 100–250 dynes/sec/$cm^5$

**Ejection Fraction (EF)** is the percentage of the total blood volume of the heart that is pumped out with each beat. Dramatically decreased values indicate heart failure.

- Normal value: 60–70%

## Preload and Afterload

**Preload** refers to the amount of elasticity in the myocardium at the end of diastole when the ventricles are filled to their maximum volume and the stretch on the muscle fibers is the greatest. The preload value is based on the volume in the ventricles. The amount of preload (stretch) affects stroke volume because as stretch increases, the resultant contraction also increases (Frank-Starling Law). Preload may decrease because of dehydration, diuresis, or vasodilation. Preload may increase because of increased venous return, controlling fluid loss, transfusion, or intravenous fluids.

**Afterload** refers to the amount of systemic vascular resistance to left ventricular ejection of blood and pulmonary vascular resistance to right ventricular ejection of blood. Determinants of afterload include the size and elasticity of the great vessels and the functioning of the pulmonic and aortic valves. Afterload increases with hypertension, stenotic valves, and vasoconstriction.

## Minimally/Non-Invasive Hemodynamic Monitoring

Hemodynamic monitoring and evaluation of cardiac function is an important component of the care of the critically ill patient. **Minimally or non-invasive** alternatives to traditional invasive means of hemodynamic monitoring (such as the use of a pulmonary artery catheter) include esophageal Doppler, arterial pressure based cardiac output monitoring, and impedance cardiography. **Esophageal Doppler** is a minimally invasive option used in surgical patients to monitor descending aortic blood flow and estimate cardiac output. A probe is inserted into the esophagus and then connected to a monitor, where waveform shapes produced by aortic blood flow are displayed.

Arterial pressure based cardiac output monitors (APCO's) use an algorithm to estimate cardiac output through the analysis of the arterial pressure waveform. The radial or femoral artery is accessed using a standard arterial catheter and no external calibration is needed.

**Impedance cardiography** is a non-invasive method of hemodynamic monitoring in which sensors placed on the body use electrical signals to measure the level of change in impedance in the thoracic fluid. A waveform is generated and is then used to calculate cardiac output and stroke volume, as well as ten additional hemodynamic parameters.

## Intraarterial Blood Pressure Monitoring

Intraarterial blood pressure monitoring uses a catheter to measure systolic, diastolic, and mean arterial pressures (MAP) continuously. Before catheter insertion, collateral circulation must be assessed by Doppler or the Allen test (radial). Complications include arterial vasospasm, hematoma formation, hemorrhage (accidental disconnect), catheter occlusion, compartment syndrome, retroperitoneal bleed (femoral site), and thrombus/embolus.

**Set up**: The line should be connected to the monitor as well as a pressure bag set at 300 mmHg with no longer than 3 feet of stiff, noncompliant tubing to ensure accuracy. The transducer is leveled at the phlebostatic axis of the patient. The line should be kept free of any air or bubbles, and re-zeroed every four hours and with a change of patient position.

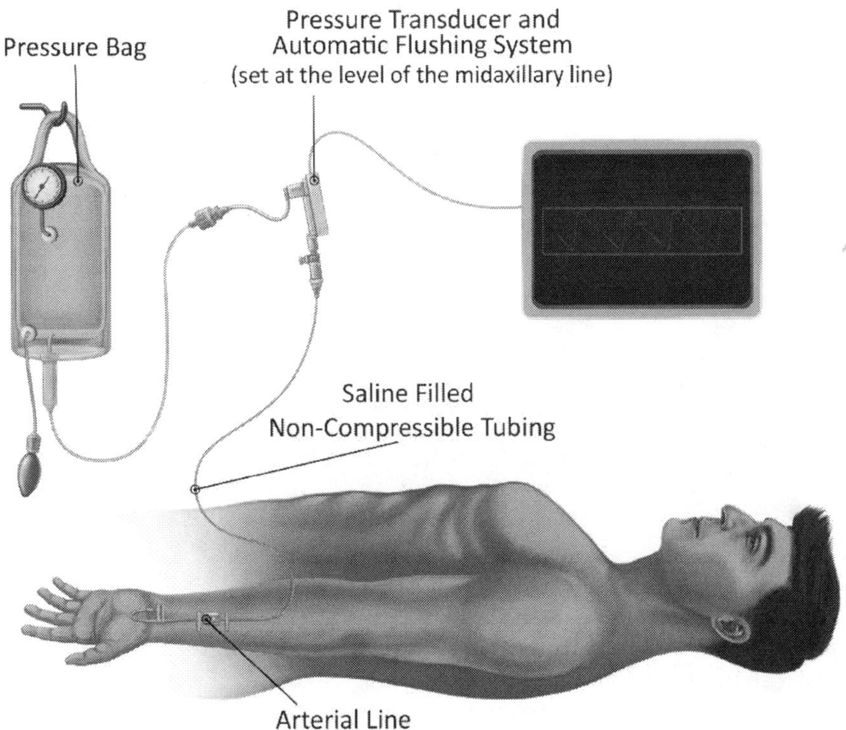

**Waveform**: A normal ABP waveform should be smooth and regular, with a dicrotic notch. To test, perform a "square-wave" or "Fast Flush" test; flush the line while watching the monitor. There should be a square shape, followed by two oscillations and a return to normal waves. A missing dicrotic notch indicates a blockage of some kind (thrombus, plaque, and vasospasm) or low pressure in the bag. Too many oscillations or an increased sharpness of the wave indicates under dampening and is caused by increased SVR or too long of tubing.

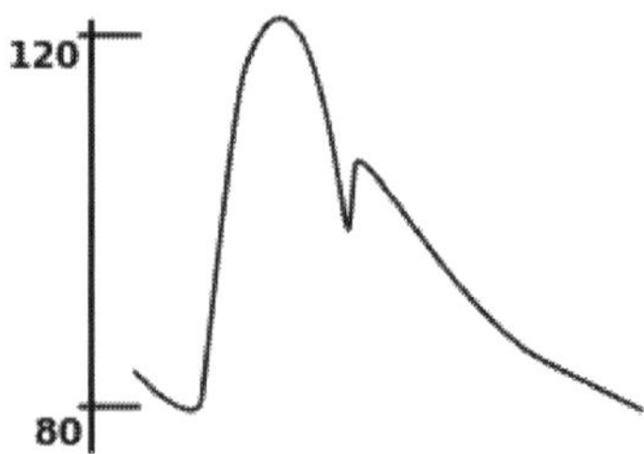


## Assessing Jugular Venous Pressure

**Jugular venous pressure** (neck-vein) is used to assess the cardiac output and pressure in the right heart as the pulsations relate to changes in pressure in the right atrium. This procedure is usually not accurate if the pulse rate is >100. This is a non-invasive estimation of central venous pressure and waveform. Measurement should be done with the internal jugular if possible; if not, the external jugular may be used.

- **Elevate** the patient's head to 45° (and to 90° if necessary) with patient's head turned to the right.
- Position a **light** at an angle to illuminate veins and shadows.
- Measure the height of the **jugular vein pulsation** above the sternal joint, using a ruler.
    - Normal height is ≤4 cm above sternal angle.

Increased pressure (>4 cm) indicates increased pressure in the right atrium, and right heart failure. It may also indicate pericarditis or tricuspid stenosis. Laughing or coughing may trigger the Valsalva response and also cause an increase in pressure.

## Additional Cardiac Assessments

The **stress test**, also called an exercise tolerance test, is a commonly used assessment to screen for ischemic heart disease. In this test, the patient is put through exercise with increasing rigor, generally on a treadmill, while attached to an ECG to monitor their heart's rhythm. The patient is assessed for chest pain and dizziness as the rigor level is increased, which is a reflection of the heart's capacity to handle increasing workloads effectively. The stress test is not diagnostic on its own, but provides feedback on the direction of additional testing.

**Water-hammer pulse** is characterized by the alternation between a bounding heartbeat that is strong and forceful, and then collapse. This could be the result of a heightened stroke volume, decreased peripheral resistance, or these two factors together. To assess for this pulse, the patient is seated and one arm is raised vertically. Upon palpation of the radial pulse in the raised arm, the pulse resembles a tapping in the muscles of the forearm. This is often an indication of aortic regurgitation.

## Perfusion Pressure and Pulse Pressure

**Perfusion pressure** directly affects coronary blood flow, and coronary perfusion occurs during diastole. Coronary artery perfusion pressure is equal to the diastolic blood pressure minus the pulmonary artery occlusion pressure. Normal values are 60–80 mmHg. During the cardiac cycle, *aortic pressure* causes the coronaries to be perfused, while *ventricular pressure* compresses the coronaries during systole, decreasing perfusion.

The **pulse pressure** is the difference between systolic and diastolic pressures, and this can be an important indicator. For example, with a decrease in cardiac output, vasoconstriction takes place in the body's attempt to maintain the blood pressure. In this case, the MAP may remain unchanged, but the pulse pressure narrows. Patients should be assessed for changes in pulse pressure that may be precipitated by medications, such as diuretics that alter fluid volume.

## Assessment of Lower Extremities

Assessment of lower extremities includes a number of different elements:

- **Appearance** includes comparing limbs for obvious differences or changes in skin or nails as well as evaluating for edema, color changes in skin, such as pallor or rubor. Legs that are thin, pale, shiny, and hairless indicate peripheral arterial disease.
- **Perfusion** should be assessed by checking venous filling time and capillary refill, skin temperature (noting changes in one limb or between limbs), bruits (indicating arterial narrowing), pulses (comparing both sides in a proximal to distal progression), ankle-brachial index and toe-brachial index.
- **Sensory function** includes the ability to feel pain, temperature, and touch.
- **Range of motion** of the ankle must be assessed to determine if the joint flexes past 90° because this is necessary for unimpaired walking and aids venous return in the calf.
- **Pain** is an important diagnostic feature of peripheral arterial disease, so the location, intensity, duration, and characteristics of pain are important.

### *Assessment of Pulse and Bruit*

Evaluation of the pulses of the **lower extremities** is an important part of assessment for peripheral arterial disease/trauma. Pulses should be first evaluated with the patient in supine position and then again with the legs dependent, checking bilaterally and proximal to distal to determine if intensity of pulse decreases distally. Pedal pulses should be examined at both the posterior tibialis and the dorsalis pedis. The pulse should be evaluated as to the rate, rhythm, and intensity, which is usually graded on a 0 to 4 scale:

0 = pulse absent
1 = weak, difficult to palpate
2 = normal as expected
3 = full
4 = strong and bounding

Pulses may be **palpable** or **absent** with peripheral arterial disease. Absence of pulse on both palpation and Doppler probe does indicate peripheral arterial disease.

**Bruits** may be noted by auscultating over major arteries, such as femoral, popliteal, peroneal, and dorsalis pedis, indicating peripheral arterial disease.

### *Assessing Perfusion of Lower Extremities*

Assessment of perfusion can indicate venous or arterial abnormalities:

- **Venous refill time**: Begin with the patient lying supine for a few moments and then have the patient sit with the feet dependent. Observe the veins on the dorsum of the foot and count the seconds before normal filling. Venous occlusion is indicated with times greater than 20 seconds.
- **Capillary refill**: Grasp the toenail bed between the thumb and index finger and apply pressure for several seconds to cause blanching. Release the nail and count the seconds until the nail regains normal color. Arterial occlusion is indicated with times of more than 2 to 3 seconds. Check both feet and more than one nail bed.

- **Skin temperature**: Using the palm of the hand and fingers, gently palpate the skin, moving distally to proximally and comparing both legs. Arterial disease is indicated by decreased temperature (coolness) or a marked change from proximal to distal. Venous disease is indicated by increased temperature about the ankle.

## ABI

### Procedure

The ankle-brachial index **(ABI) examination** is done to evaluate peripheral arterial disease of the lower extremities.

1. Apply BP cuff to one arm, palpate brachial pulse, and place conductivity gel over the artery.
2. Place the tip of a Doppler device at a 45-degree angle into the gel at the brachial artery and listen for the pulse sound.
3. Inflate the cuff until the pulse sound ceases and then inflate 20 mmHg above that point.
4. Release air and listen for the return of the pulse sound. This reading is the brachial systolic pressure.
5. Repeat the procedure on the other arm and use the higher reading for calculations.
6. Repeat the same procedure on each ankle with the cuff applied above the malleoli and the gel over the posterior tibial pulse to obtain the ankle systolic pressure.
7. Divide the ankle systolic pressure by the brachial systolic pressure to obtain the ABI.

Sometimes, readings are taken both before and after 5 minutes of walking on a treadmill.

### Interpreting Results

Once the ABI examination is completed, the ankle systolic pressure must be divided by the brachial systolic pressure. Ideally, the BP at the ankle should be equal to that of the arm or slightly higher. With peripheral arterial disease the ankle pressure falls, affecting the ABI. Additionally, some conditions that cause calcification of arteries, such as diabetes, can cause a false elevation.

**Calculation** is simple:

$$\text{ABI} = \frac{\text{Ankle systolic}}{\text{Brachial systolic}}$$

The degree of disease relates to the **score**:

- >1.4: Abnormally high, may indicate calcification of vessel wall
- 1.0–1.4: Normal reading, asymptomatic
- 0.9–1.0: Low reading, but acceptable unless there are other indications of PAD
- 0.8–0.9: Likely some arterial disease is present
- 0.5–0.8: Moderate arterial disease
- < 0.5: Severe arterial disease

# Cardiovascular Diagnostics

## CARDIAC ENZYMES

### *CK AND CK-MB*

**Creatine kinase (CK) and CK-MB levels** are evaluated every 6–8 hours in a suspected myocardial injury. Total CK and CK-MB (specific to cardiac cells) initially rise within the first 4–6 hours of an MI. A normal range would be 30 IU/L to 180 IU/L for CK and CK-MB totaling 0–5% of the CK level.

Assuming no further damage is sustained, peak levels (in excess of 6 times the normal range) are reached 12–24 hours after the injury. CK levels will return to normal within 3–4 days of the event. Small spikes in CK level might also occur following invasive cardiac procedures.

### *TROPONIN I AND T*

Troponin, which is found in cardiac and skeletal muscle, is a type of protein. Both troponin I and T (isolates of troponin) are found in the myocardium, but troponin T is also found in skeletal muscle, so it is less specific than troponin I. Troponin I, therefore, may be used to detect a myocardial infarction after non-cardiac surgery and to detect acute coronary syndrome. Troponin is released into the bloodstream when injury to the tissue (such as the myocardium) occurs and causes damage to the cell membranes, as occurs with myocardial injury.

- **Troponin I** (<0.05 ng/mL): Appears in 2-6 hours, peaks at 15-20 hours and returns to normal in 5-7 days. Exhibits a second but lower peak at 60-80 hours (biphasic).
- **Troponin T** (<0.2 ng/mL): Increases 2-6 hours after MI and stays elevated. Returns to normal in 7 days. (Less specific than troponin I)

## ECHOCARDIOGRAPHY

Echocardiography is a non-invasive ultrasound technology that is very useful for assessing and diagnosing anatomic heart abnormalities, blood flow, and valvular lesions:

- The **standard "2D Echo"** is used best for basic structural imaging, such as valvular lesions and assessment of pericardial disorders.
- The **transesophageal (TEE)** probe is an improved version of echocardiography, which allows better visualization of the left atrium and more precise evaluation of the valvular structure. TEE is also the best modality for evaluation of the thoracic aorta in the setting of suspected aortic dissection or aneurysm.
- **Doppler imaging** is used to measure blood flow, often in the context of velocity across a valve and a pressure gradient.
- **Bubble study** is an addition to echocardiography allowing the study to determine if there is right to left blood flow through a patent foramen ovale or a more distal intrapulmonary shunt of blood.

## STRESS ECHOCARDIOGRAPHY

Basic **cardiac stress testing** consists of exercise EKG testing (EET) and exercise imaging testing. The exercise imaging testing may be broken down into exercise, or "stress" echocardiography, and exercise myocardial perfusion imaging.

**Exercise imaging testing** is usually performed with echocardiography. Stress echocardiography is performed similarly to exercise EKG testing and also requires that the patient meet at least 85% maximum heart rate in order to attain optimum sensitivity and specificity. (The maximum heart rate formula is 220 minus the person's age.) Of note, chemicals may substitute for exercise during the "stress" portion of the test. This may be performed with dobutamine (beta-1-agonist: cannot be used after beta-blocker administration) or adenosine (causes diffuse coronary dilatation, leading to decreased perfusion pressure and unmasking of defects, and cannot be used with asthma). Stress imaging allows the study to determine the actual area of ischemia and whether or not this is a reversible defect. Additional information obtained during echocardiography is cardiac output and measurement of viability.

# Cardiovascular Pathophysiology

## Acute Coronary Syndromes

Acute coronary syndrome (ACS) is the impairment of blood flow through the coronary arteries, leading to ischemia of the cardiac muscle. Angina frequently occurs in ACS, manifesting as crushing pain substernally, radiating down the left arm or both arms. However, in females, elderly, and diabetics, symptoms may appear less acute and include nausea, shortness of breath, fatigue, pain/weakness/numbness in arms, or no pain at all (*silent ischemia*). There are multiple **classifications of angina**:

- **Stable angina**: Exercise-induced, short lived, relieved by rest or nitroglycerin. Other precipitating events include decrease in environmental temperature, heavy eating, strong emotions (such as fright or anger), or exertion, including coitus.
- **Unstable angina** (preinfarction or crescendo angina): A change in the pattern of stable angina, characterized by an increase in pain, not responding to a single nitroglycerin or rest, and persisting for >5 minutes. May cause a change in EKG, or indicate rupture of an atherosclerotic plaque or the beginning of thrombus formation. Treat as a medical emergency, indicates impending MI.
- **Variant angina** (Prinzmetal's angina): Results from spasms of the coronary arteries. Associated with or without atherosclerotic plaques and is often related to smoking, alcohol, or illicit stimulants, but can occur cyclically and at rest. Elevation of ST segments usually occurs with variant angina. Treatment is nitroglycerin or calcium channel blockers.

**Review Video: Coronary Artery Disease**
Visit mometrix.com/academy and enter code: 950720

## Myocardial Infarctions

### *NSTEMI and STEMI*

**Non–ST-segment elevation MI (NSTEMI)**: ST elevation on the electrocardiogram (ECG) occurs in response to myocardial damage resulting from infarction or severe ischemia. The absence of ST elevation may be diagnosed as unstable angina or NSTEMI, but cardiac enzyme levels increase with NSTEMI, indicating partial blockage of coronary arteries with some damage. Symptoms are consistent with unstable angina, with chest pain or tightness, pain radiating to the neck or arm, dyspnea, anxiety, weakness, dizziness, nausea, vomiting, and heartburn. Initial treatment may include nitroglycerin, β-blockers, antiplatelet agents, or antithrombotic agents. Ongoing treatment may include β-blockers, aspirin, statins, angiotensin-converting enzyme inhibitors, angiotensin-receptor blockers, and clopidogrel. Percutaneous coronary intervention is not recommended.

**ST-segment elevation MI (STEMI)**: This more severe type of MI involves complete blockage of one or more coronary arteries with myocardial damage, resulting in ST elevation. Symptoms are those of acute MI. As necrosis occurs, Q waves often develop, indicating irreversible myocardial damage, which may result in death, so treatment involves immediate reperfusion before necrosis can occur.

**Review Video: Myocardial Infarction**
Visit mometrix.com/academy and enter code: 148923

## Q-Wave and Non-Q-Wave Myocardial Infarctions

Formerly classified as transmural or non-transmural, myocardial infarctions are now classified as Q-wave or non-Q-wave:

- **Q-Wave**
    - Characterized by a series of abnormal Q waves (wider and deeper) on ECG, especially in the early morning (related to adrenergic activity).
    - Infarction is usually prolonged and results in necrosis.
    - Coronary occlusion is complete in 80-90% of cases.
    - Q-wave MI is often, but not always, transmural.
    - Peak CK levels occur in about 27 hours.
- **Non-Q-Wave**
    - Characterized by changes in ST-T wave with ST depression (usually reversible within a few days).
    - Usually reperfusion occurs spontaneously, so infarct size is smaller. Contraction necrosis related to reperfusion is common.
    - Non-Q-wave MI is usually non-transmural.
    - Coronary occlusion is complete in only 20-30%.
    - Peak CK levels occur in 12-13 hours.
    - Reinfarction is common.

## Locations and Types

Myocardial infarctions are also classified according to their location and the extent of injury. Q-wave infarctions involve the full thickness of the heart muscle, often producing a series of Q waves on ECG. While an MI most frequently damages the left ventricle and the septum, the right ventricle may be damaged as well, depending upon the area of the occlusion:

- **Anterior** ($V_2$ to $V_4$): Occlusion in the proximal left anterior descending (LAD) or left coronary artery. Reciprocal changes found in leads II, III, $aV_F$.
- **Lateral** (I, $aV_L$, $V_5$, $V_6$): Occlusion of the circumflex coronary artery or branch of left coronary artery. Often causes damage to anterior wall as well. Reciprocal changes found in leads II, III, $aV_F$.
- **Inferior/diaphragmatic** (II, III, $aV_F$): Occlusion of the right coronary artery and causes conduction malfunctions. Reciprocal changes found in leads I and $aV_L$.
- **Right ventricular** ($V_{4R}$, $V_{5R}$, $V_{6R}$): Occlusion of the proximal section of the right coronary artery and damages in the right ventricle and the inferior wall. No reciprocal changes should be noted on an ECG.
- **Posterior** ($V_8$, $V_9$): Occlusion in the right coronary artery or circumflex artery and may be difficult to diagnose. Reciprocal changes found in $V_1$-$V_4$.

## Clinical Manifestations and Diagnosis

Clinical manifestations of myocardial infarction may vary considerably. More than half of all patients present with acute MIs with no prior history of cardiovascular disease.

**Signs/symptoms**: Angina with pain in chest that may radiate to neck or arms, palpitations, hypertension or hypotension, dyspnea, pulmonary edema, dependent edema, nausea/vomiting, pallor, skin cold and clammy, diaphoresis, decreased urinary output, neurological/psychological disturbances: anxiety, light-headedness, headache, visual abnormalities, slurred speech, and fear.

**Diagnosis** is based on the following:

- ECG obtained immediately to monitor heart changes over time. Typical changes include T-wave inversion, elevation of ST segment, abnormal Q waves, tachycardia, bradycardia, and dysrhythmias.
- Echocardiogram: decreased ventricular function is possible, especially for transmural MI.

- Labs:
  - **Troponin**: Increases within 3–6 hours, peaks 14–20; elevated for up to 1-2 weeks.
  - **Creatinine kinase (CK-MB)**: Increases 4–8 hours and peaks at about 24 hours (earlier with thrombolytic therapy or PTCA).
  - **Ischemia Modified Albumin (IMA)**: Increase within minutes, peak 6 hours and return to baseline; verify with other labs.
  - **Myoglobin**: Increases in 0.5–4.0 hours, peaks 6–7 hours. While an increase is not specific to an MI, a failure to increase can be used to rule out an MI.

### *Papillary Muscle Rupture*

Papillary muscle rupture is a rare but often deadly complication of myocardial ischemia/infarct. It most commonly occurs with inferior infarcts. The papillary muscles are part of the cardiac wall structure. Attached to the lower portion of the ventricles, they are responsible for the opening and closing of the tricuspid and mitral valve and preventing prolapse during systole. Rupture of the papillary muscle can occur with myocardial infarct or ischemia in the area of the heart surrounding the papillary muscle. Since the papillary muscles support the mitral valve, rupture will cause severe mitral regurgitation that may result in cardiogenic shock and subsequent death. Rupture of the papillary muscle may be partial or complete and is considered a life-threatening emergency.

**Signs and symptoms**: Acute heart failure, pulmonary edema, and cardiogenic shock (tachycardia, diaphoresis, loss of consciousness, pallor, tachypnea, mental status changes, weak or thready pulse, and decreased urinary output).

**Diagnosis**: Transesophageal echocardiography (TEE) to visualize the papillary muscles, color flow Doppler, echocardiogram, and physical assessment. In patients with papillary muscle rupture, a holosystolic murmur starting at the apex and radiating to the axilla may be present.

**Treatment**: Emergent surgical intervention to repair the mitral valve.

In the cases of complete rupture, patients often experience the rapid development of cardiogenic shock and subsequent death.

## Aortic Aneurysms

### *Types*

A **dissecting aortic aneurysm** occurs when the wall of the aorta is torn and blood flows between the layers of the wall, dilating and weakening it until it risks rupture (which has a 90% mortality). Aortic aneurysms are more than twice as common in males as females, but females have a higher mortality rate, possibly due to increased age at diagnosis.

**Abdominal aortic aneurysms (AAA)** are usually related to atherosclerosis, but may also result from Marfan syndrome, Ehlers-Danlos disease, and connective tissue disorders. Rupture usually does not allow time for emergent repair, so identifying and correcting before rupture is essential. Different classification systems are used to describe the type and degree of dissection. Common classification:

- **DeBakey classification** uses anatomic location as the focal point:
  - Type I begins in the ascending aorta but may spread to include the aortic arch and the descending aorta (60%). This is also considered a proximal lesion or Stanford type A.
  - Type II is restricted to the ascending aorta (10-15%). This is also considered a proximal lesion or Stanford type A.
  - Type III is restricted to the descending aorta (25-30%). This is considered a distal lesion or Stanford type B.
- Types I and II are thoracic, and type III is abdominal.

### *Diagnosis and Treatment*

Aortic aneurysms are often asymptomatic, but when symptomatic, patients present with substernal pain, back pain, dyspnea and/or stridor (from pressure on trachea), cough, distention of neck veins, palpable and pulsating abdominal mass, edema of neck and arms.

**Diagnosis**: x-ray, CT, MRI, Cardiac catheterization, TEE/transthoracic echocardiogram.

**Treatment** includes:

- **Anti-hypertensives** to reduce systolic BP, such as β-blockers (esmolol) or Alpha-β-blocker combinations (labetalol) to reduce force of blood as it leaves the ventricle to reduce pressure against the aortic wall. IV vasodilators (sodium nitroprusside) may also be needed.
- **Intubation and ventilation** may be required if the patient is hemodynamically unstable.
- **Analgesia/sedation** to control anxiety and pain.
- **Surgical repair**: Types I and II are usually repaired surgically because of the danger of rupture and cardiac tamponade. Type III (abdominal) is often followed medically and surgically only if the aneurysm is >5.5cm or rapidly expanding. There are two types of surgical repair:
    - **Open**: Patient is placed on cardiopulmonary bypass, and through an abdominal incision the damaged portion is removed, and a graft is sutured in place.
    - **Endovascular**: A stent graft is fed through the arteries to line the aorta and exclude the aneurysm.

**Complications**: Myocardial infarction, renal injury, and GI hemorrhage/ischemic bowel, which may occur up to years after surgery. Endo-leaks can occur with a stent graft, increasing risk of rupture.

## Aortic Rupture

Aortic rupture is a catastrophic breakage of the aorta, generally as the result of trauma or rupture of an aortic aneurysm. **Aortic rupture** (spontaneous) most commonly occurs in the abdominal aorta. The patient typically experiences a severe tearing pain and loses consciousness from hypovolemic shock as the blood pours out of the aorta. Tachycardia occurs and the patient may exhibit cyanosis. An ecchymotic area may appear in the flank area because of retroperitoneal pooling of blood. Diagnostic tests include ultrasound or CT. Survival depends on the size of the tear, the amount of blood loss, and the length of time until surgical repair. About 90% of patients die prior to surgery. An aortic occlusion balloon to stem bleeding may be placed temporarily in order to stabilize the patient. Surgical repair may be via an open procedure or endovascular therapy. Risk factors include male gender, older age, smoking, history of MI, family history of abdominal aortic aneurysm, peripheral arterial disease, and hypertension.

## Cardiogenic Shock

In cardiogenic shock**,** the heart fails to pump enough blood to provide adequate circulation and oxygen to the body. The primary cause of cardiogenic shock is acute myocardial infarction, especially an anterior wall MI. Other causes include papillary muscle/ventricular septal rupture, pericarditis/myocarditis, prolonged tachyarrhythmia, and hypotensive medications.

**Signs/Symptoms**: Hypotension, altered mental status secondary to decreased cerebral circulation, oliguria, tachypnea or tachycardia, cool extremities, jugular venous distension, and pulmonary edema possible.

**Diagnosis**: ABGs: metabolic acidosis, hypoxia, hypocapnia; lactic acidosis, BNP, BUN and K elevated; EKG: arrhythmias, specifically SVT/V-tach, Sinus bradycardia, AV block and IVCDs possible; however, the EKG may be normal.

- Pulmonary artery catheter (Swan-Ganz catheter) values: CI <1.8 L/min, PCWP >18 mmHg, SBP <90, MAP <60, Increased CVP and PAP

**Treatment** includes:

- Dobutamine IV to increase cardiac contractility
- Norepinephrine IV if SBP <70
- Morphine can be given for pain; while potential for hypotension, it will decrease SNS response and decrease HR and $MVO_2$
- Treat underlying cause (e.g., papillary rupture = valve replacement)
- Intra-aortic balloon pump (IABP): Increases cardiac blood flow
- Re-vascularization if secondary to acute MI (CABG or PCI)

## Obstructive Shock

Obstructive shock occurs when the preload (diastolic filling of the RV) of the heart is obstructed in one or several ways. There can be obstruction to the great vessels of the heart (such as from pulmonary embolism), there can be excessive afterload because the flow of blood out of the heart is obstructed (resulting in decreased cardiac output), or there can be direct compression of the heart, which can occur when blood or air fills the pericardial sac with cardiac tamponade or tension pneumothorax. Other causes include aortic dissection, vena cava syndrome, systemic hypertension, and cardiac lesions. Obstructive shock is often categorized with cardiogenic shock because of their similarities. **Signs and symptoms** of obstructive shock may vary depending on the underlying cause but typically include:

- Decrease in oxygen saturation
- Hemodynamic instability with hypotension and tachycardia, muffled heart sounds
- Chest pain
- Neurological impairment (disorientation, confusion)
- Dyspnea
- Impaired peripheral circulation (cool extremities, pallor)
- Generalized pallor and cyanosis

**Treatment** depends on the cause and may include oxygen, pericardiocentesis, needle thoracostomy or chest tube, and fluid resuscitation.

## Cardiomyopathy

### *Dilated Cardiomyopathy*

Dilated cardiomyopathy (DCM) occurs when some precipitating factor leads to decreased cardiac perfusion. The resulting ischemic cardiac tissue is replaced with scar tissue, and the healthy cells are forced to over-compensate, causing hypertrophy and over stretching. Eventually, the muscle cells become stretched beyond compensation, and dilated and weak chamber results, unable to properly contract. This causes a decrease in stroke volume and cardiac output, with the end result being enlargement of the mitral and tricuspid valves and severe valve regurgitation. While DCM is the most common form of cardiomyopathy, causes include:

- **Vascular**: Cardiac ischemia, hypertension, atherosclerosis
- **Metabolic**: Diabetes, uremia, thyrotoxicosis, and acromegaly, muscular dystrophy
- **Genetics** (familial DCM), and childbirth (peripartum DCM)
- **Viral infections**, particularly adenovirus, Varicella zoster, HIV, and Hepatitis C may cause DCM
- **Alcohol poisoning or cocaine addiction**
- **Radiation or heavy metal poisoning**, specifically cobalt

**Signs/Symptoms**: Dyspnea, SOB, tachycardia, S3/S4 heart sounds, holosystolic murmur, wheezes/crackles, pleural effusions, edema, JVD, ascites

**Diagnosis**: EKG (tachycardia/T wave changes), chest x-ray (cardiomegaly), 2D Echocardiogram (valve regurgitation/EF).

**Treatment** includes:

- Treat underlying cause if possible; supportive care
- Heart transplant if patient is a candidate and damage is permanent

### *Hypertrophic Cardiomyopathy*

Hypertrophic cardiomyopathy (HCM) is a genetic disorder that causes idiopathic thickening of the heart muscle, primarily involving the ventricular septum and portions of the left ventricle. Patients with HCM produce abnormal sarcomeres and misalignment of muscle cells (myocardial disarray). Basically, HCM is characterized by ventricular hypertrophy, an asymmetrical septum, forceful systole, cardiac dysrhythmias, and myocardial disarray. Because the abnormal cells develop over time, it is common for HCM to remain undiagnosed until middle or late adulthood.

**Signs/Symptoms**: Exertional or atypical chest pain, dyspnea at rest, syncope, frequent palpitations (common due to reoccurring dysrhythmias).

**Diagnosis**: 2D echo (structure and EF), EKG (pathological Q waves and dysrhythmias), x-ray (cardiomegaly), Family history (especially cardiac death, reoccurring dysrhythmias, or myocardial hypertrophy).

**Treatment** includes:

- **Surgery**: Septal myectomy is gold standard: high mortality (3-10%), but increases cardiac output and quality of life.
- **Alcohol-based septal ablation**: Ethanol 100% injected into a branch of the LAD, creating a controlled area of infarction and consequently thinning the septum.

### *Restrictive Cardiomyopathy*

Restrictive cardiomyopathy (RCM) occurs when the ventricles become stiff and noncompliant, resulting in decreased end-diastolic cardiac refill volume. The ventricular stiffening is caused by the infiltration of fibroelastic tissue into the cardiac muscle (such as in amyloidosis or sarcoidosis). Atrial enlargement can be seen in most cases of RCM as a result of the increased effort required to push blood from the atria into the ventricles. It is not uncommon for a patient to be in atrial fibrillation secondary to atrial enlargement. In advanced cases, ventricular dysrhythmias may also be seen.

**Signs/Symptoms**: Exercise intolerance/fatigue, edema, crackles, elevated CVP, S3/S4, murmur, SOB at rest

**Diagnosis**: 2D echo (enlarged atria, decreased compliance of ventricle), hemodynamic monitoring (increased right atrial pressure and pulmonary wedge pressure, and SVR), x-ray (cardiomegaly), EKG (atrial fibrillation), endomyocardial biopsy (to differentiate from constrictive pericarditis).

**Treatment** includes:

- **Medications**: β-blockers increase ventricular filling; antiarrhythmics may be ordered
- **Surgical**: Heart transplant, if patient is a candidate

## Dysrhythmias

### Sinus Bradycardia

There are 3 primary types of **sinus node dysrhythmias**: sinus bradycardia, sinus tachycardia, and sinus arrhythmia**. Sinus bradycardia (SB)** is caused by a decreased rate of impulse from sinus node. The pulse and ECG usually appear normal except for a slower rate.

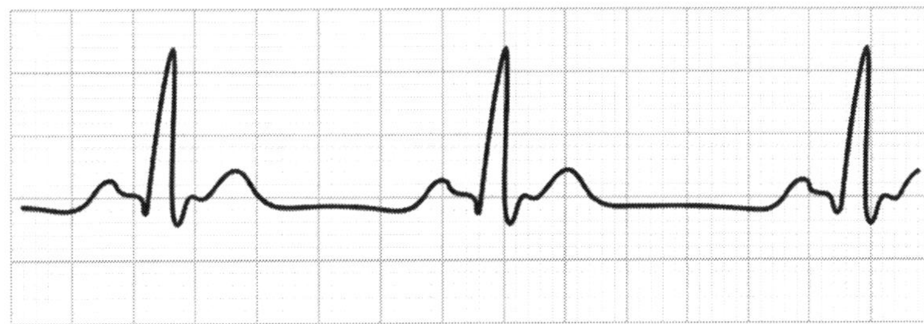

SB is characterized by a regular pulse <50-60 bpm with P waves in front of QRS, which are usually normal in shape and duration. PR interval is 0.12-0.20 seconds, QRS interval is 0.04-0.11 seconds, and P:QRS ratio of 1:1. SB may be caused by several factors:

- May be normal in athletes and older adults; generally not treated unless symptomatic
- Conditions that lower the body's metabolic needs, such as hypothermia or sleep
- Hypotension and decrease in oxygenation
- Medications such as calcium channel blockers and β-blockers
- Vagal stimulation that may result from vomiting, suctioning, defecating, or certain medical procedures (carotid stent placement, etc.)
- Increased intracranial pressure
- Myocardial infarction

**Treatment**: involves eliminating cause if possible, such as changing medications. Atropine 0.5-1.0 mg may be given IV to block vagal stimulation or increase rate if symptomatic.

### Sinus Tachycardia

Sinus tachycardia (ST) occurs when the sinus node impulse increases in frequency. ST is characterized by a regular pulse >100 with P waves before QRS but sometimes part of the preceding T wave. QRS is usually of normal shape and duration (0.04-0.11 seconds) but may have consistent irregularity. PR interval is 0.12-0.20 seconds and P:QRS ratio of 1:1.

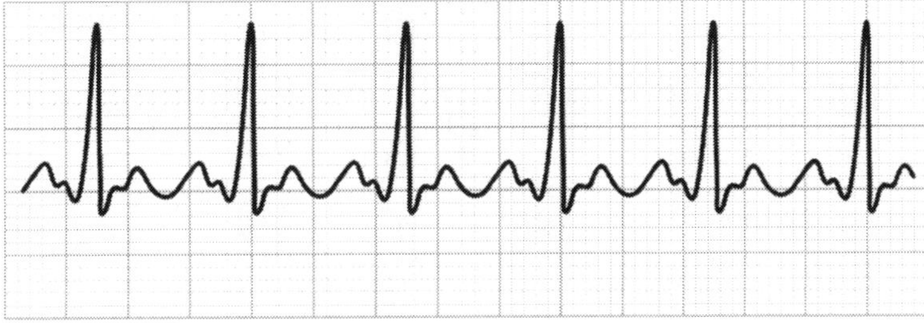

The rapid pulse decreases diastolic filling time and causes reduced cardiac output with resultant hypotension. Acute pulmonary edema may result from the decreased ventricular filling if untreated. ST may be **caused** by a number of factors:

- Acute blood loss, shock, hypovolemia, anemia
- Sinus arrhythmia, hypovolemic heart failure
- Hypermetabolic conditions, fever, infection

- Exertion/exercise, anxiety, stress
- Medications, such as sympathomimetic drugs

**Treatment**: eliminating precipitating factors, calcium channel blockers and β-blockers to reduce heart rate.

### *Supraventricular Tachycardia*

Supraventricular tachycardia (SVT) (>100 BPM) may have a sudden onset and result in congestive heart failure. Rate may increase to 200–300 BMP, which will significantly decrease cardiac output due to decreased filling time. SVT originates in the atria rather than the ventricles but is controlled by the tissue in the area of the AV node rather than the SA node. Rhythm is usually rapid but regular. The P wave is present but may not be clearly defined as it may be obscured by the preceding T wave, and the QRS complex appears normal. The PR interval is 0.12-0.20 seconds and the QRS interval is 0.04-0.11 seconds with a P:QRS ratio of 1:1.

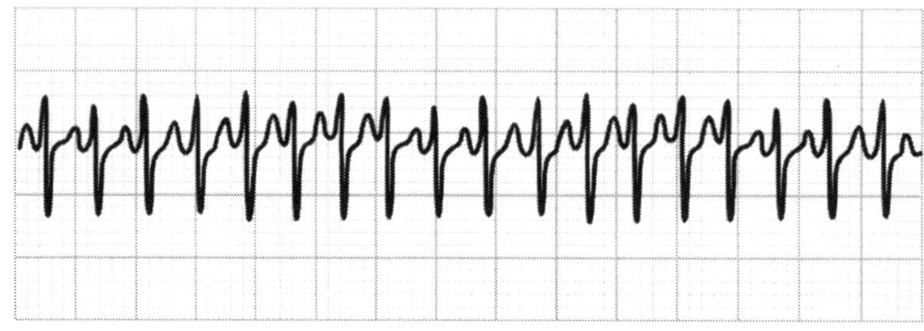

SVT may be episodic with periods of normal heart rate and rhythm between episodes of SVT, so it is often referred to as paroxysmal SVT (PSVT).

**Treatment**: Adenosine, digoxin (Lanoxin), Verapamil (Calan, Verelan), vagal maneuvers, cardioversion.

### *Sinus Arrhythmia*

Sinus arrhythmia (SA) results from irregular impulses from the sinus node, often paradoxical (increasing with inspiration and decreasing with expiration) because of stimulation of the vagal nerve during inspiration and rarely causes a negative hemodynamic effect. These cyclic changes in the pulse during respiration are quite common in both children and young adults and often lesson with age but may persist in some adults. Sinus arrhythmia can, in some cases, relate to heart or valvular disease and may be increased with vagal stimulation for suctioning, vomiting, or defecating. Characteristics of SA include a regular pulse 50-100 BPM, P waves in front of QRS with duration (0.04-0.11 seconds) and shape of QRS usually normal, PR interval of 0.12-0.20 seconds, and P:QRS ratio of 1:1.

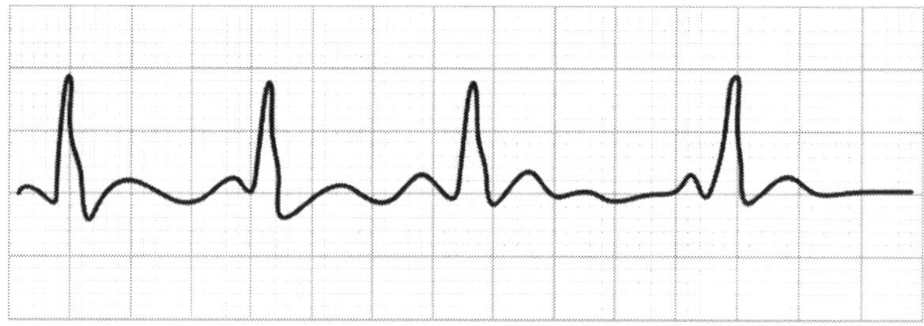

**Treatment** is usually not necessary unless it is associated with bradycardia.

### *Premature Atrial Contraction*

There are 3 primary types of **atrial dysrhythmias**: premature atrial contraction, atrial flutter, and atrial fibrillation. Premature atrial contraction (PAC) is essentially an extra beat precipitated by an electrical impulse to the atrium before the sinus node impulse. The extra beat may be caused by alcohol, caffeine, nicotine, hypervolemia, hypokalemia, hypermetabolic conditions, atrial ischemia, or infarction. Characteristics include an irregular pulse because of extra P waves, the shape and duration of QRS is usually normal (0.04-0.11 seconds) but may be abnormal, PR interval remains between 0.12-0.20, and P:QRS ratio is 1:1. Rhythm is irregular with varying P-P and R-R intervals.

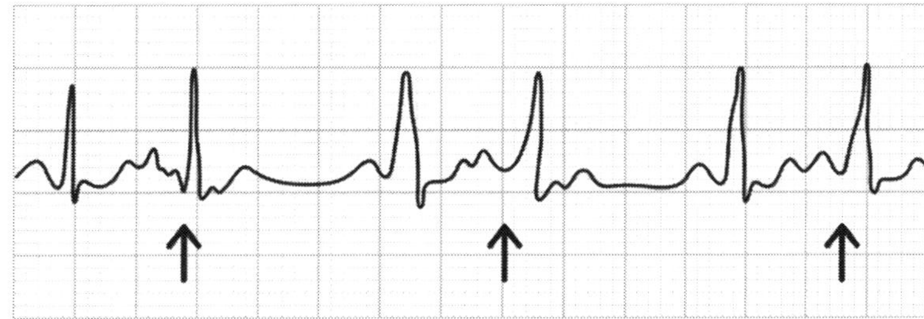

PACs can occur in an essentially healthy heart and are not usually cause for concern unless they are frequent (>6 per hr) and cause severe palpitations. In that case, atrial fibrillation should be suspected.

### *Atrial Flutter*

Atrial flutter (AF) occurs when the atrial rate is faster, usually 250-400 beats per minute, than the AV node conduction rate so not all of the beats are conducted into the ventricles. The beats are effectively blocked at the AV node, preventing ventricular fibrillation although some extra ventricular impulses may pass though. AF is caused by the same conditions that cause A-fib: coronary artery disease, valvular disease, pulmonary disease, heavy alcohol ingestion, and cardiac surgery. AF is characterized by atrial rates of 250-400 with ventricular rates of 75-150, with ventricular rate usually being regular. P waves are saw-toothed (referred to as F waves), QRS shape and duration (0.04-0.11 seconds) are usually normal, PR interval may be hard to calculate because of F waves, and the P:QRS ratio is 2:1 to 4:1. Symptoms include chest pain, dyspnea, and hypotension.

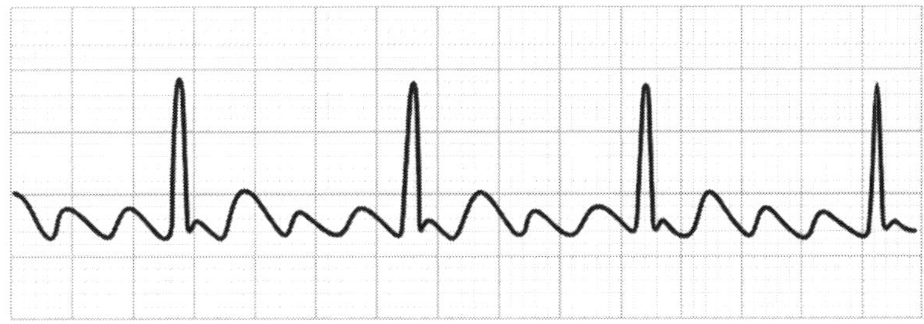

**Treatment** includes:

- Emergent cardioversion if condition is unstable
- Medications to slow ventricular rate and conduction through AV node: non-dihydropyridine calcium channel blockers (Cardizem, Calan) and beta blockers
- Medications to convert to sinus rhythm: Corvert, Tikosyn, Amiodarone; also used in practice: Cardioquin, Norpace, Cordarone

### *Atrial Fibrillation*

Atrial fibrillation (A-fib) is rapid, disorganized atrial beats that are ineffective in emptying the atria, so that blood pools in the chambers. This can lead to thrombus formation and emboli. The ventricular rate increases with a decreased stroke volume, and cardiac output decreases with increased myocardial ischemia, resulting in palpitations and fatigue. A-fib is caused by coronary artery disease, valvular disease, pulmonary disease, heavy alcohol ingestion, infection, and cardiac surgery; however, it can also be idiopathic. A-fib is characterized by a very irregular pulse with atrial rate of 300-600 and ventricular rate of 120-200, shape and duration (0.04-0.11

seconds) of QRS is usually normal. Fibrillatory (F) waves are seen instead of P waves. The PR interval cannot be measured and the P:QRS ratio is highly variable.

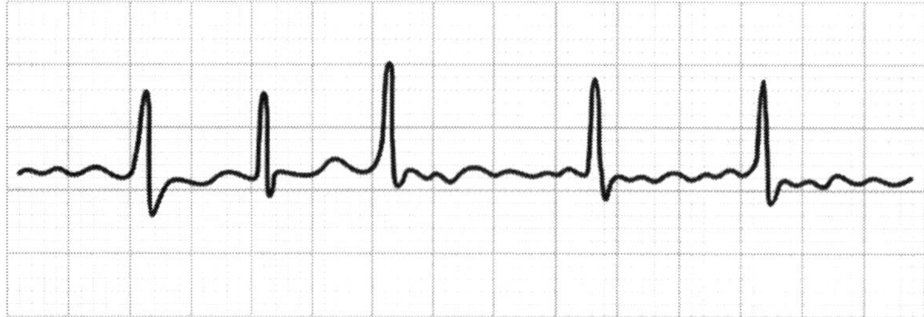

**Treatment** is the same as atrial flutter.

**Review Video: EKG Interpretation: Afib and Aflutter**
Visit mometrix.com/academy and enter code: 263842

### *Premature Junctional Contraction*

The area around the AV node is the junction, and dysrhythmias that arise from that area are called junctional dysrhythmias. Premature junctional contraction (PJC) occurs when a premature impulse starts at the AV node before the next normal sinus impulse reaches the AV node. PJC is similar to premature atrial contraction (PAC) and generally requires no treatment although it may be an indication of digoxin toxicity. The ECG may appear basically normal with an early QRS complex that is normal in shape and duration (0.04-0.11 seconds). The P wave may be absent or it may precede, be part of, or follow the QRS with a PR interval of 0.12 seconds. The P:QRS ratio may vary from <1:1 to 1:1 (with inverted P wave). The underlying rhythm is usually regular at a heart rate of 60-100. Significant symptoms related to PJC are rare.

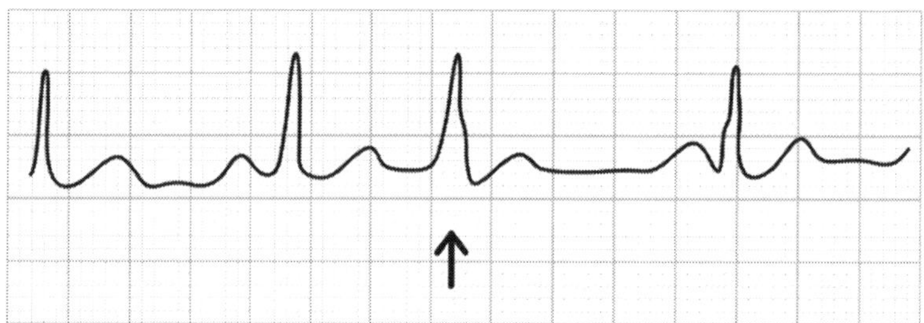

### *Junctional Rhythms*

Junctional rhythms occur when the AV node becomes the pacemaker of the heart. This can happen because the sinus node is depressed from increased vagal tone or a block at the AV node prevents sinus node impulses from being transmitted. While the sinus node normally sends impulses 60-100 beats per minute, the AV node junction usually sends impulses at 40-60 beats per minute. The QRS complex is of usual shape and duration (0.04-0.11 seconds). The P wave may be inverted and may be absent, hidden or after the QRS. If the P wave precedes the QRS, the PR interval is <0.12 seconds. The P:QRS ratio is <1:1 or 1:1. The junctional escape rhythm is a protective mechanism preventing asystole with failure of the sinus node. An **accelerated**

**junctional rhythm** is similar, but the heart rate is 60-100. **Junctional tachycardia** occurs with heart rate of >100.

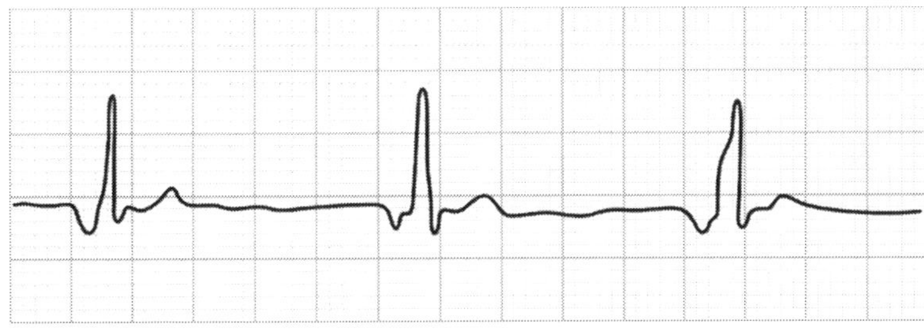

## *AV Nodal Reentry Tachycardia*

AV nodal reentry tachycardia occurs when an impulse conducts to the area of the AV node and is then sent in a rapidly repeating cycle back to the same area and to the ventricles, resulting in a fast ventricular rate. The onset and cessation are usually rapid. AV nodal reentry tachycardia (also known as paroxysmal atrial tachycardia or supraventricular tachycardia if there are no P waves) is characterized by atrial rate of 150-250 with ventricular rate of 75-250, P wave that is difficult to see or absent, QRS complex that is usually normal and a PR interval of <0.12 if a P wave is present. The P:QRS ratio is 1-2:1. Precipitating factors include nicotine, caffeine, hypoxemia, anxiety, underlying coronary artery disease and cardiomyopathy. Cardiac output may be decreased with a rapid heart rate, causing dyspnea, chest pain, and hypotension.

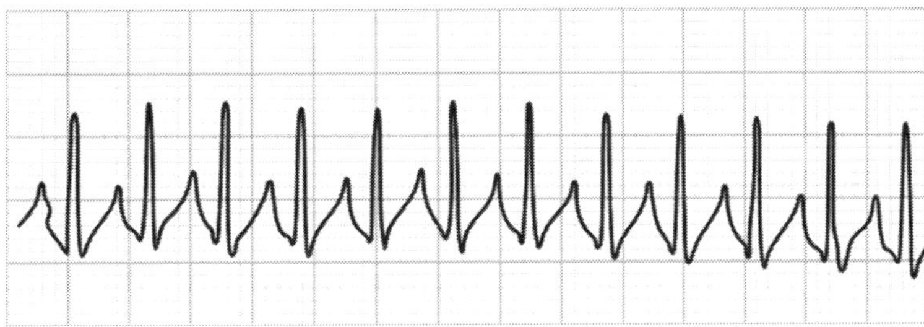

**Treatment** includes:

- Vagal maneuvers (carotid sinus massage, gag reflex, holding breath/bearing down)
- Medications (adenosine, verapamil, or diltiazem)
- Cardioversion if other methods unsuccessful

## *Premature Ventricular Contractions*

Premature ventricular contractions (PVCs) are those in which the impulse begins in the ventricles and conducts through them prior to the next sinus impulse. The ectopic QRS complexes may vary in shape, depending upon whether there is one site (unifocal) or more (multifocal) that stimulates the ectopic beats. PVCs usually cause no morbidity unless there is underlying cardiac disease or an acute MI. PVCs are characterized by an irregular heartbeat, QRS that is ≥0.12 seconds and oddly shaped. PVCs are often not treated in otherwise healthy people. PVCs may be precipitated by electrolyte imbalances, caffeine, nicotine, or alcohol. Because PVCs may occur with any supraventricular dysrhythmia, the underlying rhythm must be noted as well as the PVCs. If there are more than six PVCs in an hour, that is a risk factor for developing ventricular tachycardia.

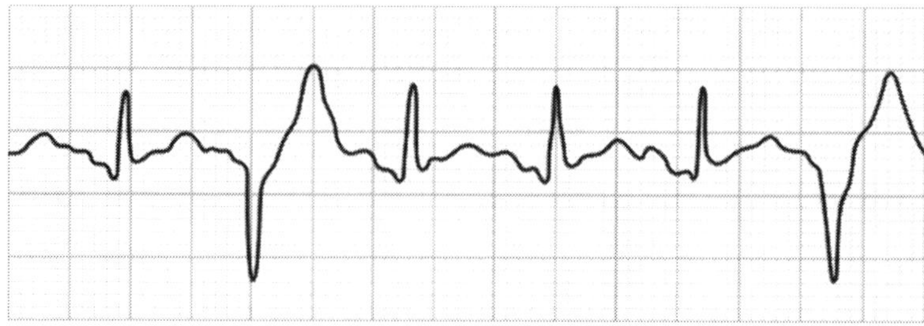

**Bigeminy** is a rhythm where every other beat is a PVC. **Trigeminy** is a rhythm where every third beat is a PVC.

**Ventricular bigeminy** is a rhythm where every other beat is a PVC. **Ventricular trigeminy** is a rhythm where every third beat is a PVC.

**Treatment**: Lidocaine (affects the ventricles, may cause CNS toxicity with nausea and vomiting), Procainamide (affects the atria and ventricles and may cause decreased BP and widening of QRS and QT); treat underlying cause.

### *Ventricular Tachycardia*

Ventricular tachycardia (VT) is greater than 3 PVCs in a row with a ventricular rate of 100-200 beats per minute. Ventricular tachycardia may be triggered by the same factors as PVCs and often is related to underlying coronary artery disease. The rapid rate of contractions makes VT dangerous as the ineffective beats may render the person unconscious with no palpable pulse. A detectable rate is usually regular and the QRS complex is ≥0.12 seconds and is usually abnormally shaped. The P wave may be undetectable with an irregular PR interval if P wave is present. The P:QRS ratio is often difficult to ascertain because of the absence of P waves.

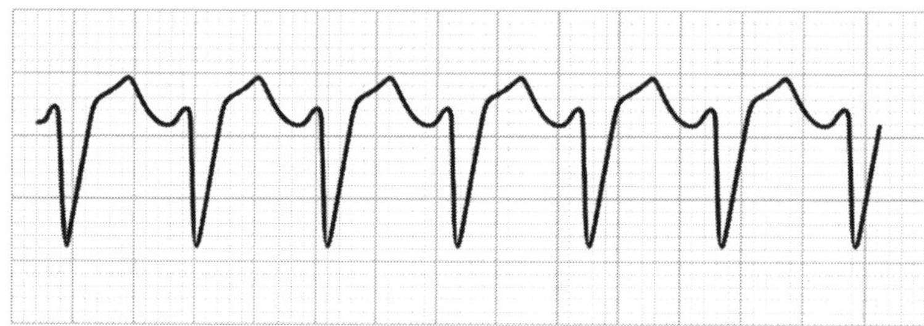

**Treatment** is as follows:

- With pulse: Synchronized cardioversion, adenosine
- No pulse: Same as ventricular fibrillation

### Narrow Complex and Wide Complex Tachycardias

Tachycardias are classified as narrow complex or wide complex. Wide and narrow refer to the configuration of the QRS complex.

- **Wide complex tachycardia (WCT)**: About 80% of cases of WCT are caused by ventricular tachycardia. WCT originates at some point below the AV node and may be associated with palpitations, dyspnea, anxiety, diaphoresis, and cardiac arrest. Wide complex tachycardia is diagnosed with more than 3 consecutive beats at a heart rate >100 BPM and QRS duration ≥0.12 seconds.

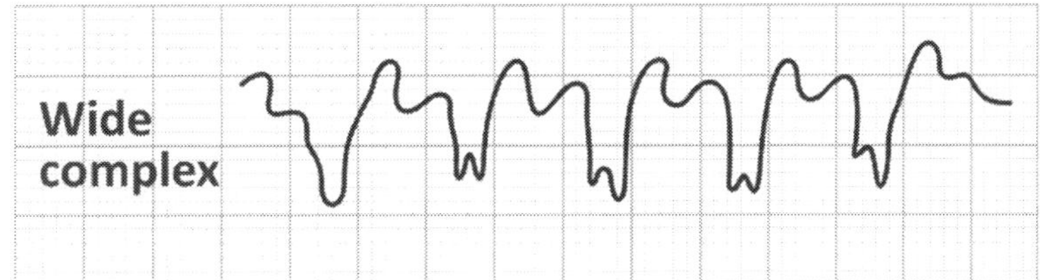


- **Narrow complex tachycardia (NCT)**: NCT is associated with palpitations, dyspnea, and peripheral edema. NCT is generally supraventricular in origin. Narrow complex tachycardia is diagnosed with ≥3 consecutive beats at heart rate of >100 BPM and QRS duration of <0.12 seconds.

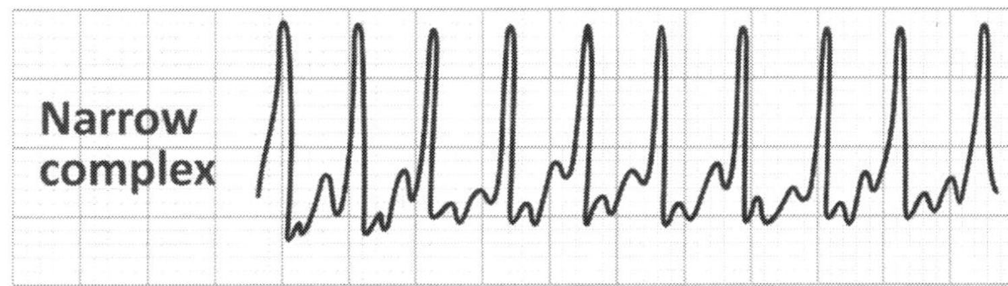


### *Ventricular Fibrillation*

Ventricular fibrillation (VF) is a rapid, very irregular ventricular rate >300 beats per minute with no atrial activity observable on the ECG, caused by disorganized electrical activity in the ventricles. The QRS complex is not recognizable as ECG shows irregular undulations. The causes are the same as for ventricular tachycardia and asystole. VF is accompanied by lack of palpable pulse, audible pulse, and respirations and is immediately life threatening without defibrillation.

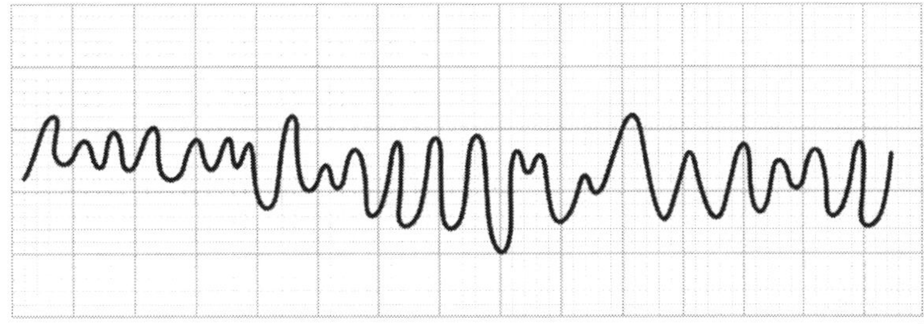

**Treatment** includes:

- Emergency defibrillation, the cause should be identified and treated
- Epinephrine 1 mg q 3-5minutes then amiodarone 300mg (2nd dose: 150mg) IV push

**Review Video: EKG Interpretation: Ventricular Arrythmias**
Visit mometrix.com/academy and enter code: 933152

### *Idioventricular Rhythm*

Ventricular escape rhythm (idioventricular) occurs when the Purkinje fibers below the AV node create an impulse. This may occur if the sinus node fails to fire or if there is blockage at the AV node so that the impulse does not go through. Idioventricular rhythm is characterized by a regular ventricular rate of 20-40 BPM. Rates >40 BPM are called accelerated idioventricular rhythm. The P wave is missing and the QRS complex has a very bizarre and abnormal shape with duration of ≥0.12 seconds. The low ventricular rate may cause a decrease in cardiac output, often making the patient lose consciousness. In other patients, the idioventricular rhythm may not be associated with reduced cardiac output.

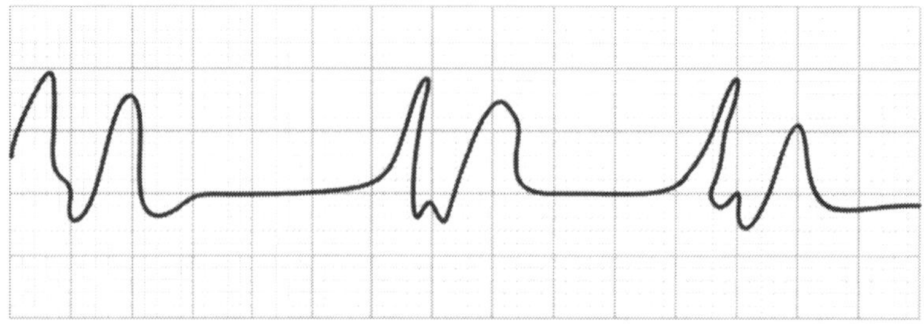

### *Ventricular Asystole*

Ventricular asystole is the absence of audible heartbeat, palpable pulse, and respirations, a condition often referred to as "cardiac arrest." While the ECG may show some P waves initially, the QRS complex is absent although there may be an occasional QRS "escape beat" (agonal rhythm). Cardiopulmonary resuscitation is required with intubation for ventilation and establishment of an intravenous line for fluids. Without immediate treatment, the patient will suffer from severe hypoxia and brain death within minutes. Identifying the cause is critical for the patient's survival. Consider the "Hs & Ts": hypovolemia, hypoxia, hydrogen ions (acidosis), hypo/hyperkalemia, hypothermia, tension pneumothorax, tamponade (cardiac), toxins, and thrombosis (pulmonary or coronary). Even with immediate treatment, the prognosis is poor and ventricular asystole is often a sign of impending death.

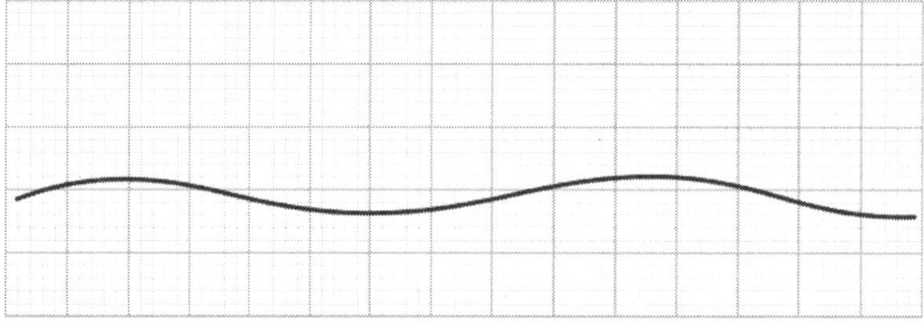

**Treatment** includes:

- CPR only; Asystole is not a shockable rhythm therefore defibrillation is not indicated
- Epinephrine 1 mg q 3-5 minutes

### Sinus Pause

Sinus pause occurs when the sinus node fails to function properly to stimulate heart contractions, so there is a pause on the ECG recording that may persist for a few seconds to minutes, depending on the severity of the dysfunction. A prolonged pause may be difficult to differentiate from cardiac arrest. During the sinus pause, the P wave, QRS complex and PR and QRS intervals are all absent. P:QRS ratio is 1:1 and the rhythm is irregular. The pulse rate may vary widely, usually 60-100 BPM. Patients with frequent pauses may complain of dizziness or syncope. The patient may need to undergo an electrophysiology study and medication reconciliation to determine the cause. If measures such as decreasing medication are not effective, a pacemaker is usually indicated (if symptomatic).

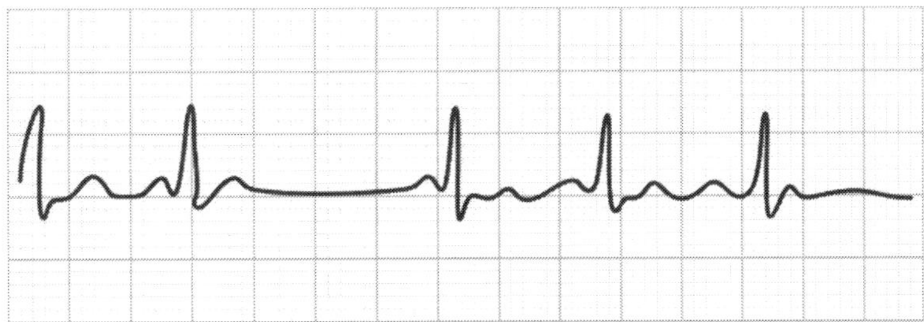

### First-Degree AV Block

First-degree AV block occurs when the atrial impulses are conducted through the AV node to the ventricles at a rate that is slower than normal. While the P and QRS are usually normal, the PR interval is >0.20 seconds, and the P:QRS ratio is 1:1. A narrow QRS complex indicates a conduction abnormality only in the AV node, but a widened QRS indicates associated damage to the bundle branches as well. *Chronic* first-degree block may be caused by fibrosis/sclerosis of the conduction system related to coronary artery disease, valvular disease, cardiac myopathies and carries little morbidity, thus is often left untreated. *Acute* first-degree block, on the other hand, is of much more concern and may be related to digoxin toxicity, β-blockers, amiodarone, myocardial infarction, hyperkalemia, or edema related to valvular surgery.

**Treatment**: involves eliminating cause if possible, such as changing medications. Atropine 0.5-1.0 mg may be given IV if rate falls.

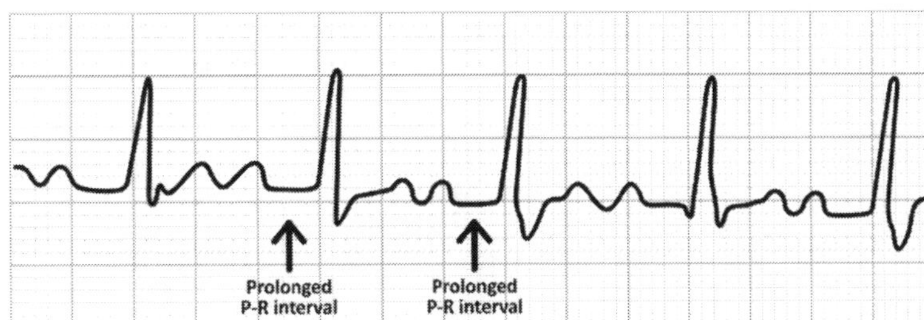

## Second-Degree AV Block

Second-degree AV block occurs when some of the atrial beats are blocked. Second-degree AV block is further subdivided according to the patterns of block.

### Type I

Mobitz type I block (Wenckebach) occurs when each atrial impulse in a group of beats is conducted at a lengthened interval until one fails to conduct (the PR interval progressively increases), so there are more P waves than QRS complexes, but the QRS complex is usually of normal shape and duration. The sinus node functions at a regular rate, so the P-P interval is regular, but the R-R interval usually shortens with each impulse. The P:QRS ratio varies, such as 3:2, 4:3, 5:4. This type of block by itself usually does not cause significant morbidity unless associated with an inferior wall myocardial infarction.

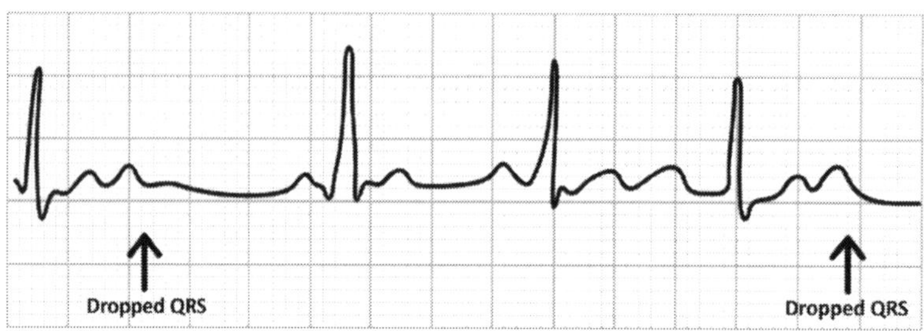


### Type II

In Mobitz type II, only some of the atrial impulses are conducted unpredictably through the AV node to the ventricles, and the block always occurs below the AV node in the bundle of His, the bundle branches, or the Purkinje fibers. The PR intervals are the same if impulses are conducted, and the QRS complex is usually widened. The P:QRS ratio varies 2:1, 3:1, and 4:1. Type II block is more dangerous than Type I because it may progress to complete AV block and may produce Stokes-Adams syncope. Additionally, if the block is at the Purkinje fibers, there is no escape impulse. Usually, a transcutaneous cardiac pacemaker and defibrillator should be at the patient's bedside. **Symptoms** may include chest pain if the heart block is precipitated by myocarditis or myocardial ischemia.

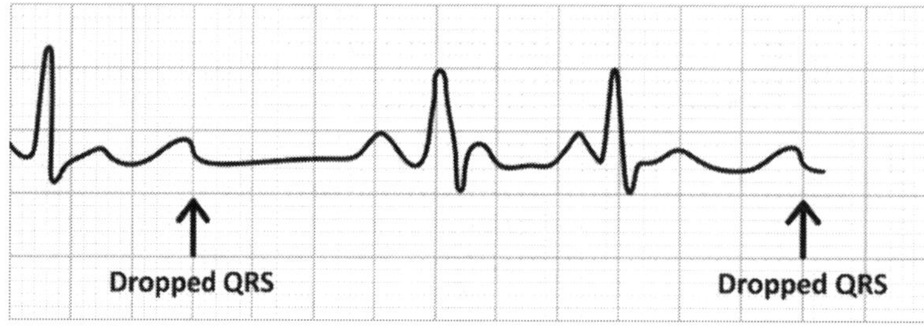

### THIRD-DEGREE

With third-degree AV block, there are more P waves than QRS complexes, with no clear relationship between them. The atrial rate is 2-3 times the pulse rate, so the PR interval is irregular. If the SA node malfunctions, the AV node fires at a lower rate, and if the AV node malfunctions, the pacemaker site in the ventricles takes over at a bradycardic rate; thus, with complete AV block, the heart still contracts, but often ineffectually. With this type of block, the atrial P (sinus rhythm or atrial fibrillation) and the ventricular QRS (ventricular escape rhythm) are stimulated by different impulses, so there is AV dissociation.

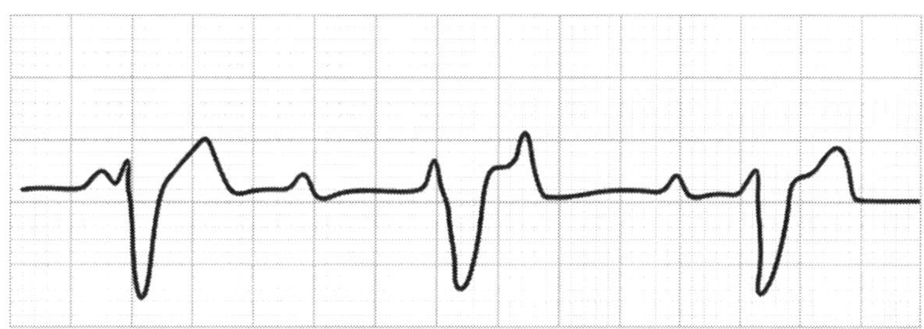

The heart may compensate at rest but can't keep pace with exertion. The resultant bradycardia may cause congestive heart failure, fainting, or even sudden death, and usually conduction abnormalities slowly worsen. **Symptoms** include dyspnea, chest pain, and hypotension, which are treated with IV atropine. Transcutaneous pacing may be needed. Complete persistent AV block normally requires implanted pacemakers, usually dual chamber.

**Review Video: AV Heart Blocks**
Visit mometrix.com/academy and enter code: 487004

### *BUNDLE BRANCH BLOCKS*

A **right bundle branch block (RBBB)** occurs when conduction is blocked in the right bundle branch that carries impulses from the Bundle of His to the right ventricle. The impulse travels through the left ventricle instead, and then reaches the right ventricle, but this causes a slight delay in contraction of the right ventricle. A RBBB is characterized by normal P waves (as the right atrium still contracts appropriately), but the QRS complex is widened and notched (referred to as an "RSR pattern" that resembles the letter "M") in lead V1, which is a reflection of the asynchronous ventricular contraction. The PR interval is normal or prolonged, and the QRS interval is > 0.12 seconds. P:QRS ratio remains 1:1 with regular rhythms.

A **left bundle branch block (LBBB)** occurs when there is a delay in conduction between the left atrium and left ventricle. It is also characterized by normal or inverted P waves, but the QRS complex may be widened with a deep S wave and an interval of >0.12 seconds (in lead V1) that resembles a "W." The PR interval may be normal or prolonged. The P:QRS ratio is 1:1 and the rhythm is regular.

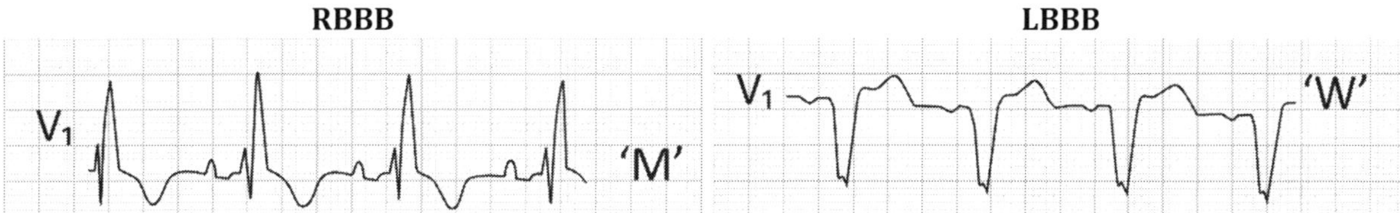


## HEART FAILURE

Heart failure (formerly congestive heart failure) is a cardiac disease that includes disorders of contractions (systolic dysfunction) or filling (diastolic dysfunction) or both and may include pulmonary, peripheral, or systemic edema. The most common causes are coronary artery disease, systemic or pulmonary hypertension, cardiomyopathy, and valvular disorders. The incidence of chronic heart failure correlates with age. The 2 main types of HF are systolic and diastolic. HF is classified according to symptoms and prognosis:

- **Class I**: The patient is essentially asymptomatic during normal activities with no pulmonary congestion or peripheral hypotension. There is no restriction on activities, and prognosis is good.
- **Class II**: Symptoms appear with physical exertion but are usually absent at rest, resulting in some limitations of activities of daily living (ADLs). Slight pulmonary edema may be evident by basilar rales. Prognosis is good.
- **Class III**: Obvious limitations of ADLs and discomfort on any exertion. Prognosis is fair.
- **Class IV**: Symptoms at rest. Prognosis is poor.

**Treatment** may include:

- Careful monitoring of **fluid balance** and **weight** to determine changes in fluid retention
- **Low sodium diet**
- **Restriction of activity**
- **Medications** may include diuretics, vasodilators, or ACE inhibitors to decrease the heart's workload, digoxin may be given to increase contractibility
- **Anticoagulant therapy** if distended atria, enlarged ventricles, or atrial fibrillation to decrease the danger of thromboembolic

**Review Video: Congestive Heart Failure**
Visit mometrix.com/academy and enter code: 924118

### *Systolic Heart Failure*

Systolic heart failure is the typical "left-sided" failure and reduces the amount of blood ejected from the ventricles during contraction (decreased ejection fraction). This stimulates the SNS to produce catecholamines to support the myocardium, which eventually causes down regulation, the destruction of beta and adrenergic receptor sites, and ultimately further myocardial damage. Because of reduced perfusion, the R-A-A pathway (renin, angiotensin I&II, aldosterone) is initiated by the kidneys, causing sodium and fluid retention. The end result of these processes is increased preload and afterload, thus increased workload on the ventricles. They begin to lose contractibility and blood begins to pool inside, stretching the myocardium (ventricular remodeling). The heart compensates by thickening the muscle (hypertrophy) without an adequate increase in capillary blood supply, leading to ischemia.

**Symptoms**: Activity intolerance, dyspnea/orthopnea (sleeping in a recliner is a classic symptom), cough (frothy sputum), edema, heart sounds S3 and S4, hepatomegaly, JVD, LOC changes, and tachycardia.

**Treatment** includes:

- Medication
- **Surgery**: Heart transplant (if a candidate)
- **Lifestyle modification**: Low-sodium diet, supplemental oxygen, daily weights (report >3 lb/day or 5 lb/week weight gain to physician)

### *Diastolic Heart Failure*

Diastolic heart failure may be difficult to differentiate from systolic heart failure based on clinical symptoms, which are similar. With diastolic heart failure, the myocardium is unable to sufficiently relax to facilitate filling of the ventricles. This may be the end result of systolic heart failure as myocardial hypertrophy stiffens the muscles, and the causes are similar. Diastolic heart failure is more common in females >75. Typically, intra-cardiac pressures at rest are within normal range but increase markedly on exertion. Because the relaxation of the heart is delayed, the ventricles do not expand enough for the fill-volume, and the heart cannot increase stroke volume during exercise, so symptoms (dyspnea, fatigue, pulmonary edema) are often pronounced on exertion. Ejection fractions are usually >40-50% with increase in left ventricular end-diastolic pressure (LVEDP) and decrease in left ventricular end-diastolic volume (LVEDV).

The major goal with all types of heart failure is to prevent further damage and remodeling, prevent exacerbations, and improve the patient's long-term prognosis.

### *Acute Heart Failure*

Acute decompensated heart failure occurs when the body cannot compensate for the heart's inability to provide adequate perfusion. Cardiac output is no longer sufficient to meet the metabolic demands of the body. Acute heart failure occurs suddenly and can be precipitated by dysrhythmias, illness, noncompliance with medications, acute ischemia, fluid overload or hypertensive crisis. Acute heart failure is most commonly related to left ventricular systolic or diastolic dysfunction. It requires immediate treatment to restore adequate perfusion and is often life-threatening.

**Signs and symptoms**: Dyspnea, cough, edema, ascites and elevated jugular venous pressure, fatigue, cool extremities, hypotension and altered mental status

**Diagnostic testing**: Chest x-ray, electrocardiogram, physical exam; labs—basic metabolic panel, BUN, creatinine, and B-natriuretic peptide (BNP)

**Treatment**: Rapid assessment and stabilization of the patient. The physical assessment should include a thorough evaluation of the patient's respiratory status and supplemental oxygen and potentially ventilator support may be necessary. Medications: Diuretics to decrease fluid volume; vasodilators to decrease pulmonary congestion. Cardiac monitoring, urine output monitoring, sodium restriction, and venous thromboembolism prophylaxis may also be utilized.

### *Acute Cardiac-Related Pulmonary Edema*

Acute cardiac-related pulmonary edema occurs when heart failure results in fluid overload, leading to third-spacing of fluid into the interstitial spaces of the lungs. Pulmonary edema may result from MI, chronic HF, volume overload, ischemia, or mitral stenosis.

**Symptoms** include severe dyspnea, cough with blood-tinged frothy sputum, wheezing/rales/crackles on auscultation, cyanosis, and diaphoresis.

**Diagnosis**: Auscultation, chest x-ray, and echocardiogram.

**Treatment** includes:

- Sitting position with 100% oxygen by mask to achieve $PO_2$ >60%
- Non-invasive pressure support ventilation (BiPAP) or endotracheal intubation and mechanical ventilation
- Morphine sulfate 2-8 mg (IV for severe cases), repeated every 2-4 hours as needed—decreases pre-load and anxiety
- IV diuretics (furosemide ≥40 mg or bumetanide ≥1 mg) to provide venous dilation and diuresis
- Nitrates as a bolus with an infusion—decreases pre-load
- Inhaled β-adrenergic agonists or aminophylline for bronchospasm
- Digoxin IV for tachycardia
- ACE inhibitors, nitroprusside to reduce afterload

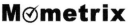

## Myocardial Conduction System Abnormalities

### *Prolonged QT Interval*

The normal **QT interval** is 400-460 ms in females and 400-440 ms in males. QT interval value greater than 500 ms increases risk of cardiac abnormalities. If the QT interval extends greater than half the RR, it is prolonged. Long QT syndrome occurs when depolarization and repolarization is prolonged between beats and can result in torsades de points or VT. "R-on-T" phenomenon can trigger these dangerous arrhythmias and is a serious risk with long QT intervals, as the chance of a PVC (specifically the ventricular depolarization of the PVC) falling on the t-wave is what induces the arrhythmia. The longer the QT interval, the greater the chance of this phenomenon occurring. Long QT syndrome may be a genetic condition or may be acquired and associated with electrolyte imbalances, some medications (antidepressants, diuretics, antibiotics), and some conditions (anorexia nervosa). Continuous QT interval monitoring measures from the QRS complex (depolarization) to the end of the T wave (repolarization).

- Newly diagnosed with bradyarrhythmia
- Receiving anti-arrhythmic drugs or other drugs associated with torsade de pointes (a life-threatening dysrhythmia)
- Overdosing on agents or receiving antipsychotics or drugs that may cause arrhythmias
- With electrolyte imbalances (hypokalemia, hypomagnesemia) that may cause arrhythmias
- With acute neurological events, such as stroke

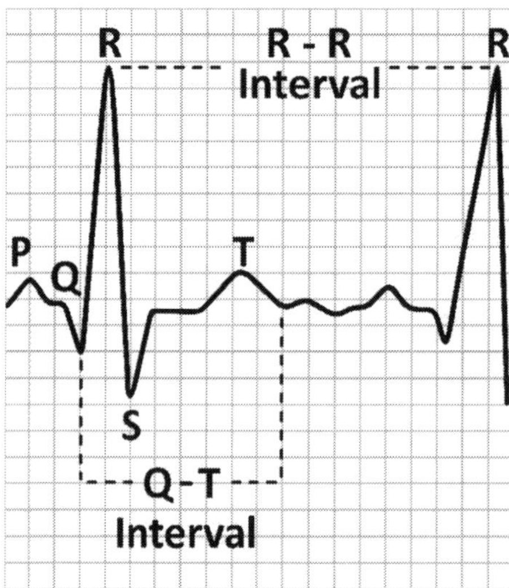


### *Wolff-Parkinson-White Syndrome*

The Wolff-Parkinson-White syndrome (a preexcitation syndrome) is characterized by a short PR interval and a delta wave, which appears as a slurred upstroke into the QRS complex, so the PR interval is missing. The QRS complex is prolonged because of the delta wave. The rhythm is very irregular and the rate is often 250-300 bpm. The delta wave is produced because of premature depolarization of part of the ventricles. With preexcitation syndromes, electrical stimulation of the ventricles occurs through an accessory (in this case Kent's bundle) pathway while the impulse also travels through the AV node, and this can lead to rapid paroxysmal tachyarrhythmias (usually AV reentry tachycardia—AVRT). About 40% develop atrial fibrillation.

Medications, such as amiodarone and sotalol may be used to slow conduction, but cardioversion may be necessary. WPW syndrome is most common in children and young adults.

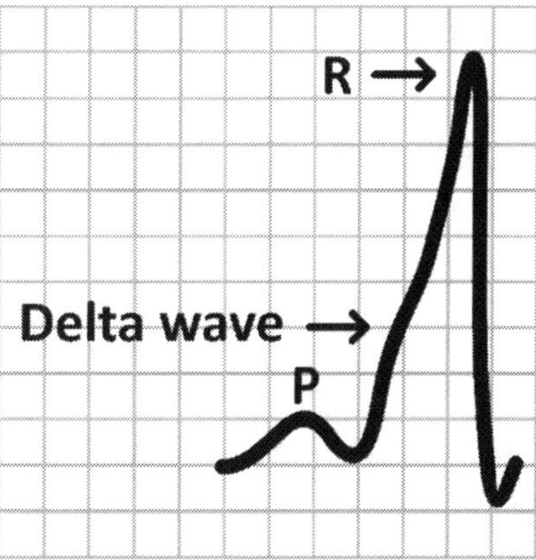


## ENDOCARDITIS

Endocarditis is an infection of the lining of the heart that covers the heart valves and contains Purkinje fibers, known as the endocardium. Risk factors include being over 60 years of age, being male, IV drug use, and dental infections. Staphylococcal aureus is the most common cause of infective endocarditis. Etiology includes subacute bacterial endocarditis (often related to dental procedures), prosthetic valvular endocarditis (following valve replacement), and right sided endocarditis (often related to catheter infections and IV drug use). Organisms enter the bloodstream from portals of entry (surgery, catheterization, IV drug abuse) and migrate to the heart, growing on the endothelial tissue and forming vegetations (verrucae), collagen deposits, and platelet thrombi. With endocarditis, the valves frequently become deformed, but the pathogenic agents may also invade other tissues, such as the chordae tendineae. The lesions may invade adjacent tissue and break off, becoming emboli. The mitral valve is the most common valve affected, followed by aortic, tricuspid, and the pulmonary valve being the least often affected. Positive blood cultures, widened pulse pressures, ECG, murmurs, and vegetations seen on a transesophageal echocardiogram are used to make the diagnosis. After diagnosis is made, antibiotics are used for treatment, and when unsuccessful or when heart failure is present, valve repair may be warranted. Serious complications from endocarditis include emboli, sepsis, and heart failure. Untreated endocarditis is fatal.

### *DIAGNOSIS AND TREATMENT*

Diagnosis of endocarditis is made on the basis of clinical presentation and **diagnostic procedures** that may include:

- **Blood cultures** should be done with 3 sets for both aerobic and anaerobic bacteria. Diagnosis is definitive if 2 cultures are positive, but a negative culture does not preclude bacterial endocarditis.
- **Echocardiogram** may identify vegetation on valves or increasing heart failure
- **ECG** may demonstrate prolonged PR interval
- **Anemia** (normochromic, normocytic)
- Elevated **white blood cell count**
- Elevated **erythrocyte sedimentation rate** (ESR) and **C-reactive protein** (CRP)

**Treatment** includes general management of symptoms and the following:

- **Antimicrobials** specific to the pathogenic organism, usually administered IV for 4 to 6 weeks
- **Surgical replacement** of aortic and/or mitral valves may be necessary (in 30% to 40% of cases) if there is no response to treatment and/or after infection is controlled if there are severe symptoms related to valve damage

### *Clinical Symptoms*

Clinical symptoms of endocarditis usually relate to the response to infection, the underlying heart disease, emboli, or immunological response. Typical **symptoms** include:

- Slow onset with unexplained low-grade and often intermittent **fever**
- **Anorexia** and weight loss, difficulty feeding
- General **lassitude** and malaise
- **Splenomegaly** present in 60% of patients; **hepatomegaly** may also be present
- **Anemia** is present in almost all patients
- Sudden **aortic valve insufficiency** or mitral valve insufficiency
- **Cyanosis** with clubbing of fingers
- **Embolism** of other body organs (brain, liver, bones)
- **Congestive heart failure**
- **Dysrhythmias**
- New or change in **heart murmur**
- **Immunological responses**
- **Janeway lesions**: painless areas of hemorrhage on palms of hands and soles of feet
- **Splinter hemorrhages**: thin, brown-black lines on nails of fingers and toes
- **Petechiae**: pinpoint-sized hemorrhages on oral mucous membranes, as well as hands and trunk
- **Roth spots**: retinal hemorrhagic lesions caused by emboli on nerve fibers
- **Glomerulonephritis**: microscopic hematuria

## Myocarditis

Myocarditis is inflammation of the cardiac myocardium (muscle tissue), usually triggered by a viral infection, such as the influenza virus, Coxsackie virus, and HIV. Myocarditis can also be caused by bacteria, fungi, or parasites, or an allergic response to medications. In some cases, it is also a complication of endocarditis. It may also be triggered by chemotherapy drugs and some antibiotics. Myocarditis can result in dilation of the heart, development of thrombi on the heart walls (known as mural thrombi), and infiltration of blood cells around the coronary vessels and between muscle fibers, causing further degeneration of the muscle tissue. The heart may become enlarged and weak, as the ability to pump blood is impaired, leading to congestive heart failure. Symptoms depend upon the extent of damage but may include fatigue, dyspnea, pressure and discomfort in chest or epigastric area, and palpitations.

### *Diagnosis and Treatment*

Diagnosis of myocarditis depends upon the clinical picture, as there is no test specific for myocarditis, although a number of tests may be done to verify the **clinical diagnosis**:

- **Chest radiograph** may indicate cardiomegaly or pulmonary edema.
- **ECG** may show nonspecific changes.
- **Echocardiogram** may indicate cardiomegaly and demonstrate defects in functioning.
- **Cardiac catheterization** and **cardiac biopsy** will yield confirmation in 65% of cases, but not all of the heart muscle may be affected, so a negative finding does not rule out myocarditis.
- **Viral cultures** of nasopharynx and rectal may help to identify organism.
- **Viral titers** may increase as disease progresses.
- **Polymerase chain reaction** (PCR) of biopsy specimen may be most effective for diagnosis.

**Treatment**:

- As indicated for underlying cause (such as antibiotics)
- Restriction of activities
- Careful **monitoring** for heart failure and medical treatment as indicated (e.g., diuretics, digoxin)

- **Oxygen** as needed to maintain normal oxygen saturation
- **IV gamma globulin** for acute stage

## Acute Pericarditis

Pericarditis is inflammation of the pericardial sac with or without increased pericardial fluid. It may be an isolated process or the effect of an underlying disease. If the underlying cause is autoimmune or related to malignancy of some sort, the patient usually presents with symptoms that relate to that disorder. However, most cases are related to a viral etiology, and therefore usually present with flu-like symptoms. Patients that have idiopathic pericarditis or viral pericarditis have a good prognosis with medication alone.

**Signs/Symptoms**: Sharp chest pain, worsened with inspiration and relieved by leaning forward or sitting up (most common symptom; "Mohammad's Sign"), pericardial effusion, respiratory distress, auscultated friction rub, ST elevation/PR depression (progresses to flattened T, inverted T, then return to normal); risk of pericardial effusion.

**Diagnosis**: Echocardiogram, ECG, pericardiocentesis or pericardial biopsy, cardiac enzymes (may be mildly elevated), WBC/ESR/CRP all elevated.

**Treatment** includes:

- **Medications**: NSAIDs for pain/inflammation, Colchicine 0.5 mg twice a day for six months is often prescribed in adjunct to NSAID therapy, as it decreases the incidence of recurrence
- **Surgery**: Pericardiectomy only in extreme cases

## Mitral Stenosis

Mitral stenosis is a narrowing of the mitral valve that allows blood to flow from the left atrium to the left ventricle. Pressure in the left atrium increases to overcome resistance, resulting in enlargement of the left atrium and increased pressure in the pulmonary veins and capillaries of the lung (pulmonary hypertension). Mitral stenosis can be caused by infective endocarditis, calcifications, or tumors in the left atrium.

**Signs/Symptoms**: Exertional dyspnea, orthopnea/nocturnal dyspnea, right-sided heart failure, loud $S_1$ and $S_2$, and mid-diastolic murmur.

**Diagnosis**: Cardiac catheterization, chest x-ray, echocardiogram, ECG.

**Treatment** includes:

- **Medications**: Antiarrhythmic, anticoagulant, and antihypertensive medications
- **Surgical**: Open/closed commissurotomy, balloon valvuloplasty, and mitral valve replacement

## Mitral Valve Insufficiency

Mitral valve insufficiency occurs when the mitral valve fails to close completely so that there is backflow into the left atrium from the left ventricle during systole, decreasing cardiac output. It may occur with mitral stenosis or independently. Mitral valve insufficiency can result from damage caused by rheumatic fever, myxomatous degeneration, infective endocarditis, collagen vascular disease (Marfan's syndrome), or cardiomyopathy/left heart failure. There are **three phases** of the disease:

- **Acute**: May occur with rupture of a chordae tendineae or papillary muscle causing sudden left ventricular flooding and overload.
- **Chronic compensated**: Enlargement of the left atrium to decrease filling pressure, and hypertrophy of the left ventricle.
- **Chronic decompensated**: Left ventricle fails to compensate for the volume overload; decreased stroke volume and increased cardiac output.

**Symptoms**: Orthopnea/dyspnea, split $S_2/S_3/S_4$ heart sounds, systolic murmur, palpitations, right-sided heart failure, fatigue, angina (rare).

**Diagnosis**: Cardiac catheterization, chest x-ray, echocardiogram, ECG.

**Treatment** includes:

- **Medications**: Antiarrhythmic, anticoagulant, and antihypertensive medications.
- **Surgical**: Annuloplasty or valvuloplasty, and mitral valve replacement.

## AORTIC STENOSIS

Aortic stenosis is a stricture (narrowing) of the aortic valve that controls the flow of blood from the left ventricle. This causes the left ventricular wall to thicken as it increases pressure to overcome the valvular resistance, increasing afterload and increasing the need for blood supply from the coronary arteries. This condition may result from a birth defect or childhood rheumatic fever, and tends to worsen over the years as the heart grows.

**Symptoms**: Angina, exercise intolerance, dyspnea, split $S_1$ and $S_2$, systolic murmur at base of carotids, hypotension on exertion, syncope, left-sided heart failure; sudden death can occur.

**Diagnosis**: Cardiac catheterization, chest x-ray, echocardiogram, ECG.

**Treatment** includes:

- **Medications**: Antiarrhythmic, anticoagulant, and antihypertensive medications
- **Surgical**: Balloon valvuloplasty, and aortic valve replacement

## PULMONIC STENOSIS

Pulmonic stenosis is a stricture of the pulmonary blood that controls the flow of blood from the right ventricle to the lungs, resulting in right ventricular hypertrophy as the pressure increases in the right ventricle and decreased pulmonary blood flow. The condition may be asymptomatic or symptoms may not be evident until adulthood, depending upon the severity of the defect. Pulmonic stenosis may be associated with a number of other heart defects.

**Symptoms**: May be asymptomatic; dyspnea on exertion, systolic heart murmur, right-sided heart failure.

**Diagnosis**: Cardiac catheterization, chest x-ray, echocardiogram, ECG.

**Treatment** includes:

- **Medications**: Antiarrhythmic, anticoagulant, and antihypertensive medications
- **Surgical**: Balloon valvuloplasty, valvotomy, valvectomy with or without transannular patch, and pulmonary valve replacement

## BLUNT CARDIAC TRAUMA AND TRAUMATIC INJURY TO THE GREAT VESSELS

Blunt cardiac trauma most often occurs as the result of motor vehicle accidents, falls, or other blows to the chest. This can result in respiratory distress, rupture of the great vessels, and cardiac tamponade/increasing intrathoracic pressure. The right atrium and right ventricle are the most commonly injured because they are anterior to the rest of the heart. While not definitive, echocardiogram in conjunction with CPK MB levels is useful in predicting complications. Because diagnosis is challenging until complications appear, every patient with suspected blunt chest trauma should receive an ECG upon admission/STAT. If abnormalities are present, continuous cardiac monitoring should be done for 24-48 hours. Decreased cerebral perfusion/anoxia may result in severe agitation with combative behavior.

Traumatic injuries to the great vessels most commonly result from severe decelerating blunt force or penetrating injuries, with aortic trauma the most common. If the aorta is torn, it will result in almost instant death, but in some cases, there is an incomplete laceration to the intimal lining (innermost membrane) of the aorta, causing an aortic hematoma or bulging. This lining, the adventitia, is quite strong and often will contain the rupture long enough to allow surgical repair.

**Diagnosis**: Chest x-ray or CT; transesophageal echocardiogram to verify

**Treatment**: STAT surgical repair to avoid eventual rupture, during which other vessels are examined for clotting or internal injuries

## Penetrating Cardiac Injuries

The incidence of penetrating cardiac injuries has been on the rise, primarily associated with gunshot injuries and stabbings. The extent of damage caused by a stab wound is often easier to assess than gunshot wounds, which may be multiple and often result in unpredictable and widespread damage not only to the heart but other structures. Mortality rates are very high in the first hour after a penetrating cardiac injury, so it is imperative that the patient be taken immediately to a trauma center rather than attempts be made to stabilize the person at the site. NEVER attempt to remove the object in the field/without a physician present.

The primary **complications**:

- **Exsanguination** is frequently related to gunshot wounds, and prognosis is very poor. This may lead to hemothorax and hemorrhagic shock.
- **Cardiac tamponade** is more common with knife wounds, but prognosis is fairly good with surgical repair. Cardiac tamponade often presents with three classic symptoms, known as Beck's triad that should be quickly recognized: muffled heart sounds, low arterial blood pressure, and jugular vein distention.
- **Pneumothorax**: Deviated trachea, increasing SVR, tachypnea and anxiety all may indicate tension pneumothorax, which is a medical emergency. It is treated by emergent insertion of a chest tube or needle aspiration of trapped air. Open wounds can be emergently dressed with a three-sided dressing until a chest tube can be inserted to create a "flutter valve" effect and allow trapped air to escape.

**Nursing Considerations**: Management includes controlling bleeding, giving fluids and vasopressors for blood pressure, preparing patient for surgery, and monitoring for the above-mentioned complications.

## Carotid Artery Stenosis

The common carotid artery branches from the subclavian artery and then bifurcates into the external carotid and internal carotid arteries. This point of bifurcation is a common site for the development of plaques, causing **carotid artery stenosis** that interferes with cranial blood flow. When stenosis develops slowly, collateral vessels may form to aid circulation, but sudden occlusion can cause permanent brain damage and death. Most stenosis is caused by atherosclerosis, with increasing incidence with age. Most ischemia relates to an embolism or thrombus formation.

**Symptoms** of occlusion are often asymptomatic; however, they include severe pain, anxiety, and those symptoms common to brain attacks (hemiparesis, confusion, aphasia, and diplopia).

**Diagnosis**: Duplex ultrasound (combining conventional ultrasound with Doppler, determines blood flow and obstruction), CT scan, MRA or angiogram (will indicate degree of blockage).

**Treatment** may include:

- Medications: Anticoagulants and thrombolytics.
- Carotid endarterectomy (recommended if stenosis >60%): poses the danger of a post-procedure stroke due to plaque dislodgement or increased blood flow to narrowed vessels, so the benefits must be carefully weighed.
- Carotid stents/angioplasty (newer non-invasive approaches).

## CARDIAC TAMPONADE

Cardiac tamponade occurs with pericardial effusion, causing pressure against the heart. It may be a complication of trauma, pericarditis, cardiac surgery, pneumothorax, or heart failure. About 50 mL of fluid normally circulates in the pericardial area to reduce friction, and a sudden increase in this volume or air in the pericardial sac can compress the heart, causing a number of cardiac responses such as:

- Increased end-diastolic pressure in both ventricles
- Decrease in venous return
- Decrease in ventricular filling

Symptoms may include pressure or pain in the chest, dyspnea, and pulsus paradoxus >10 mmHg. Beck's triad (increased CVP, distended neck veins, muffled heart sounds, and hypotension) is common. A sudden decrease in chest tube drainage can occur as fluid and clots accumulate in the pericardial sac, preventing the blood from filling the ventricles and decreasing cardiac output and perfusion of the body, including the kidneys (resulting in decreased urinary output). X-ray may show change in cardiac silhouette and mediastinal shift (in 20%). Treatment includes pericardiocentesis with large bore needle or surgical repair to control bleeding and relieve cardiac compression. Risk factors include cardiac surgery, cardiac tumors, MI, and chest trauma.

## HYPERTENSIVE CRISES

Hypertensive crises are marked elevations in blood pressure that can cause severe organ damage if left untreated. Hypertensive crises may be caused by endocrine/renal disorders (pheochromocytoma), dissection of an aortic aneurysm, pulmonary edema, subarachnoid hemorrhage, stroke, eclampsia, and medication noncompliance. There are two **classifications**:

- **Hypertensive emergency** occurs when acute hypertension, usually >220 systolic and 120 mmHg diastolic, must be treated immediately to lower blood pressure in order to prevent damage to vital organs.
- **Hypertensive urgency** occurs when acute hypertension must be treated within a few hours but the vital organs are not in immediate danger. Blood pressure is lowered more slowly to avoid hypotension, ischemia of vital organs, or failure of autoregulation.
    - 1/3 reduction in 6 hours
    - 1/3 reduction in next 24 hours
    - 1/3 reduction over days 2-4

**Symptoms**: Basilar HA, blurred vision, chest pain, N/V, SOB, seizures, ruddy pallor, and anxiety

**Diagnostics**: ECG, Chest x-ray, CBC, BMP, Urinalysis (+ blood and casts)

**Treatment** includes:

- Medications: Vasodilators (Cardene, Nitro, etc.) and diuretics
- Nursing Interventions: Raise HOB to 90°, supplemental $O_2$, frequent neuro checks, teach concerning medication compliance

## Congenital Heart Defects Seen in Adulthood

Congenital heart defects are often identified in infancy or early childhood; however, diagnosis may be delayed until adulthood due to the lack of signs and symptoms. Atrial septal and ventricular septal defects are common congenital anomalies that can present at any age. An atrial septal defect occurs when part of the atrial septum does not form properly, leaving a hole in the septum. A ventricular septal defect results from a hole in the septum separating the ventricles. Patent ductus arteriosus, coarctation of the aorta and Ebstein's anomaly are other types of congenital defects that are less commonly diagnosed in adulthood.

**Signs and symptoms**: Murmurs, cyanosis, clubbing of the fingernails, shortness of breath, fatigue, syncope, palpitations, and edema. Heart failure and endocarditis may also occur.

**Diagnosis**: Physical assessment, EKG, Chest x-ray, transesophageal echocardiogram, CT, and MRI.

**Treatment**: Treatment options depend on the size and location of the defect. Most commonly the anomaly will be corrected by open surgical repair; however percutaneous intervention may be an option in some patients.

## Peripheral Arterial and Venous Insufficiency

Characteristics of peripheral arterial and venous insufficiency are listed below:

- **Arterial insufficiency**
  - **Pain**: Ranging from intermittent claudication to severe and constant shooting pain
  - **Pulses**: Weak or absent
  - **Skin**: Rubor on dependency, but pallor of foot on elevation; pale, shiny, and cool skin with loss of hair on toes and foot; nails thick and ridged
  - **Ulcers**: Painful, deep, circular, often necrotic ulcers on toe tips, toe webs, heels, or other pressure areas
  - **Edema**: Minimal
- **Venous insufficiency**
  - **Pain**: Aching/cramping
  - **Pulses**: Strong/present
  - **Skin**: Brownish discoloration around ankles and anterior tibial area
  - **Ulcers**: Varying degrees of pain in superficial, irregular ulcers on medial or lateral malleolus and sometimes the anterior tibial area
  - **Edema**: Moderate to severe

## Acute Peripheral Vascular Insufficiency

Acute peripheral arterial insufficiency can occur when sudden occlusion of a blood vessel causes tissue ischemia, ultimately leading to cellular death and necrosis. This can occur as a result of traumatic injury or non-traumatic events such as arterial thrombus or embolism, vasospasm, or severe swelling (compartment syndrome). Risk factors for acute peripheral arterial insufficiency include age, tobacco use, diabetes mellitus, hyperlipidemia, and hypertension.

- **Signs and symptoms**: Classic 6 P's: Pain (extreme, unrelieved by narcotics), pallor, pulselessness, poikilothermia (the inability to regulate body temperature; extremity is room temperature), paresthesias, and paralysis (late).
- **Diagnosis**: Ultrasound, angiography, and physical exam; labs—coagulation studies, CBC, BMP, creatinine phosphokinase
- **Treatment**: Re-establishment of blood flow to the affected area
- **Arterial thrombus or embolism**: Mechanical thrombolysis may be performed to remove the clot occluding the vessel.

- **Trauma**: Surgical repair of the severed/injured vessels. Fasciotomy may be performed in the event of compartment syndrome to relieve pressure.
- **Other treatment options**: Hyperbaric oxygen therapy, anti-platelet therapy for the prevention of arterial thrombosis and anti-coagulant therapy for the prevention of venous thrombosis

## Acute Venous Thromboembolism

Acute venous thromboembolism (VTE) is a condition that includes both deep vein thrombosis (DVT) and pulmonary emboli (PE). VTE may be precipitated by invasive procedures, lack of mobility, and inflammation, so it is a common complication in critical care units. **Virchow's triad** comprises common risk factors: blood stasis, injury to endothelium, and hypercoagulability. Some patients may be initially asymptomatic, but **symptoms** may include:

- Aching or throbbing pain
- Positive Homan's sign (pain in calf when foot is dorsiflexed)
- Unilateral erythema and edema
- Dilation of vessels
- Cyanosis

**Diagnosis**: ultrasound and/or D-dimer test, which tests the serum for cross-linked fibrin derivatives. A CT scan, pulmonary angiogram, and ventilation-perfusion lung scan may be used to diagnose pulmonary emboli.

**Treatment** includes:

- Medications: IV heparin, tPA, or other anticoagulation; analgesia for pain
- Surgical: May have to surgically remove clot if large
- Bed rest, elevation of affected limb; stockings on ambulation

**Prevention**: Use of sequential compression devices (SCDs) or foot pumps, routine anticoagulant use for those at highest risk (Heparin SQ), early and frequent ambulation

# Cardiovascular Procedures and Interventions

## CARDIOVERSION

Cardioversion sends a timed electrical stimulation to the heart to convert a tachydysrhythmia (such as atrial fibrillation) to a normal sinus rhythm. Usually, anticoagulation therapy is done for at least 3 weeks prior to elective cardioversion to reduce the risk of emboli, and digoxin is discontinued for at least 48 hours prior. During the procedure, the patient is usually sedated and/or anesthetized. Electrodes in the form of gel-covered paddles or pads are placed in the anteroposterior position and then connected by leads to a computerized ECG and cardiac monitor with a defibrillator. The defibrillator is synchronized with the ECG so that the electrical current is delivered during ventricular depolarization (QRS). The timing must be precise in order to prevent ventricular tachycardia or ventricular fibrillation. Sometimes, drug therapy is used in conjunction with cardioversion; for example, antiarrhythmics (Cardizem, Cordarone) may be given before the procedure to slow the heart rate.

| Arrhythmia | Beginning Monophasic Shock | Beginning Biphasic Shock |
|---|---|---|
| Atrial Fibrillation | 50-100 J | 25 J |
| Atrial Flutter | 25-50 J | 15 J |
| Ventricular Tachycardia | 100-200 J | 50 J |

## EMERGENCY DEFIBRILLATION

Emergency defibrillation delivers a non-synchronized shock that is given to treat acute ventricular fibrillation, pulseless ventricular tachycardia, or polymorphic ventricular tachycardia with a rapid rate and decompensating hemodynamics. **Defibrillation** can be given at any point in the cardiac cycle. It causes depolarization of myocardial cells, which can then repolarize to regain a normal sinus rhythm. Defibrillation delivers an electrical discharge through pads/paddles. In an acute care setting, the preferred position to place the pads is the anteroposterior position. In this position, one pad is placed to the right of the sternum about the second to third intercostal space, and the other pad is placed between the left scapula and the spinal column. This decreases the chances of damaging implanted devices, such as pacemakers, and this positioning has also been shown to be more effective for external cardioversion (if indicated at some point during resuscitation). There are two main types of defibrillator shock waveforms: monophasic and biphasic. Biphasic defibrillators deliver a shock in one direction for half of the shock, and then in the return direction for the other half, making them more effective and able to be used at lower energy levels. Monophasic defibrillation is given at 200-360 J and biphasic defibrillation is given at 100-200 J.

## PERICARDIOCENTESIS

Pericardiocentesis is done with ultrasound guidance to diagnose pericardial effusion or with ECG and ultrasound guidance to relieve cardiac tamponade. **Pericardiocentesis** may be done as treatment for cardiac arrest or with presentation of PEA with increased jugular venous pressure. Non-hemorrhagic tamponade may be relieved in 60-90% of cases, but hemorrhagic tamponade requires thoracotomy, as blood will continue to accumulate until the cause of the hemorrhage is corrected. Resuscitation equipment must be available, including a defibrillator, intravenous line in place, and cardiac monitoring.

The **procedure** is as follows:

- Elevate the chest 45° to bring the heart closer to the chest wall, pre-medicate with atropine, and insert a nasogastric tube if indicated.
- Cleanse the skin with chlorhexidine or another appropriate cleanser.
- After insertion of the needle using ultrasound guidance, remove the obturator and attach a syringe for aspiration.
- The needle can often be replaced with a catheter after removal for drainage.
- A post-procedure chest x-ray should be done to check for pneumothorax.

**Possible Complications:** Pneumo/hemothorax, coronary artery rupture, hepatic injury, dysrhythmias, and false negative/positive aspiration.

## PACEMAKERS

Pacemakers are used to stimulate the heart when the normal conduction system of the heart is defective. **Pacemakers** may be used temporarily or be permanently implanted. Temporary pacemakers for external cardiac pacing are commonly used in the emergency setting. Temporary pacemakers may be used prophylactically or therapeutically to treat a cardiac abnormality. Clinical uses include:

- To treat persistent **dysrhythmias** not responsive to medications
- To increase **cardiac output** with bradydysrhythmia by increasing rate
- To decrease **ventricular or supraventricular tachycardia** by "overdrive" stimulation of contractions
- To treat **secondary heart block** caused by myocardial infarction, ischemia, and drug toxicity
- To improve **cardiac output** after cardiac surgery
- To provide **diagnostic information** through electrophysiology studies, which induce dysrhythmias for purposes of evaluation
- To provide **pacing** when a permanent pacemaker malfunctions

**Review Video: Pacemaker Care**
Visit mometrix.com/academy and enter code: 979075

### *TRANSCUTANEOUS PACING*

Transcutaneous pacing is used temporarily in an emergency situation to treat symptomatic bradydysrhythmias that don't respond to medications (atropine) and result in hemodynamic instability. Generally, the patient is provided oxygen and some sort of mild sedation before the pacing. The placement of pacing pads is usually one pacing pad (negative) on the left chest, inferior to the clavicle, and the other (positive) on the left back, inferior to the scapula, so the heart is sandwiched between the two. Lead wires attach the pads to the monitor. The rate of pacing is usually set around 80 bpm. The current is increased slowly until capture occurs—a spiking followed by QRS sequence—then the current is readjusted downward if possible just to maintain capture, keeping it 5-10 mA above the pacing threshold. Both demand and fixed modes are available, but demand mode is preferred. The patient should be warned that the shocks may induce pain.

### *EPICARDIAL PACING*

Epicardial pacing wires may be attached directly to the exterior atria, ventricles, or both at the conclusion of surgery for CPB or valve repair in the event that postoperative pacing support is required or for those with risk of AV block because of medications used to control atrial fibrillation. Cold cardioplegia may precipitate the transient sinus node or AV node dysfunction. While some surgeons avoid placing epicardial pacing wires because of concerns about bleeding and cardiac tamponade on removal, recommendations include placing at least one ventricular pacing wire. A typical configuration for pacing wires is atrial pacing wires placed in a plastic disk that is sutured low on the right atrium. The two ventricular wires are attached over the right ventricular wall. Atrial pacing wires may be used to record atrial activity and, and with standard ECG, can help to distinguish atrial and junctional arrhythmias and ventricular arrhythmias. Pacing wires can also be used therapeutically to increase the heart rate to about 90 bpm in order to achieve optimal hemodynamics. The epicardial leads are intended for use of 7 days or less and may be less reliable if used for extended periods. The wires are removed by applying gentle traction.

### *TEMPORARY TRANSVENOUS PACEMAKERS*

Transvenous pacemakers, comprised of a catheter with a lead at the end, may be used prophylactically or therapeutically on a temporary basis to treat symptomatic bradycardias or heart blocks when other methods have failed. The catheter has a balloon tip that must be checked for leaks prior to insertion – this is usually done by inflating the catheter tip while submersed in normal saline and checking for bubbles. After the balloon's integrity is verified, the catheter is inserted through the femoral or jugular vein and the balloon is inflated. The catheter is then attached to an external pulse generator, and the settings are adjusted to achieve capture. The balloon is then deflated, and placement can be verified via ultrasound or chest x-ray.

Complications are similar to those of PCI and permanent pacemaker insertion, including infection, hemorrhage, catheter migration, perforation, embolism, thrombosis, and pacemaker syndrome.

### TRANSVENOUS PACER SETTINGS

Temporary transvenous pacing utilizes bipolar leads with two tails, positive/proximal and negative/distal, and these must be connected properly to the pulse generator, with the distal end of the pacing lead to the negative terminal and the proximal end to the positive terminal. Once the transvenous pacing wire is inserted and the leads are connected to the pulse generator, it must be set to the patient's needs:

- **Rate**: The beats per minute are usually set between 70 and 80 (allowable range is generally 50-90), but this may vary according to individual needs.
- **Sensitivity**: The myocardial voltage needed for the pacing electrode to detect P or R waves. The sensitivity is usually set at 2 mV and then adjusted as needed to ensure capture. Most pacemakers can sense 0.3-10.0 mV from the atria and 0.8-29.0 mV from the ventricles, but setting it relatively low prevents oversensing.
- **Output**: The current or pulse produced by the pulse generator is usually set at 5 mA. The current is delivered rapidly, in about 0.6 ms.

### PROBLEMS RELATED TO TRANSVENOUS PACING

With transvenous pacing (usually per a pulse generator connected to a pacing cable and a pacing wire, which is inserted into the right internal jugular to the right ventricle for ventricular pacing and right atrium for atrial pacing), sensing refers to the ability to detect electrical activity of the heart. Capture occurs when an artificial stimulus (the pulse generator) depolarizes the heart, indicated by a pacer spike followed by the QRS complex. **Problems** include:

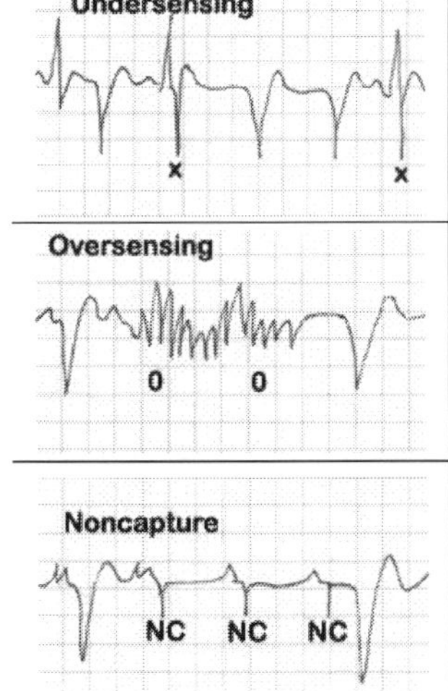


**Undersensing**:
The sensitivity is too low to detect cardiac depolarizations, and triggers unneeded contractions, competing with the patient's native rhythm. This may be related to the dislodging of the lead, incorrect positioning of the lead, or a low-amplitude cardiac signal.

**Oversensing**:
The sensitivity is too high and misinterprets artifacts (such as muscle contractions) and non-depolarization events as contractions and fails to trigger, resulting in decreased cardiac output because of the interruption in contractions. This may result from damage or disconnection of the lead.

**Noncapture**:
The pacemaker does not trigger contractions. This may be related to settings, lead disconnection, low battery, or metabolic changes.

## *PACEMAKER COMPLICATIONS*

Pacemakers, transvenous and permanent, are invasive foreign bodies and, as such, can cause a number of different **complications**:

- Infection, bleeding, or hematoma may occur at the entry site of leads for temporary pacemakers or at the subcutaneous area of implantation for permanent generators.
- Puncture of the subclavian vein or internal mammary artery may cause a hemothorax.

- The endocardial electrode may irritate the ventricular wall, causing ectopic beats or tachycardia.
- Dislodgement of the transvenous lead may lead to malfunction or perforation of the myocardium. This is one of the most common early complications.
- Dislocation of leads may result in phrenic nerve or muscle stimulation (which may be evidenced by hiccupping).
- Cardiac tamponade may result when the epicardial wires of temporary pacing are removed.
- General malfunctioning of the pacemaker may indicate dislodgement, dislocation, interference caused by electromagnetic fields, and the need for new batteries or a new generator.
- Pacemaker syndrome

### *PACEMAKER SYNDROME*

Pacemaker syndrome can occur with any type of pacemaker if there is inadequate synchronicity between the contractions of the atria and ventricles, resulting in a decrease in cardiac output and inadequate atrial contribution to the filling of the ventricles. Total peripheral vascular resistance may increase to maintain blood pressure, but hypotension occurs after decompensation.

- **Mild**:
  - Pulsations evident in the neck and abdomen
  - Cardiac palpitations
  - Headache and feeling of anxiety
  - General malaise and unexplained weakness
  - Pain or feeling of fullness in jaw and/or chest
- **Moderate**:
  - Increasing dyspnea on exertion with accompanying orthopnea
  - Dizziness, vertigo, and increasing confusion
  - Feeling of choking
- **Severe**:
  - Increasing pulmonary edema with dyspnea even at rest
  - Crackling rales
  - Syncope
  - Heart failure

## AUTOMATIC ICD

The **automatic implantable cardioverter-defibrillator (AICD)** is similar to the pacemaker and is implanted in the same way, with one or more leads to the ventricular myocardium or the epicardium, but it is used to control tachycardia and/or fibrillation. Most AICDs consist of a pacing/sensing electrode, a pulse generator, and defibrillation electrodes. Severe tachycardia may be related to electrical disturbances, cardiomyopathy, or postoperative response to the repair of congenital disease. In some cases, it is not responsive to medications. When the pulse reaches a certain preset rate, then the device automatically provides a small electrical impulse to the atrial or ventricular myocardium to slow the heart. If fibrillation occurs, a higher energy shock is delivered. It takes 5-15 seconds for the device to detect abnormalities in the pulse rate, and more than one shock may be required so fainting can occur. Contemporary devices can function as both a pacemaker and an ICD, which is especially important for those who have episodes of both bradycardia and tachycardia. The use of adjunctive antiarrhythmics or ablation is important to prevent AICD shocks.

## Closure Devices with PCI

**Percutaneous catheter intervention (PCI)** is often the treatment choice for patients with symptomatic coronary artery disease. Percutaneous transluminal coronary angioplasty (PTCA), arthrectomy, and stent insertion are common types of percutaneous catheter intervention procedures. While historically, manual compression has been utilized to achieve hemostasis after PCI, different types of devices exist to assist in achieving hemostasis post-procedure. Passive devices such as hemostasis pads and compression devices help to enhance hemostasis. Active devices are used at the femoral access site after the sheath used for the procedure is removed. There are different types of active devices, including percutaneous suture mediated devices, that use needles and sutures to suture the artery closed after the procedure. Collagen plugs are another type of closure, where collagen is injected into the supra-arterial space until hemostasis is achieved. These devices may be used independently or in combination. Clip devices such as implantable clips can be used to pull the edges of the arteriotomy together for closure. Active devices shorten the time to achieve hemostasis as well as the time the patient must remain hospitalized post-procedure.

**Complications**: Persistent coronary artery spasms, dissection of the coronary artery, thrombosis, bleeding, and hematoma formation. Other complications may arise depending on the type of closure device utilized. For example, the use of clip devices may result in arterial laceration, occlusion of the artery, or arterial stenosis.

## PTCA and Stent Insertion

**Percutaneous transluminal coronary angioplasty (PTCA)** is a procedure done to reperfuse coronary arteries blocked by plaque or an embolus. Cardiac catheterization is done with a hollow catheter (sheath), usually inserted into the femoral vein or artery and fed through the vessels to the coronary arteries. When the atheroma is verified by fluoroscopy, a balloon-tipped catheter is fed over the sheath and the balloon is inflated with a contrast agent to a specified pressure to compress the atheroma. The balloon may be inflated a number of times to ensure that residual stenosis is <20%. Laser angioplasty using the excimer laser is also used to vaporize plaque. **Stents** may be inserted during the angioplasty to maintain patency. Stents may be flexible plastic or wire mesh and are typically placed over the catheter, which is inflated to expand the stent against the arterial wall. All patients with a stent must be discharged on aspirin, an antiplatelet, and a statin.

**Complications** include:

- **Intraoperative**: Perforation/dissection of the coronary artery, arrythmias, and vasospasm
- **Postoperative**: Hemorrhage/hematoma at insertion site, thrombus/embolus, arteriovenous fistula/pseudoaneurysm, retroperitoneal bleed, and failure of angioplasty

## IABP

The **intra-aortic balloon pump (IABP)** is a catheter with an inflatable balloon at the tip, which is inserted through the femoral artery and threaded into the descending thoracic aorta. The balloon inflates during diastole to increase circulation to the coronary arteries and then deflates during systole to decrease afterload. It is indicated in patients experiencing cardiogenic/septic shock, acute heart failure, unstable angina, and papillary or ventricular septal rupture.

**Contraindications**: Aortic valve stenosis and large aortic aneurysms.

**Complications**: Stroke, peripheral ischemia, renal injury, air embolus, and arrhythmias.

**Nursing considerations** are as follows:

- **Placement:**
  - Too high: occludes the left subclavian artery, which results in dizziness and decreased radial pulse.
  - Too low: occludes the renal artery, which results in flank pain and a sudden decrease in urine output.

- Preventing displacement: the patient cannot bend his or her knees, sit up, or flex the hips more than 45°. Patient should remain in a supine position.

- **Timing**: In ECG mode, the balloon should inflate in the T-wave and deflate with the R. Do site checks, I&O, neuro-checks, and vascular checks every hour.
- If a **gas-leak alarm sounds** OR **blood is visible in the catheter**, this indicates balloon rupture/damage to the catheter. Immediately shut down the machine, place the patient in the Trendelenburg position, and notify the physician.
- **Weaning**: Decrease balloon volume/frequency to wean. Use the flutter function to prevent embolus while the catheter is still in place. After removal, the physician will allow bleeding for five seconds to eject clots.

### CAROTID ENDARTERECTOMY

A carotid endarterectomy involves clamping the carotids, opening the occluded artery, and removing the plaque that is occluding the artery. A shunt may be inserted during the procedure to ensure blood supply to the brain. Postoperative **complications** may include:

- **Hematoma:** May obstruct respiration; watch closely for increased respiratory effort and swelling near the airway.
- **Hypertension:** Especially in the first 48 postoperative hours, may increase risk of neurologic impairment and hematoma.
- **Hypotension:** Usually resolves in 24-48 hours, but may indicate myocardial infarction.
- **Hyperperfusion syndrome:** Caused by inadequate vasoconstriction of vessels dilated from long-term diminished blood flow. It can cause hemorrhage and edema, usually identified by severe unilateral headache relieved by raising the head.
- **Hemorrhage:** May be fatal or cause severe impairment.
- **Stroke:** Risk of plaque dislodging and forming an embolus; frequent neurological checks are crucial.

## CABG

**Coronary artery bypass graft (CABG)** is a surgical procedure for the treatment of angina that does not respond to medical treatment, unstable angina, blockage of >60% in the left main coronary artery, blockage of multiple coronary arteries that include the proximal left anterior descending artery, left ventricular dysfunction, and previous unsuccessful PCIs. The surgery is performed through a midsternal incision that exposes the heart, which is chilled and placed on cardiopulmonary bypass with blood going from the right atrium to the machine and back to the body while the aorta is clamped to keep the surgical field free of blood. Bypass grafts are sutured into place to bypass areas of occluded coronary arteries. Grafts may be obtained from various sites: gastroepiploic artery, internal mammary artery, radial artery, or saphenous vein (commonly used, especially for emergency procedures).

**Complications:** Arrhythmias, infection, cardiac tamponade, cardiogenic shock, embolus/stroke, and renal or pulmonary dysfunction

### *MIDCAB AND PORT ACCESS CORONARY ARTERY BYPASS GRAFT*

**Minimally-invasive direct coronary artery bypass (MIDCAB)** applies a bypass graft through a 10 cm incision in the mid-chest without using cardiopulmonary bypass. Because the incision must be over the bypass area, this procedure is suitable only for bypass of one or two coronary arteries, usually on the left side of the heart. A small portion of rib is removed to allow access to the heart, and the internal mammary artery is used for grafting. Special instruments, such as a heart stabilizer, are used to limit movement of the heart during suturing. Surgery usually takes 2-3 hours and recovery time is decreased as patients have less pain. Because anastomosis is difficult on a beating heart, complications such as ischemia may occur during surgery, so a cardiopulmonary bypass machine must be available.

**Port access coronary artery bypass graft** is an alternative form of CABG that utilizes a number of small incisions (ports) along with cardiopulmonary bypass (CPB) and cardioplegia to do a video-assisted surgical repair. Usually, 3 or more incisions are required, with one in the femoral area to allow access to the femoral artery for a multipurpose catheter that is threaded through to the ascending aorta to return blood from the CPB, block the aorta with a balloon, provide a cardioplegic solution, and vent air. Another catheter is threaded through the femoral vein to the right atrium to carry blood to the CPB. An incision is also needed for access to the jugular vein for catheters to the pulmonary artery and the coronary sinus. One to three thoracotomy incisions are made for the insertion of video imaging equipment and instruments. While the midsternal incision is avoided, multiple incisions pose the potential for possible increased morbidity.

## Cardiac Surgical Options for Repair of Cardiac Valves

There are a number of different surgical options for the repair of cardiac valves:

- **Valvotomy/Valvuloplasty** is usually done through cardiac catheterization. A valvotomy/valvuloplasty involves releasing valve leaflet adhesions or opening a stenosed valve. In balloon valvuloplasty, a catheter with an inflatable balloon is positioned in the stenotic valve and inflated and deflated a number of times to dilate the opening. Risks include stroke from a broken-off calcified valve and worsened valvular insufficiency/rupture.
- **Aortic valve replacement** is an open-heart procedure with cardiopulmonary bypass. Aortic valves are tricuspid (3 leaflets) and repair is usually not possible, so defective valves must be replaced with either mechanical (metal, plastic, or pyrolytic carbon) or biological (porcine or bovine) grafts.
- **Aortic homograft** uses part of a donor's aorta with the aortic valve attached to replace the recipient's faulty aortic valve and part of the ascending aorta.
- **Ross procedure** uses the patient's pulmonary artery with the pulmonary valve to replace the aortic valve and part of the aorta and then uses a donor graft to replace the pulmonary artery.

### *TAVR*

**Transcatheter aortic valve replacement (TAVR)** is usually reserved for patients with advanced symptomatic stenosis of the aortic valve who are unable to tolerate open-heart surgery or are at high risk with the procedure. Symptoms of aortic stenosis include chest pain, peripheral edema, dyspnea, fainting, weakness, and heart failure. With a TAVR, patients generally receive a general anesthesia, and a catheter is inserted, usually transfemoral (most common), transaortic, or transapical. Two types of replacement valves are available in the US: a balloon-expandable valve (Sapien XT) or a self-expanding valve (CoreValue). Once the catheter with a balloon device and the replacement valve attached is in place in the aortic valve, the balloon is inflated to secure the replacement valve, then the balloon is deflated and the catheter is removed. With the self-expanding valve, the valve is attached to the catheter and expanded when it is in place in the stenotic valve and the catheter is removed.

## Postoperative Care for Cardiac Surgery

The **recovery period** is discussed below:

- 2:1 nursing ratio; monitor hemodynamics closely (check vitals every 5-15 minutes).
- Warm patient according to policy; monitor ECG closely for arrhythmias during rewarming.
- Maintain MAP between 70-110 mmHg to prevent inadequate perfusion or graft rupture/hemorrhage; urine output should be >30 mL/hr.
- The patient will have multiple chest tubes; ensure output is not excessive (>200 mL/hr = hemorrhage) and does not suddenly stop/decrease.
- Auscultate heart sounds and evaluate extremities frequently to assess perfusion; hourly urine output should be 30 mL/hr OR 1 mL/kg/hr (gold standard).
- Monitor ABGS (every 2-4 hr during recovery) and adjust ventilator settings accordingly.

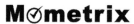

- Close blood sugar control (will probably be on insulin drip) and prophylactic cephalosporin to prevent infection.
- Monitor CMP and replace electrolyte imbalances as ordered.

**Monitor for the following complications:**

- Cardiac Tamponade: bleeding from graft sites into the pericardial sac
- Hypotension/shock: decreased cardiac output
- Arrhythmias: due to blood flow changes and cardioplegic solution – be prepared for epicardial pacing and defibrillation if needed
- Stroke (clots from grafts), infection (surgical site), etc.

**Nursing considerations** are as follows:

- Educate patient: recovery, possibility of Dressler's Syndrome and postoperative depression; adequate pain management and splinting.

## ARTERIAL LINE INSERTION

Indications for an **arterial line** include hemodynamic instability, frequent ABG monitoring, placement of IABP, monitoring arterial pressure, and medication administration when venous access cannot be obtained. Sterile technique is utilized for arterial line insertion. Insertions sites include radial (most common), femoral (second choice), brachial, or dorsalis pedis arteries.

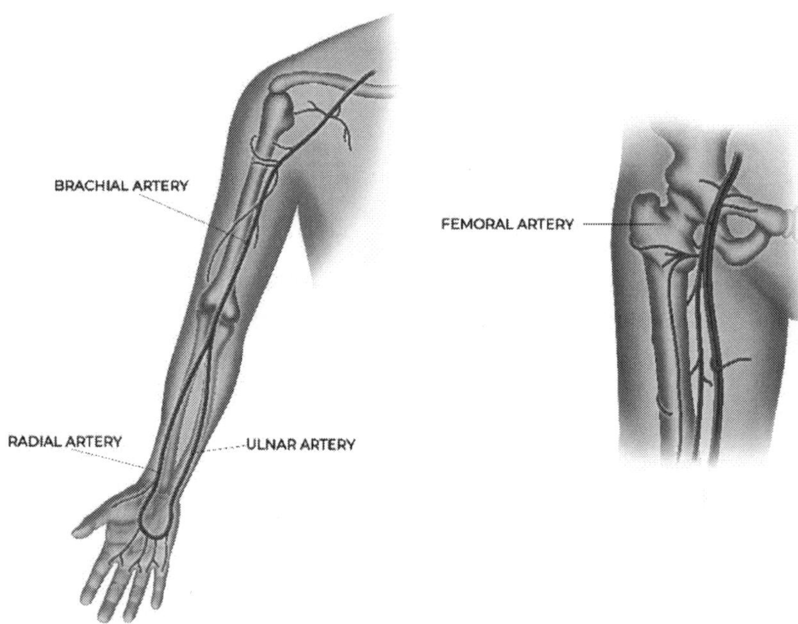


**Procedure**:

- Verify adequate perfusion and position.
    - Radial: Perform modified Allen test and position wrist in dorsiflexion with an arm board.
    - Femoral: Place the patient in a supine position with the leg on the insertion side slightly abducted and extended.
- Prep and drape. Apply 1% lidocaine if the patient is conscious.
- Insert needle.

- Over-the-needle catheter insertion: Needle is inserted at a 30-45° degree angle and decreased to a 10-15° angle when blood returns, catheter advanced into vessel, needle removed, and catheter connected to transducer.
- Over-wire catheter insertion: Needle is inserted into the artery at a 30-45° angle until blood returns. A wire is then inserted and advanced through the needle, and needle removed, leaving the wire in place. A catheter is then advanced over the wire, wire removed, and catheter connected to transducer system.

- A small incision is made at insertion site and catheter sutured into place.

**Complications** include bleeding, coagulopathy, thrombosis (especially with larger catheters or smaller arteries), advanced atherosclerosis, and infection.

**Review Video: Nursing Care of Arterial Lines**
Visit mometrix.com/academy and enter code: 561047

## Central Line Insertion

Central lines allow rapid administration of large volumes of fluid, blood testing, and CVP measuring. Central lines may be placed into the internal jugular vein (right preferred), subclavian vein, or femoral vein (usually avoided). The insertion site is located through an ultrasound. The patient is positioned, supine Trendelenburg (or legs elevated) for interior jugular, using sterile technique. Following skin prep, the CVC kit is placed on a sterile field and opened, the equipment is prepared, and the insertion site is again verified by a probe (covered with sterile cover). Topical anesthetic (lidocaine) is administered and the needle inserted with the triangulation or spear method, always pulling back on the plunger of the syringe so that blood returns when entering the vein. The syringe is removed and the guidewire inserted into needle ≤20 cm. The needle is then removed and the wire position verified with ultrasound. A small incision is made at the insertion site, and a dilator is applied over the wire and inserted about 2.5-3.5 cm. The catheter is placed over the wire and advanced into the vein (13-17 cm). The wire is then removed, the lines are flushed, and the catheter is sutured in place and dressing is applied. Long (24-inch) PICCs may be inserted in the basilic or cephalic veins and advanced into central circulation.

## Intraosseous Infusion

Intraosseous (IO) infusion is an alternative to IV access for neonates, pediatric emergencies, and adult emergencies when rapid temporary access is necessary or when peripheral or vascular access can't be achieved. It is often used in pediatric cardiac arrest. Because yellow marrow replaces red marrow, access in those older than 5 is more difficult. Preferred sites are based on age, though across all ages, the **proximal tibia is preferred**. Additional sites include:

- 0-1: Distal femur
- 1-12: Distal tibia or fibula
- 12-18: Distal tibia or fibula, sternum
- 18 and older: Distal tibia or fibula, proximal humerus, sternum

IO infusion is used to administer fluids and anesthesia and to obtain blood samples. Equipment requires a special needle (13-20 gauge) as standard needles may bend. The bone injection gun (BIG) with a loaded spring facilitates insertion. The FAST needle is intended for use in the sternum of adults and prevents accidental puncture of the thoracic cavity. Knowledge of bony landmarks and correct insertion angle and site is important. The position is confirmed by aspiration of 5-10 mL of blood and marrow before infusion.

## VASCULAR INTERVENTIONS

Vascular interventions are required when a patient has a condition that is decreasing blood flow to the limbs, causing ischemia-related damage. Conditions that require a vascular intervention include acute occlusion (embolus), severe unresponsive vascular disease, ruptured/dissecting aneurysm, damaged vessels, or congenital defect.

- **Bypass grafts:** The MD uses a harvested vein from another part of the body (saphenous usually) or synthetic graft to bypass the occlusion. Because veins have valves, they must be reversed or stripped of valves prior to attachment; however, synthetic grafts have a higher failure rate. A common peripheral bypass is the femoropopliteal (Fem-pop) bypass, extending from the femoral artery around the blockage to the popliteal artery.
- **Embolectomy:** A catheter is inserted into the blocked artery and threaded through the thrombus. Then a balloon on the tip is inflated, and the physician removes the catheter, removing the clot with it.
- **Aortic aneurysm repair:** This is an intense procedure, requiring an open incision and the patient to be placed on cardiopulmonary bypass. The affected area is resected and replaced with a vascular or Dacron graft.

**Nursing considerations:** Monitor and control blood pressure carefully to protect the patency and integrity of the grafts. Neurologic and renal function should also be carefully monitored, as emboli could block the renal or cerebral artery. Frequent neuro, urine output, vascular, and dressing checks.

**Possible complications:** Pulmonary infection, graft-site infection, renal dysfunction, occlusion, hemorrhage, and embolus/thrombus.

## PERIPHERAL STENTS

**Peripheral vascular stenting** may be utilized as an intervention in the treatment of peripheral vascular insufficiency. Often performed in interventional radiology, the interventionalist uses balloon angioplasty to unblock the vessel under fluoroscopic guidance. A small balloon attached to a catheter is inserted into the occluded vessel and inflated to expand the arterial wall and compress the blockage. A small metal tube (stent) is then placed to support the vessel and maintain its patency. Stents are primarily made of stainless steel or a metal alloy. This intervention helps to restore circulation to the affected area and prevent restenosis of the vessel. There are different types of stents available based on the type of vessel affected and the type of lesion. Stenting may be used in both peripheral and coronary arteries.

- **Indications**: Stenting may be the initial choice of intervention in patients with iliac, renal, subclavian, or carotid stenosis. Stenting may be indicated in patients with severe claudication, non-healing ulcers of the extremities, ischemic pain with rest, and in patients who have a high operative risk. Peripheral stenting often results in shorter hospital stays and shorter recovery times in comparison with surgical intervention.
- **Complications**: Complications that may occur in patients undergoing peripheral stenting include bleeding, infection, arterial spasm or rupture, dissection of the vessel, restenosis or thrombus formation within the vessel, and intravascular fracture of the stent.

## FEM-POP BYPASS

**Femoropopliteal (Fem-Pop) bypass** is used for femoral artery disease in order to bypass an occluded femoral artery above or below the knee. Either a man-made or a vein graft (such as the saphenous vein) is used and is sewn above the blocked area to the femoral artery and below to the popliteal artery, allowing the blood to bypass the occluded area. In addition to the incisions in the affected leg, if a vein graft is obtained from the other leg, the patient may also have a long incision where the vein was removed. Edema in the surgical sites is common and may persist for up to 3 months. Femoral popliteal bypass surgery is indicated for peripheral vascular insufficiency that does not respond to medical treatment, causes severe intermittent claudication and/or ischemic resting pain, and results in gangrene or other non-healing wounds, especially if the limb is at risk for amputation because of impaired oxygenation. The limb(s) must be monitored carefully in the postoperative period for color, sensation, warmth, and ability to move.

# Cardiovascular Pharmacology

## Anti-Hypertensive Medications

The classes of anti-hypertensive medications are as follows: Diuretics, sympatholytics, vasodilators, calcium channel blockers, and angiotensin-converting enzyme inhibitors (ACE inhibitors).

- Diuretics include hydrochlorothiazide, chlorthalidone, chlorothiazide, indapamide, metolazone, amiloride, spironolactone, triamterene, furosemide, bumetanide, ethacrynic acid, and torsemide.
- Sympatholytics are clonidine, methyldopa, guanabenz, guanadrel, guanethidine, reserpine, labetalol, prazosin, and terazosin.
- Vasodilators include diazoxide, hydralazine, minoxidil, and nitroprusside sodium.
- Calcium channel blockers include amlodipine, nimodipine, isradipine, nicardipine, nifedipine, bepridil, diltiazem, and verapamil.
- ACE inhibitors include benazepril, captopril, enalapril, fosinopril, lisinopril, moexipril, quinapril, ramipril, and losartan.

## Diuretics

Diuretics increase **renal perfusion and filtration**, thereby reducing preload and decreasing peripheral and pulmonary edema, hypertension, CHF, diabetes insipidus, and osteoporosis. There are different types of diuretics: loop, thiazide, and potassium sparing.

### *Loop Diuretics*

Loop diuretics inhibit the reabsorption of sodium and chloride (primarily) in the ascending loop of Henle. They also cause increased secretion of other electrolytes, such as calcium, magnesium, and potassium, and this can result in imbalances that cause dysrhythmias. Other side effects include frequent urination, postural hypotension, and increased blood sugar and uric acid levels. They are short-acting so are less effective than other diuretics for control of hypertension.

- **Bumetanide** (Bumex) is given intravenously after surgery to reduce preload or orally to treat heart failure.
- **Ethacrynic acid** (Edecrin) is given intravenously after surgery to reduce preload.
- **Furosemide** (Lasix) is used for the control of congestive heart failure as well as renal insufficiency. It is used after surgery to decrease preload and to reduce the inflammatory response caused by cardiopulmonary bypass (post-perfusion syndrome).

**Review Video: Diuretics**
Visit mometrix.com/academy and enter code: 373276

### *Thiazide Diuretics*

Thiazide diuretics inhibit the **reabsorption of sodium and chloride** primarily in the early distal tubules, forcing more sodium and water to be excreted. Thiazide diuretics increase secretion of potassium and bicarbonate, so they are often given with supplementary potassium or in combination with potassium-sparing diuretics. Thiazide diuretics are the first line of drugs for treatment of **hypertension**. They have a long duration of action (12-72 hours, depending on the drug) so they are able to maintain control of hypertension better than short-acting drugs. They may be given daily or 3–5 days per week. There are numerous thiazide diuretics, including:

- Chlorothiazide (Diuril)
- Bendroflumethiazide (Naturetin)
- Chlorthalidone (Hygroton)
- Trichlormethiazide (Naqua)

Side effects include, dizziness, lightheadedness, postural hypotension, headache, blurred vision, and itching, especially during initial treatment. Thiazide diuretics cause sensitivity to sun exposure, so people should be counseled to use sunscreen.

### *POTASSIUM-SPARING DIURETICS*

Potassium-sparing diuretics inhibit the **reabsorption of sodium** in the late distal tubule and collecting duct. They are weaker than thiazide or loop diuretics, but do not cause a reduction in potassium level; however, if used alone, they may cause an increase in potassium, which can cause weakness, irregular pulse, and cardiac arrest. Because potassium-sparing diuretics are less effective alone, they are often given in a combined form with a thiazide diuretic (usually chlorothiazide), which mitigates the potassium imbalance. Typical side effects include dehydration, blurred vision, nausea, insomnia, and nasal congestion, especially in the first few days of treatment.

- **Spironolactone** (Aldactone) is a synthetic steroid diuretic that increases the secretion of both water and sodium and is used to treat congestive heart failure. It may be given orally or intravenously.
- **Eplerenone** is an antimineralocorticoid similar to spironolactone but with fewer side effects.

## ANTIDYSRHYTHMIC DRUGS

Antidysrhythmic drugs include a number of drugs that act on the conduction system, the ventricles and/or the atria to control dysrhythmias. There are four classes of drugs that are used as well as some that are unclassified:

- **Class I:** 3 subtypes of sodium channel blockers (quinidine, lidocaine, procainamide)
- **Class II:** β-receptor blockers (esmolol, propranolol)
- **Class III:** Slows repolarization (amiodarone, ibutilide)
- **Class IV**: Calcium channel blockers (diltiazem, verapamil)
- **Unclassified:** Miscellaneous drugs with proven efficacy in controlling arrhythmias (adenosine, electrolyte supplements)

## SMOOTH MUSCLE RELAXANTS

Smooth muscle relaxants decrease peripheral vascular resistance, but may cause hypotension and headaches.

- Sodium nitroprusside (Nipride) dilates both arteries and veins; rapid-acting and used for reduction of hypertension and afterload reduction for heart failure.
- Nitroglycerin (Tridil) primarily dilates veins and is used sublingual or IV to reduce preload for acute heart failure, unstable angina, and acute MI. Nitroglycerin may also be used prophylactically after PCIs to prevent vasospasm.
- Hydralazine (Apresoline) dilates arteries and is given intermittently to reduce hypertension.

## CALCIUM CHANNEL BLOCKERS

Calcium channel blockers are primarily arterial vasodilators that may affect the peripheral and/or coronary arteries.

- Side effects: Lethargy, flushing, edema, ascites, and indigestion:
- Nifedipine (Procardia) and nicardipine (Cardene) are primarily arterial vasodilators, used to treat acute hypertension. Diltiazem (Cardizem) and Verapamil (Calan, Isoptin) dilate primarily coronary arteries and slow the heart rate, thus are used for angina, atrial fibrillation, and SVT. *Note:* Nifedipine (Procardia) should be avoided in older adults due to increased risk of hypotension and myocardial ischemia.

**Review Video: Ca Channel Blockers**
Visit mometrix.com/academy and enter code: 942825

## Additional Vasodilators

**B-type natriuretic peptide (BNP)** (Nesiritide [Natrecor]) is type of vasodilator (non-inotropic), which is a recombinant form of a peptide of the human brain. It decreases filling pressure, vascular resistance, and increases U/O.

- May cause hypotension, headache, bradycardia, and nausea. It is used short term for worsening decompensated CHF; contraindicated in SBP<90, cardiogenic shock, contrictive pericarditis, or valve stenosis.

**Alpha-adrenergic blockers** block alpha receptors in arteries and veins, causing vasodilation.

- May cause orthostatic hypotension and edema from fluid retention.
- Labetalol (Normodyne) is a combination peripheral alpha-blocker and cardiac β-blocker that is used to treat acute hypertension, acute stroke, and acute aortic dissection.
- Phentolamine (Regitine) is a peripheral arterial dilator that reduces afterload. It is used for HTN crisis in patients with pheochromocytoma, as well as a subcutaneous injection for extravasation of vessicants.

**Selective specific dopamine DA-1-receptor agonists:**

- Fenoldopam (Corlopam) is a peripheral dilator affecting renal and mesenteric arteries and can be used for patients with renal dysfunction or those at risk of renal insufficiency.

## Inotropic Agents

Inotropic agents are drugs used to increase cardiac output and improve contractibility. IV inotropic agents may increase the risk of death, but may be used when other drugs fail. Oral forms of these drugs are less effective than intravenous. Inotropic agents include:

- **β-Adrenergic agonists**:
  - **Dobutamine** improves cardiac output, treats cardiac decompensation, and increases blood pressure. It helps the body to utilize norepinephrine. Side effects include increased or labile blood pressure, increased heart rate, PVCs, N/V, and bronchospasm.
  - **Dopamine** improves cardiac output, blood pressure, and blood flow to the renal and mesenteric arteries. Side effects include tachycardia or bradycardia, palpitations, BP changes, dyspnea, nausea and vomiting, headache, and gangrene of extremities.
- **Phosphodiesterase III inhibitors**:
  - **Milrinone** (Primacor) increases strength of contractions and cause vasodilation. Side effects include ventricular arrhythmias, hypotension, and headaches.
- **Digoxin (Lanoxin)** increases contractibility and cardiac output and prevents arrhythmias.

## Medications for Heart Failure

A patient with heart failure may be prescribed with one or multiple of the drugs below:

- **ACE inhibitors:** Captopril (Capoten), enalapril (Vasotec), and lisinopril (Prinivil). Decrease afterload/preload and reverse ventricular remodeling; they also prevent neuropathy in DM. Contraindicated with renal insufficiency, renal artery stenosis, and pregnancy.
  - Side effects include cough (#1), hyperkalemia, hypotension, angioedema, dizziness, and weakness.
- **Angiotensin receptor blockers (ARBs):** Losartan (Cozaar) and valsartan (Diovan). Decrease afterload/preload and reverse ventricular remodeling, causing vasodilation and reducing blood pressure. They are used for those who cannot tolerate ACE inhibitors.

- Side effects include cough (less common than with ACE inhibitors), hyperkalemia, hypotension, headache, dizziness, metallic taste, and rash.
- **β-Blockers:** Metoprolol (Lopressor), carvedilol (Coreg) and esmolol (Brevibloc). Slow the heart rate, reduce hypertension, prevent dysrhythmias, and reverse ventricular remodeling. Contraindicated in bradyarrythmias, decompensated HF, uncontrolled hypoglycemia/diabetes mellitus, and airway disease.
    - Side effects: bradycardia, hypotension, bronchospasm, may mask signs of hypoglycemia.
- **Aldosterone agonist:** Spironolactone (Aldactone). Decreases preload and myocardial hypertrophy and reduces edema and sodium retention but may increase serum potassium.
- **Furosemide (Lasix)** is used for the control of congestive heart failure as well as renal insufficiency. It is used after surgery to decrease preload and to reduce the inflammatory response caused by cardiopulmonary bypass (post-perfusion syndrome).

## Digoxin (Lanoxin)

Digitalis drugs, most commonly administered in the form of digoxin (Lanoxin), are derived from the foxglove plant and are used to increase myocardial contractility, left ventricular output, and slow conduction through the AV node, decreasing rapid heart rates and promoting diuresis. Digoxin does not affect mortality, but increases tolerance to activity and reduces hospitalizations for heart failure. Therapeutic levels (0.5-2.0 ng/mL) should be maintained to avoid digitalis toxicity, which can occur even if digoxin levels are within therapeutic range, so observation of symptoms is critical. Because patients with heart failure are often on diuretics which decrease potassium levels, they are at increased risk for toxicity.

**Symptoms of toxicity** are as follows:

- Early signs: Increasing fatigue, lethargy, depression, and nausea and vomiting; progress to severe diarrhea, blurred vision/yellow or green halos around lights, fatigue/weakness
- Arrythmias: SA or AV block, VT/VF, PVCs, and bradycardia

**Treatment** consists of the following:

- Monitor serum levels and symptoms.
- Digoxin immune FAB (Digibind) may be used to bind to digoxin and inactivate it if necessary.

## Glycoprotein IIB/IIIA Inhibitors

Glycoprotein IIB/IIIA Inhibitors are drugs that are used to inhibit platelet binding and prevent clots prior to and following invasive cardiac procedures, such as angioplasty and stent placement. These medications are used in combination with anticoagulant drugs, such as heparin and aspirin for the following:

- Acute coronary syndromes (ACS), such as unstable angina or myocardial infarctions
- Percutaneous coronary intervention (PCI), such as angioplasty and stent placement

These medications are contraindicated in those with a low platelet count or active bleeding:

- **Eptifibatide (Integrilin)**: Used with both heparin and aspirin for ACS and PCI and affects platelet binding for 6-8 hours after administration. Should not be used in patients with renal problems.
- **Tirofiban (Aggrastat)**: Used with heparin for PCI patients with reduced dosage for those with renal problems and affects platelet binding for only 4-8 hours after administration.

## Pharmacologic Measures to Maximize Perfusion

The primary focus of pharmacologic measures to **maximize perfusion** is to reduce the risk of **thromboses**:

- **Antiplatelet agents**, such as aspirin, Ticlid, and Plavix, which interfere with the function of the plasma membrane, interfering with clotting. These agents are ineffective to treat clots but prevent clot formation.
- **Vasodilators** may divert blood from ischemic areas, but some may be indicated, such as Pletal, which dilates arteries and decreases clotting, and is used for control of intermittent claudication.
- **Antilipemic**, such as Zocor and Questran, slow progression of atherosclerosis.
- **Hemorheologic agents**, such as Trental, reduce fibrinogen, reducing blood viscosity and rigidity of erythrocytes; however, clinical studies show limited benefit. It may be used for intermittent claudication.
- **Analgesics** may be necessary to improve quality of life. Opioids may be needed in some cases.
- **Thrombolytics** may be injected into a blocked artery under angiography to dissolve clots.
- **Anticoagulants**, such as Coumadin and Lovenox, prevent blood clots from forming.

### *Administration of Fibrinolytic (Thrombolytic) Infusions for MI*

Fibrinolytic infusion is indicated for acute myocardial infarction under these conditions:

- Symptoms of MI, <6-12 hours since onset of symptoms
- ≥1 mm elevation of ST in ≥2 contiguous leads
- No contraindications and no cardiogenic shock

**Fibrinolytic agents** should be administered as soon as possible, within 30 minutes is best. All agents convert plasminogen to plasmin, which breaks down fibrin, dissolving clots:

- Streptokinase and anistreplase (1st generation)
- Alteplase or tissue plasminogen activator (tPA) (2nd generation)
- Reteplase and tenecteplase (3rd generation)

**Contraindications**

- Present or recent bleeding or history of severe bleeding
- History of intracranial hemorrhage
- History of stroke (<3 months unless within 3 hours)
- Aortic dissection or pericarditis
- Intracranial/intraspinal surgery or trauma within 3 months or neoplasm, aneurysm, or AVM

**Relative contraindications**

- Active peptic ulcer
- >10 minutes of CPR
- Advanced renal or hepatic disease
- Pregnancy
- Anticoagulation therapy
- Acute uncontrolled hypertension or chronic poorly controlled hypertension
- Recent (2–4 weeks) internal bleeding
- Non-compressible vascular punctures

# Respiratory Emergencies

## Respiratory Assessment

### Assessment of the Respiratory System

If significant respiratory distress is present, one must stabilize the patient before doing a **respiratory history** or ask family if available:

- Question the patient about risk factors, such as smoking, exposure to smoke or other inhaled toxins, past lung problems, and allergies.
- Ask the patient about symptoms of respiratory problems, such as dyspnea, cough, sputum production, fatigue, ability to do ADLs and IADLs, and chest pain.
- Determine how long symptoms have been present, the length of periods of dyspnea, aggravating and alleviating factors, and the severity of symptoms.

When performing a **physical assessment**, one should assess vital signs, posture, pulse oximetry, check nails for clubbing, do a skin assessment, listen to lung sounds via auscultation and percussion, and look for accessory muscle use, signs of anxiety, and edema. Depending on condition, blood may be drawn for arterial blood gases, electrolytes, and CBC. Sputum cultures may be obtained.

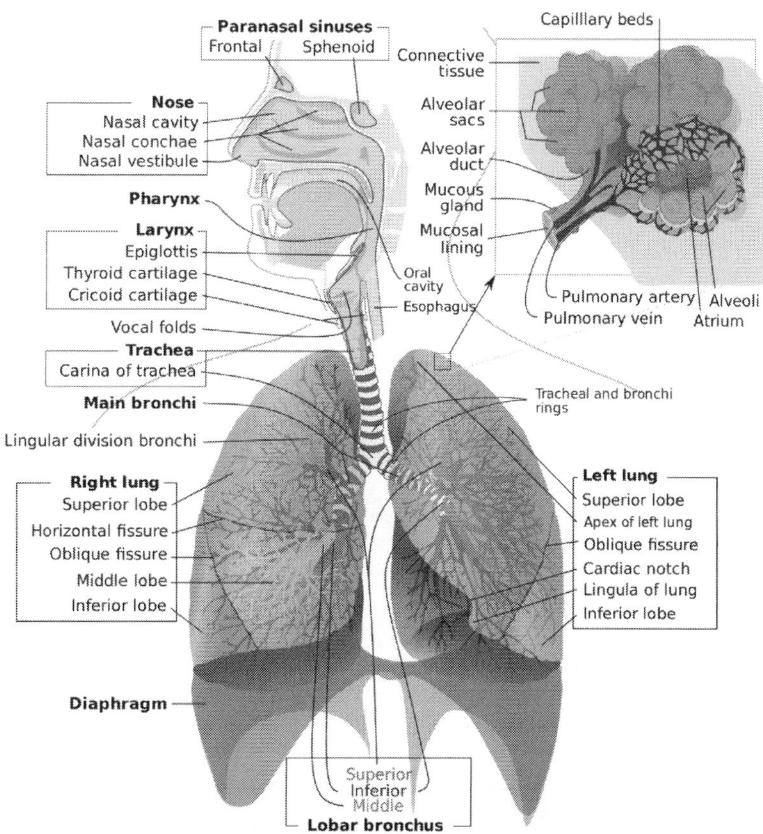


**Review Video: Respiratory System**
Visit mometrix.com/academy and enter code: 783075

## Primary and Secondary Muscles Used for Breathing

Muscles used for breathing are separated into primary and secondary muscle groups.

- The **primary muscle groups** are those that are used in normal, quiet breathing. When patients are in respiratory distress and breathing is more difficult, secondary muscle groups become activated. The muscles considered primary for breathing are the diaphragm and the external intercostal muscles. These muscles act by changing the pressure gradient, allowing the lungs to expand and air to flow in and out.
- The **secondary muscle groups** include the sternocleidomastoid, scaleni, internal intercostals, obliques, and abdominal muscles. These secondary muscle groups work when breathing is difficult, both in inspiration and expiration, in cases such as obstructions or bronchoconstriction. Use of these secondary muscle groups can often be seen on exam and may be described as see-saw or abdominal breathing (when the abdominal muscles are being used during exhalation) or retractions as the muscles activate and can be seen between rigid structures such as bone.

## Normal Physiological Airway Clearance

**Normal airway clearance** is caused by various aspects of the respiratory system. A thin layer of mucus lines the airways as a protective mechanism against debris and helps trap foreign objects before they enter the lower airways. Proper hydration keeps the mucosa adequately moist so it can trap foreign debris. As this debris lands in the mucus, the cilia in the respiratory tract act as an "elevator" to push the debris up to the larynx, where it can either be coughed up or swallowed and digested. An intact cough reflex is necessary for the debris to stimulate the cough, and normal muscle strength and nerve innervation of the diaphragm is required to produce a sufficiently forceful cough.

## Ventilation/Perfusion Ratio

In order to maintain homeostasis, the respiratory and cardiac systems need to maintain a careful balance. The **ventilation/perfusion ratio** indicates that ventilation of the lungs and perfusion to the lungs are within a normal balance. A normal ventilation/perfusion ratio is equal to 0.8. A ventilation/perfusion ratio higher than normal is indicative of ventilation that is too high, perfusion that is too low, or some combination of the two. This can occur because of hyperventilation (either physiological or caused by healthcare practitioners due to incorrect ventilator settings), pulmonary embolism, or hypotension. Essentially, a high ventilation/perfusion ratio means that there is more ventilation than perfusion. If the ventilation/perfusion ratio is lower than normal, then ventilation is too low, perfusion is too high, or some combination of the two. This can be caused by atelectasis, pneumonia, or lung disease. Whatever the cause, a low ventilation/perfusion ratio indicates that there is more perfusion than ventilation.

## Normal and Abnormal Breath Sound Terms

Normal breath sounds can be divided into three types. Vesicular breath sounds are low, soft sounds that can normally be heard over the peripheral lung space. Bronchovesicular breath sounds are moderate pitch breath sounds that are normally heard in the upper lung fields. Tracheal breath sounds are higher in pitch and heard over the trachea. Abnormal breath sounds are also known as adventitious lung sounds. Wheezes are high-pitched, expiratory sounds caused by air flowing through an obstructed airway. Stridor is also high-pitched, but is usually heard on inspiration in the upper airways. Coarse crackles are caused by an excessive amount of secretions in the airway and can be heard on inspiration and expiration. Fine crackles occur late in the expiratory phase and usually occur when the peripheral airways are being "popped" back open.

**Review Video: Lung Sounds**
Visit mometrix.com/academy and enter code: 765616

## Diagnostic Procedures and Tools Used During Pulmonary Assessment

The diagnostic procedures and tools used during assessment of **pulmonary and thoracic trauma/disease** will vary according to the type and degree of injury/disease, but may include:

- **Thorough physical examination** including cardiac and pulmonary status, assessing for any abnormalities.
- **Electrocardiogram** to assess for cardiac arrhythmias.
- **Chest x-ray** should be done for all those with injuries to check for fractures, pneumothorax, major injuries, and placement of intubation tubes. X-rays can be taken quickly and with portable equipment so they can be completed quickly during the initial assessment.
- **Computerized tomography** may be indicated after initial assessment, especially if there is a possibility of damage to the parenchyma of the lungs.
- **Oximetry and atrial blood gases** as indicated.
- **12-lead electrocardiogram** may be needed if there are arrhythmias for more careful observation.
- **Echocardiogram** should be done if there is apparent cardiac damage.

## Capnography with End-Tidal $CO_2$ Detector

**Capnometry** utilizes an **end-tidal $CO_2$ (ETCO) detector** that measures the concentration of $CO_2$ in expired air, usually through pH sensitive paper that changes color (commonly purple to yellow). Typically, the capnometer is attached to the ETT and a bag-valve-mask (BVM) ventilator attached. The capnogram provides data in the shape of a waveform that represents the partial pressure of exhaled gas. It is often used to confirm placement of endotracheal tubes as clinical assessment is not always sufficient, and it is a noninvasive mode of monitoring carbon dioxide in the respiratory cycle. Information provided by the capnogram includes:

- $PaCO_2$ level
- Type and degree of bronchial obstruction, such as COPD (waveform changes from rectangular to a fin-like)
- Air leaks in the ventilation system
- Rebreathing precipitated by need for new $CO_2$ absorber
- Cardiac arrest
- Hypothermia or reduced metabolism

The normal capnogram is a waveform that represents the varying $CO_2$ level throughout the breath cycle:

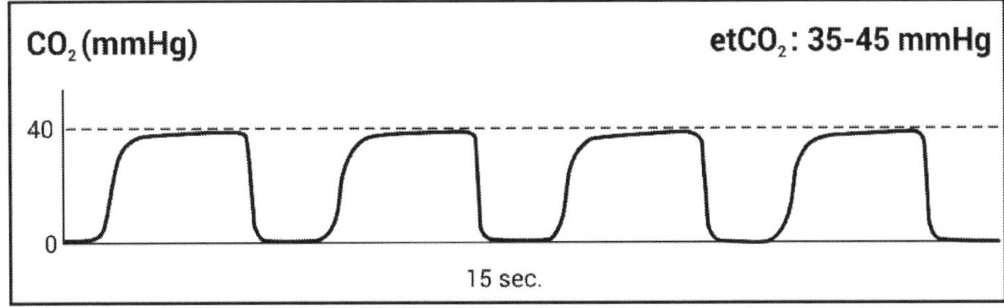


## Arterial Blood Gases

**Arterial blood gases** (ABGs) are monitored to assess effectiveness of oxygenation, ventilation, and acid-base status and to determine oxygen flow rates. Partial pressure of a gas is that exerted by each gas in a mixture of gases, proportional to its concentration, based on total atmospheric pressure of 760 mmHg at sea level. Normal values include:

- Acidity/alkalinity (pH): 7.35-7.45
- Partial pressure of carbon dioxide ($PaCO_2$): 35-45 mmHg

- Partial pressure of oxygen ($PaO_2$): ≥80 mmHg
- Bicarbonate concentration ($HCO_3^-$): 22-26 mEq/L
- Oxygen saturation ($SaO_2$): ≥95%

The relationship between these elements, particularly the $PaCO_2$ and the $PaO_2$ indicates respiratory status. For example, $PaCO_2$ >55 and the $PaO_2$ <60 in a patient previously in good health indicates respiratory failure. There are many issues to consider. Ventilator management may require a higher $PaCO_2$ to prevent barotrauma and a lower $PaO_2$ to reduce oxygen toxicity.

# Respiratory Pathophysiology

## ACUTE PULMONARY EMBOLISM

Acute pulmonary embolism occurs when a pulmonary artery or arteriole is blocked, cutting off blood supply to the pulmonary vessels and subsequent oxygenation of the blood. While most pulmonary emboli are from thrombus formation, they can also be caused by air, fat, or septic embolus (from bacterial invasion of a thrombus). Common originating sites for thrombus formation are the deep veins in the legs, the pelvic veins, and the right atrium. Causes include stasis related to damage to endothelial wall and changes in blood coagulation factors. Atrial fibrillation poses a serious risk because blood pools in the right atrium, forming clots that travel directly through the right ventricle to the lungs. The obstruction of the artery/arteriole causes an increase in alveolar dead space in which there is ventilation but impairment of gas exchange because of the ventilation/perfusion mismatching or intrapulmonary shunting. This results in hypoxia, hypercapnia, and the release of mediators that cause bronchoconstriction. If more than 50% of the vascular bed becomes excluded, pulmonary hypertension occurs.

### *SYMPTOMS AND DIAGNOSIS*

Clinical manifestations of acute pulmonary embolism (PE) vary according to the size of the embolus and the area of occlusion.

**Symptoms** include:

- Dyspnea with tachypnea
- Cyanosis; may turn grey or blue from nipple line up (massive PE)
- Anxiety and restlessness, feeling of doom
- Chest pain, tachycardia, may progress to arrhythmias (PEA)
- Fever
- Rales
- Cough (sometimes with hemoptysis)
- Hemodynamic instability

**Diagnostic tests** are as follows:

- ABG analysis may show hypoxemia (decreased $PaO_2$), hypocarbia (decreased $PaCO_2$) and respiratory alkalosis (increased pH).
- D-dimer will show elevation with PE but is not definitively diagnostic without a CT scan.
- ECG may show sinus tachycardia or other abnormalities.
- Echocardiogram can show emboli in the central arteries and can assess the hemodynamic status of the right side of the heart.
- Spiral CT may provide definitive diagnosis.
- V/Q scintigraphy can confirm diagnosis.
- Pulmonary angiograms also can confirm diagnosis.

### *MEDICAL MANAGEMENT*

Medical management of pulmonary embolism starts with preventive measures for those at risk, including leg exercises, elastic compression stockings, and anticoagulation therapy. Most pulmonary emboli present as medical emergencies, so the immediate task is to stabilize the patient. **Medical management** may include:

- **Oxygen** to relieve hypoxemia
- **Intravenous infusions:** Dobutamine (Dobutrex) or dopamine (Intropin) to relieve hypotension
- **Cardiac monitoring** for dysrhythmias and issues due to right sided heart failure
- **Medications** as indicated: digitalis glycosides, diuretic, and antiarrhythmics
- Intubation and mechanical ventilation may be required

- **Analgesics** (such as morphine sulfate) or sedation to relieve anxiety
- **Anticoagulants** to prevent recurrence (although it will not dissolve clots already present), including heparin and warfarin (Coumadin)
- **Placement of percutaneous venous filter** (Greenfield) in the inferior vena cava to prevent further emboli from entering the lungs, if anticoagulation therapy is contraindicated
- **Thrombolytic therapy,** recombinant tissue-type plasminogen activator (rt-PA) or streptokinase, for those severely compromised, but these treatments have limited success and pose the danger of bleeding

## Traumatic Asphyxia

**Asphyxia** may relate to a number of different injuries:

- **Traumatic asphyxia** most commonly involves a crush injury of the thorax and possibly traumatic injuries to multiple organs. Crush injuries are characterized by petechiae in the area of compression although tight-fitting clothing, such as a woman's bra, may prevent petechiae from forming.
- **Manual strangulation** may involve crush injuries to the throat, such as hyoid fracture. Often the face appears cyanotic while the rest of the body does not. Petechiae may be present on the face as well. Bruising may be noted about the throat.
- **Ligature strangulation** is similar to manual although throat markings are different, with an indented area surrounding the neck.
- **Hanging** produces a V-shaped marking on the throat and does not encircle the neck.
- **Choking** obstructs the airway. (May require bronchoscopy to remove foreign object).

In all cases, immediate establishment of airway, breathing, and circulation (ABCs) takes precedence. Surgical intervention may be needed for traumatic crush injuries.

## Submersion Asphyxia

Submersion (near-drowning) asphyxiation can cause profound damage to the central nervous system, pulmonary dysfunction related to aspiration, cardiac hypoxia with life-threatening arrhythmias, fluid and electrolyte imbalances, and multi-organ damage, so treatment can be complex. Hypothermia related to near drowning has some protective affect because blood is shunted to the brain and heart. **Treatment** includes:

- Immediate establishment of airway, breathing and circulation (ABCs)
- NG tube and gastric decompression to reduce risk of aspiration
- Neurological evaluation
- Pulmonary management includes monitoring for ≥72 hours for respiratory deterioration. Ventilation may need positive-end expiratory pressure (PEEP), but this poses danger to cardiac output and can cause barotrauma, so use should be limited.
- In patients that are symptomatic but do not yet need intubation, use supplemental oxygen to keep $SpO_2 > 94\%$
- Monitoring of cardiac output and function
- Neurological care to reduce cerebral edema and increased intracranial pressure and prevent secondary injury
- Rewarming if necessary (0.5-1.0 °C/hr)

## Acute Lung Injury and Acute Respiratory Distress Syndrome

Acute lung injury (ALI) comprises a syndrome of respiratory distress culminating in acute respiratory distress syndrome (ARDS). ARDS is a dangerous, potentially fatal respiratory condition, always caused by an illness or injury to the lungs. Lung injury causes fluid to leak into the spaces between the alveoli and capillaries, increasing pressure on the alveoli, causing them to collapse. With increased fluid accumulation in the lungs, the ability of the lungs to move oxygen into the blood is decreased, resulting in hypoxemia. Lung injury also causes a release of cytokines, a type of inflammatory protein, which then brings neutrophils to the lung. These proteins and cells leak into nearby blood vessels and cause inflammation throughout the body. This immune response, in combination with low levels of blood oxygen, can lead to organ failure. Symptoms are characterized by respiratory distress within 72 hours of surgery or a serious injury to a person with otherwise normal lungs and no cardiac disorder. Untreated, the condition results in respiratory failure, MODS, and a mortality rate of 5-30%.

**Symptoms** include:

- Refractory hypoxemia (hypoxemia not responding to increasing levels of oxygen)
- Crackling rales/wheezing in lungs
- Decrease in pulmonary compliance which results in increased tachypnea with expiratory grunting
- Cyanosis/skin mottling
- Hypotension and tachycardia
- Symptoms associated with volume overload are missing (3rd heart sound or JVD)
- Respiratory alkalosis initially but, as the disease progresses, replaced with hypercarbia and respiratory acidosis
- Normal x-ray initially but then diffuse infiltrates in both lungs, while the heart and vessels appear normal

### *Management*

The management of acute respiratory distress syndrome (ARDS) involves providing adequate gas exchange and preventing further damage to the lung from forced ventilation.

**Treatment** includes:

- Mechanical ventilation to maintain oxygenation and ventilation
- Corticosteroids (may increase mortality rates in some patient populations, though this is the most commonly given treatment), nitrous oxide, inhaled surfactant, and anti-inflammatory medications
- Treatment of the underlying condition is the only proven treatment, especially identifying and treating an infection with appropriate antibiotics, as sepsis is most common etiology for ARDS, but prophylactic antibiotics are not indicated.
- Conservative fluid management is indicated to reduce days on the ventilator, but does not reduce overall mortality.

**Pharmacologic preventive care**: Enoxaparin 40 mg subcutaneously QD, sucralfate 1 g NGT four times daily or omeprazole 40 mg IV QD, and enteral nutrition support within 24 hours of ICU admission or intubation.

### *Ventilation Management*

Ventilation management in ARDS consists of the following:

- $O_2$ therapy by nasal prongs, cannula, or mask may be sufficient in very mild cases to maintain oxygen saturation above 90%. Oxygen should be administered at 100% because of the mismatch between ventilation (V) and perfusion (Q), which can result in hypoxia on position change.
- ARDS oxygenation goal is $PaO_2$ 55-80 mmHg or $SpO_2$ 88-95%.
- Endotracheal intubation may be needed if $SpO_2$ falls or $CO_2$ levels rise.
- The ARDS Network recommends low tidal volumes (6 mL/kg) and higher PEEP (12 $cmH_2O$ or more).
- The low tidal volume ventilation described above is referred to as lung protective ventilation, and it has been shown to reduce mortality in patients with ARDS.
- Placing patients with severe ARDS in prone position for 18-24 hours per day with chest and pelvis supported and abdomen unsupported allows the diaphragm to move posteriorly, increasing functional residual capacity (FRC) in many patients.

## Acute Respiratory Failure

### *Cardinal Signs*

The cardinal signs of respiratory failure include:

- Tachypnea
- Tachycardia
- Anxiety and restlessness
- Diaphoresis

**Symptoms** may vary according to the cause. An obstruction may cause more obvious respiratory symptoms than other disorders.

- Early signs may include changes in the depth and pattern of respirations with flaring nares, sternal retractions, expiratory grunting, wheezing, and extended expiration as the body tries to compensate for hypoxemia and increasing levels of carbon dioxide.
- Cyanosis may be evident.
- Central nervous depression, with alterations in consciousness occurs with decreased perfusion to the brain.
- As the hypoxemia worsens, cardiac arrhythmias, including bradycardia, may occur with either hypotension or hypertension.
- Dyspnea becomes more pronounced with depressed respirations.
- Eventually stupor, coma, and death can occur if the condition is not reversed.

### *Hypoxemic and Hypercapnic Respiratory Failure*

**Hypoxemic respiratory failure** occurs suddenly when gaseous exchange of oxygen for carbon dioxide cannot keep up with demand for oxygen or production of carbon dioxide:

- $PaO_2$ <60 mmHg
- $PaCO_2$ >40 mmHg
- Arterial pH <7.35

Hypoxemic respiratory failure can be the result of low inhaled oxygen, as at high elevations or with smoke inhalation. The following ventilatory mechanisms may be involved:

- Alveolar hypotension
- Ventilation-perfusion mismatch (the most common cause)
- Intrapulmonary shunts
- Diffusion impairment

**Hypercapnic respiratory failure** results from an increase in $PaCO_2$ >45-50 mmHg associated with respiratory acidosis and may include:

- Reduction in minute ventilation, total volume of gas ventilated in one minute (often related to neurological, muscle, or chest wall disorders, drug overdoses, or obstruction of upper airway)
- Increased dead space with wasted ventilation (related to lung disease or disorders of chest wall, such as scoliosis)
- Increased production of $CO_2$ (usually related to infection, burns, or other causes of hypermetabolism)
- Oxygen saturation normal or below normal

### UNDERLYING CAUSES

There are a number of underlying causes for respiratory failure:

- **Airway obstruction:** Obstruction may result from an inhaled object or from an underlying disease process, such as cystic fibrosis, asthma, pulmonary edema, or infection.
- **Inadequate respirations:** This is a common cause among adults, especially related to obesity and sleep apnea. It may also be induced by an overdose of sedation medications such as opioids.
- **Neuromuscular disorders:** Those disorders that interfere with the neuromuscular functioning of the lungs or the chest wall, such as muscular dystrophy or spinal cord injuries can prevent adequate ventilation.
- **Pulmonary abnormalities:** Those abnormalities of the lung tissue, found in pulmonary fibrosis, burns, ARDS, and reactions to drugs, can lead to failure.
- **Chest wall abnormalities:** Disorders that impact lung parenchyma, such as severe scoliosis or chest wounds can interfere with lung functioning.

**Nursing interventions** to help prevent respiratory issues:

- Turn, position, and ambulate the patient.
- Have the patient cough and breathe deeply.
- Use vibration and percussion treatments.
- Hydrate the patient to help hydrate the airway secretions, and incentive spirometry.

### MANAGEMENT

Respiratory failure must be **treated** immediately before severe hypoxemia causes irreversible damage to vital organs.

- **Identifying and treating** the underlying cause should be done immediately because emergency medications or surgery may be indicated. Medical treatments will vary widely depending upon the cause; for example, cardiopulmonary structural defects may require surgical repair, pulmonary edema may require diuresis, inhaled objects may require surgical removal, and infections may require aggressive antimicrobials.
- **Intravenous lines/central lines** are inserted for testing, fluids, and medications.
- **Oxygen therapy** should be initiated to attempt to reverse hypoxemia; however, if refractory hypoxemia occurs, then oxygen therapy alone will not suffice. Oxygen levels must be titrated carefully.
- **Intubation and mechanical ventilation** are frequently required to maintain adequate ventilation and oxygenation. Positive end expiratory pressure (PEEP) may be necessary with refractory hypoxemia and collapsed alveoli.
- **Respiratory status** must be monitored constantly, including arterial blood gases and vital signs.

## PNEUMONIA

Pneumonia is inflammation of the lung parenchyma, filling the alveoli with exudate. It is common throughout childhood and adulthood. Pneumonia may be a primary disease or may occur secondary to another infection or disease, such as lung cancer. Pneumonia may be caused by bacteria, viruses, parasites, or fungi. Common causes for community-acquired pneumonia (CAP) include:

- *Streptococcus pneumoniae*
- *Legionella* species
- *Haemophilus influenzae*
- *Staphylococcus aureus*
- *Mycoplasma pneumoniae*
- Viruses

Pneumonia may also be caused by chemical damage. Pneumonia is characterized by **location**:

- **Lobar** involves one or more lobes of the lungs. If lobes in both lungs are affected, it is referred to as bilateral or double pneumonia.
- **Bronchial/lobular** involves the terminal bronchioles, and exudate can involve the adjacent lobules. Usually, the pneumonia occurs in scattered patches throughout the lungs.
- **Interstitial** involves primarily the interstitium and alveoli where white blood cells and plasma fill the alveoli, generating inflammation and creating fibrotic tissue as the alveoli are destroyed.

**Review Video: Pneumonia**
Visit mometrix.com/academy and enter code: 628264

### *Hospital-Acquired Pneumonia*

Hospital-acquired pneumonia (HAP) is defined as pneumonia that did not appear to be present on admission that occurs at least 48 hours after admission to a hospital. **Healthcare-associated pneumonia (HCAP)** is defined as pneumonia that occurs in a patient within 90 days of being hospitalized for 2 or more days at an acute care hospital or LTAC. **Ventilator-associated pneumonia (VAP)** is one type of hospital acquired pneumonia that a patient acquires more than 48 hours after having an ETT placed. The most common way that the patient is infected is via aspiration of bacteria that is colonized in the upper respiratory tract. It is estimated that close to 75% of patients that are critically ill will be colonized with multidrug resistant bacteria within 48 hours of entering an ICU. Aspiration occurs at a rate of about 45% in patients with no health problems and the rate is much higher in those with HAP, HCAP, and VAP. The frequency of patients developing these types of pneumonia is increasing, with those at highest risk being those with immunosuppression, septic shock, currently hospitalized for more than five days, and those who have had antibiotics for another infection within the previous three months. These types of pneumonia should be considered if a patient already hospitalized has purulent sputum or a change in respiratory status such as deoxygenating, in combination with a worsening or new chest x-ray infiltrate.

**Treatment** includes:

- Antibiotic therapy
- Using appropriate isolation and precautions with infected patients
- Preventive measures including maintaining ventilated patients in 30° upright positions, frequent oral care for vent patients, and changing ventilator circuits as per protocol

Antibiotic treatment options for HAP, HCAP, and VAP should take into account many factors, including culture data (when available), patient's comorbidities, flora in the unit, any recent antibiotics by the patient, and whether the patient is at high risk for having multidrug resistant bacteria. As most critical care patients are at high risk, due to factors such as being in an ICU setting, ventilators, and comorbidities, antibiotic recommendations to follow are for coverage for patients with risk factors for multidrug resistant bacteria.

**One** of the following:

- Ceftazidime 2 g every 8 hours IV **OR**
- Cefepime 2 g every 8 hours IV **OR**
- Imipenem 500 mg every 6 hours IV **OR**
- Piperacillin-tazobactam 4.5 g every 6 hours IV

**AND one** of the following:

- Ciprofloxacin 400 mg every 8 hours IV **OR**
- Levaquin 750 mg every 24 hours IV

## Aspiration Pneumonitis/Pneumonia

Aspiration pneumonitis/pneumonia may occur as the result of any type of aspiration, including foreign objects. The aspirated material creates an inflammatory response, with the irritated mucous membrane at high risk for bacterial infection secondary to the aspiration, causing pneumonia. Gastric contents and oropharyngeal bacteria are commonly aspirated. Gastric contents can cause a severe chemical pneumonitis with hypoxemia, especially if the pH is <2.5. Acidic food particles can cause severe reactions. With acidic damage, bronchospasm and atelectasis occur rapidly with tracheal irritation, bronchitis, and alveolar damage with interstitial edema and hemorrhage. Intrapulmonary shunting and V/Q mismatch may occur. Pulmonary artery pressure increases. Non-acidic liquids and food particles are less damaging, and symptoms may clear within 4 hours of liquid aspiration or granuloma may form about food particles in 1-5 days. Depending upon the type of aspiration, pneumonitis may clear within a week, ARDS or pneumonia may develop, or progressive acute respiratory failure may lead to death.

There are a number of risk factors that can lead to **aspiration pneumonitis/pneumonia:**

- Altered level of consciousness related to illness or sedation
- Depression of gag, swallowing reflex
- Intubation or feeding tubes
- Ileus or gastric distention
- Gastrointestinal disorders, such as gastroesophageal reflux disorders (GERD)

**Diagnosis** is based on clinical findings, ABGs showing hypoxemia, infiltrates observed on x-ray, and elevated WBC if infection is present.

**Symptoms:** Similar to other pneumonias:

- Cough often with copious sputum
- Respiratory distress, dyspnea
- Cyanosis
- Tachycardia
- Hypotension

**Treatment** includes:

- Suctioning as needed to clear upper airway
- Supplemental oxygen
- Antibiotic therapy as indicated after 48 hours if symptoms not resolving
- Symptomatic respiratory support

## Foreign Body Aspiration

Foreign body aspiration can cause obstruction of the pharynx, larynx, or trachea, leading to acute dyspnea or asphyxiation, and the object may also be drawn distally into the bronchial tree. With adults, most foreign bodies migrate more readily down the right bronchus. Food is the most frequently aspirated, but other small objects, such as coins or needles, may also be aspirated. Sometimes the object causes swelling, ulceration, and general inflammation that hampers removal.

**Symptoms** include:

- **Initial***:* Severe coughing, gagging, sternal retraction, wheezing. Objects in the larynx may cause inability to breathe or speak and lead to respiratory arrest. Objects in the bronchus cause cough, dyspnea, and wheezing.
- **Delayed***:* Hours, days, or weeks later, an undetected aspirant may cause an infection distal to the aspirated material. Symptoms depend on the area and extent of the infection.

**Treatment** includes:

- Removal with laryngoscopy or bronchoscopy (rigid is often better than flexible)
- Antibiotic therapy for secondary infection
- Surgical bronchotomy (rarely required)
- Symptomatic support

## Chronic Bronchitis

Chronic bronchitis is a pulmonary airway disease characterized by severe cough with sputum production for at least 3 months a year for at least 2 consecutive years. Irritation of the airways (often from smoke or pollutants) causes an inflammatory response, increasing the number of mucus-secreting glands and goblet cells while ciliary function decreases so that the extra mucus plugs the airways. Additionally, the bronchial walls thicken, alveoli near the inflamed bronchioles become fibrotic, and alveolar macrophages cannot function properly, increasing susceptibility to infections. Chronic bronchitis is most common in those >45 years old and occurs twice as frequently in females as males.

**Symptoms** include:

- Persistent cough with increasing sputum
- Dyspnea
- Frequent respiratory infections

**Treatment** includes:

- Bronchodilators
- Long term continuous oxygen therapy or supplemental oxygen during exercise
- Pulmonary rehabilitation to improve exercise and breathing
- Antibiotics during infections
- Corticosteroids for acute episodes

## Emphysema

Emphysema, the primary component of COPD, is characterized by abnormal distention of air spaces at the ends of the terminal bronchioles, with destruction of alveolar walls so that there is less and less gaseous exchange and increasing dead space with resultant hypoxemia, hypercapnia, and respiratory acidosis. The capillary bed is damaged as well, altering pulmonary blood flow and raising pressure in the right atrium (cor pulmonale) and pulmonary artery, leading to cardiac failure. Complications include respiratory insufficiency and failure. There are two primary types of emphysema (and both forms may be present):

- **Centrilobular** (the most common form) involves the central portion of the respiratory lobule, sparing distal alveoli, and usually affects the upper lobes. Typical symptoms include abnormal ventilation-perfusion ratios, hypoxemia, hypercapnia, and polycythemia with right-sided heart failure.
- **Panlobular** involves enlargement of all air spaces, including the bronchiole, alveolar duct, and alveoli, but there is minimal inflammatory disease. Typical symptoms include hyperextended rigid barrel chest, marked dyspnea, weight loss, and active expiration.

# COPD

### *Stages*

Functional dyspnea, body mass index (BMI), and spirometry are used to assess the **stages of chronic obstructive pulmonary disease (COPD)**. Spirometry measures used are the ratio of forced expiratory volume in the first second of expiration ($FEV_1$) after full inhalation to total forced vital capacity (FVC). Normal lung function decreases after age 35; so normal values are adjusted for height, weight, gender, and age:

- **Stage I** (mild): Minimal dyspnea with or without cough and sputum. $FEV_1$ is ≥80% of predicted rate and $FEV_1$:FVC <70%.
- **Stage 2** (moderate): Moderate to severe chronic exertional dyspnea with or without cough and sputum. $FEV_1$ is 50-80% of predicted rate and $FEV_1$:FVC <70%.
- **Stage 3** (severe): Same as stage 2 but with repeated episodes with increased exertional dyspnea and condition impacting quality of life. $FEV_1$ is 30-50% of predicted rate and $FEV_1$:FVC <70%.
- **Stage 4** (very severe): Severe dyspnea and life-threatening episodes that severely impact quality of life. $FEV_1$ is 30% of predicted rate or <50% with chronic respiratory failure and $FEV_1$:FVC <70%.

### *Management*

COPD is not reversible, so management aims at slowing its progression, relieving symptoms, and improving quality of life:

- Smoking cessation is the primary means to slow progression and may require smoking cessation support in the form of classes or medications, such as Zyban, nicotine patches or gum, clonidine, or nortriptyline.
- Bronchodilators, such as albuterol (Ventolin) and salmeterol (Serevent), relieve bronchospasm and airway obstruction.
- Corticosteroids, both inhaled (Pulmicort, Vanceril) and oral (prednisone) may improve symptoms but are used mostly for associated asthma.
- Oxygen therapy may be long term continuous or used during exertion.
- Bullectomy (for bullous emphysema) to remove bullae (enlarged airspaces that do not ventilate).
- Lung volume reduction surgery may be done if involvement in the lung is limited; however, mortality rates are high.
- Lung transplantation is a definitive high-risk option.
- Pulmonary rehabilitation includes breathing exercises, muscle training, activity pacing, and modification of activities.

## Chronic Ventilatory Failure

Chronic ventilatory failure occurs when alveolar ventilation fails to increase in response to increasing levels of carbon dioxide, usually associated with chronic pulmonary diseases, such as asthma and COPD, drug overdoses, or diseases that impair respiratory effort, such as Guillain-Barré and myasthenia gravis. Normally, the ventilatory system is able to maintain $PCO_2$ and pH levels within narrow limits, even though $PO_2$ levels may be more variable, but with ventilatory failure, the body is not able to compensate for the resultant hypercapnia and pH falls, resulting in respiratory acidosis. Symptoms include increasing dyspnea with tachypnea, gasping respirations, and use of accessory muscles. Patients may become confused as hypercapnia causes increased intracranial pressure. If pH is <7.2, cardiac arrhythmias, hyperkalemia, and hypotension can occur as pulmonary arteries constrict and the peripheral vascular system dilates. Diagnosis is per symptoms, ABGs consistent with respiratory acidosis ($PCO_2$ >50 and pH <7.35), pulse oximetry, and chest x-ray. Treatment can include non-invasive PPV (BiPAP), endotracheal mechanical ventilation, corticosteroids, and bronchodilators.

## Chronic Asthma

The three primary symptoms of chronic asthma are cough, wheezing, and dyspnea. In cough-variant asthma, a severe cough may be the only symptom, at least initially. Chronic asthma is characterized by recurring bronchospasm and inflammation of the airways resulting in airway obstruction. Asthma affects the bronchi and not the alveoli. While no longer considered part of COPD because airway obstruction is not constant and is responsive to treatment, over time fibrotic changes in the airways can result in permanent obstruction, especially if asthma is not treated adequately. **Symptoms** of chronic asthma include nighttime coughing, exertional dyspnea, tightness in the chest, and cough. Acute exacerbations may occur, sometimes related to triggers, such as allergies, resulting in increased dyspnea, wheezing, cough, tachycardia, bronchospasm, and rhonchi. **Treatment** of chronic asthma includes chest hygiene, identification and avoidance of triggers, prompt treatment of infections, bronchodilators, long-acting β-2 agonists, and inhaled glucocorticoids.

## STATUS ASTHMATICUS

### *PATHOPHYSIOLOGY*

Status asthmaticus is a severe acute attack of asthma that does not respond to conventional therapy. An acute attack of asthma is precipitated by some stimulus, such as an antigen that triggers an allergic response, resulting in an inflammatory cascade that causes edema of the mucous membranes (swollen airway), contraction of smooth muscles (bronchospasm), increased mucus production (cough and obstruction), and hyperinflation of airways (decreased ventilation and shunting). Mast cells and T lymphocytes produce cytokines, which continue the inflammatory response through increased blood flow coupled with vasoconstriction and bronchoconstriction, resulting in fluid leakage from the vasculature. Epithelial cells and cilia are destroyed, exposing nerves and causing hypersensitivity. Sympathetic nervous system receptors in the bronchi stimulate bronchodilation.

### *CLINICAL SYMPTOMS*

The person with status asthmaticus will often present in acute distress, non-responsive to inhaled bronchodilators. **Symptoms** include:

- Signs of airway obstruction
- Sternal and intercostal retractions
- Tachypnea and dyspnea with increasing cyanosis
- Forced prolonged expirations
- Cardiac decompensation with increased left ventricular afterload and increased pulmonary edema resulting from alveolar-capillary permeability. Hypoxia may trigger an increase in pulmonary vascular resistance with increased right ventricular afterload.
- Pulsus paradoxus (decreased pulse on inspiration and increased on expiration) with extra beats on inspiration detected through auscultation but not detected radially. Blood pressure normally decreases slightly during inspiration, but this response is exaggerated. Pulsus paradoxus indicates increasing severity of asthma.
- Hypoxemia (with impending respiratory failure)
- Hypocapnia followed by hypercapnia (with impending respiratory failure)
- Metabolic acidosis

### *INDICATIONS FOR MECHANICAL VENTILATION FOR STATUS ASTHMATICUS*

Mechanical ventilation (MV) for status asthmaticus should be avoided, if possible, because of the danger of increased bronchospasm as well as barotrauma and decreased circulation. However, there are some absolute indications for the use of intubation and ventilation and a number of other indications that are evaluated on an individual basis.

The following are **absolute indications for MV:**

- Cardiac and/or pulmonary arrest
- Markedly depressed mental status (obtundation)
- Severe hypoxia and/or apnea

The following are **relative indications for MV:**

- Exhaustion/muscle fatigue from exertion of breathing
- Sharply diminished breath sounds and no audible wheezing
- Pulse paradoxus >20-40 mmHg; absent = imminent respiratory arrest
- $PaO_2$ <70 mmHg on 100% oxygen
- Dysphonia
- Central cyanosis
- Increased hypercapnia
- Metabolic/respiratory acidosis: pH <7.20

In this patient population, ventilator goal is to minimize airway pressures while oxygenating the patient. Vent settings include: low tidal volume (6-8 mL/kg), low respiratory rate (10-14 respirations/minute), and high inspiratory flow rate (80-100 L/min).

**Review Video: Mechanical Ventilation**
Visit mometrix.com/academy and enter code: 679637

## Air Leak Syndromes

Air leak syndromes may result in significant respiratory distress. Leaks may occur spontaneously or secondary to some type of trauma (accidental, mechanical, iatrogenic) or disease. As pressure increases inside the alveoli, the alveolar wall pulls away from the perivascular sheath and subsequent alveolar rupture allows air to follow the perivascular planes and flow into adjacent areas. There are two categories:

- **Pneumothorax:**
  - Air in the pleural space causes a lung to collapse.
- **Barotrauma/volutrauma** with air in the interstitial space (usually resolve over time):
  - Pneumoperitoneum is air in the peritoneal area, including the abdomen and occasionally the scrotal sac of male infants.
  - Pneumomediastinum is air in the mediastinal area between the lungs.
  - Pneumopericardium is air in the pericardial sac that surrounds the heart.
  - Subcutaneous emphysema is air in the subcutaneous tissue planes of the chest wall.
  - Pulmonary interstitial emphysema (PIE) is air trapped in the interstitium between the alveoli.

### *Pneumothorax*

Pneumothorax occurs when there is a leak of air into the pleural space, resulting in complete or partial collapse of a lung.

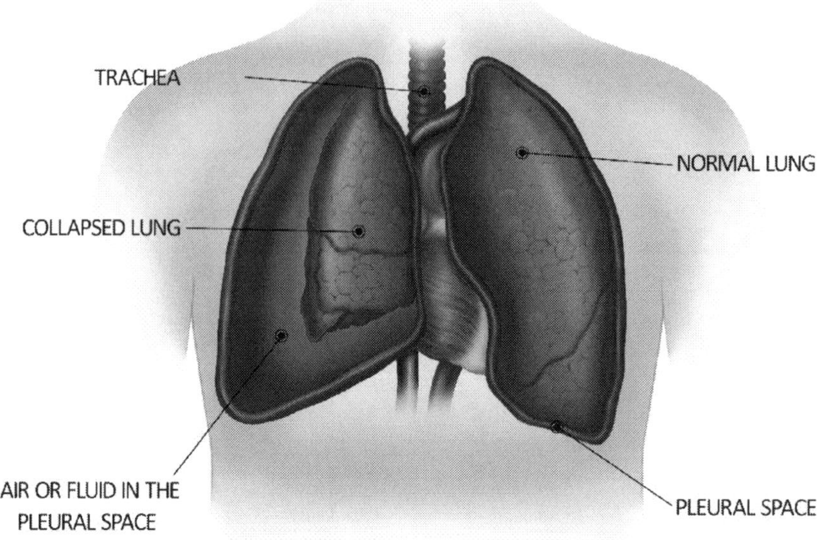


**Symptoms:** Vary widely depending on the cause and degree of the pneumothorax and whether or not there is an underlying disease. Symptoms include acute pleuritic pain (95%), usually on the affected side, and decreased breath sounds. In a *tension pneumothorax,* symptoms include tracheal deviation and hemodynamic compromise.

**Diagnosis:** Clinical findings; radiograph: 6-foot upright posterior-anterior; ultrasound may detect traumatic pneumothorax.

**Treatment:** Chest-tube thoracostomy with underwater seal drainage is the most common treatment for all types of pneumothorax.

- Tension pneumothorax: Immediate needle decompression and chest tube thoracostomy
- Small pneumothorax, patient stable: Oxygen administration and observation for 3-6 hours. If no increase is shown on repeat x-ray, patient may be discharged with another x-ray in 24 hours.
- Primary spontaneous pneumothorax: Catheter aspiration or chest tube thoracostomy

## Pleural Effusion and Empyema

**Pleural effusion** is the accumulation of fluid in the pleural space, usually secondary to other disease processes, such as heart failure, TB, neoplasms, nephrotic syndrome, and viral respiratory infections. The fluid may be serous, bloody, or purulent (empyema) and transudative or exudative. Signs and symptoms depend on underlying condition but includes dyspnea, from mild to severe. Tracheal deviation away from the affected side may be evident. Diagnosis includes chest x-ray, lateral decubitus x-ray, CT, thoracentesis, and pleural biopsy. Treatment includes treating underlying cause, thoracentesis to remove fluid, insertion of chest tube, pleurodesis, or pleurectomy or pleuroperitoneal shunt (primarily with malignancy).

**Review Video: Pleural Effusions**
Visit mometrix.com/academy and enter code: 145719

**Empyema** is a pleural effusion in which the collection of pleural fluid is thick and purulent, usually as a result of bacterial pneumonia or penetrating chest trauma. Empyema may also occur as a complication of thoracentesis or thoracic surgery. Signs and symptoms include acute illness with fever, chills, pain, cough, and dyspnea. Diagnosis is per chest CT and thoracentesis with culture and sensitivity. Treatment includes antibiotics and drainage of pleural space per needle aspiration, tube thoracostomy, or open chest drainage with thoracotomy.

## Pulmonary Fibrosis

Pulmonary fibrosis is a progressive disease of the lungs in which scarring of the tissue causes the lining of the lungs to thicken. This thickening prevents adequate oxygen exchange from occurring. The cause of pulmonary fibrosis is unknown, however environmental toxins such as asbestos, infections, smoking and occupational exposure to wood or metal dust may be contributing factors. The disease is more prevalent in males and the average age at the time of diagnosis is between 40 and 70. There may also be a genetic predisposition in the development of pulmonary fibrosis. The median survival for patients diagnosed with pulmonary fibrosis is less than five years.

**Signs and symptoms**: Shortness of breath, dry cough, fatigue, weight loss, and clubbing of the finger tips and nails.

**Diagnosis**: Physical assessment, chest x-ray and/or computed tomography, pulmonary function tests, arterial blood gases and lung biopsy.

**Treatment**: There is no cure for pulmonary fibrosis and treatment options are minimal. Anti-inflammatory medications such as corticosteroids may be used for symptom management as well as supplemental oxygen therapy. Lung transplantation may be an option for some patients based on age and advancement of disease. Some patients may be eligible for participation in a clinical trial, as there are research efforts focused on treatment options to halt the progression of the disease.

## Pulmonary Hypertension and Pulmonary Arterial Hypertension

Pulmonary arterial hypertension (PAH) is a progressive disease of the pulmonary arteries that can severely compromise cardiovascular patients. It may involve multiple processes. Usually, the pulmonary vasculature adjusts easily to accommodate blood volume from the right ventricle. If there is increased blood flow, the low resistance causes vasodilation and vice versa. However, sometimes the pulmonary vascular bed is damaged or obstructed, and this can impair the ability to handle changing volumes of blood. In that case, an increase in flow will increase the pulmonary arterial pressure, increasing pulmonary vascular resistance (PVR). This in turn, increases pressure on the right ventricle (RV) with increased RV workload and eventually causes RV hypertrophy with displacement of the intraventricular septum and tricuspid regurgitation (cor pulmonale). Over time, this leads to right heart failure and death. Pulmonary hypertension is usually diagnosed by right-sided heart catheterization and is indicated by systolic pulmonary artery pressure >30 mmHg and mean pulmonary artery pressure >25 mmHg. Non-invasive testing may include echocardiogram to look for cardiac changes.

### *Types*

Pulmonary hypertension or pulmonary arterial hypertension (PAH) may be classified as primary (idiopathic) or secondary.

- **Primary (idiopathic) PAH** may result from changes in immune responses, pulmonary emboli, sickle cell disease, collagen diseases, Raynaud's, and the use of contraceptives. The cause may be unknown or genetic.

- **Secondary PAH** may result from pulmonary vasoconstriction brought on by hypoxemia related to COPD, sleep-disordered breathing, kyphoscoliosis, obesity, smoke inhalation, altitude sickness, interstitial pneumonia, and neuromuscular disorders. It may also be caused by a decrease in pulmonary vascular bed of 50-75%, which may result from pulmonary emboli, vasculitis, tumor emboli, and interstitial lung disease, such as sarcoidosis. Primary cardiac disease, such as congenital defects in infants, and acquired disorders, such as rheumatic valve disease, mitral stenosis, and left ventricular failure may also contribute to PAH.

### *Treatment Options for PAH*

Medical treatment for pulmonary arterial hypertension (PAH) aims to identify and treat any underlying cardiac or pulmonary disease, control symptoms, and prevent complications:

- **Oxygen therapy** may be needed, especially supplemental oxygen during exercise.
- **Calcium channel blockers** may provide vasodilation for some patients.
- **Pulmonary vascular dilators**, such as IV epoprostenol (Flolan) and subcutaneous treprostinil sodium (Remodulin) and oral bosentan (Tracleer) help to control symptoms and prolong life.
- **Anticoagulants**, such as warfarin (Coumadin) are an important part of therapy because of recurrent pulmonary emboli. Studies have shown that anticoagulation increases survival rates.
- **Diuretics**, such as furosemide (Lasix) may be needed to relieve edema and restrict fluids, especially with right ventricular hypertrophy.

In some patients who cannot be managed adequately through medical treatment, a heart-lung transplant may be considered as the only effective treatment for long-term survival.

## Management of Pulmonary and Thoracic Trauma

### *Pulmonary Hemorrhage*

Pulmonary hemorrhage is an acute life-threatening injury that often results in death prior to arrival at the hospital; however, those presenting with traumatic pulmonary hemorrhage, as from a blunt or penetrating injury, require immediate surgical repair. Even with immediate surgery, survival after serious injury to a major pulmonary vessel is rare. It is important that a large bore IV be immediately inserted and fluid replacement begun while blood is typed and cross matched. The patient should be evaluated for shock and treatment, including colloid solutions, crystalloids, or blood, provided as indicated. Pulmonary hemorrhage may result in hemothorax. In some cases, pneumothorax may also be present, resulting in mediastinal shift that increases the difficulty of identifying and repairing the bleeding vessel. If the patient is stabilized, computed tomography may provide accurate diagnosis to isolate the area of hemorrhage.

### *Tracheal Perforation/Injury*

Tracheal perforation/injury may result from external injury, such as from trauma from a vehicle accident or from an assault, such as a gunshot or knife wound, or in some cases a laceration as a complication of percutaneous dilation tracheostomy (PDT) or other endotracheal tubes. In some cases, an inhaled foreign object may become lodged in the trachea and eventually erode the tissue. If the injury is severe, respiratory failure may cause death in a very short period of time, so rapid diagnosis and treatment is critical.

**Symptoms** include:

- Severe respiratory distress
- Hemoptysis
- Strider with progressive dysphonia
- Pneumothorax, pneumomediastinum
- Subcutaneous emphysema from air leaking from the pleural space into the tissues of the chest wall, neck, face, and even into the upper extremities

**Treatment** includes:

- Intubation and non-surgical healing for small lacerations
- Surgical repair for larger wounds or severe respiratory distress

### *PULMONARY CONTUSION*

Pulmonary contusion is the result of direct force to the lung, resulting in parenchymal injury, bleeding, and edema that impact the capillary-alveoli juncture, resulting in intrapulmonary shunting as the alveoli and interstitium fill with fluid. Parenchymal injury reduces compliance and impairs ventilation. **Diagnosis** may be more difficult if other injuries, such as fractured ribs or pneumothorax, are also present because they may all contribute to respiratory distress. CT scans provide the best diagnostic tool.

**Symptoms** vary widely depending upon the degree of injury:

- Mild dyspnea
- Severe progressive dyspnea
- Hemoptysis
- Acute respiratory failure

**Treatment** varies according to the injury:

- Close monitoring of arterial blood gases and respiratory status
- Supplemental oxygen
- Intubation and mechanical ventilation with positive-end expiratory pressure (PEEP) for more severe respiratory distress
- Fluid management and diuretics to control pulmonary edema
- Respiratory physiotherapy to clear secretions

### *FRACTURED RIBS*

Fractured ribs are usually the result of severe trauma, such as blunt force from a motor vehicle accident or physical abuse. Underlying injuries should be expected according to the area of fractures:

- Upper 2 ribs: Injuries to trachea, bronchi, or great vessels
- Right-sided ≥ rib 8: Trauma to liver
- Left-sided ≥ rib 8: Trauma to spleen

Pain, often localized or experienced on respirations or compression of chest way may be the primary symptom of rib fractures, resulting in shallow breathing that can lead to atelectasis or pneumonia.

**Diagnosis**: Chest x-ray or CT scan.

**Treatment** is primarily supportive as rib fractures usually heal in about 6 weeks: however, preventing pulmonary complications (pneumothorax, hemothorax) often necessitates adequate pain control. Underlying injuries are treated according to the type and degree of injury:

- Supplemental oxygen
- Analgesia may include NSAIDs, intercostal nerve blocks, and narcotics
- Pulmonary physiotherapy
- Rib belts
- Surgical fixation (ORIF) only in those requiring thoracotomy for underlying injuries
- Splinting

### *Flail Chest*

Flail chest is a more common injury in adults and older teens than children. It occurs when at least 3 adjacent ribs are fractured, both anteriorly and posteriorly, so that they float free of the rib cage. There may be variations, such as the sternum floating with ribs fractured on both sides. Flail chest results in a failure of the chest wall to support changes in intrathoracic pressure so that paradoxical respirations occur with the flail area contracting on inspiration and expanding on expiration. The lungs are not able to expand properly, decreasing ventilation, but the degree of respiratory distress may relate to injury to underlying structures more than the flail chest alone. **Treatment**:

- Initial stabilization with tape, one side only, don't wrap chest
- Give analgesia for pain relief
- Respiratory physiotherapy is done to prevent atelectasis
- Mechanical ventilation is usually not indicated unless needed for underlying injuries
- Surgical fixation is usually done only in those who require thoracotomy for underlying injuries

### *Hemothorax*

Hemothorax occurs with bleeding into the pleural space, usually from major vascular injury such as tears in intercostal vessels, lacerations of great vessels, or trauma to lung parenchyma. A small bleed may be self-limiting and seal, but a tear in a large vessel can result in massive bleeding, followed quickly by hypovolemic shock. The pressure from the blood may result in the inability of the lung to ventilate and a mediastinal shift. Often a hemothorax occurs with a pneumothorax, especially in severe chest trauma. Further symptoms include severe respiratory distress, decreased breath sounds, and dullness on auscultation.

**Treatment** includes placement of a chest tube to drain the hemothorax, but with large volumes, the pressure may be preventing exsanguination, which can occur abruptly as the blood drains and the pressure is reduced, so a large bore intravenous line should be in place before placement of the chest tube and typed and cross-matched blood immediately available. Autotransfusion may be used, but it is contraindicated if the wound is older than three hours and has the possibility of bowel/stomach contamination, liver failure, and malignancy. Thoracotomy may be indicated after chest tube insertion if there is still hemodynamic instability, tension hemothorax, more than 1500 mL blood initially on insertion, or bleeding continues at a rate of >300 mL/hr.

# Respiratory Procedures and Interventions

## Non-Invasive Ventilation

### *Nasal Cannula*

A nasal cannula can be used to deliver supplemental oxygen to a patient, but it is only useful for flow rates ≤6 L/min as higher rates are drying of the nasal passages. As it is not an airtight system, some ambient air is breathed in as well so oxygen concentration ranges from about 24-44%. The nasal cannula does not allow for control of respiratory rate, so the patient must be able to breathe independently.

### *Non-Rebreather Mask*

A non-rebreather mask can be used to deliver higher concentrations (60-90%) of oxygen to those patients who are able to breathe independently. The mask fits over the nose and mouth and is secured by an elastic strap. A 1.5 L reservoir bag is attached and connects to an oxygen source. The bag is inflated to about 1 liter at a rate of 8-15 L/min before the mask is applied as the patient breathes from this reservoir. A one-way exhalation valve prevents most exhaled air from being rebreathed.

### *Non-Invasive Positive Pressure Ventilators*

Non-invasive positive pressure ventilators provide air through a tight-fitting nasal or face mask, usually pressure cycled, avoiding the need for intubation and reducing the danger of hospital-acquired infection and mortality rates. It can be used for acute respiratory failure and pulmonary edema. There are 2 types of non-invasive positive pressure ventilators:

- **CPAP (Continuous positive airway pressure)** provides a steady stream of pressurized air throughout both inspiration and expiration. CPAP improves breathing by decreasing preload for patients with congestive heart failure. It reduces the effort required for breathing by increasing residual volume and improving gas exchange.
- **Bi-PAP (Bi-level positive airway pressure)** provides a steady stream of pressurized air as CPAP but it senses inspiratory effort and increases pressure during inspiration. Bi-PAP pressures for inspiration and expiration can be set independently. Machines can be programmed with a backup rate to ensure a set number of respirations per minute.

**NEVER place a patient in wrist restraints while wearing these devices. If the patient vomits, they need to be able to remove the mask to prevent aspiration.*

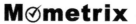

### *Face Mask*

Ensuring that a face mask (Ambu bag) is the correct fit and type is important for adequate ventilation, oxygenation, and prevention of aspiration. Difficulties in management of face mask ventilation relate to risk factors: >55 years, obesity, beard, edentulous, and history of snoring. In some cases, if dentures are adhered well, they may be left in place during induction. The face mask is applied by lifting the mandible (jaw thrust) to the mask and avoiding pressure on soft tissue. Oral or nasal airways may be used, ensuring that the distal end is at the angle of the mandible. There are a number of steps to prevent mask airway leaks:

- Increasing or decreasing the amount of air to the mask to allow better seal
- Securing the mask with both hands while another person ventilates
- Accommodating a large nose by using the mask upside down
- Utilizing a laryngeal mask airway if excessive beard prevents seal

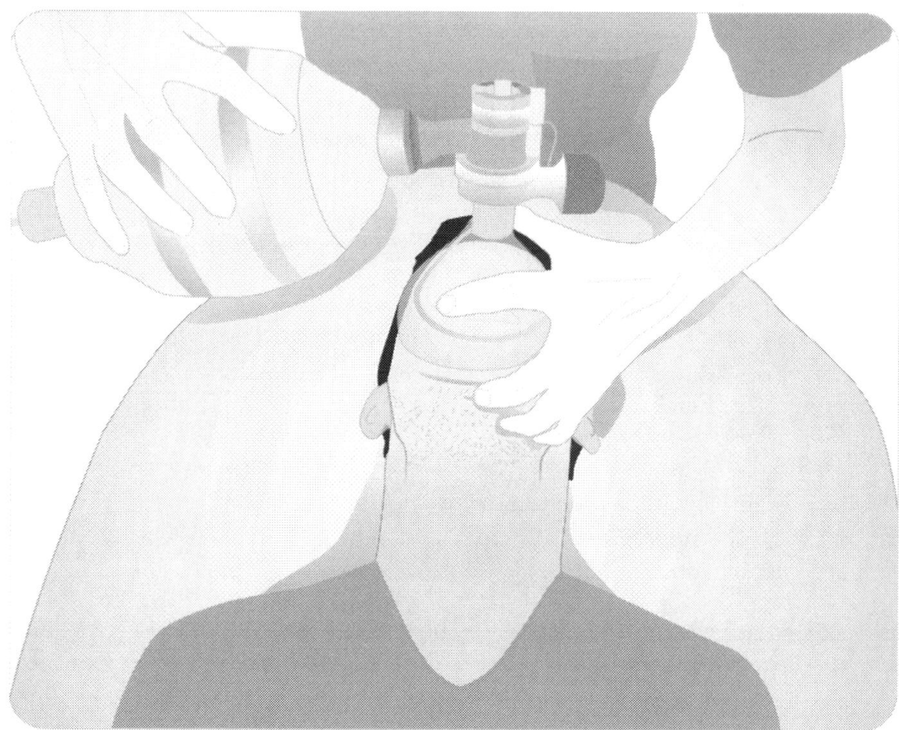

### *High and Low Flow Oxygen Delivery*

**High flow** oxygen delivery devices provide oxygen at flow rates higher than the patient's inspiratory flow rate at specific medium to high $FiO_2$, up to 100%. However, a flow of 100% oxygen actually provides only 60-80% $FiO_2$ to the patient because the patient also breathes in some room air, diluting the oxygen. The actual amount of oxygen received depends on the type of interface or mask. Additionally, the flow rate is actually less than the inspiratory flow rate upon actual delivery. High flow oxygen delivery is usually not used in the sleep center. Humidification is usually required because the high flow is drying.

**Low flow** oxygen delivery devices provide 100% oxygen at flow rates lower than the patient's inspiratory flow rate, but the oxygen mixes with room air, so the $FiO_2$ varies. Humidification is usually only required if flow rate is >3L/min. Much oxygen is wasted with exhalation, so a number of different devices to conserve oxygen are available. Interfaces include transtracheal catheters and cannulae with reservoirs.

## Airway Devices

### Oropharyngeal, Nasopharyngeal, and Tracheostomy Tubes

**Airways** are used to establish a patent airway and facilitate respirations:

- **Oropharyngeal**: This plastic airway curves over the tongue and creates space between the mouth and the posterior pharynx. It is used for anesthetized or unconscious patients to keep tongue and epiglottis from blocking the airway.
- **Nasopharyngeal** (trumpet): This smaller flexible airway is more commonly used in conscious patients and is inserted through one nostril, extending to the nasopharynx. It is commonly utilized in patients who need frequent suctioning.
- **Tracheostomy tubes**: Tracheostomy may be utilized for mechanical ventilation. Tubes are inserted into the opening in the trachea to provide a conduit and maintain the opening. The tube is secured with ties around the neck. Because the air entering the lungs through the tracheostomy bypasses the warming and moistening effects of the upper airway, air is humidified through a room humidifier or through the delivery of humidified air through a special mask or mechanical ventilation. If the tracheostomy is going to be long-term, eventually a stoma will form at the site, and the tube can be removed.

### Laryngeal Mask Airway

The laryngeal-mask airway (LMA) is an intermediate airway allowing ventilation but not complete respiratory control. The LMA consists of an inflatable cuff (the mask) with a connecting tube. It may be used temporarily before tracheal intubation or when tracheal intubation can't be done. It can also be a conduit for later blind insertion of an endotracheal tube. The head and neck must be in neutral position for insertion of the LMA. If the patient has a gag reflex, conscious sedation or topical anesthesia (deep oropharyngeal) is required. The LMA is inserted by sliding along the hard palate, using the finger as a guide, into the pharynx, and the ring is inflated to create a seal about the opening to the larynx, allowing ventilation with mild positive-pressure. The ProSeal LMA has a modified cuff that extends onto the back of the mask to improve seal. LMA is contraindicated in morbid obesity, obstructions or abnormalities of oropharynx, and non-fasting patients, as some aspiration is possible even with the cuff seal inflated.

### Esophageal-Tracheal Combitube

The esophageal tracheal Combitube (ETC) is an intermediate airway that contains two lumens and can be inserted into either the trachea or the esophagus (≤91%). The twin-lumen tube has a proximal cuff providing a seal of the oropharynx and a distal cuff providing a seal about the distal tube. Prior to insertion, the Combitube cuffs should be checked for leaks (15 mL of air into distal and 85 mL of air into proximal). The patient should be non-responsive and with absent gag reflex with head in neutral position. The tube is passed along the tongue and into the pharynx, utilizing markings on the tube (black guidelines) to determine depth by aligning the ETC with the upper incisors or alveolar ridge. Once in place the distal cuff is inflated (10-15 mL) and then placement in the trachea or esophagus should be determined, so the proper lumen for ventilation can be used. The proximal cuff is inflated (usually to 50-75 mL) and ventilation begun. A capnogram should be used to confirm ventilation.

## MECHANICAL VENTILATION

### ENDOTRACHEAL INTUBATION

Endotracheal intubation is often necessary with respiratory failure for control of hypoxemia, hypercapnia, hypoventilation, and/or obstructed airway. Equipment should be assembled and tubes and connections checked for air leaks with a 10 mL syringe. The mouth and/or nose should be cleaned of secretions and suctioned if necessary. The patient should be supine with the patient's head level with the lower sternum of the clinician. With orotracheal/endotracheal intubation, the clinician holds the laryngoscope (in left hand) and inserts it into right corner of mouth, the epiglottis is lifted and the larynx exposed. A thin flexible intubation stylet may be used and the endotracheal tube (ETT) (in right hand) is inserted through the vocal cords and into the trachea, cuff inflated to minimal air leak (10 mL initially until patient stabilizes), and placement confirmed through capnometry or esophageal detection devices. The correct depth of insertion is verified: 21 cm (female), 23 cm (male). After insertion, the tube is secured.

**Review Video: Mechanical Ventilation**
Visit mometrix.com/academy and enter code: 679637

### RAPID SEQUENCE INTUBATION (RSI)

Rapid sequence intubation (RSI) is the simultaneous giving of a sedative and a paralytic in order to facilitate emergency intubation and is considered to be the standard of care for emergency airway management (except in patients with anticipated difficult intubation or in those with contraindications to sedatives/paralytics).

Initial preparation includes inserting 2 IV lines and establishing cardiac monitoring, oximetry, and capnography. The patient should be preoxygenated (100%) for at least 3 minutes, but without pressure ventilation that may cause aspiration of stomach contents. Procedure includes:

- **Induction agent**: Thiopental, ketamine, etomidate, propofol
- **Paralysis**: Succinylcholine, rocuronium, other NMBAs
- **Sellick's maneuver** (pressure applied externally with thumb and index finger to cricoid) to close off the esophagus and prevent aspiration
- **Suction** to clear mouth if necessary
- **Laryngoscopy** to visual vocal cords
- **EET** inserted, cuff inflated, and ETT secured

Proper placement verified by capnometer or capnograph. Breath sounds should be auscultated. Post intubation chest x-ray to assess depth of tube and check for any trauma or issue. Induction agents and use of additional sedation may vary from one institution to another, but the primary goal is to safely anesthetize and intubate while preventing regurgitation of stomach contents.

### CONFIRMING CORRECT PLACEMENT OF ENDOTRACHEAL TUBES

There are a number of methods to **confirm correct placement** of endotracheal tubes. Clinical assessment alone is not adequate.

- **Capnometry** utilizes an end-tidal $CO_2$ ($ETCO_2$) detector that measures the concentration of $CO_2$ in expired air, usually through pH sensitive paper that changes color (commonly purple to yellow). The capnometer is attached to the ETT and a bag-valve-mask (BVM) ventilator is also attached. The patient is provided 6 ventilations and the $CO_2$ concentration is checked.
- **Capnography** is attached to the ETT and provides a waveform graph, showing the varying concentrations of $CO_2$ in real time throughout each ventilation (with increased $CO_2$ on expiration) and can indicate changes in respiratory status.

- **Esophageal detection devices** fit over the end of the ETT so that a large syringe can be used to attempt to aspirate. If the ETT is in the esophagus, the walls collapse on aspiration and resistance occurs, whereas the syringe fills with air if the ETT is in the trachea. A self-inflating bulb (Ellik device) may also be used.
- **Chest x-ray** provides visual confirmation of placement.

### *Ventilator Management*

There are many types of ventilators now in use, and the specific directions for each type must be followed carefully, but there are general principles that apply to all **ventilator management**. The following should be monitored:

- **Type of ventilation:** Volume-cycled, pressure-cycled, negative-pressure, HFJV, HFOV, CPAP, Bi-PAP
- **Control mode**: Controlled ventilation, assisted ventilation, synchronized intermittent mandatory (allows spontaneous breaths between ventilator-controlled inhalation/exhalation), positive end-expiratory pressure (PEEP), CPAP, Bi-PAP
- **Tidal volume** (TV) range should be set in relation to respiratory rate
- **Inspiratory-expiratory ratio** (I:E) usually ranges from 1:2-1:5, but may vary
- **Respiratory rate** will depend upon TV and $PaCO_2$ target
- **Fraction of inspired oxygen** ($FiO_2$) [percentage of oxygen in the inspired air], usually ranging from 21-100%, usually maintained <40% to avoid toxicity
- **Sensitivity** determines the effort needed to trigger inspiration
- **Pressure** controls the pressure exerted in delivering TV
- **Rate of flow** controls the L/min speed of TV

### *High Frequency Jet Ventilation*

High frequency jet ventilation (HFJV) (Life Pulse) directs a high velocity stream of air into the lungs in a long spiraling spike that forces carbon dioxide against the walls, penetrating dead space and providing gas exchange by using small tidal volumes of 1-3 mL/kg, much smaller than with conventional mechanical ventilation. Because the jet stream technology is effective for short distances, the valve and pressure transducer must be placed by the person's head. Inhalation is controlled while expiration is passive, but the rate of respiration is up to 11 per second ("panting" respirations). HFJV may be used in conjunction with low-pressure conventional ventilation to increase flow to alveoli. HFJV reduces barotrauma because of the low tidal volume and low pressure. HFJV is used for numerous conditions, including evolving chronic lung disease, pulmonary interstitial emphysema, bronchopulmonary dysplasia, and hypoxemic respiratory failure. It reduces mean airway pressure (MAP) and the oxygenation index. Treatment with HFJV may reduce the need for ECMO.

### *High Frequency Oscillatory Ventilation*

High frequency oscillatory ventilation (HFOV) provides pressurized ventilation with tidal volumes approximately equal to dead space at about 150 breaths per minutes (BPM). Pressure is usually higher with HFOV than HFJV in order to maintain expansion of the alveoli and to keep the airway open during gas exchange. Oxygenation is regulated separately. HFOV has both an active inspiration and expiration, so the respiratory cycle is completely controlled. HFOV reduces pulmonary vascular resistance and improves ventilation-perfusion matching and oxygenation without injuring the lung, reducing the risk of barotrauma. HFOV is used for respiratory distress syndrome, persistent pulmonary hypertension, more commonly for infants and children, but there is increasing interest in using HFOV with adults because of the smaller tidal volume that prevents overinflation of the lungs and atelectasis of those with ARDS.

### *Positive Pressure Ventilators*

Positive pressure ventilators assist respiration by applying pressure directly to the airway, inflating the lungs, forcing expansion of the alveoli, and facilitating gas exchange. Generally, endotracheal intubation or tracheostomy is necessary to maintain positive pressure ventilation for extended periods. There are 3 basic kinds of positive pressure ventilators:

- **Pressure cycled:** This type of ventilation is usually used for short-term treatment in adolescents or adults. The IPPB machine is the most common type. This delivers a flow of air to a preset pressure and then cycles off. Airway resistance or changes in compliance can affect volume of air and may compromise ventilation.
- **Time cycled**: This type of ventilation regulates the volume of air the patient receives by controlling the length of inspiration and the flow rate.
- **Volume cycled**: This type of ventilation provides a preset flow of pressurized air during inspiration and then cycles off and allows passive expiration, providing a fairly consistent volume of air.

### *Tracheostomy*

Tracheostomy, surgical tracheal opening, may be utilized for mechanical ventilation. Tracheostomy tubes are inserted directly into an opening in the trachea to provide a conduit and maintain the opening. Tracheostomy tubes are usually silastic or plastic, and may have permanent of disposable inner cannulas. The tube is secured with ties around the neck. Because the air entering the lungs through the tracheostomy bypasses the warming and moistening effects of the upper airway, air is humidified through a room humidifier or through delivery of humidified air through a special mask or mechanical ventilation. The patient with a tracheostomy must have continuous monitoring of vital signs and respiratory status to ensure patency of tracheostomy. The inner cannula should be cleaned/replaced regularly (every 8-24 hours and PRN). Regular suctioning is needed, especially initially, to remove secretions:

- Suction catheter should be 50% the size of the tracheostomy tube to allow ventilation during suctioning
- Vacuum pressure: 80-100 mmHg
- Catheter should only be inserted ≤0.5 cm beyond tube to avoid damage to tissues or perforation
- Catheter should be inserted without suction and intermittent suction on withdrawal

### *Ventilation-Induced Lung Injury*

Ventilation-induced lung injury (VILI) is damage caused by mechanical ventilation. It is common in acute distress syndrome (ARDS) but can affect any mechanically ventilated patient. VILI comprises four interrelated elements:

- **Barotrauma**: Damage to the lung caused by excessive pressure
- **Volutrauma**: Alveolar damage related to high tidal volume ventilation
- **Atelectotrauma**: Injury caused by repetitive forced opening and closing of alveoli
- **Biotrauma**: Inflammatory response

In VILI, essentially the increased pressure and tidal volume over-distends the alveoli, which rupture, and air moves into the interstitial tissue resulting in pulmonary interstitial emphysema. With continued ventilation, the air in the interstitium moves into the subcutaneous tissue and may result in pneumopericardium and pneumomediastinum, or rupture the pleural sac which can cause tension pneumothorax and mediastinal shift, which can cause respiratory failure and cardiac arrest. VILI has caused a change in ventilation procedures with lower tidal volumes and pressures used as well as newer forms of ventilation, HFJV and HFOV, preferred to traditional mechanical ventilation for many patients.

### *Preventing Complications from Ventilators*

Methods to prevent complications from mechanical ventilation ("ventilator bundle") include:

- Elevate patient's head and chest to 30° to prevent aspiration and ventilation-associated pneumonia.
- Reposition patient every 2 hours.

- Provide DVT prophylaxis, such as external compression support and/or heparin (5000 u sq 2-3 times daily).
- Administer famotidine or pantoprazole PO/IV daily to prevent gastrointestinal stress-ulcers/bleeding.
- Decrease and eliminate sedation/analgesia as soon as possible—regular sedation vacations to assess neurological status.
- Follow careful protocols for pressure settings to prevent barotrauma. Tidal volumes are usually maintained at 8-12 mL/kg PBW (per AACN guidelines), but in incidences of high probability of ARDS, volumes should be less (6 mL/kg) to avoid lung injury.
- Monitor for pneumothorax or evidence of barotrauma.
- Conduct nutritional assessment (including lab tests) to prevent malnutrition.
- Monitor intake and output carefully and administer IV fluids to prevent dehydration.
- Do daily spontaneous breathing trials and discontinue ventilation as soon as possible.

### *Ventilator Weaning*

Ventilator weaning has three phases: Changing settings of the ventilator to allow the patient to demonstrate the ability to breath on their own (standby mode), extubation, and finally removal of supportive oxygen. Criteria for ventilator weaning include:

- Vital capacity 10-15 mL/kg
- Maximum (negative) inspiratory pressure of at least -20 $cmH_2O$
- Tidal volume (TV) of 7-9 mL/kg
- Minute ventilation of about 6L/min (Respiratory rate x TV)
- Rapid shallow breathing index <100 breaths/min/L
- $PaO_2$ >60 mmHg
- $FiO_2$ <40%

If these criteria are met and the patient passes a spontaneous breathing trial (SBT), then extubation can be done. Various protocols are followed in weaning patients off of ventilators, including the use of intermittent mandatory ventilation (IMV) and synchronized intermittent mandatory ventilation (SIMV), which can be used with pressure support ventilation (PSV).

**Criteria for oxygen weaning**:

- $FiO_2$ reduced until $PaO_2$ 70-100 mmHg on room air
- Supplemental $O_2$ necessary with $PaO_2$<70 mmHg (Medicare requires $PaO_2$ 55 mmHg for reimbursement for home oxygen use)

### *Spontaneous Breathing Trial as Preparation for Extubation*

A spontaneous breathing trial (SBT) is when a patient is taken off mechanical ventilation while remaining intubated (usually by changing the ventilator settings to CPAP) for a short period of time to assess readiness to extubate. SBT should be used prior to extubating a patient if the patient is not agitated and has no evidence of myocardial ischemia or increased ICP. The patient should exhibit some spontaneous triggering of respirations and should not be receiving large doses of vasopressor or inotropic agent. $SpO_2$ should be ≥88% with $FiO_2$ of 0.50 and PEEP at 7.5 $cmH_2O$ prior to the SBT. The SBT should be done in the morning for a prescribed period (usually 30-120 minutes). The ventilator rate is adjusted to 0 and pressure support decreased to 0–7. The SBT should be discontinued if the following occur:

- Respiratory rate >35 or <8 for at least 5 minutes
- Mental status changes
- $SpO_2$ <88% for >15 minutes
- Respiratory distress (HR >130 BPM or <60 BPM, marked dyspnea, diaphoresis, increased use of accessory respiratory muscles, respiratory arrest)

Patients who pass the SBT have an 85-90% chance of breathing successfully after extubation. Patients who repeatedly fail daily SBT may require tracheostomy.

### *Failure to Wean from Mechanical Ventilation*

Failure to wean from mechanical ventilation can occur in approximately 20-30% of ventilated patients. Many factors affect a patient's ability to wean from mechanical ventilation including physical, psychological, and situational factors. Before discontinuation of ventilation can be considered, the patient must be able to protect his/her airway, be hemodynamically stable and have resolution of the clinical problem that initiated the need for mechanical ventilation. Weaning protocols use clinical criteria such as oxygen saturation, blood pressure, respiratory rate, and tidal volume to determine the patient's tolerance of lessening mechanical ventilator support. Failure to wean is demonstrated by multiple daily spontaneous breathing trial failures or the need for reintubation within 48 hours of extubation. Failure to resolve the clinical problem(s) that initiated mechanical ventilation, insufficient ventilator drive, respiratory muscle weakness, co-morbidities, and/or the development of new clinical problems (e.g., infection) may contribute to the inability to wean.

**Signs and symptoms**: Decreased tidal volume, increased respiratory rate, increased $PaCO_2$, oxygen desaturation, anxiety, diaphoresis, fatigue, changes in blood pressure or heart rate, mental status changes, and hemodynamic changes.

**Treatment**: The initial treatment strategy for patients who experience a dysfunctional ventilator weaning response is identification and treatment of the underlying cause(s) of the weaning failure. In addition, other treatment strategies may include psychological preparation of the patient for further weaning attempts, readiness testing and respiratory muscle training.

## Sedation/Analgesia with Mechanical Ventilation

Patients intubated for mechanical ventilation are usually given **sedation and/or analgesia** initially, but medications should be reduced and given in boluses rather than with continuous IV drip with a goal of stopping sedation as it prolongs ventilation time. Typical sedatives include midazolam, propofol, and lorazepam. Narcotic analgesics include fentanyl and morphine sulfate. Uses of sedation include:

- Controlling agitation and excessive movement that may interfere with ventilation
- Reduce pain and discomfort associated with ventilation
- Control respiratory distress

Triglyceride levels must be checked periodically if propofol is administered for more than 24–48 hours. Neuromuscular blocking agents are rarely used because they may cause long-term weakness and increase length of ventilation although they may be indicated in some cases, such as with excessive shivering or cardiac arrest. Many patients are able to tolerate mechanical ventilation without sedation, and sedation should always be decreased to the minimal amount necessary as excess sedation may delay extubation. An ideal level of sedation will keep the patient calm and compliant with the ventilator but still alert and able to follow commands.

### *Conscious Sedation*

Conscious sedation is used to decrease sensations of pain and awareness caused by a surgical or invasive procedure, such a biopsy, chest tube insertion, fracture repair, and endoscopy. It is also used during presurgical preparations, such as insertion of central lines, catheters, and use of cooling blankets. Conscious sedation uses a combination of analgesia and sedation so that patients can remain responsive and follow verbal cues but have a brief amnesia preventing recall of the procedures. The patient must be monitored carefully, including pulse oximetry, during this type of sedation. The most commonly used drugs include:

- Midazolam (Versed): This is a short-acting water-soluble sedative, with onset of 1-5 minutes, peaking in 30, and duration usually about 1 hour (up to 6 hours).
- Fentanyl: This is a short-acting opioid with immediate onset, peaking in 10-15 minutes and with a duration of about 20-45 minutes. Monitor respiratory function.

The fentanyl/midazolam combination provides both sedation and pain control. Conscious sedation usually requires 6 hours fasting prior to administration.

### *Therapeutic Gases*

**Carbon dioxide** is a potent stimulator of respirations, but it is rarely used therapeutically because it can depress respirations if hypercarbia or respiratory acidosis is present. $CO_2$ may be administered at times as part of anesthesia, but it is most commonly used for insufflation for laparoscopic/endoscopic procedures.

**Nitric oxide** (NO) is used as a pulmonary vessel dilator to improve oxygenation by decreasing pulmonary artery pressure and pulmonary vascular resistance. NO is FDA-approved for use for neonatal PPH but is sometimes used for adults, although studies have not shown it an effective treatment for ARDS. NO should be delivered at 0.1-50 ppm to avoid toxicity that can occur over 50 ppm. Toxic reactions include methemoglobinemia and platelet inhibition with resultant bleeding.

**Heliox** is helium mixed with oxygen that is used to reduce airway resistance during mechanical ventilation and for pulmonary function tests. Heliox may also be used to treat respiratory obstruction and is used during laser surgery on the airway because it readily conducts heat away from the surgical site, reducing tissue damage. Heliox is sometimes used for COPD patients as it increases hyperventilation and reduces carbon dioxide levels.

## Thoracentesis

A thoracentesis (aspiration of fluid or air from pleural space) is done to make a diagnosis, relieve pressure on the lung caused by pleural effusion, or instill medications. A chest x-ray is done prior to the procedure. A sedative may be given. The patient is in a sitting position, leaning onto a padded bedside stand, straddling a chair with head supported on the back of the chair, or lying on the opposite side with the head of the bed elevated 30-45° to ensure that fluid remains at the base. The patient should avoid coughing or moving during the procedure. The chest x-ray or ultrasound determines needle placement. After a local anesthetic is administered, a needle (with an attached 20-mL syringe and 3-way stopcock with tubing and a receptacle) is advanced intercostally into the pleural space. Fluid is drained, collected, examined, and measured. The needle is removed and a pressure dressing applied. A chest x-ray is done to ensure there is no pneumothorax. The patient is monitored for cough, dyspnea, and hypoxemia.

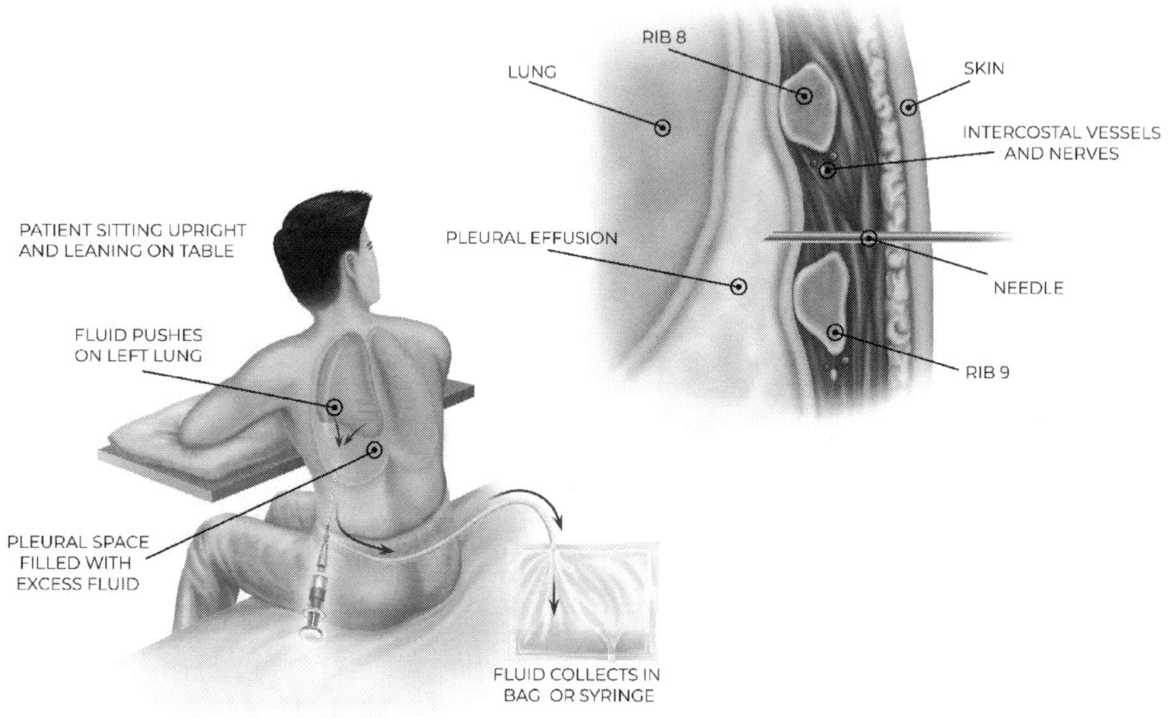

## Bronchoscopy

Bronchoscopy utilizes a thin, flexible fiberoptic bronchoscope to inspect the larynx, trachea, and bronchi for diagnostic purposes. It is also used to collect specimens, obtain biopsies, remove foreign bodies or secretions, treat atelectasis, and to excise lesions. The patient is in supine position during the procedure. The Mallampati classification may be used to determine difficulty of airway. The patient receives local anesthesia to the nares (lidocaine gel) and oropharynx (lidocaine gel, spray, or nebulizer), and usually receives a benzodiazepine (commonly midazolam or lorazepam), an opioid (fentanyl or meperidine), or propofol. Medications are usually given in small incremental doses throughout the procedure and may be combined. Over-sedation may cause physiologic depression, but undersedation may result in recall and agitation with sympathetic activation. The tube is advanced through the nares and down the trachea to the bronchi. Airway patency, respiratory rate, and oxygen saturation must be constantly monitored. Complications can include bleeding, arrhythmias, obstruction, laryngospasm, and respiratory failure.

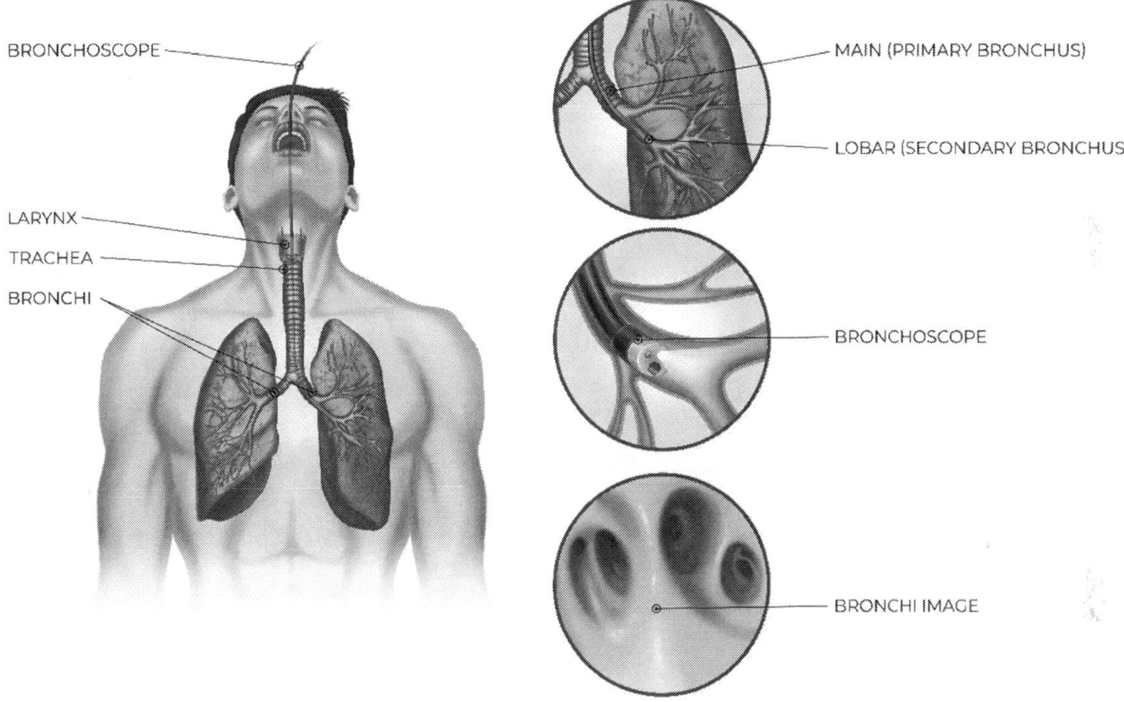


## Chest Tubes

Chest tubes with a closed drainage system are usually left in place after thoracic surgery or pneumothorax to drain air or fluid. Nursing interventions during insertion include ensuring the patient receives adequate pain control, attending to sterile technique, assisting the physician with suturing as needed, attaching the tube to the chest tube drainage device, placing an occlusive dressing, and confirming placement.

Chest tube drainage systems have three major parts: suction control, water seal, and a chamber for collection. The system should have no bubbling in the water seal area (such would indicate a leak), but a subtle rise and fall of the water seal corresponding with respirations, and gentle bubbling in the suction control chamber.

Nursing interventions after chest tube is in place: in most circumstances, report drainage >100 mL/hr, assess tubing after position changes for occlusion, maintain sterile dressing, avoid stripping the tubing, and assessing the insertion site for drainage or crepitus, the tubing, the patency of the entire system, and the output (including color, amount, and any other traits). The nurse should be knowledgeable about specimen collection, replacing the system, and dealing with clots.

**Review Video: Chest Tubes**
Visit mometrix.com/academy and enter code: 696975

## Thoracic Surgery

### *Lung Volume Reduction*

Lung volume reduction surgery (LVRS) usually involves removing about 20-35% of lung tissue that is not functioning adequately in order to reduce the lung size so that the lungs work more effectively. This procedure is most commonly used with adult emphysematous COPD patients. In adults, surgery is usually bilateral; however, some patients are not candidates for bilateral surgery because of cardiac disease or emphysema affecting only one lung. Unilateral surgery has been shown to be effective. Surgical removal of part of the lung improves ventilation and gas exchange and does not require the immunosuppressant therapy required for lung transplantation. Studies have shown that those with low risk for the surgery and with emphysematous changes in the upper lobes can benefit from the surgery, but high-risk patients with more widespread emphysematous changes have increased mortality rates. The surgery may be done through an open-chest thoracotomy or through a less invasive video-assisted thoracotomy.

### *Pneumonectomy*

Pneumonectomy is the surgical removal of one of the lungs. There are 2 surgical procedures:

- **Simple**: removal of just the lung
- **Extrapleural**: removal not only of the lung but also part of the diaphragm on the affected side and the pericardium on that same side

During the operative procedure, much care must be taken to prevent contamination of the remaining lung, including the use of bronchus blockers or prone position during surgery.

Removal of the lung is indicated for a number of conditions, including:

- Cancerous lesions (the most common reason for surgery)
- Severe bronchiectasis from chronic suppurative pneumonia, resulting in dilation of terminal bronchioles
- Severe hypoplasia
- Unilateral lung destruction with pulmonary hypertension
- Pulmonary hemorrhage
- Lobar emphysema
- Chronic pulmonary infections with destruction of lung tissue

Because the lung capacity is reduced, persistent shortness of breath may occur with exertion even many months after surgery.

### *Lobectomy and Other Procedures to Remove Partial Lung Tissue*

Lobectomy removes one or more lobes of a lung (which has 2 on the left and 3 on the right) and is usually done for lesions or trauma that is confined to one lobe, such as tubercular lesions, abscesses or cysts, cancer (usually non-small cell in early stages), traumatic injury, or bronchiectasis. Surgery is usually done through an open thoracotomy or video-assisted thoracotomy. Complications can include hemorrhage, post-operative infection with or without abscess formation, and pneumothorax. Usually, 1-2 chest tubes are left in place in the immediate post-surgical period to remove air and/or fluid.

- **Segmental resection** removes a bronchovascular segment and is used for small lesions in the periphery, bronchiectasis or congenital cysts or blebs.
- **Wedge resection** removes a small wedged-shape portion of the lung tissue and is used for small peripheral lesions, granulomas, or blebs.
- **Bronchoplastic (sleeve) reconstruction** removes part of bronchus and lung tissue with reanastomosis of bronchus and is used for small lesions of the carina or bronchus.

# Respiratory Pharmacology

## Pharmacological Agents Used for Asthma

Numerous pharmacological agents are used for control of asthma, some that are long-acting to prevent attacks and others that are short-acting to provide relief for acute episodes. Listed with each are the standard med and dosage used for urgent care:

- **β-Adrenergic agonists** include both long-acting and short-acting preparations used for relaxation of smooth muscles and bronchodilation, reducing edema, and aiding clearance of mucus. Medications include salmeterol (Serevent), sustained-release albuterol (Volmax ER) and short-acting albuterol (Proventil), and levalbuterol (Xopenex). Albuterol 2.5-5.0 mg every 20 minutes, 3 doses by nebulizer.
- **Anticholinergics** aid in preventing bronchial constriction and potentiate the bronchodilating action of β-Adrenergic agonists. The most commonly used medication is ipratropium bromide (Atrovent) 500 mcg every 20 minutes, 3 doses by nebulizer.
- **Corticosteroids** provide anti-inflammatory action by inhibiting immune responses and decreasing edema, mucus, and hyper-responsiveness. Because of numerous side effects, glucocorticosteroids are usually administered orally or parenterally for ≤5 days (prednisone, prednisolone, methylprednisolone) and then switched to inhaled steroids. If a person receives glucocorticoids for more than 5 days, then dosages are tapered. Methylprednisolone 60-125 mg IV is the standard dose for respiratory failure. The Global Initiative for Asthma (GINA) recommends daily inhaled corticosteroids for all individuals with severe asthma to reduce the risk of exacerbations.
- **Methylxanthines** are used to improve pulmonary function and decrease the need for mechanical ventilation. Medications include aminophylline and theophylline.
- **Magnesium sulfate** is used to relax smooth muscles and decrease inflammation. If administered intravenously, it must be given slowly to prevent hypotension and bradycardia. When inhaled, it potentiates the action of albuterol. Standard dosage: 2 g (8 mmol), 1 dose by IV over 20 minutes.
- **Heliox** (helium-oxygen) is administered to decrease airway resistance with airway obstruction, thereby decreasing respiratory effort. Heliox improves oxygenation of those on mechanical ventilation.
- **Leukotriene inhibitors** are used to inhibit inflammation and bronchospasm for long-term management. Medications include montelukast (Singulair).

## Additional Pulmonary Pharmacology

There is a wide range of agents used for pulmonary pharmacology, depending upon the type and degree of pulmonary disease. Agents include:

- **Opioid analgesics:** Used to provide both pain relief and sedation for those on mechanical ventilation to reduce sympathetic response. Medications may include fentanyl (Sublimaze) or morphine sulfate (MS Contin).
- **Neuromuscular blockers:** Used for induced paralysis of those who have not responded adequately to sedation, especially for intubation and mechanical ventilation. Medications may include pancuronium (Pavulon) and vecuronium (Norcuron). However, there is controversy about the use of such blockers, as induced paralysis has been linked to increased mortality rates, sensory hearing loss (pancuronium), atelectasis, and ventilation-perfusion mismatch.
- **Human B-type natriuretic peptides:** Used to reduce pulmonary capillary wedge pressure. Medications include nesiritide (Natrecor).
- **Surfactants**: Reduces surface tension to prevent the collapse of alveoli. Beractant (Survanta) is derived from bovine lung tissue and calfactant (Infasurf) from calf lung tissue. They are administered as inhalants.
- **Alkalinizers**: Used to treat metabolic acidosis and reduce pulmonary vascular resistance by achieving an alkaline pH. Medications include sodium bicarbonate and tromethamine (THAM).

- **Pulmonary vasodilator (inhaled nitric oxide):** Used to relax the vascular muscles and produce pulmonary vasodilation. Some studies show it reduces the need for extracorporeal membrane oxygenation (ECMO).
- **Methylxanthines:** Used to stimulate muscle contractions of the chest and stimulate respirations. Medications include aminophylline (Aminophylline), caffeine citrate (Cafcit), and doxapram (Dopram).
- **Diuretics**: Used to reduce pulmonary edema. Medications include loop diuretics such as furosemide (Lasix) and metolazone (Mykrox).
- **Nitrates**: Used for vasodilation to reduce preload and afterload, which in turn reduces myocardial need for oxygen. Medications include nitroglycerin (Nitro-Bid) and nitroprusside sodium (Nitropress).
- **Antibiotics**: Used for treatment of respiratory infections, including pneumonia. Medications are used according to the pathogenic agent and may include macrolides such as azithromycin (Zithromax) and erythromycin (E-Mycin).
- **Antimycobacterials**: Used for treatment of TB and other mycobacterial diseases. Medications include isoniazid (Laniazid, Nydrazid), ethambutol (Myambutol), rifampin (Rifadin), streptomycin sulfate, and pyrazinamide.
- **Antivirals**: Used to inhibit replication of a virus early in a viral infection. Effectiveness decreases as time passes because the replication process has already begun. Medications include ribavirin (Virazole) and zanamivir (Relenza).

# Neurological Emergencies

## Neurological Assessment

### Assessment of the Neurological System

Assessment of the neurological system includes:

- Assess the **health history** for any trauma, falls, alcoholism, drug abuse, medications taken, and family history of neurological problems.
- Ask about any presenting **neurological symptoms**, the circumstances in which they occur, whether they fluctuate, and any associated factors, such as seizures, pain, vertigo, weakness, abnormal sensations, visual problems, loss of consciousness, changes in cognition, and motor problems.

Assessment includes determining the level of consciousness and cognition. Posture and movements are assessed for abnormalities. Facial expression and movement are noted. Cranial nerve assessment is done. The patient is assessed for strength, coordination, and balance and the ability to perform ADLs. One should assess for clonus and test all reflexes, including Babinski, gag, blink, swallow, upper and lower abdominal, cremasteric in males, plantar, perianal, biceps, triceps, brachioradialis, patellar and ankle. Peripheral sensation is tested by touching the patient with cotton balls and the sharp and dull ends of a broken tongue blade.

**Review Video: Nervous System**
Visit mometrix.com/academy and enter code: 708428

### Assessing Functional Status

**Functional abilities** include the acts needed to meet basic needs and perform *activities of daily living* (ADLs), such as eating and elimination, as well as those *activities that are essential to independent living* (IADLs), such as shopping. A thorough assessment of the patient's functional abilities will identify areas that should be concentrated upon during rehabilitation. One should observe the patient as he/she performs these functions and record the following:

- Degree of independence shown
- Ability to complete activity without rest
- Nerve function
- Muscle function and strength
- Motion
- Coordination
- Cardiac status
- Respiratory status
- Assistance required to complete activity

The facility usually provides one of the tools available to record a functional assessment. The most common tool used is the Functional Independence Measure (FIM). Other tools available include the Barthel Index, the PULSES Profile, and the Patient Evaluation Conference System.

## American Stroke Association Classification System for the Extent of Brain Attack Injury

The American Stroke Association developed a **brain attack outcome classification system** to standardize descriptions of stroke injuries:

- **Number of impaired domains** (Potentially affected neurological domains: motor, sensory, vision, language, cognition, and affect): Level 0: no domains impaired; Level 1: one domain impaired; Level 2: two domains impaired; Level 3: greater than 2 domains impaired.
- **Severity of impairment**: A (minimal or no neurological deficit due to stroke); B (mild/moderate deficit); or C (severe deficit). Note: When more than one domain is affected, severity is measured by the domain with the most impairment.

Assessment of function determines the ability to **live independently**:

- **I**: Independent in basic activities of daily living (BADL), such as bathing, eating, toileting, and walking; and instrumental activities of daily living (IADL), such as telephoning, shopping, maintaining a household, socializing, and using transportation
- **II**: Independent in BADL but partially dependent in IADL
- **III**: Partially dependent in BADL (less than 3 areas) and IADL
- **IV**: Partially dependent in BADL (3 or more areas)
- **V**: Completely dependent in BADL (5 or more areas) and IADL

Level III requires much assistance and Levels IV and V cannot live independently.

## Administration of the NIHSS

The **National Institutes of Health Stroke Scale (NIHSS)** is administered with careful attention to directions. The examiner should record the answers and avoid coaching or repeating requests, although demonstration may be used with aphasic patients. The scale comprises 11 sections, with scores for each section ranging from 0 (normal) to 2, 3, or 4:

- **Level of consciousness**: Response to noxious stimulation (0-3), request for month and his/her age (0-2), request to open and close eyes, grip and release unaffected hand (0-2)
- **Best gaze**: Horizontal eye movement (0-2)
- **Visual**: Visual fields (0-3)
- **Facial palsy**: Symmetry when patient shows teeth, raises eyebrows, and closes eyes (0-3)
- **Motor, arm**: Drift while arm extended with palms down (0-4)
- **Motor, leg**: Leg drift at 30 degrees while patient supine (0-4)
- **Limb ataxia**: Finger-nose and heel-shin (0-2)
- **Sensory**: Grimace or withdrawal from pinprick (0-2)
- **Best language**: Describes action of pictures (0-3)
- **Dysarthria**: Reads or describes words on list (0-2)
- **Distinction and inattention**: Visual spatial neglect (0-2)

## Glasgow Coma Scale

The Glasgow coma scale (GCS) measures the depth and duration of coma or impaired level of consciousness and is used for post-operative assessment. The GCS measures three parameters: best eye response, best verbal response, and best motor response, with a total possible score that ranges from 3 to 15:

| | |
|---|---|
| **Eye opening** | 4: Spontaneous<br>3: To verbal stimuli<br>2: To pain (not of face)<br>1: No response |

| | |
|---|---|
| **Verbal** | 5: Oriented<br>4: Conversation confused, but can answer questions<br>3: Uses inappropriate words<br>2: Speech incomprehensible<br>1: No response |
| **Motor** | 6: Moves on command<br>5: Moves purposefully respond pain<br>4: Withdraws in response to pain<br>3: Decorticate posturing (flexion) in response to pain<br>2: Decerebrate posturing (extension) in response to pain<br>1: No response |

Injuries/conditions are classified according to the total score: 3-8 Coma; ≤8 Severe head injury likely requiring intubation; 9-12 Moderate head injury; 13-15 Mild head injury.

**Review Video: Glasgow Coma Scale**
Visit mometrix.com/academy and enter code: 133399

## Cranial Nerves

| | Name | Function | PE Test |
|---|---|---|---|
| I | Olfactory | Smell | Test olfaction |
| II | Optic | Visual acuity | Snellen eye chart; Accommodation |
| III | Oculomotor | Eye movement/ pupil | Pupillary reflex; Eye/eyelid motion |
| IV | Trochlear | Eye movement | Eye moves down & out |
| V | Trigeminal | Facial motor/ sensory | Corneal reflex; Facial sensation; Mastication |
| VI | Abducens | Eye movement | Lateral eye motion |
| VII | Facial | Facial expression; Taste | Moves forehead, closes eyes, smile/frown, puffs cheeks; Taste |
| VIII | Vestibulo-cochlear (Acoustic) | Hearing; Balance | Hearing (Weber/Rinne tests); Nystagmus |
| IX | Glosso-pharyngeal | Pharynx motor/sensory | Gag reflex; Soft palate elevation |
| X | Vagus | Visceral sensory, motor | Gag, swallow, cough |
| XI | Accessory | Sternocleidomastoid and trapezius (motor) | Turns head & shrugs shoulders against resistance |
| XII | Hypoglossal | Tongue movement | Push out tongue; move tongue from side to side |

## ICP and Monroe-Kellie Hypothesis

Increasing **intracranial pressure (ICP)** is a frequent complication of brain injuries, tumors, or other disorders affecting the brain, so monitoring the ICP is very important. Increased ICP can indicate cerebral edema, hemorrhage, and/or obstruction of cerebrospinal fluid. The **Monroe-Kellie hypothesis** states that in order to maintain a normal ICP, a change in volume in one compartment must be compensated by a reciprocal change in volume in another compartment. There are 3 compartments in the brain: the brain tissue, cerebrospinal fluid (CSF), and blood. The CSF and blood can change more easily to accommodate changes in pressure than tissue, so medical intervention focuses on cerebral blood flow and drainage. Normal ICP is 1-15 mmHg on transducer or 13.6–203.9 mmH$_2$O on manometer. As intracranial pressure increases, **symptoms** include:

- Headache
- Alterations in level of consciousness
- Restlessness

- Slowly reacting or nonreacting dilated or pinpoint pupils
- Seizures
- Motor weakness
- Cushing's triad (late sign):
    - Increased systolic pressure with widened pulse pressure
    - Bradycardia in response to increased pressure
    - Decreased respirations

### *ICP Monitoring Devices*

The intracranial pressure (ICP) **monitoring device** may be placed during surgery or a ventriculostomy performed in which a burr hole is drilled into the frontal area of the scalp and an **intraventricular catheter** threaded into the lateral ventricle. The intraventricular catheter may be used to monitor ICP and to drain excess CSF. Other monitoring devices include:

- **Intracranial pressure monitor bolt** (subarachnoid bolt) is applied through a burr hole with the distal end of the monitor probe resting in the subarachnoid space.
- **Epidural monitors** are placed into the epidural space.
- **Fiberoptic monitors** may be placed inside the brain.

The intraventricular catheter is the most accurate. CSF may be drained continuously or intermittently and must be monitored hourly for amount, color, and character. For ICP measurement, the patient's head must be elevated to 30-45° and the transducer leveled to the tragus of the ear or outer canthus of the eye, depending on facility policy.

## Cerebral Blood Flow, MAP, and CPP

**Cerebral blood flow,** or the blood supply to the brain at any given moment, is influenced directly by one's **mean arterial pressure** (MAP). A MAP of greater than 60 mmHg is required to perfuse vital organs, including the brain. A MAP that falls below 60 mmHg risks ischemia and infarction. An excessively high MAP (greater than 100 mmHg) can also cause damage. A high MAP can result in increased oxygen demands by the heart, vascular injury, end organ damage, and stroke.

**Cerebral perfusion pressure** (CPP) is the pressure required to maintain adequate blood flow to the brain. CPP is based on mean arterial pressure (MAP) and intracranial pressure (ICP). Elevated ICP can be associated with a reduction in CPP.

$$\text{CPP} = \text{MAP} - \text{ICP}$$

- Normal CPP: 60-100 mmHg.
- <60 mmHg: Hypoperfusion occurs , resulting in focal or global ischemia.
- <30 mmHg: Hypoperfusion is marked and incompatible with life.
- >100 mmHg: Leads to hypertensive encephalopathy and cerebral edema (particularly if CPP >120 mmHg); Patients with chronic hypertension tolerate a higher level of CPP.

## Neurological Motor Testing and Testing for Nuchal Rigidity

**Neurological motor testing** requires careful observation for involuntary or spastic movements and examination of muscles for lack of symmetry or atrophy with observation of gait. Muscle tone is examined by flexing and extending the upper and lower extremities, observing for flaccid or spastic changes. Muscle strength is examined by having the patient press fingers, wrists, elbows, hips, knees, ankles, and plantar area against resistance, graded 0 (no movement) to 5 (normal).

Pronator drift is an indication of disease of the upper motor neurons. The patient stands with eyes closed and both arms extended horizontally in front with the palms facing upwards (supination). The patient should be told to hold the arms still and not move them while the examiner taps downward on the arm. If motor neuron disease is present, the patient's arms will drift downward and hands will drift toward pronation.

**Nuchal rigidity** is tested by placing the hands behind the patient's head and flexing the neck gently to determine if there is increased resistance.

# Neurological Diagnostics

## LUMBAR PUNCTURE

The lumbar puncture (spinal tap) is done between the 3rd and 4th or between the 4th and 5th lumbar vertebrae. The patient is in the lateral recumbent position with knees drawn toward the chest during the procedure. A local anesthetic is applied to prevent pain when the needle is inserted into the subarachnoid space to withdraw CSF and measure CSF pressure, which should be 70-200 $mmH_2O$.

**Queckenstedt's test**: Compress jugular veins on each side of the neck during the procedure. Note pressure and then release the veins and note pressure in 10-second intervals. Pressure should rise quickly with compression and fall quickly with release. Slower or no response indicates blockage of subarachnoid pathways.

Normal values (CSF analysis):

- Clear and colorless
- Protein: 15-45 mg/dL
- Glucose: 60-80 mg/dL
- Lactic acid: <25.2 mg/dL
- Culture: Negative
- RBCs: 0
- WBCs: 0.5/mL

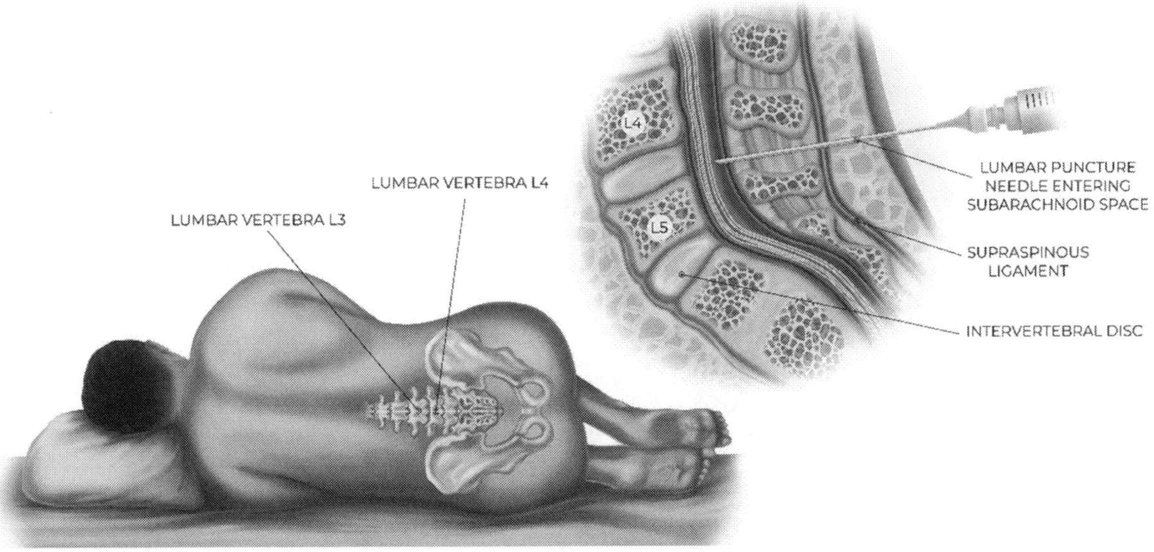

## Avoiding Complications After Lumbar Puncture and Use of Epidural Blood Patch

After a lumbar puncture, the patient should remain in the prone position for at least 3 hours to ensure that the needle puncture sites through the dural and arachnoid areas remain separate in order to reduce the chance of CSF leakage. If >20 mL of CSF is removed, then the patient should remain prone for 2 hours, side-lying (flat) for 2-3 hours, and supine or prone for 6 additional hours. Relieving intracranial pressure by withdrawing CSF may cause herniation of the brain, so lumbar puncture should be done with care in the presence of increased ICP. The most common complaint is of spinal headache, which may occur within a few hours or several days of the procedure. Increased fluid intake may reduce risk of headache. If headache occurs, it may be treated with analgesics, fluids, and bed rest; however, if the headache is severe or persistent, an **epidural blood patch** may be done, with venous blood withdrawn and then injected into the epidural space at the site of the puncture to seal the leaking opening.

# Neurological Pathophysiology

## ENCEPHALOPATHIES

### *HYPERTENSIVE ENCEPHALOPATHY WITH CEREBRAL EDEMA*

Hypertensive encephalopathy can occur as part of a hypertensive crisis. With chronic hypertension, the brain adapts to higher pressures to regulate blood flow, but in a hypertensive crisis, autoregulation of the blood-brain barrier is overwhelmed and the capillaries leak fluid into the tissue and vasodilation takes place with resultant cerebral edema. Damage to arterioles occurs, causing increasing neurological deficits and papilledema. Hypertensive encephalopathy is relatively rare, but carries a high mortality rate and is most common in middle-aged males with long-standing hypertension. **Symptoms** usually develop over 1-2 days and include:

- Non-specific neurological deficits, such as weakness and visual abnormalities
- Alterations in mental status, including confusion
- Headache, often constant
- Nausea and vomiting
- Seizures
- Coma

### *TREATMENT FOR HYPERTENSIVE ENCEPHALOPATHY WITH CEREBRAL EDEMA*

Hypertensive encephalopathy with cerebral edema requires prompt treatment in order to prevent neurological damage.

**Treatment** includes identifying and treating the underlying causes for the hypertensive crisis and taking steps to lower the blood pressure:

- **Nitroprusside sodium (Nitropress)** is usually used initially to lower BP. However, caution must be used not to lower the blood pressure too quickly, as this can lead to cerebral ischemia.
- **Positioning** of the patient to prevent obstruction of venous return from the head
- **Monitoring blood gas** and maintaining $PaCO_2$ at 33-37 mmHg to facilitate vasoconstriction of cerebral arteries
- **Preventing hyperthermia** with antipyretics and cooling devices
- **BP monitoring** and maintenance
- **Seizure control** with phenobarbital and/or phenytoin
- **Lidocaine** through endotracheal tube or intravenously prior to nasotracheal suctioning
- **Diuretics**, such as osmotic agents (mannitol) and loop diuretics (furosemide) to control fluid volume
- **Controlling metabolic demand** by measures to increase pain control and reduce stimulation
- **Barbiturates** (pentobarbital, thiopental) in high doses may be used if other treatments fail to decrease intracranial pressure

### *HYPOXIC ENCEPHALOPATHY*

Cerebral hypoxia (hypoxic encephalopathy) occurs when the oxygen supply to the brain is decreased. If hypoxia is mild, the brain compensates by increasing cerebral blood flow, but it can only double in volume and cannot compensate for severe hypoxic conditions. Hypoxia may be the result of insufficient oxygen in the environment, inadequate exchange at the alveolar level of the lungs, or inadequate circulation to the brain. Brain cells may begin dying within 5 minutes if deprived of adequate oxygenation, so any condition or trauma that interferes with oxygenation can result in brain damage:

- Near-drowning
- Asphyxia
- Cardiac arrest

- High altitude sickness
- Carbon monoxide
- Diseases that interfere with respiration, such as myasthenia gravis and amyotrophic lateral sclerosis
- Anesthesia complications

**Symptoms** include increasing neurological deficits, depending upon the degree and area of damage, with changes in mentation that range from confusion to coma. Prompt identification of the cause and increase in perfusion to the brain is critical for survival.

### *Metabolic Encephalopathy*

Metabolic encephalopathy (hepatic encephalopathy) is damage to the brain resulting from a disturbance in metabolism, primarily hepatic failure to remove toxins from the blood. There may be impairment in cerebral blood flow, cerebral edema, or increased intracranial pressure. It can occur as the result of the ingestion of drugs or toxins which can have a direct toxic effect on neurons, but it can also occur with liver disease, especially when stressed by co-morbidities, such as hemorrhage, hypoxemia, surgery, trauma, renal failure with dialysis, or electrolyte imbalances.

**Symptoms** may vary:

- Irritability and agitation
- Alterations in consciousness
- Dysphonia
- Lack of coordination, spasticity
- Seizures are common and may be the presenting symptom
- Disorientation progressing to coma

Prompt diagnosis is important because the condition may be reversible if underlying causes are identified and treated before permanent neuronal damage occurs.

**Treatment** varies according to the underlying cause.

### *Infectious Encephalopathy*

Infectious encephalopathy is an encompassing term describing encephalopathies caused by a wide range of bacteria, viruses, or prions. Common to all infections are altered brain function that results in alterations in consciousness and personality, cognitive impairment, and lethargy. A wide range of neurological symptoms may occur: myoclonus, seizures, dysphagia, and dysphonia, neuromuscular impairment with muscle atrophy and tremors or spasticity. **Treatment** depends on the underlying cause and response to treatment. Prion infections are not treatable, but bacterial infections may respond to antibiotic therapy, and viral infections may be self-limiting. HIV-related encephalopathy results from opportunistic infections as immune responses decrease, usually indicated by CD4 counts <50. Aggressive antiretroviral treatment and treatment of the infection may reverse symptoms if permanent damage has not occurred for HIV-related encephalopathy. Treatment for other infectious encephalopathies varies according to the type of infection and underlying causes.

## Cerebral Aneurysms

Cerebral aneurysms, the weakening and dilation of a cerebral artery, are usually congenital (90%) while the remaining (10%) result from direct trauma or infection. Aneurysms are usually 2-7 mm in size and occur in the

Circle of Willis at the base of the brain. A rupturing aneurysm may decrease perfusion as well as increasing pressure on surrounding brain tissue. Cerebral aneurysms are classified as follows:

- **Berry/saccular:** The most common congenital type occurs at a bifurcation and grows from the base on a stem, usually at the Circle of Willis.
- **Fusiform**: Large and irregular (>2.5 cm) and rarely ruptures but causes increased intracranial pressure. Usually involves the internal carotid or vertebrobasilar artery.
- **Mycotic**: Rare type that occurs secondary to bacterial infection and aseptic emboli.
- **Dissecting**: Wall is torn apart and blood enters layers. This may occur during angiography or secondary to trauma or disease.
- **Traumatic Charcot-Bouchard (pseudoaneurysm):** Small lesion resulting from chronic hypertension.

## Arteriovenous Malformation

Arteriovenous malformation (AVM) is a congenital abnormality within the brain consisting of a tangle of dilated arteries and veins without a capillary bed. AVMs can occur anywhere in the brain and may cause no significant problems. Usually the AVM is "fed" by one or more cerebral arteries, which enlarge over time, shunting more blood through the AVM. The veins also enlarge in response to increased arterial blood flow because of the lack of a capillary bridge between the two. Because vein walls are thinner and lack the muscle layer of an artery, the veins tend to rupture as the AVM becomes larger, causing a subarachnoid hemorrhage. Chronic ischemia that may be related to the AVM can result in cerebral atrophy. Sometimes small leaks, usually accompanied by headache and nausea and vomiting, may occur before rupture. AVMs may cause a wide range of neurological symptoms, including changes in mentation, dizziness, sensory abnormalities, confusion, increasing ICP, and dementia.

**Treatment** includes:

- Supportive management of symptoms
- Surgical repair or focused irradiation (definitive treatments)

## Intracranial/Intraventricular Hemorrhage

### *Epidural and Subdural*

**Epidural hemorrhage** is bleeding between the dura and the skull that pushes the brain downward and inward. The hemorrhage is usually caused by arterial tears, so bleeding is often rapid, leading to severe neurological deficits and respiratory arrest.

**Subdural hemorrhage** is bleeding between the dura and the cerebrum, usually from tears in the cortical veins of the subdural space. It tends to develop more slowly than epidural hemorrhage and can result in a subdural hematoma. If the bleeding is acute and develops within minutes or hours of injury, the prognosis is poor. Subacute hematomas that develop more slowly cause varying degrees of injury. Subdural hemorrhage is a common injury related to trauma but it can also result from coagulopathies or aneurysms. Symptoms of acute injury may occur within 24-48 hours, but subacute bleeding may not be evident for up to 2 weeks after injury. Chronic hemorrhage occurs primarily in the elderly. Symptoms vary and may include bradycardia, tachycardia, hypertension, and alterations in consciousness. Older children and adults usually require surgical evacuation of the hematoma.

### *Subarachnoid*

**Subarachnoid hemorrhage (SAH)** may occur after trauma but is a common result of rupture of a berry aneurysm or an arteriovenous malformation (AVM). However, there are a number of disorders that may be implicated: neoplasms, sickle cell disease, infection, hemophilia, and leukemia. The first presenting symptom may be complaints of severe headache, nausea and vomiting, nuchal rigidity, palsy related to cranial nerve compression, retinal hemorrhages, and papilledema. Late complications include hyponatremia and hydrocephalus. **Symptoms** worsen as intracranial pressure rises. SAH from aneurysm is classified as follows:

- **Grade I:** No symptoms or slight headache and nuchal rigidity
- **Grade II:** Moderate to severe headache with nuchal rigidity and cranial nerve palsy
- **Grade III**: Drowsy, progressing to confusion or mild focal deficits
- **Grade IV:** Stupor, with hemiparesis (moderate to severe), early decerebrate rigidity, and vegetative disturbances
- **Grade V**: Coma state with decerebrate rigidity

**Treatment** includes:

- Identifying and treating underlying cause
- Observing for re-bleeding
- Anti-seizure medications (such as levetiracetam or phenytoin) to control seizures
- Antihypertensives
- Surgical repair if indicated

## Cerebral Vasospasm

Cerebral vasospasm, a luminal narrowing of cerebral arteries, occurs in about 70% of patients after aneurysmal subarachnoid hemorrhage, resulting in ischemic stroke or death in about 15-20%. Onset is usually 4-12 days after initial rupture. The most common sign of vasospasm is new onset lethargy, which requires a STAT transcranial doppler. If progressive neurological decline is noted, a STAT angiogram will be needed. The cause is unclear but may relate to narrowing caused by pressure of the clot on the arteries. The large arteries are usually affected, causing decreased perfusion to large cerebral areas. A number of therapies are under study, but three common approaches include:

- **Hypertensive hypervolemic hemodilution therapy** (HHH) involves using vasoactive drugs to increase systolic BP to 150-160 while diluting the blood with intravenous fluids and volume expanders in order to improve perfusion. However, if done prior to clipping of the aneurysm, this poses a danger of rebleeding. Cerebral edema, increased intracranial pressure, cardiac failure, and electrolyte imbalance may also occur.
- **Nimodipine** every 4 hours for 21 days reduces/prevents vasospasm. IV magnesium and milrinone may also be used.
- **Cerebral angioplasty** may be done if medical approaches fail but poses a danger of perforation, thromboembolism, and stenosis.

## Hydrocephalus

### *Communicating and Noncommunicating*

The ventricular system produces and circulates cerebrospinal fluid (CSF). The right and left lateral ventricles open into the third ventricle at the interventricular foramen (foramen of Monro). The aqueduct of Sylvius connects the third and fourth ventricles. The fourth ventricle, anterior to the cerebellum, supplies CSF to the subarachnoid space and the spinal cord (dorsal surface). The CSF circulates and then returns to the brain and is absorbed in the arachnoid villi. **Hydrocephalus** occurs when there is an imbalance between production and absorption of cerebrospinal fluid in the ventricles, resulting from impaired absorption or obstruction, which may be congenital or acquired. There are two common types of hydrocephalus:

- **Communicating:** CSF flows (communicates) between the ventricles but is not absorbed in the subarachnoid space (arachnoid villi).
- **Noncommunicating:** CSF is obstructed (non-communicating) between the ventricles, with the obstruction most often due to stenosis of the aqueduct of Sylvius.

### Symptoms

**Symptoms** of hydrocephalus depend on the age of onset. In *early infancy*, before closure of cranial sutures, head enlargement is the most common presentation, but in adults with less elasticity in the skull, neurological symptoms usually relate to increasing pressure on structures of the brain. Hydrocephalus may occur at any age, but the type that occurs in *young/middle-aged adults* is different than that common in children or those >50. Hydrocephalus in young and middle-aged adults may result from a congenital defect, hydrocephalus of infancy with shunt failure, or trauma and is characterized by:

- Headache relieved by vomiting
- Papilledema
- Lack of bladder control
- Strabismus and other visual disorders
- Ataxia
- Irritability
- Lethargy
- Confusion and impairment of cognitive abilities

With **adult-onset normal pressure hydrocephalus** (>50) cerebrospinal fluid increases and dilates the ventricles, but frequently without increasing intracranial pressure. The cause is often unclear. Symptoms include gait disturbance, bladder control issues, and mild dementia

### Treatment

Hydrocephalus is diagnosed through CT and MRI scans, which help to determine the cause. **Treatment** may vary somewhat depending upon the underlying disorder. For example, if obstruction is caused by a tumor, surgical excision to directly remove the obstruction is required. Generally, however, most hydrocephalus is treated with shunts:

- **Ventricular-peritoneal shunt:** This procedure is the most common and consists of placing a ventricular catheter directly into the ventricles (usually lateral) at one end with the other end in the peritoneal area to drain away excess CSF. There is a one-way valve near the proximal end that prevents backflow but opens when pressure rises to drain fluid. In some cases, the distal end drains into the right atrium.
- **Third ventriculostomy:** A small opening is made in the base of the third ventricle so CSF can bypass an obstruction. This procedure is not common and is done with a small endoscope.

## Neurologic Infectious Disease

### Bacterial Meningitis

Bacterial meningitis may be caused by a wide range of bacteria, including *Streptococcus pneumoniae* and *Neisseria meningitidis.* Bacteria can enter the CNS from distant infection, surgical wounds, invasive devices, nasal colonization, or penetrating trauma. The infective process includes inflammation, exudates, WBC accumulation, and brain tissue damage with hyperemia and edema. Purulent exudate covers the brain and invades and blocks the ventricles, obstructing CSF and leading to increased intracranial pressure. **Symptoms** include abrupt onset, fever, chills, severe headache, nuchal rigidity, and alterations of consciousness with seizures, agitation, and irritability. Antibodies specific to bacteria don't cross the blood brain barrier, so immune response is poor. Some may have photophobia, hallucinations, and/or aggressive behavior or may become stuporous and lapse into coma. Nuchal rigidity may progress to opisthotonos. Reflexes are variable but Kernig and Brudzinski signs are often positive. Signs may relate to particular bacteria, such as rashes, sore joints, or a draining ear. **Diagnosis** is usually based on lumbar puncture examination of cerebrospinal fluid and symptoms. **Treatment** includes IV antibiotics and supportive care: fluids, a dark and calm environment, measures to reduce ICP, etc.

### *Fungal Meningitis*

Fungal meningitis is the least common cause of meningitis. It occurs when a fungal organism enters into the subarachnoid space, cerebral spinal fluid, and meninges. Immune deficient patients such as those with HIV, cancer, or immunodeficiency syndromes are most at risk for the development of fungal meningitis. The most common organisms causing fungal meningitis are candida albicans and Cryptococcus neoformans. Fungal meningitis caused by candida may occur in immunosuppressed patients, in those who have had a ventricular shunt placed, or in those that have had a lumbar puncture performed. Cryptococcus is a fungus found in soil throughout the world and does not usually affect people with a healthy immune system. Cryptococcal meningitis is most commonly seen in patients with HIV/AIDS and is one of the leading causes of death in HIV/AIDS patients in certain parts of Africa.

**Signs and symptoms**: Headache, fever, nausea and vomiting, stiff neck, photophobia, and mental status changes.

**Diagnosis**: Lumbar puncture with subsequent culture of cerebral spinal fluid. In addition, blood cultures may be obtained as well as a CT of the head.

**Treatment**: The treatment of fungal meningitis involves a long course of anti-fungal medications, including Amphotericin B, flucytosine, and fluconazole. Anticonvulsants may be administered for seizure control.

### *Viral Infections That Can Impact the Neurological System*

Many different types of viral infections can impact the neurological system either by direct infection transmitted through the bloodstream or by spreading along the nerve pathways (such as rabies). Common viral infections affecting the neurological system include:

- **Viral encephalitis**: Arboviral infections are transmitted from an animal host to an arthropod (typically a mosquito or tick) to humans, who are typically dead-end hosts. Arboviral infections include western equine encephalitis, eastern equine encephalitis, St. Louis encephalitis, Powassan encephalitis, Colorado tick fever and La Crosse encephalitis. West Nile virus may also invade the CNS and cause encephalitis.
- **Viral meningitis**: Viral meningitis is usually self-limiting within 7 to 10 days and is less severe than bacterial meningitis.
- **Herpes virus**: Herpes simplex virus can invade the nervous system and cause herpes simplex encephalitis, which has a high mortality rate.
- **HIV**: Inflammation may affect the CNS and interfere with neuronal functions.

## Neuromuscular Disorders

### *Multiple Sclerosis*

Multiple sclerosis is an autoimmune disorder of the CNS in which the myelin sheath around the nerves is damaged and replaced by scar tissue that prevents conduction of nerve impulses.

**Symptoms** vary widely and can include problems with balance and coordination, tremors, slurring of speech, cognitive impairment, vision impairment, nystagmus, pain, and bladder and bowel dysfunction. Symptoms may be relapsing-remitting, progressive, or a combination. Onset is usually at 20-30 years of age, with incidence higher in females. Patient may initially present with problems walking or falling or optic neuritis (30%) causing loss of central vision. Males may complain of sexual dysfunction as an early symptom. Others have dysuria with urinary retention.

**Diagnosis** is based on clinical and neurological examination and MRI. **Treatment** is symptomatic and includes treatment to shorten duration of episodes and slow progress.

- **Glucocorticoids**: Methylprednisolone
- **Immunomodulator**: Interferon beta, glatiramer acetate, natalizumab
- **Immunosuppressant**: Mitoxantrone
- **Hormone**: Estriol (for females)

**Review Video: Multiple Sclerosis**
Visit mometrix.com/academy and enter code: 417355

## ALS

Amyotrophic lateral sclerosis (ALS) is a progressive degenerative disease of the upper and lower motor neurons, resulting in progressively severe symptoms such as spasticity, hyperreflexia, muscle weakness, and paralysis that can cause dysphagia, cramping, muscular atrophy, and respiratory dysfunction. ALS may be sporadic or familial (rare). Speech may become monotone; however, cognitive functioning usually remains intact. Eventually, patients become immobile and cannot breathe independently.

**Diagnosis** is based on history, electromyography, nerve conduction studies, and MRI. Treatment includes riluzole to delay progression of the disease. Patients in the ED usually have been diagnosed and have developed an acute complication, such as acute respiratory failure, aspiration pneumonia, or other trauma.

**Treatment** includes:

- Nebulizer treatments with bronchodilators and steroids
- Antibiotics for infection
- Mechanical ventilation

If **ventilatory assistance** is needed, it is important to determine if the patient has a living will expressing the wish to be ventilated or not or has assigned power of attorney for health matters to someone to make this decision.

## Parkinson's Disease

Parkinson's disease (PD) is an extrapyramidal movement motor system disorder caused by loss of brain cells that produce dopamine. Typical symptoms include tremor of face and extremities, rigidity, bradykinesia, akinesia, poor posture, and a lack of balance and coordination causing increasing problems with mobility, talking, and swallowing. Some may suffer depression and mood changes. Tremors usually present unilaterally in an upper extremity.

**Diagnosis** includes:

- **Cogwheel rigidity test**: The extremity is put through passive range of motion, which causes increased muscle tone and ratchet-like movements.
- **Physical and neurological exam**
- **Complete history** to rule out drug-induced Parkinson akinesia

**Treatment** includes:

- Symptomatic support
- Dopaminergic therapy: Levodopa, amantadine, and carbidopa
- Anticholinergics: Trihexyphenidyl, benztropine
- For drug-induced Parkinson's, terminate drugs

Drug therapy tends to decrease in effectiveness over time, and patients may present with a marked increase in symptoms. Discontinuing the drugs for 1 week may exacerbate symptoms initially, but functioning may improve when drugs are reintroduced.

### *Guillain-Barré Syndrome*

Guillain-Barré syndrome (GBS) is an autoimmune disorder of the myelinated motor peripheral nervous system, causing ascending and descending paralysis. GBS is often triggered by a viral infection, but may be idiopathic in origin. Diagnosis is by history, clinical symptoms, and lumbar puncture, which often show increased protein with normal glucose and cell count although protein may not increase for a week or more.

> **Review Video: Guillain-Barre Syndrome**
> Visit mometrix.com/academy and enter code: 742900

**Symptoms** include:

- Numbness and tingling with increasing weakness of lower extremities that may become generalized, sometimes resulting in complete paralysis and inability to breathe without ventilatory support.
- Deep tendon reflexes are typically absent and some people experience facial weakness and ophthalmoplegia (paralysis of muscles controlling movement of eyes).

**Treatment** includes:

- Supportive: Fluids, physical therapy, and antibiotics for infections
- Patients should be hospitalized for observation and placed on ventilator support if forced vital capacity is reduced.
- While there is no definitive treatment, plasma exchange or IV immunoglobulin may shorten the duration of symptoms.

### *Muscular Dystrophy*

Muscular dystrophies are genetic disorders with gradual degeneration of muscle fibers and progressive weakness and atrophy of skeletal muscles and loss of mobility. **Pseudohypertrophic (Duchenne) muscular dystrophy** is the most common form and the most severe. It is an X-linked disorder in about 50% of the cases with the rest sporadic mutations, affecting males almost exclusively. Children typically have some delay in motor development with difficulty walking and have evidence of muscle weakness by about age 3. Pseudohypertrophic refers to enlargement of muscles by fatty infiltration associated with muscular atrophy, which causes contractures and deformities of joints. Abnormal bone development results in spinal and other skeletal deformities. The disease progresses rapidly, and most children are wheelchair bound by about 12 years of age. As the disease progresses, it involves the muscles of the diaphragm and other muscles needed for respiration. Mild to frank mental deficiency is common. Facial, oropharyngeal, and respiratory muscles weaken late in the disease. Cardiomegaly commonly occurs. Death most often relates to respiratory infection or cardiac failure by age 25. Treatment is supportive.

### *Cerebral Palsy*

Cerebral palsy (CP) is a non-progressive motor dysfunction related to CNS damage associated with congenital, hypoxic, or traumatic injury before, during, or ≤2 years after birth. It may include visual defects, speech impairment, seizures, and intellectual disability. There are four **types of motor dysfunction:**

- **Spastic**: Damage to the cerebral cortex or pyramidal tract. Constant hypertonia and rigidity lead to contractures and curvature of the spine.
- **Dyskinetic**: Damage to the extrapyramidal, basal ganglia. Tremors and twisting with exaggerated posturing and impairment of voluntary muscle control.

- **Ataxic**: Damage to the extrapyramidal cerebellum. Atonic muscles in infancy with lack of balance, instability of muscles, and poor gait.
- **Mixed**: Combinations of all three types with multiple areas of damage.

**Characteristics** of CP include:

- Hypotonia or hypertonia with rigidity and spasticity
- Athetosis (constant writhing motions)
- Ataxia
- Hemiplegia (one-sided involvement, more severe in upper extremities)
- Diplegia (all extremities involved, but more severe in lower extremities)
- Quadriplegia (all extremities involved with arms flexed and legs extended)

### *Myasthenia Gravis*

Myasthenia gravis is an autoimmune disorder that results in sporadic, progressive weakness of striated (skeletal) muscles because of impaired transmission of nerve impulses. Myasthenia gravis usually affects muscles controlled by the cranial nerves although any muscle group may be affected. Many patients also have thymomas.

**Signs and symptoms** include weakness and fatigue that worsens throughout the day. Patients often exhibit ptosis and diplopia. They may have trouble chewing and swallowing and often appear to have masklike facies. If respiratory muscles are involved, patients may exhibit signs of respiratory failure. Myasthenic crisis occurs when patients can no longer breathe independently.

**Diagnosis** includes electromyography and the Tensilon test (an IV injection of edrophonium or neostigmine, which improves function if the patient has myasthenia gravis, but does not improve function if the symptoms are from a different cause). CT or MRI to diagnose thymoma.

**Treatment** includes anticholinesterase drugs (neostigmine, pyridostigmine) to relieve some muscle weakness, but these drugs lose effectiveness as the disease progresses. Corticosteroids may be used. Thymectomy is performed if thymoma is present. Tracheotomy and mechanical ventilation may be needed for myasthenic crisis.

## Seizure Disorders

### *Partial Seizures*

Partial seizures are caused by electrical discharges to a localized area of the cerebral cortex, such as the frontals, temporal, or parietal lobes with seizure characteristics related to the area of involvement. They may begin in a focal area and become generalized, often preceded by an aura.

- **Simple partial:** Unilateral motor symptoms including somatosensory, psychic, and autonomic
    - Aversive: Eyes and head turned away from focal side
    - Sylvan (usually during sleep): Tonic-clonic movements of the face, salivation, and arrested speech
- **Special sensory:** Various sensations (numbness, tingling, prickling, or pain) spreading from one area. May include visual sensations, posturing or hypertonia.
- **Complex (psychomotor):** No loss of consciousness, but altered consciousness and non-responsive with amnesia. May involve complex sensorium with bad tastes, auditory or visual hallucinations, feeling of déjà vu, strong fear. May carry out repetitive activities, such as walking, running, smacking lips, chewing, or drawling. Rarely aggressive. Seizure usually followed by prolonged drowsiness and confusion. Most common ages 3 through adolescence.

### *Generalized Seizures*

Generalized seizures lack a focal onset and appear to involve both hemispheres, usually presenting with loss of consciousness and no preceding aura.

- **Tonic-clonic (Grand Mal)**: Occurs without warning
    - Tonic period (10-30 seconds): Eyes roll upward with loss of consciousness, arms flexed; stiffen in symmetric tonic contraction of body, apneic with cyanosis and salivating
    - Clonic period (10 seconds to 30 minutes, but usually 30 seconds). Violent rhythmic jerking with contraction and relaxation. May be incontinent of urine and feces. Contractions slow and then stop.

Following seizures, there may be confusion, disorientation, and impairment of motor activity, speech, and vision for several hours. Headache, nausea, and vomiting may occur. Person often falls asleep and awakens more lucid.

- **Absence (Petit Mal):** Onset is at ages 4-12 and usually ends in puberty. Onset is abrupt with brief loss of consciousness for 5-10 seconds and slight loss of muscle tone but often appears to be daydreaming. Lip smacking or eye twitching may occur.

### *Epilepsy*

Epilepsy is diagnosed based on a history of seizure activity as well as supporting EEG findings. Treatment is individualized. First line treatments include antiepileptic medications for partial and generalized tonic-clonic seizures. Usually, treatment is started with one medication, but this may need to be changed, adjusted, or an additional medication added until the seizures are under control or to avoid adverse effects, which include allergic reactions, especially skin irritations and acute or chronic toxicity. Milder reactions often subside with time or adjustment in doses. Toxic reactions may vary considerably, depending upon the medication and duration of use, so close monitoring is essential. Severe rash and hepatotoxicity are common toxic reactions that occur with many of the antiepileptic drugs. Dosages of drugs may need to be adjusted to avoid breakthrough seizures during times of stress, such as during illness or surgery. Alcohol/drug abuse and sleep deprivation may also cause breakthrough seizures. Most anticonvulsant drugs are teratogenic.

### *Status Epilepticus*

Status epilepticus (SE) is usually generalized tonic-clonic seizures that are characterized by a series of seizures with intervening time too short for regaining of consciousness. The constant assault and periods of apnea can lead to exhaustion, respiratory failure with hypoxemia and hypercapnia, cardiac failure, and death.

**Causes:** Uncontrolled epilepsy or non-compliance with anticonvulsants, infections such as encephalitis, encephalopathy or stroke, drug toxicity (isoniazid), brain trauma, neoplasms, and metabolic disorders.

**Treatment** includes:

- Anticonvulsants usually beginning with a fast-acting benzodiazepine (lorazepam), often in steps, with administration of medication every 5 minutes until seizures subside.
- If cause is undetermined, acyclovir and ceftriaxone may be administered.
- If there is no response to the first 2 doses of anticonvulsants (refractory SE), rapid sequence intubation (RSI), which involves sedation and paralytic anesthesia, may be done while therapy continues. Combining phenobarbital and benzodiazepine can cause apnea, so intubation may be necessary.
- Antiepileptic medications are added.

## Brain Tumors

Any type of brain tumor can occur in adults. Brain tumors may be primary, arising within the brain, or secondary as a result of metastasis:

- **Astrocytoma**: This arises from astrocytes, which are glial cells. It is the most common type of tumor, occurring throughout the brain. There are many types of astrocytomas, and most are slow growing. Some are operable while others are not. Radiation may be given after removal. Astrocytomas include glioblastomas, aggressively malignant tumors occurring most often in adults 45-70.
- **Glioblastoma**: This is the most common and most malignant adult brain tumor/astrocytoma. Treatment includes surgery, radiation, and chemotherapy, but survival rates are very low.
- **Brain stem glioma**: This may be fast or slow growing but is generally not operable because of location, although it may be treated with radiation or chemotherapy.
- **Craniopharyngioma**: This is a congenital, slow-growing, recurrent (especially if >5 cm) and benign cystic tumor that is difficult to resect and is treated with surgery and radiation.
- **Meningioma**: Slow growing recurrent tumors are usually benign and most often occur in women, ages 40-70; however, they can cause severe impairment/death, depending on size and location. Meningiomas are surgically removed if causing symptoms.
- **Ganglioglioma**: This can occur anywhere in the brain and is usually slow growing and benign.
- **Medulloblastoma**: There are many types of medulloblastoma, most arising in the cerebellum, malignant, and fast growing. Surgical excision is often followed by radiation and chemotherapy although recent studies show using just chemotherapy controls recurrence with less neurological damage.
- **Oligodendroglioma**: This tumor most often occurs in the cerebrum, primarily the frontal or temporal lobes, involving the myelin sheath of the neurons. It is slow growing and most common in those age 40-60.
- **Optical nerve glioma**: This slow growing tumor of the optic nerve is usually a form of astrocytoma. Optic nerve glioma is often associated with neurofibromatosis type I (NF1), occurring in 15-40% of patients with NF1. Despite surgical, chemotherapy, or radiotherapy treatment, it is usually fatal.

## Strokes

### *Hemorrhagic Strokes*

Hemorrhagic strokes account for about 20% of all strokes and result from a ruptured cerebral artery, causing not only a lack of oxygen and nutrients but also edema that causes widespread pressure and damage:

- **Intracerebral** is bleeding into the substance of the brain from an artery in the central lobes, basal ganglia, pons, or cerebellum. Intracerebral hemorrhage usually results from atherosclerotic degenerative changes, hypertension, brain tumors, anticoagulation therapy, or use of illicit drugs, such as cocaine.
- **Intracranial aneurysm** occurs with ballooning cerebral artery ruptures, most commonly at the Circle of Willis.
- **Arteriovenous malformation**. Rupture of AVMs can cause brain attack in young adults.
- **Subarachnoid hemorrhage** is bleeding in the space between the meninges and brain, resulting from aneurysm, AVM, or trauma. This type of hemorrhage compresses brain tissue.

**Treatment includes:** The patient may need airway protection/artificial ventilation if neurologic compromise is severe. Blood pressure is lowered to control rate of bleeding but with caution to avoid hypotension and resulting cerebral ischemia (Goal – CPP >70). Sedation can lower ICP and blood pressure, and seizure prophylaxis will be indicated as blood irritates the cerebral cells. An intraventricular catheter may be used in ICP management; correct any clotting disorders if identified.

### *Ischemia Strokes*

Strokes (brain attacks, cerebrovascular accidents) result when there is interruption of the blood flow to an area of the brain. The two basic types are ischemic and hemorrhagic. About 80% are **ischemic**, resulting from blockage of an artery supplying the brain:

- **Thrombosis** in a large artery, usually resulting from atherosclerosis, may block circulation to a large area of the brain. It is most common in the elderly and may occur suddenly or after episodes of transient ischemic attacks.
- **Lacunar infarct** (a penetrating thrombosis in a small artery) is most common in those with diabetes mellitus and/or hypertension.
- **Embolism** travels through the arterial system and lodges in the brain, most commonly in the left middle cerebral artery. An embolism may be cardiogenic, resulting from cardiac arrhythmia or surgery. An embolism usually occurs rapidly with no warning signs.
- **Cryptogenic** has no identifiable cause.

**Medical management** of ischemic strokes with tissue plasminogen activator (tPA) (Activase), the primary treatment, should be initiated within 3 hours (or up to 4.5 hours if inclusion criteria are met):

- **Thrombolytic,** such as tPA, which is produced by recombinant DNA and is used to dissolve fibrin clots. It is given intravenously (0.9 mg/kg up to 90 mg) with 10% injected as an initial bolus and the rest over the next hour.
- **Antihypertensives** if MAP >130 mmHg or systolic BP >220
- **Cooling** to reduce hyperthermia
- **Osmotic diuretics** (mannitol), hypertonic saline, loop diuretics (Lasix), and/or corticosteroids (dexamethasone) to decrease cerebral edema and intracranial pressure
- **Aspirin/anticoagulation** may be used with embolism
- Monitor and treat hyperglycemia
- **Surgical Intervention:** Used when other treatment fails, may go in through artery and manually remove the clot

### *Symptoms of Brain Attacks in Relation to Area of Brain Affected*

Brain attacks most commonly occur in the right or left hemisphere, but the exact location and the extent of brain damage from a brain attack affects the type of presenting symptoms. If the frontal area of either side is involved, there tends to be memory and learning deficits. Some symptoms are common to specific areas and help to identify the area involved:

- **Right hemisphere**: This results in left paralysis or paresis and a left visual field deficit that may cause spatial and perceptual disturbances, so people may have difficulty judging distance. Fine motor skills may be impacted, resulting in trouble dressing or handling tools. People may become impulsive and exhibit poor judgment, often denying impairment. Left-sided neglect (lack of perception of things on the left side) may occur. Difficulty following directions, short-term memory loss, and depression are also common. Language skills usually remain intact.
- **Left hemisphere**: Results in right paralysis or paresis and a right visual field defect. Depression is common and people often exhibit slow, cautious behavior, requiring repeated instruction and reinforcement for simple tasks. Short-term memory loss and difficulty learning new material or understanding generalizations is common. Difficulty with mathematics, reading, writing, and reasoning may occur. Aphasia (expressive, receptive, or global) is common.
- **Brain stem**: Because the brain stem controls respiration and cardiac function, a brain attack in the brain stem frequently causes death, but those who survive may have a number of problems, including respiratory and cardiac abnormalities. Strokes may involve motor or sensory impairment or both.
- **Cerebellum**: This area controls balance and coordination. Brain attacks in the cerebellum are rare but may result in ataxia, nausea and vomiting, and headaches and dizziness or vertigo.

### TIA

Transient ischemic attacks (TIAs) from small clots cause similar but short-lived (minutes to hours) symptoms. Emergent treatment includes placing patient in semi-Fowlers or Fowler's position and administering oxygen. The patient may require oral suctioning if secretions pool. The patient's circulation, airway, and breathing should be assessed and IV access line placed. Thrombolytic therapy to dissolve blood clots should be administered within 1 to 3 hours. While a patient can recover fully from a TIA, they should be educated, because having a TIA increases an individual's risk for a stroke.

## Acute Spinal Cord Injury

**Spinal cord injuries** may result from blunt trauma (such as automobile accidents), falls from a significant height, sports injuries, and penetrating trauma (such as gunshot or knife wounds). Damage results from mechanical injury and secondary responses resulting from hemorrhage, edema, and ischemia. The type of symptoms relates to the area and degree of injury. About 50% of spinal cord injuries involve the cervical spine between C4 and C7 with a 20% mortality rate, and 50% of injuries result in quadriplegia. Neurogenic shock may occur with injury above T6, with bradycardia, hypotension, and autonomic instability. Patients may develop hypoxia because of respiratory dysfunction. With high injuries, up to 70% of patients will require a tracheostomy (especially at or above C3). Patients with paralysis are at high risk for pressure sores, urinary tract infections (from catheterization), and constipation and impaction. Management varies according to the level of injury but may include mobilization, mechanical ventilation, support surfaces, ROM, assisted mobility, rehabilitation therapy, analgesia, psychological counseling, bowel training, and skin care.

## Head Trauma

### Blunt Head Trauma

Head trauma can occur as the result of intentional or unintentional blunt or penetrating trauma, such as from falls, automobile accidents, sports injuries, or violence. The degree of injury correlates with the impact force. The skull provides protection to the brain, but a severe blow can cause significant neurological damage. **Blunt trauma** can include:

- **Acceleration-deceleration injuries** are those in which a blow to the stationary head causes the elastic skull to change shape, pushing against the brain, which moves sharply backward in response, striking against the skull.
- **Bruising** can occur at the point of impact (*coup*) and the point where the brain hits the skull (*contrecoup*). So, a blow to the frontal area can cause damage to the occipital region.

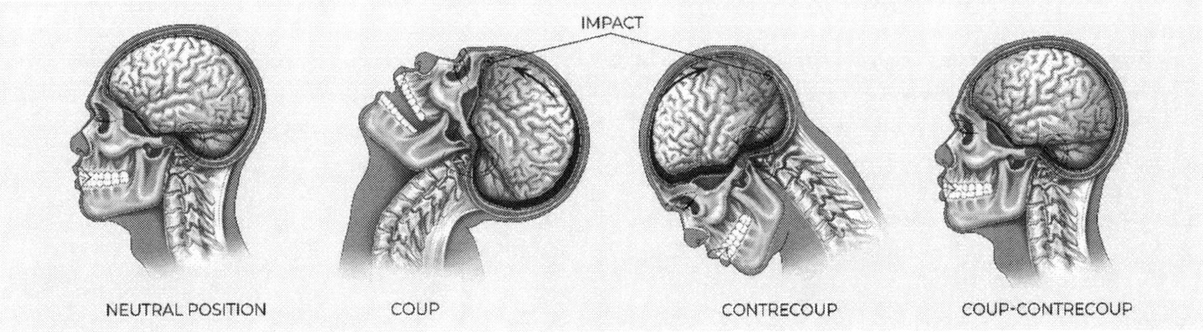


- **Shear injuries,** where vessels are torn, result from sudden movement of the brain.
- **Severe compression** may force the brain through the tentorial opening, damaging the brainstem.

### Cerebral Edema and Increased ICP Secondary to Head Trauma

Head injuries that occur at the time of trauma include fractures, contusions, hematomas, and diffuse cerebral and vascular injury. These injuries may result in hypoxia, increased intracranial pressure, and cerebral edema. Open injuries may result in infection. Patients often suffer initial hypertension, which increases intracranial pressure, decreasing perfusion. Often the primary problem with head trauma is a significant increase in swelling, which also interferes with perfusion, causing hypoxia and hypercapnia, which trigger increased blood flow. This increased volume at a time when injury impairs auto-regulation increases cerebral edema, which increases intracranial pressure and results in a further decrease in perfusion with resultant ischemia. If pressure continues to rise, the brain may herniate. Concomitant hypotension may result in hypoventilation, further complicating treatment. **Treatments** include:

- Monitoring ICP and CCP
- Providing oxygen
- Elevating the head of the bed and maintaining proper body alignment
- Giving medications: Analgesics, anticonvulsants, and anesthetics
- Providing blood/fluids to stabilize hemodynamics
- Managing airway, providing mechanical ventilation if needed
- Providing osmotic agents, such as mannitol and hypertonic saline solution, to reduce cerebral edema

### *Concussions, Contusions, and Lacerations*

A variety of different injuries can occur as a result of head trauma:

- **Concussions** are diffuse areas of bleeding in the brain and one of the most common injuries. They are usually relatively transient, causing no permanent neurological damage. They may result in confusion, disorientation, and mild amnesia, which last only minutes or hours.
- **Contusions/lacerations** are bruising and tears of cerebral tissue. There may be petechial areas at the impact site (coup) or larger bruising. Contrecoup injuries are less common in children than in adults. Areas most impacted by contusions and lacerations are the occipital, frontal, and temporal lobes. The degree of injury relates to the amount of vascular damage, but initial symptoms are similar to a concussion; however, symptoms persist and may progress, depending upon the degree of injury. Lacerations are often caused by fractures.

### *Skull Fractures*

Skull fractures are a common mechanism of penetrating wounds causing cerebral lacerations. Open fractures are those in which the dura is torn, and closed fractures are those in which the dura remain intact. While fractures by themselves do not cause neurological damage, force is needed to fracture the skull, often causing damage to underlying structures. Meningeal arteries lie in grooves on the underside of the skull, and a fracture can cause an arterial tear and hemorrhage. **Skull fractures** include:

- **Basilar**: Occurs in bones at the base of the brain and can cause severe brainstem damage. May see bruising around the ear ("Battles sign") and leaking of CSF from nose and ears ("Halo sign"—bloody fluid will develop a ring of clear fluid when placed on gauze or linens).
- **Comminuted**: Skull fractures into small pieces.
- **Compound**: Surface laceration extends to include a skull fracture.
- **Depressed**: Pieces of the skull are depressed inward on the brain tissue, often producing dural tears.
- **Linear/hairline:** Skull fracture forms a thin line without any splintering.

### *Traumatic Brain Injury*

Traumatic brain injury (TBI) occurs when an external force damages the brain, thereby causing an alteration in its function. TBIs can be classified as mild, moderate, or severe. Common causes of traumatic brain injury include falls, motor vehicle accidents, and assaults. Traumatic brain injuries are more common in males than females.

**Signs and symptoms**: Signs and symptoms of a traumatic brain injury may not be immediately present, depending on the severity of the injury. Symptoms may be subtle initially and then worsen. Symptoms include:

loss of consciousness, headache, blurred vision, confusion, nausea, vomiting, fatigue, somnolence, dizziness, loss of balance or coordination, seizures, tinnitus, slurred speech, and photosensitivity.

**Diagnosis**: X-rays of the spine, CT and MRI of the head and angiography if penetrating injury occurred. The Glasgow coma scale is most commonly used to assess neurologic status in the TBI patient.

**Treatment**: Treatment of TBI includes frequent monitoring of vital signs, fluid balance and neurologic status. Intracranial pressure may also be monitored. Mannitol and hypertonic saline may be administered to decrease intracranial pressure and cerebral edema. Antiepileptic medications may be utilized to prevent or minimize seizure activity. In cases of severe injury, decompressive craniotomy and initiation of a hypothermia protocol may be used to reduce intracranial pressure, cerebral edema, and cell death.

# Neurological Procedures and Interventions

## Clipping for Treatment of Aneurysm

**Surgical clipping** of a ruptured or large, unstable **aneurysm** is necessary because of the danger of rebleeding, 4% in the first 24 hours and 1-2% each day for the next month. Mortality rates with rebleeding are about 70%. Surgical repair is usually done within 48 hours. Clipping may be done prophylactically to prevent rupture. Clipping is done to secure the aneurysm without impairing circulation. Typically, a craniotomy is done and an incision is made into the brain to access the site of the aneurysm. When bleeding is controlled, a small spring-like clip (or sometimes multiple clips) is placed about the neck of the aneurysm. The bulging part of the aneurysm is drained with a needle to make sure that it does not refill and angiography may be done to ensure patency of the artery that feeds the aneurysm. It is possible during surgery for a clot to break away from the aneurysm with resultant extensive hemorrhage. Neurological damage may occur related to surgical manipulation, especially if access is difficult. Post-op monitoring includes frequent neurological checks—sometimes every hour, checking for signs and symptoms of stroke, hemorrhage or cerebral edema/increased ICP. An angiogram may be performed after surgery to confirm placement of clips and ensure there are no leaks.

## Embolization for Treatment of Aneurysm or AVM

Embolization is a minimally-invasive method that is an alternative to clipping for some aneurysms and is also used for AVMs. There are different types of embolization, but all use percutaneous transfemoral catheterization and fluoroscopy. The catheter is fed through the femoral and carotid artery to the area requiring repair:

- AVM repair by introducing small silastic beads or glue into the feeder vessels, allowing blood flow to carry the material to the site. This may also be done prior to surgical repair.
- AVM or aneurysm repair by placing one or more detachable balloons into the aneurysm or an AVM and inflating it with a liquid polymerizing agent that solidifies.
- Aneurysm repair with endovascular coiling involves feeding very small platinum coils through the catheter to fill the aneurysm.

Results of endovascular coiling have been very positive, with risk of death or disability at one year over 22% lower than those treated with clipping, although distal ischemia related to emboli is a possible complication.

## Surgical Excision of AVM

Surgical excision of AVM is the definitive treatment for AVMs as both embolization and radiotherapy treatment pose the risk that the abnormal vessels will recur. Sometimes, 2-3 different surgeries may be required for large AVMs. Usually, nonfunctioning brain tissue surrounds the AVM, so it is possible to remove the AVM without damaging brain tissue. However, reperfusion bleeding may occur as blood is diverted to surrounding arterials that had dilated because of chronic ischemia. The sudden increase in blood flow and pressure may cause leakage of blood from the vessels. There may be extensive blood loss during surgery, so constant monitoring of arterial pressure and multiple IV cannulas are important. Embolization may be done prior to surgery to reduce bleeding. Hyperventilation and mannitol are often used, and β-blockers may be used to prevent hypertension and cerebral edema. Postoperatively, blood pressure is kept low to prevent reperfusion bleeding.

## Evacuation of Hematomas

Evacuation of hematomas can be done in a number of different ways, including burr holes, needle aspiration, direct surgical craniotomy, or endoscopic craniotomy, but evacuation can pose considerable risks:

- **Epidural hematomas** are usually arterial but may be venous (20%) and are always medical emergencies and require craniotomy with evacuation before compression damage to the brain occurs. Prognosis is good if corrected early because underlying brain damage is rarely severe.

- **Subdural hematomas**, often from acceleration-deceleration accidents or abuse, involve damage to the brain tissue. Evacuation may be done if the hematoma is large and causing compression, but the brain tissue beneath hematomas is often extremely swollen. If the dura is opened, suddenly relieving the pressure may cause the brain to herniate through the opening, so aggressive therapy to reduce swelling preoperatively and careful surgical planning are necessary.

## Craniotomies

Craniotomies for tumors or other surgical repair (AVMs, aneurysms) are increasingly done with micro-endoscopic equipment, but the surgical opening must be large enough to allow access and the use of necessary instruments. Procedures vary widely according to the reason for craniotomy, the type of tumor, and the age and condition of the patient. Direct craniotomies through the skull are needed in some instances, but newer approaches, including transnasal and transsphenoidal endoscopy are used when possible. Some areas of the brain are not accessible with craniotomy, but may be accessible through stereotactic radiosurgery with Gamma Knife or CyberKnife. Stereotactic radiosurgery is often used as a secondary treatment after primary removal of tumor for regrowth or residual tumor. Radiosurgery may be fractionated and given in a series of treatments. These non-invasive treatments are usually done while adults are awake.

### *Postoperative Care for Craniotomy Patients*

In the post-operative period immediately following a craniotomy, the patient must be observed carefully for any **complications** or changes in condition:

- Monitor intracranial pressure
- Position the head in a midline, neutral position. HOB is elevated 30-45° for supratentorial surgery and is flat or only slightly elevated for infratentorial surgery
- Initiate anti-thromboembolism measures: Compression stockings or intermittent pneumatic compression device
- Monitor fluid balance (intake and output)
- Observe surgical wound for swelling and drainage; empty and measure drainage devices (usually bulb drains)
- Monitor oxygen saturation and ABGs to ensure proper oxygenation
- Monitor thermoregulation and prevent hyperthermia
- Administer analgesics and antiemetics routinely to maintain comfort and prevent stress or increased ICP from vomiting
- Administer corticosteroids to reduce postoperative swelling
- Administer anticoagulants (heparin) to prevent clotting
- Monitor laboratory status:
    - Complete blood count to observe for blood loss/infection
    - Electrolyte levels, especially observing for hyponatremia and/or hyperkalemia
    - Blood glucose level (may elevate with corticosteroids)

## Burr Holes

Burr holes are small holes drilled through the skull, often as an emergent procedure to relieve increased intracranial pressure (such as from subdural, epidural hematoma, or hydrocephalus), to drain blood, or to remove foreign objects. Burr holes may also be used as access points for minimally-invasive surgeries on the brain, such as to remove a brain tumor. The burr holes are generally drilled with the patient under general anesthesia, and the opening may be closed or left open with a drain in place. The patient must be monitored for indications of bleeding or other surgical complications. Perioperative complications may include increased intracranial pressure from cerebral edema, seizures, intracranial bleeding, and coma. The patient's vital signs and neurological signs should be closely monitored. If a drain is in place, the amount and character of the drainage should be monitored. The patient may receive prophylactic antibiotics to reduce the risk of infection.

## Ventricular Drains

Ventricular drains are inserted into one of the **brain's lateral ventricles** (usually on the right to prevent damage to the language center) to drain cerebrospinal fluid associated with hydrocephalus. The catheter is tunneled under the skin and sutured in place with an occlusive dressing covering the insertion site. The catheter drains into a collection chamber, which is separated from a drainage bag by a stopcock that can be opened or closed. A pressure scale (which should be leveled with zero at the tragus of the ear) is at the same level as the collection chamber. The target pressure should be determined by the neurosurgeon. The dressing should be changed only if soiled, and any indication of CSF leakage or blood in the CSF should be immediately reported. The CSF output should be measured and recorded hourly (after which the collection chamber is emptied into the drainage bag) and VS and neurological assessment at least every 4 hours. The catheter should be checked when the collection chamber is emptied to ensure it is patent and not kinked. During straining or activities that involve moving the patient, the drainage should be stopped, but for short periods only. Over drainage may result in headache.

Ventricular-peritoneal shunts may become occluded or disconnected, the catheter may be positioned incorrectly, and the valve pressure may not be adequate. If the shunt does not function properly, signs of hydrocephalus and increased intracranial pressure can occur. If there is a flush valve, this may relieve the obstruction, but obstruction may be difficult to assess with radiography, so a neurosurgical consult may be indicated for revision of the shunt.

## Lumbar Drains

A lumbar drain is inserted in the lumbar region (usually L3-L4 or L4-L5) into the arachnoid space in order to drain cerebrospinal fluid. Indications for a lumbar drain include shunt infection, increased intracranial pressure, hydrocephalus, thoracoabdominal aortic aneurysm repair, and dural fistula (traumatic/postoperative). The patient should be positioned with the head of the bed elevated to 30 degrees and the transducer leveled to the phlebostatic axis or to the right atrium. The cerebrospinal fluid pressure should be monitored continuously and recorded at least every hour for the first 72 hours as well as the volume of drainage, which should be prescribed by the neurosurgeon. Over-drainage may cause a sudden decline in ICP and subarachnoid hemorrhage. Vital signs, neuromuscular and neurovascular checks should be carried out at least every hour for 24 hours. Systolic BP should be maintained ≥140 mmHg and fluid bolus administered for hypotension. After 24 hours, the patient may sit in a chair if stable, but CSF should not be drained while the patient is out of bed. Any sign of blood in CSF should be immediately reported to the neurosurgeon. Hemoglobin should be maintained at >9 mg/dL.

## Transsphenoidal Hypophysectomy

The sella turcica is a depressed area that holds the pituitary gland (which extends down from the brain on a stalk) in the sphenoid bone at the base of the skull. Pituitary tumors < 10 mm diameter are removed in a **transsphenoidal hypophysectomy**. In addition to general anesthesia, supplemental infraorbital blocks may provide postoperative pain relief. Vasoconstrictors (such as epinephrine) with local anesthesia are usually administered intranasally to control bleeding. Microscopic surgery is done with an incision in the gingival mucosa beneath the upper lip then through the nasal septum and through the roof of the sphenoid cavity to access the base of the sella turcica and the pituitary tumor. Endoscopic surgery is done directly through the nares with removal of the mucosa but no incision. After microscopic surgery, stents are placed in the nasal septum and the nose packed. With both procedures, nasal discharge must be observed for CSF leakage ("Halo sign") and the patient cautioned not to blow the nose.

## Neuro-Endovascular Interventions

### *Coiling*

Coiling is a minimally-invasive procedure used to treat cerebral aneurysm. A catheter is inserted in the femoral area and advanced to the aneurysm. Then a microcatheter with coil attached is fed through the catheter into the aneurysm until the coil fills the aneurysm. The coil is separated with an electrical current and the catheter is removed. In some cases, more than one coil may be needed. The coil is spring like and very thin. Blood enters the aneurysm about the coils and clots so that no further blood can enter, effectively sealing the aneurysm.

### *Thrombectomy*

Thrombectomy is a procedure by which an endovascular clot is removed. Various techniques may be used, but a catheter is generally inserted into the femoral vein and advanced to the clot and then the clot may be suctioned, broken up mechanically and the pieces removed, or a helical thrombectomy device wrapped around the clot so that it can be removed. Thrombectomy is used as treatment for stroke to restore blood flow as well as for removal of clots in the arms or legs.

# Neurological Pharmacology

## Anticonvulsants

### Carbamazepine (Tegretol)

*Use*: Partial, tonic-clonic, and absence seizures; analgesia for trigeminal neuralgia

*Side effects*: Dizziness, drowsiness, nausea, and vomiting. Toxic reactions include severe skin rash, agranulocytosis, aplastic anemia, and hepatitis

### Clonazepam (Klonopin)

*Use*: Akinetic, absence, and myoclonic seizures; Lennox-Gastaut syndrome

*Side effects*: Behavioral changes, hirsutism or alopecia, headaches, and drowsiness. Toxic reactions include hepatotoxicity, thrombocytopenia, ataxia, and bone marrow failure.

### Ethosuximide (Zarontin)

*Use*: Absence seizures

*Side effects*: Headaches and gastrointestinal disorders. Toxic reactions include skin rash, blood dyscrasias (sometimes fatal), hepatitis, and lupus erythematosus.

### Felbamate (Felbatol)

*Use*: Lennox-Gastaut syndrome

*Side effects*: Headache, fatigue, insomnia, and cognitive impairment. Toxic reactions include aplastic anemia and hepatic failure. It is recommended only if other medications have failed.

### Fosphenytoin (Cerebyx)

*Use*: Status epilepticus prevention and treatment during neurosurgery

*Side effects*: CNS depression, hypotension, cardiovascular collapse, dizziness, nystagmus, and pruritus.

### Gabapentin (Neurontin)

*Use*: Partial seizures; post-herpetic neuralgia

*Side effects*: Dizziness, somnolence, drowsiness, ataxia, weight gain, and nausea. Toxic reactions include hepatotoxicity and leukopenia.

### Lamotrigine (Lamictal)

*Use*: Partial and primary generalized tonic-clonic seizures; Lennox-Gastaut syndrome

*Side effects*: Tremor, ataxia, weight gain, dizziness, headache, and drowsiness. Toxic reactions include severe rash, which may require hospitalization.

**Levetiracetam (Keppra)**

*Use*: Partial onset, myoclonic, and generalized tonic-clonic seizures

*Side effects*: Idiopathic generalized epilepsy, dizziness, somnolence, irritability, alopecia, double vision, sore throat, and fatigue. Toxic reactions include bone marrow suppression and liver failure.

**Oxcarbazepine (Trileptal)**

*Use*: Partial seizures

*Side effects*: Double or abnormal vision, tremor, abnormal gait, GI disorders, dizziness, and fatigue. A toxic reaction is hepatotoxicity.

**Phenobarbital (Luminal)**

*Use*: Tonic-clonic and cortical local seizures; acute convulsive episodes; insomnia

*Side effects*: Sedation, double vision, agitation, and ataxia. Toxic reactions include anemia and skin rash.

**Phenytoin (Dilantin)**

*Use*: Tonic-clonic and complex partial seizures

*Side effects*: Nystagmus, vision disorders, gingival hyperplasia, hirsutism, dysrhythmias, and dysarthria. Toxic reactions include collapse of cardiovascular system and CNS depression.

**Primidone (Mysoline)**

*Use*: Grand mal, psychomotor, and focal seizures

*Side effects*: Double vision, ataxia, impotence, lethargy, and irritability. Toxic reactions include skin rash.

**Tiagabine (Gabitril)**

*Use*: Partial seizures

*Side effects*: Concentration problems, weak knees, dysarthria, abdominal pain, tremor, dizziness, fatigue, and agitation.

**Topiramate (Topamax)**

*Use*: Partial and tonic-clonic seizures; migraines

*Side effects*: Anorexia, weight loss, somnolence, confusion, ataxia, and confusion. Toxic reactions include kidney stones.

**Valproate/Valproic acid (Depakote, Depakene)**

*Use*: Complex partial, simple, and complex absence seizures; bipolar disorder

*Side effects*: Weight gain, alopecia, tremor, menstrual disorders, nausea, and vomiting. Toxic reactions include hepatotoxicity, severe pancreatitis, rash, blood dyscrasias, and nephritis.

**Zonisamide (Zonegran, Excegran)**

*Use*: Partial seizures

*Side effects*: Anorexia, nausea, agitation, rash, headache, dizziness, and somnolence. Toxic reactions include leukopenia and hepatotoxicity.

## Hypertonic Saline Solution

Hypertonic saline solution (HSS) has a sodium concentration higher than 0.9% (NS) and is used to reduce intracranial pressure/cerebral edema and treat traumatic brain injury. Concentrations usually range from 2% to 23.4%. The hypertonic solution draws fluid from the tissue through osmosis. As edema decreases, circulation improves. HSS also expands plasma, increasing CPP, and counteracts hyponatremia that occurs in the brain after injury.

**Administration**:

- Peripheral lines: HSS <3% only
- Central lines: HSS ≥3%

HSS can be administered continuously at rates varying from 30-150 mL/hr. Rate must be carefully controlled. Fluid status must be monitored to prevent hypovolemia, which increases risk of renal failure. Boluses (typically 30 mL of 23.4%) may be administered over 15 minutes for acute increased ICP or transtentorial herniation.

**Laboratory monitoring** includes:

- Sodium (every 6 hours): Maintain at 145-155 mmol/L. Higher levels can cause heart/respiratory/renal failure.
- Serum osmolality (every 12 hours): Maintain at 320 mOsm/L. Higher levels can cause renal failure.

## Mannitol

Mannitol is an osmotic diuretic that increases excretion of both sodium and water and reduces intracranial pressure and brain mass, especially after traumatic brain injury. Mannitol may also be used to shrink the cells of the blood-brain barrier in order to help other medications breach this barrier. Mannitol is administered per intravenous infusion:

- 2 g/kg in a 15-25% solution over 30-60 minutes

Cerebral spinal fluid pressure should show decrease within 15 minutes. Fluid and electrolyte balances must be carefully monitored as well as intake and output and body weight. Concentrations of 20-25% require a filter. Crystals may form if the mannitol solution is too cold and the mannitol container may require heating (in 80 °C water) and shaking to dissolve crystals, but the solution should be cooled to below body temperature prior to administration. Mannitol cannot be administered in polyvinylchloride bags as precipitates form. Side effects include fluid and electrolyte imbalance, nausea, vomiting, hypotension, tachycardia, fever, and urticaria.

# Gastrointestinal, Genitourinary, Gynecology, and Obstetrical Emergencies

## Gastrointestinal

### Assessment of the Gastrointestinal System

Assessment of the gastrointestinal system includes:

- Ask about personal and family history of gastrointestinal problems and risk factors, such as alcoholism, smoking, drug and medicine use, and poor dietary habits.
- Ask about symptoms, such as GI discomfort, flatus, nausea, vomiting, diarrhea, and abdominal pain.
- Determine the defecation pattern and ask about weight fluctuations.

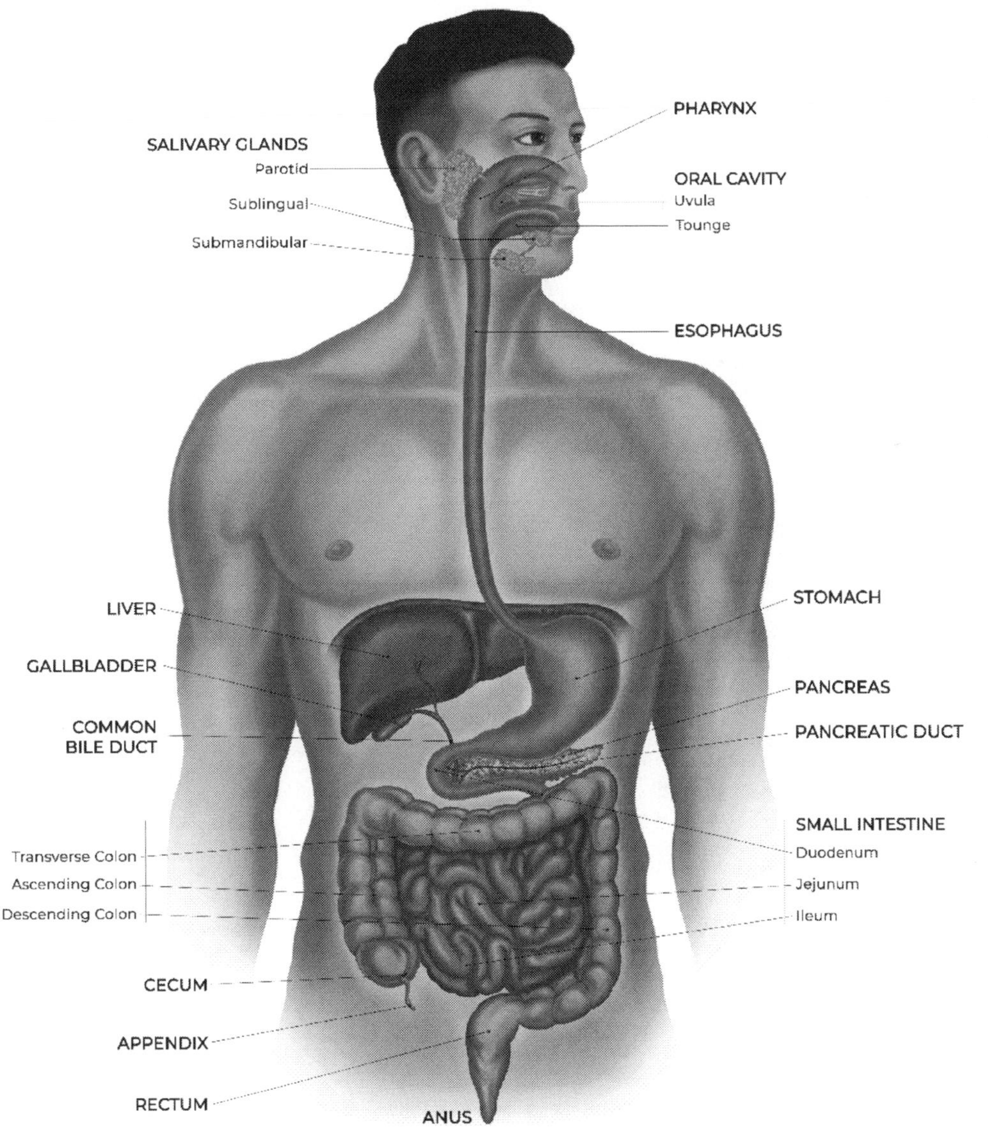

When performing a **physical assessment**, one must assess oral mucosa, tongue, teeth, pharynx, thyroid and parathyroid glands, skin color, moisture, turgor, nodules or lesions, bruises, scars, abdominal shape, and bowel sounds, assessing the abdomen in all 4 quadrants using the stethoscope diaphragm. The number of sounds heard determine if the intestines are functioning:

- **Absent**: no sounds in 3-5 minutes
- **Hypoactive**: only one sound in 2 minutes
- **Normal**: sounds heard every 5-20 seconds
- **Hyperactive**: 5-6 sounds in <30 seconds

One should examine the anal region for fissures, inflammation, tears, and dimples. Blood may be drawn for liver function studies, lipid profile, iron studies, CBC.

**Review Video: Gastrointestinal System**
Visit mometrix.com/academy and enter code: 378740

## Assessment for Gallbladder and Pancreatic Disease

Gallbladder and pancreatic assessments are prompted by the appearance of symptoms. Symptoms of gallbladder disease include epigastric discomfort following fatty food intake, abdominal distension, right upper quadrant pain, which may be colicky, nausea, and vomiting. Pain may occur intermittently.

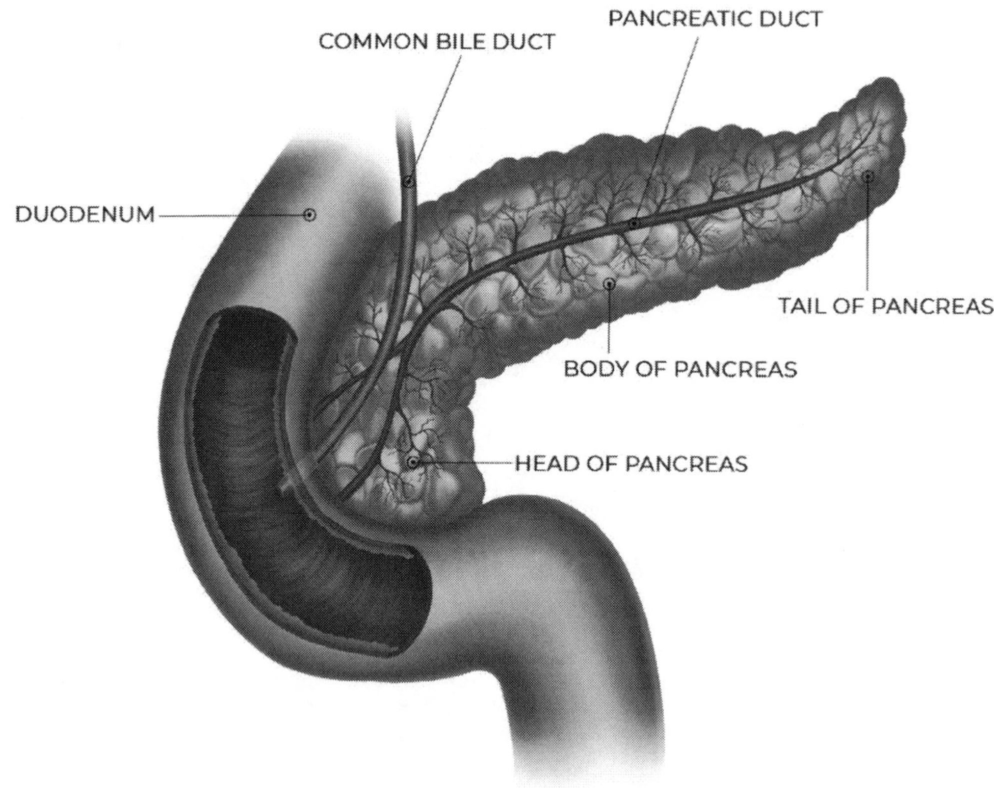

The patient with pancreatitis may have acute onset of severe abdominal pain, back pain, extensive vomiting, and dyspnea. Pancreatitis is most often related to gallstones or alcoholism, so history of alcohol use and examination for gallstones must be done:

- Assess for RUQ tenderness and mass, bowel sounds, and abdominal guarding.
- Assess the vital signs for hypotension, tachycardia, or fever and note any anxiety, agitation, or confusion.
- Note signs of hypoxia.
- Assess the skin for jaundice and bruising on the flanks and near the umbilicus.
- Blood is drawn to assess amylase and lipase, CBC, calcium, glucose, and bilirubin.

## Assessment for Liver Disease

The liver must be 70% damaged before lab tests show abnormalities. Assessment of risk factors and early symptoms are important to identify early disease. Risk factors for liver disease include alcoholism and drug abuse, risky sexual practices, exposure to infection or environmental toxins, and travel to countries with poor sanitation. One should question the patient about symptoms of liver disease, such as fatigue, itching, abdominal pain, anorexia, weight gain, fever, blood in stools or black stools, sleep problems, lack of menstruation, and lack of libido. Physical assessment includes checking vital signs and skin for scratches, pallor, jaundice, dryness, bruising, petechiae, abdominal veins and spider angiomas, and red palms:

- Assess for gynecomastia, abdominal distension, fluid waves, bowel sounds, liver margins, tenderness, consistency, and hardness and sharpness of the edge.
- Examine extremities for wasting, edema, and weakness.
- Assess neurological system for cognitive status, tremors, balance problems, slurred speech.
- Identify testicular atrophy.
- Blood should be drawn for serum enzymes and proteins, bilirubin, ammonia, clotting factors, and lipid profile.

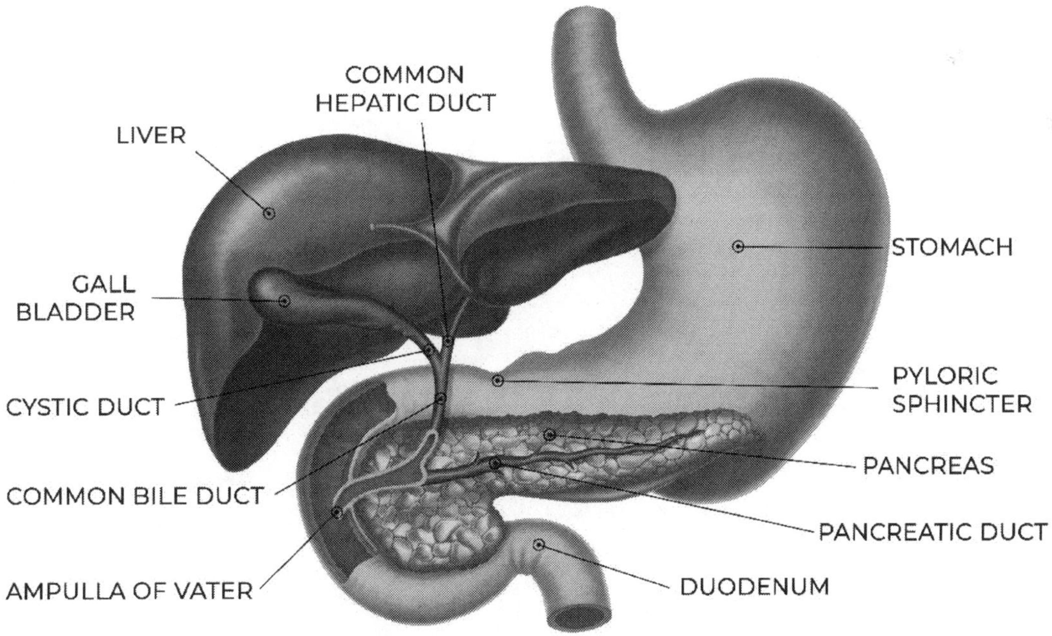

## Assessment of Nutritional Status

Assessment of nutritional status begins with an assessment of the patient's intake. The patient is asked to report intake for the previous 24 hours. This may indicate the need for a **food diary** over a period of time:

- Compare the patient's nutritional intake with the requirements of the USDA's MyPlate.
- Measure height and weight and check against a BMI table to help determine nutritional status.
- Measure waist circumference.
- Assess the patient for physical signs of poor nutrition such as muscle wasting, obesity, hair breakage and loss, poor skin turgor, ulcers, bruising, and loss of subcutaneous tissue.
- Assess mucous membranes and condition of teeth, abdomen, extremities, and thyroid gland.

Nutritional status is connected to endocrine disease, infections, other acute and chronic diseases, digestion, absorption, excretion, and storage of nutrients, so these areas must also be assessed. Blood testing should include proteins, transferrin, electrolytes, vitamins A and C, carotene, and CBC. Test urine for creatinine, thiamine, riboflavin, niacin, albumin, and iodine.

### *Assessing Nutritional Status of Hospitalized Patients*

Assessing the nutritional status of the hospital inpatient is an important part of forming a care plan. The two screening tools that are most commonly used are the **Subjective Global Assessment (SGA)** and the **Prognostic Nutritional Index (PNI)**. The SGA provides a nutritional assessment based on both the patient history and current symptoms. The patient is asked about any changes in weight and is also asked questions about his or her diet. The presence of symptoms that may lead to weight loss and poor nutritional status, such as diarrhea, nausea, and vomiting, as well as water retention (edema) and muscle wasting (cachexia), is also included in the SGA. The PNI is also used as an indicator of malnutrition and is especially helpful in determining how well a patient will recover from surgery. The PNI assesses nutritional status through the measurement of serum proteins such as albumin and transferrin combined with a skinfold measurement and a cutaneous hypersensitivity test as an indicator of immune function.

## Liver Function Studies

Liver function studies are described below:

- **Bilirubin:** Determines the ability of the liver to conjugate and excrete bilirubin, direct 0.0–0.3 mg/dL, total 0.0–0.9 mg/dL, and urine bilirubin, which should be 0
- **Total protein:** Normal: 6.0–8.0 g/dL (Albumin: 4.0–5.5 g/dL, Globulin: 1.7–3.3 g/dL); normal albumin/globulin (A/G) ratio: 1.5:1 to 2.5:1, measured by serum protein electrophoresis
- **Prothrombin time (PT):** 100% or clot detection in 10-14 seconds; PT increases with liver disease
    - International normalized ratio (PT result/normal average): <2 for those not receiving anticoagulation, 2-3 for those receiving anticoagulation, critical value >3 in patients receiving anticoagulation therapy
- **Alkaline phosphatase:** 36–93 units/L in adults (normal values vary with method); indicates biliary tract obstruction if no bone disease
- **AST (SGOT):** 10–40 units (increases with liver cell damage)
- **ALT (SGPT):** 5–35 units (increases with liver cell damage)
- **GGT, GGTP:** 5–55 µ/L females, 5–85 µ/L males (increases with alcohol abuse)
- **LDH:** 100–200 units (increases with alcohol abuse)
- **Serum ammonia:** 150–250 mg/dL (increases with liver failure)
- **Cholesterol:** Increases with bile duct obstruction and decrease with parenchymal disease

## Nutritional Lab Monitoring

### *Total Protein and Albumin*

**Total protein** levels can be influenced by many factors, including stress and infection, but it may be monitored as part of an overall nutritional assessment. Protein is critical for general health and wound healing, and because metabolic rate increases in response to a wound, protein needs increase:

- Normal values: 6–8 g/dL
- Diet requirements for wound healing: 1.25–1.5 g/kg/day

**Albumin** is a protein that is produced by the liver and is a necessary component for cells and tissues. Levels decrease with renal disease, malnutrition, and severe burns. Albumin levels are the most common screening to determine protein levels. Albumin has a half-life of 18–20 days, so it is sensitive to long-term protein deficiencies more than short-term.

- Normal values: 3.5–5.5 g/dL
- Mild deficiency: 3.0–3.5 g/dL
- Moderate deficiency: 2.5–3.0 g/dL
- Severe deficiency: <2.5 g/dL

Levels below 3.2 correlate with increased morbidity and death. Dehydration (poor intake, diarrhea, or vomiting) elevates levels, so adequate hydration is important to ensure meaningful results.

### *Prealbumin*

Prealbumin (transthyretin) is most commonly monitored for acute changes in nutritional status because it has a half-life of only 2–3 days. Prealbumin is a protein produced in the liver, so it is often decreased with liver disease. Oral contraceptives and estrogen can also decrease levels. Levels may rise with Hodgkin's disease or the use of steroids or NSAIDS. Prealbumin is necessary for transportation of both thyroxine and vitamin A throughout the body, so if **prealbumin levels** fall, both thyroxine and vitamin A utilization are also affected:

- Normal values: 16–40 mg/dL
- Mild deficiency: 10–15 mg/dL
- Moderate deficiency: 5–9 mg/dL
- Severe deficiency: <5 mg/dL

Prealbumin is a good measurement because it quickly decreases when nutrition is inadequate and rises quickly in response to increased protein intake. Protein intake must be adequate to maintain levels of prealbumin. Death rates increase with any decrease in prealbumin levels.

### *Transferrin*

Transferrin, which transports about one-third of the body's iron, is a protein produced by the liver. It transports **iron** from the intestines to the bone marrow where it is used to produce **hemoglobin**. The half-life of transferrin is about 8–10 days. It is sometimes used as a measure of nutritional status; however, transferrin levels are sensitive to many factors. Levels rapidly decrease with protein malnutrition. Liver disease and anemia can also depress levels, but a decrease in iron, commonly found with inadequate protein, stimulates the liver to produce more transferrin, which increases transferrin levels but also decreases production of albumin and prealbumin. Transferrin levels may also increase with pregnancy, use of oral contraceptives, and polycythemia. Thus, **transferrin levels** alone are not always reliable measurements of nutritional status:

- Normal values: 200–400 mg/dL
- Mild deficiency: 150–200 mg/dL
- Moderate deficiency: 100–150 mg/dL
- Severe deficiency: <100 mg/dL

## EGD

**Esophagogastroduodenoscopy (EGD)** with a flexible fiberscope equipped with a lighted fiberoptic lens allows direct inspection of the mucosa of the esophagus, stomach, and duodenum. The scope has a still or video camera attached to a monitor for viewing during the procedure. The scope may be used for biopsies or therapeutically to dilate strictures or treat gastric or esophageal bleeding. The patient is positioned on the left side (head supported) to allow saliva drainage. Conscious sedation (midazolam, propofol) is commonly used along with a topical anesthetic spray or gargle to facilitate placing the lubricated tube through the mouth into the esophagus. Atropine reduces secretions. A bite guard in the mouth prevents the patient from biting the scope. The airway must be carefully monitored through the procedure (which usually takes about 30 minutes), including oximeter to measure oxygen saturation. While perforation, bleeding, or infection may occur, most complications are cardiopulmonary in nature and relate to drugs (conscious sedation) used during the procedure, so reversal agents (flumazenil, naloxone) should be available.

**Review Video: GI Diagnostic Procedures**
Visit mometrix.com/academy and enter code: 645436

### ABDOMINAL TRAUMA

#### *SPLENIC INJURIES*

The **spleen** is the most frequently injured solid organ in blunt trauma. Injuries to the spleen are the most common because the spleen is not well protected by the rib cage and is very vascular. Symptoms may be very non-specific. Kehr sign (radiating pain in left shoulder) indicates intra-abdominal bleeding and Cullen sign (ecchymosis around umbilicus) indicates hemorrhage from ruptured spleen. Some may have right upper abdominal pain although diffuse abdominal pain often occurs with blood loss, associated with hypotension. Splenic injuries are **classified** according to the degree of injury:

- I: Tear in splenic capsules or hematoma
- II: Laceration of parenchyma (<3 cm)
- III: Laceration of parenchyma (≥3cm)
- IV: Multiple lacerations of parenchyma or burst-type injury

**Treatment**: Because removing the spleen increases the risk of life-threatening infections, every effort (bed rest, transfusion, reduced activity for at least 8 weeks) is done to avoid surgery (argon gas, fibrin "glue", or therapeutic ultrasound). Lab testing for the absence of Howell-Jolly bodies indicates the spleen in functioning properly. If conservative efforts fail (usually occurs in first 72 hours), a splenectomy is performed. After surgery, the patient has an increased risk for infection and thrombosis. Lifetime anticoagulation therapy and vaccinations (combo of pneumonia/meningitis/influenza B vaccine) should be administered.

#### *HEPATIC INJURIES*

Hepatic injury is the most common cause of death from abdominal trauma. It is particularly dangerous as hematoma rupture can occur hours to 6 weeks after the time of injury. Because hepatic injury is often associated with multiple organ damage, symptoms may be non-specific and difficult to diagnose. Therefore, elevation in liver transaminase levels or elevation of right hemidiaphragm on x-ray in trauma patients indicates damage that may require further examination. Liver injuries are classified according to the **degree of injury**:

- I: Tears in capsule with hematoma
- II: Laceration(s) of parenchyma (<3 cm)
- III: Laceration(s) of parenchyma (≥3 cm)
- IV: Destruction of 25-75% of lobe from burst injury
- V: Destruction of >75% of lobe from burst injury
- VI: Avulsion [tearing away]

Hemodynamically stable patients are managed medically, but surgical repair may be necessary if the patient is unstable or bleeding. Hemorrhage is a common complication of hepatic injury and may require ligation of hepatic arteries or veins. **Treatment** often includes intravenous fluids for fluid volume deficit as well as blood products (plasma, platelets) for coagulopathies. Surgical or angiographic embolization of the tear may be indicated in severe injury.

### *Abdominal Compartment Syndrome*

Abdominal trauma with pronounced shock increases risk of **compartment syndrome**, in which the pressure in the abdomen increases to the point of acute ischemia and anoxia of the tissues. Causes include edema of the intestines (trauma/surgical manipulation), reduced expansion of abdominal cavity (burns), hemorrhage, and capillary leakage after excessive fluid resuscitation.

**Signs/Symptoms:** Increased airway pressures and acute respiratory distress syndrome, decreased U/O, and cerebral edema.

**Diagnosis:** Increased intra-abdominal pressure (>20 $cmH_2O$), measured by a Foley catheter or NG tube with a pressure transducer or water-column manometry; elevated CVP and ICP, decreased CO and GFR.

**Treatment** includes:

- Medications: Sudden release of pressure and reperfusion may cause acidosis, hyperkalemia, vasodilation, and cardiac arrest. The patient should be given crystalloid solutions before decompression. Treatment may also include milrinone, dopamine, and mannitol.
- Surgical decompression

**Prevention**: If risk for compartment syndrome exists, the wound should not be closed, but left open and covered with a sterile dressing. Negative-pressure wound therapy may be used to decrease risk.

## Peritonitis

Peritonitis (inflammation of the peritoneum) may be primary (from infection of blood or lymph) or, more commonly, secondary, related to perforation or trauma of the gastrointestinal tract. Common causes include perforated bowel, ruptured appendix, abdominal trauma, abdominal surgery, peritoneal dialysis or chemotherapy, or leakage of sterile fluids, such as blood, into the peritoneum.

**Symptoms:** Diffuse abdominal pain with rebound tenderness (Blumberg's sign), abdominal rigidity, paralytic ileus, fever (with infection), nausea and vomiting, and sinus tachycardia.

**Diagnosis:** Increased WBC (>15,000), abdominal x-ray/CT, paracentesis, blood and peritoneal fluid culture.

**Treatment** includes:

- Intravenous fluids and electrolytes
- Broad-spectrum antibiotics
- Laparoscopy as indicated to determine cause of peritonitis and effect repair

## Appendicitis

Appendicitis is inflammation of the appendix often caused by luminal obstruction and pressure within the lumen; secretions build up and can eventually perforate the appendix. Diagnosis can be made difficult by the fact that there is some variation in the exact location of the appendix in some patients. Appendicitis can occur in all ages, but children younger than 2 years usually present with peritonitis or sepsis because of difficulty in early diagnosis. **Symptoms** include:

- Acute abdominal pain, which may be epigastric, periumbilical, right lower quadrant, or right flank with rebound tenderness
- Anorexia
- Nausea and vomiting
- Positive psoas and obturator signs
- Fever may develop after 24 hours
- Malaise
- Bowel irregularity and flatulence

**Diagnosis** is based on clinical presentation, CBC (although leukocytosis may not be present), urinalysis, and imaging studies (usually an abdominal CT with contrast).

## Cholecystitis

Cholecystitis can result in obstruction of the bile duct related to calculi as well as pancreatitis from obstruction of the pancreatic duct. In acute cholecystitis, there is fever, leukocytosis, right upper quadrant abdominal pain, and inflammation of the gallbladder. The disease is most common in overweight women 20-40 years of age, but can occur in pregnant women and people of all ages, especially those who are diabetic or elderly. Cholecystitis may develop secondary to cystic fibrosis, obesity, or total parenteral nutrition. Many times, cholecystitis may resolve in about 7-10 days on its own, but acute cholecystitis may need surgical intervention to prevent complications such as gangrene in the gallbladder or perforation. Diagnosis is confirmed by ultrasound of gallbladder showing thickening of gallbladder walls or positive Murphy's sign, or a HIDA scan showing failure to fill.

**Symptoms:**

- Severe right upper quadrant or epigastric pain (ranging from 2-6 hours per episode)
- Nausea and vomiting
- Jaundice
- Altered mental status
- Positive Murphy's sign

**Treatment**:

- Antibiotics for sepsis/ascending cholangitis
- Antispasmodic agents (glycopyrrolate) for biliary colic and vomiting
- Analgesics (note that opioids result in increased sphincter of Oddi pressure)
- Antiemetics
- Surgical consultation for possible laparoscopic or open cholecystectomy

## Erosive vs. Nonerosive Gastritis

Gastritis is inflammation of the epithelium or endothelium of the stomach. Types include:

- **Erosive**: Typically caused by alcohol, NSAIDs, illness, portal hypertension, and/or stress. Risk factors include severe illness, mechanical ventilation, trauma, sepsis, organ failure, and burns. Patients may be essentially asymptomatic but may have hematemesis or "coffee ground" emesis. Treatment depends on cause and severity but often includes a proton pump inhibitor (such as omeprazole 20-40 mg per day). Some may receive an H2-rceptor (such as famotidine). Those with portal hypertension may respond to propranolol or nadolol or portal decompression.

- **Nonerosive**: Typically caused by Helicobacter pylori infection or pernicious anemia. H. pylori infection can lead to gastric and duodenal ulcers. Treatment for H. pylori is per antibiotics and proton pump inhibitors with standard triple or standard quadruple therapy. Pernicious anemia is treated with vitamin B-12. Gastritis may also be caused by a wide range of pathogens, including parasites, so treatment depends on the causative agent.

## GASTROENTERITIS

### *VIRAL GASTROENTERITIS*

Viral gastroenteritis (commonly referred to as stomach flu) is characterized by nausea, vomiting, abdominal cramping, watery (may become bloody) diarrhea, headache, muscle aches, and fever. Viral gastroenteritis is spread through the fecal-oral route. Common **causes** include:

- **Norovirus**: Symptoms generally include diarrhea and vomiting with symptoms persisting for 1-3 days. Most people do not require treatment, but if diarrhea or vomiting is severe, an antiemetic or antidiarrheal may be prescribed if the patient is younger than 65. If severe dehydration occurs, the patient may require intravenous fluids until she is able to resume adequate oral intake.
- **Rotavirus**: Symptoms include watery diarrhea, nausea, vomiting, abdominal pain and cramping, lack of appetite and fever. Patients may become easily dehydrated and require rehydration with Pedialyte or Rice-Lyte or IV fluids. Medications are usually not needed but the rotavirus vaccine prevents severe rotavirus-related diarrhea and is given in 3 doses (2 months, 4 months, and 6 months).

### *BACTERIAL GASTROENTERITIS*

Bacterial gastroenteritis generally results in cramping, nausea, and severe diarrhea. Some bacteria cause gastroenteritis because of enterotoxins that adhere to the mucosa of the intestines and others because of exotoxins that remain in contaminated food. Some bacteria directly invade the intestinal mucosa. Bacterial gastroenteritis is commonly **caused** by:

- ***Salmonella***: Sudden onset of bloody diarrhea, abdominal cramping, nausea, and vomiting, leading to dehydration. Infection may become systemic and life-threatening. Treatment is supportive although antibiotics may be administered to those at risk.
- ***Campylobacter***: Bloody diarrhea, cramping, fever, for up to 7 days that usually resolves but may become systemic in those who are immunocompromised. Treatment is primarily supportive with antibiotics only for those at risk.
- ***Shigella* spp.**: Most common in children <5 and presents with fever, abdominal cramping, and bloody diarrhea, persisting 5-7 days. Treatment is primarily supportive (rehydration) although those at risk (very young, old, immunocompromised) may receive antibiotics because the disease may become systemic.
- ***Escherichia coli***: Different strains are associated with traveler's diarrhea and food-borne illnesses, and severity varies. Most result in diarrhea, nausea, vomiting, and cramping, but some strains (O157) may develop into life-threatening hemolytic uremic syndrome (HUS). Treatment is supportive. Antibiotics increase risk of developing HUS.

### *Parasitic Gastroenteritis*

Parasitic gastroenteritis is generally caused by infection with protozoa (one-celled pathogens):

- ***Giardia intestinalis***: Common cause of waterborne (drinking and recreational) disease and non-bacterial diarrhea, resulting from fecal contamination. Symptoms include diarrhea, abdominal cramping, flatulence, greasy floating stools, nausea and vomiting as well as weight loss. Symptoms usually persist for up to 3 weeks although some develop chronic disease. Metronidazole is the drug of choice: Adults, 250 mg TID for 5-7 days. Pediatrics, 15 mg/kg/day in 3 doses for 5-7 days.
- ***Cryptosporidium parvum***: About 10,000 cases occur in the US each year, usually from contact with fecal-contaminated water. Symptoms include watery diarrhea, abdominal pain, nausea, vomiting, weight loss, and fever and persist for up to 2 weeks although a severe chronic infection may occur in those who are immunocompromised. Treatment for non-HIV-infected patients (medications ineffective for HIV patients): Adults and children >11, Nitazoxanide 500 mg BID for 3 days. Pediatrics, 1-3 years 100 mg BID for 3 days; 4-11 years 200 mg BID for 3 days.

## Constipation and Impaction

**Constipation** is a condition with bowel movements less frequent than normal for a person, or hard, small stool that is evacuated fewer than 3 times weekly. Food moves through the GI from the small intestine to the colon in semi-liquid form. Constipation results from the colon, where fluid is absorbed. If too much fluid is absorbed, the stool can become too dry. People may have Abdominal distension and cramps and need to strain for defecation.

**Fecal impaction** occurs when the hard stool moves into the rectum and becomes a large, dense, immovable mass that cannot be evacuated even with straining, usually as a result of chronic constipation. In addition to abdominal cramps and distention, the person may feel intense rectal pressure and pain accompanied by a sense of urgency to defecate. Nausea and vomiting may also occur. Hemorrhoids will often become engorged. Fecal incontinence, with liquid stool leaking about the impaction, is common.

### *Medical Procedures to Evaluate Causes of Constipation*

Medical procedures to evaluate causes of constipation should be preceded by a careful history as this may help to define the type and guide the choice of diagnostic procedures. Most tests are necessary only for severe constipation that does not respond to treatment. Medical **diagnostic procedures** may include the following:

- **Physical exam** should include rectal exam and abdominal palpation to assess for obvious hard stool or impaction.
- **Blood tests** can identify hypothyroidism and excess parathyroid hormone.
- **Abdominal x-ray** may show large amounts of stool in the colon.
- **Barium enema** can indicate tumors or strictures causing obstruction.
- **Colonic transit studies** can show defects of the neuromuscular system.
- **Defecography** shows the defecation process and abnormalities of anatomy.
- **Anorectal manometry studies** show malfunction of anorectal muscles.
- **Colonic motility studies** measure the pattern of colonic pressure.
- **Colonoscope** allows direct visualization of the lumen of the rectum and colon.

## Bowel Obstructions

Bowel obstruction occurs when there is a mechanical obstruction of the passage of intestinal contents because of constriction of the lumen, occlusion of the lumen, adhesion formation, or lack of muscular contractions (paralytic ileus). **Symptoms** include abdominal pain, rigidity, and distention, n/v, dehydration, constipation, respiratory distress from the diaphragm pushing against the pleural cavity, sepsis, and shock. **Treatment** includes strict NPO, insertion of naso/orogastric tube, IV fluids and careful monitoring; may correct spontaneously, severe obstruction requires surgery.

## Bowel Infarctions

Bowel infarction is ischemia of the intestines related to severely restricted blood supply. It can be the result of a number of different conditions, such as strangulated bowel or occlusion of arteries of the mesentery, and may follow untreated bowel obstruction. Patients present with acute abdomen and shock, and mortality rates are very high even with resection of infarcted bowel. **Treatment** includes replacing volume, correcting the underlying issue, improving blood flow to the mesentery, insertion of NGT, and/or surgery.

## Intestinal Perforation

Intestinal perforation is a partial or complete tear in the intestinal wall, leaking intestinal contents into the peritoneum. Causes include trauma, NSAIDs (elderly, patients with diverticulitis), acute appendicitis, PUD, iatrogenic (laparoscopy, endoscopy, colonoscopy, radiotherapy), bacterial infections, IBS, and ingestion of toxic substances (acids) or foreign bodies (toothpicks). The danger posed by infection after perforation varies depending upon the site. The stomach and proximal portions of the small intestine have little bacteria, but the distal portion of the small intestine contains aerobic bacteria, such as *E. coli,* as well as anaerobic bacteria.

**Signs/Symptoms:** (appear within 24-48 hours): Abdominal pain and distention and rigidity, fever, guarding and rebound tenderness, tachycardia, dyspnea, absent bowel sounds/paralytic ileus with nausea and vomiting; Sepsis and abscess or fistula formation can occur.

**Diagnosis:** Labs: elevated WBC; lactic acid and pH change as late signs. X-ray and CT will show free air in abdominal cavity.

**Treatment** includes:

- Prompt antibiotic therapy and surgical repair with peritoneal lavage
- The abdominal wound may be left open to heal by secondary intention and to prevent compartment syndrome

## Gastroesophageal Reflux

Gastroesophageal reflux (GER) occurs when the lower esophageal sphincter fails to remain closed, allowing the contents of the stomach to back into the esophagus. This reflux of the acid containing contents of the stomach may cause irritation of the lining of the esophagus. Over time, damage to the lining of the esophagus can occur. In some patients, this may lead to the formation of Barrett's esophagus. In Barrett's esophagus, the lining of the esophagus begins to resemble the tissue lining the intestine. Patients with Barrett's esophagus have an increased risk of developing esophageal adenocarcinoma.

**Signs and symptoms**: Heartburn, dysphagia, belching, water brash, sore throat, hoarseness, and chest pain.

**Diagnosis**: Clinical signs/symptoms, ambulatory esophageal reflux monitoring (this test uses a thin pH probe that is placed in the esophagus). Data is collected on the amount of acid entering the esophagus along with the presence of clinical symptoms. Endoscopy may be used in the diagnosis of GERD in patients with persistent or progressive symptoms.

**Treatment**: GER is often treated with proton pump inhibitors (inhibit gastric acid secretion). Surgical therapy may be utilized if medical management is unsuccessful. Patients are taught to eliminate foods that trigger symptoms (chocolate, caffeine, alcohol, and highly acidic foods). In addition, patients with GERD should avoid meals 2-3 hours before bed and may find it helpful to sleep with the head of the bed elevated to alleviate symptoms.

## Peptic Ulcer Disease

Peptic ulcer disease (PUD) includes both ulcerations of the duodenum and stomach. They may be primary (usually duodenal) or secondary (usually gastric). Gastric ulcers are commonly associated with ***H. pylori*** infections (80%) but may be caused by aspirin and NSAIDs. *H. pylori* are spread in the fecal-oral route from person to person or contaminated water and cause a chronic inflammation and ulcerations of the gastric mucosa. PUD is 2 to 3 times more common in males and is associated with poor economic status that results in a crowded, unhygienic environment, although it can occur in others. Usually, other family members have a history of ulcers as well.

**Symptoms** include abdominal pain, nausea, vomiting, and GI bleeding in children younger than 6 years with epigastric and postprandial pain and indigestion in older children and adults.

**Treatment** includes:

- Antibiotics for *H. pylori*: amoxicillin, clarithromycin, metronidazole
- Proton pump inhibitors: lansoprazole or omeprazole
- Bismuth
- Histamine-receptor antagonists: cimetidine or famotidine

**Review Video: Peptic Ulcers and GERD**
Visit mometrix.com/academy and enter code: 184332

## Inflammatory Bowel Disease

### *Ulcerative Colitis*

Ulcerative colitis is superficial inflammation of the mucosa of the colon and rectum, causing ulcerations in the areas where inflammation has destroyed cells. These ulcerations, ranging from pinpoint to extensive, may bleed and produce purulent material. The mucosa of the bowel becomes swollen, erythematous, and granular. Patients may present emergently with **severe ulcerative colitis** (having >6 blood stools a day, fever, tachycardia, anemia) or with **fulminant colitis** (>10 blood stools per day, severe bleeding, and toxic symptoms) These patients are at high risk for megacolon and perforation. For patients with severe and fulminant ulcerative colitis:

**Symptoms:**

- Abdominal pain
- Anemia
- F&E depletion
- Bloody diarrhea/rectal bleeding
- Diarrhea
- Fecal urgency
- Tenesmus
- Anorexia
- Weight loss
- Fatigue
- Systemic disorders: Eye inflammation, arthritis, liver disease, and osteoporosis as immune system triggers generalized inflammation

**Treatment:**

- Glucocorticoids
- Aminosalicylates
- Antibiotics if signs/symptoms of toxicity
- D/C anticholinergics, NSAIDS, and antidiarrheals

- If fulminant: Admitted & monitored for deterioration. Kept NPO, and given IV F&E replacement. NGT for decompression if intestinal dilation is present. Knee-elbow position to reposition gas in bowel. Colectomy for those with megacolon or who are unresponsive to therapy.

**Review Video: Ulcerative Colitis**
Visit mometrix.com/academy and enter code: 584881

### *Crohn's Disease*

Crohn's disease manifests with inflammation of the GI system. Inflammation is transmural (often leading to intestinal stenosis and fistulas), focal, and discontinuous with aphthous ulcerations progressing to linear and irregular-shaped ulcerations. Granulomas may be present. Common sites of inflammation are the terminal ileum and cecum. The condition is chronic, but patients with severe or fulminant disease (fevers, persistent vomiting, abscess, obstruction) often present emergently for treatment.

**Symptoms:**

- Perirectal abscess/fistula in advanced disease
- Diarrhea
- Watery stools
- Rectal hemorrhage
- Anemia
- Abdominal pain (commonly RLQ)
- Cramping
- Weight loss
- Nausea and vomiting
- Fever
- Night sweats

**Treatment:**

- Triamcinolone for oral lesions, aminosalicylates, glucocorticoids, antidiarrheals, probiotics, avoid lactose, and identify and eliminate food triggers.
- For patients who present with toxic symptoms: hospitalization for careful monitoring, IV glucocorticoids, aminosalicylates, antibiotics, and bowel rest. Parenteral nutrition for the malnourished.
- For repeated relapses (refractory):
    - Immunomodulatory agents (azathioprine, mercaptopurine, methotrexate) or Biologic therapies (infliximab). Bowel resection if unresponsive to all treatment or with ischemic bowel.

## Diverticular Disease

Diverticular disease is a condition in which diverticula (saclike pouchings of the bowel lining that extend through a defect in the muscle layer) occur anywhere within the GI tract. About 20% of patients with diverticular disease will develop acute diverticulitis, which occurs as diverticula become inflamed when food or bacteria are retained within the diverticula. This may result in abscess, obstruction, perforation, bleeding, or fistula. Diagnosis is best confirmed by abdominal CT with contrast (showing a localized thickening of the bowel wall, increased density of soft tissue, and diverticula in the colon). Many patients have normal lab studies, but some present with leukocytosis, elevated serum amylase, and pyuria on urinalysis.

**Symptoms** (similar to appendicitis):

- Steady pain in left lower quadrant
- Change in bowel habits

- Tenesmus
- Dysuria from irritation
- Recurrent urinary infections from fistula
- Paralytic ileus from peritonitis or intra-abdominal irritation
- Toxic reactions: fever, severe pain, leukocytosis

**Treatment**:

- Rehydration and electrolytes per IV fluids
- Nothing by mouth initially
- Antibiotics, broad spectrum (IV if toxic reactions)
- NG suction if necessary, for obstruction
- Careful observation for signs of perforation or obstruction

## Acute Gastrointestinal Hemorrhage

Gastrointestinal (GI) hemorrhage may occur in the upper or lower gastrointestinal track. The primary cause (50-70%) of GI hemorrhage is gastric and duodenal ulcers, generally caused by stress, NSAIDs or infection with *Helicobacter pylori.*

**Symptoms:** Abdominal pain and distention, coffee-ground emesis/hematemesis, bloody or tarry stools, hypotension with tachycardia.

**Diagnosis:** Stool occult blood (Guaiac test), EGD, colonoscopy, GI Bleed scan.

**Treatment** includes:

- Medications: Fluid replacement with blood transfusions if necessary, antibiotic therapy for *Helicobacter pylori,* continuous pantoprazole IV to prevent further irritation
- Endoscopic thermal therapy to cauterize or injection therapy (hypertonic saline, epinephrine, ethanol) to cause vasoconstriction
- Arteriography with intra-arterial infusion of vasopressin and/or embolizing agents, such as stainless-steel coils, platinum microcoils, or Gelfoam pledgets
- Vagotomy and pyloroplasty if bleeding persists

**Prevention**: Prophylactic medications (pantoprazole [Protonix] IV is common).

## Hepatic Cirrhosis

### *Compensated*

Cirrhosis is a chronic hepatic disease in which normal liver tissue is replaced by the fibrotic tissue that impairs liver function. There are three **types**:

- **Alcoholic** (from chronic alcoholism) is the most common type and results in fibrosis about the portal areas. The liver cells become necrotic, replaced by fibrotic tissue, with areas of normal tissue projecting in between, giving the liver a hobnail appearance.
- **Post-necrotic** with broad bands of fibrotic tissue is the result of acute viral hepatitis.
- **Biliary**, the least common type, is caused by chronic biliary obstruction and cholangitis, with resulting fibrotic tissue about the bile ducts.

Cirrhosis may be either compensated or decompensated. **Compensated** cirrhosis usually involves non-specific symptoms, such as intermittent fever, epistaxis, ankle edema, indigestion, abdominal pain, and palmar erythema. Hepatomegaly and splenomegaly may also be present.

### *DECOMPENSATED*

Decompensated cirrhosis occurs when the liver can no longer adequately synthesize proteins, clotting factors, and other substances so that portal hypertension occurs.

**Symptoms:**

- Hepatomegaly
- Chronic elevated temperature
- Clubbing of fingers
- Purpura resulting from thrombocytopenia, with bruising and epistaxis
- Portal obstruction resulting in jaundice and ascites
- Bacterial peritonitis with ascites
- Esophageal varices
- Edema of extremities and presacral area resulting from reduced albumin in the plasma. Vitamin deficiency from interference with formation, use, and storage of vitamins, such as A, C, and K
- Anemia from chronic gastritis and decreased dietary intake
- Hepatic encephalopathy with alterations in mentation
- Hypotension
- Atrophy of gonads

**Treatment** varies according to the symptoms and is supportive rather than curative as the fibrotic changes in the liver cannot be reversed:

- Dietary supplements and vitamins
- Diuretics (potassium sparing), such as Aldactone and Dyrenium, to decrease ascites
- Colchicine to reduce fibrotic changes
- Liver transplant (the definitive treatment)

## FULMINANT HEPATITIS

Fulminant hepatitis is a severe acute infection of the liver that can result in hepatic necrosis, encephalopathy, and death within 1 to 2 weeks. Most hepatitis is caused by infection with hepatitis viruses A, B, C, D, or E, but it can also be caused by numerous viruses, toxic chemicals (carbon tetrachloride), metabolic diseases (Wilson disease), and drugs, such as acetaminophen. Fulminant hepatitis can result from any of these factors. Fulminant hepatitis can be divided into three stages according to the duration from jaundice to encephalopathy:

0 to 7 days = Hyperacute liver failure
7 to 28 days = Acute liver failure
28 to 72 days = Subacute liver failure

**Symptoms**:

- Poor feeding/anorexia
- Increased intracranial pressure with cerebral edema and encephalopathy
- Coagulopathies
- Renal failure
- Electrolyte imbalances

**Treatment**:

- Identify and treat underlying cause
- Intracranial pressure monitoring and treatment

- Diuresis; liver transplantation may be necessary
- Survival rates vary from 50-85%

## Portal Hypertension

Portal hypertension occurs when obstructed blood flow increases blood pressure throughout the portal venous system, preventing the liver from filtering blood and causing the development of collateral blood vessels that return unfiltered blood to the systemic circulation. Increasing serum aldosterone levels cause sodium and fluid retention in the kidneys, resulting in hypervolemia, ascites and esophageal varices. Portal hypertension can be caused by any liver disease, especially cirrhosis and inherited or acquired coagulopathies that cause thrombosis of the portal vein.

**Symptoms:** Ascites with distended abdomen, esophageal varices with bleeding, dyspnea, abdominal discomfort, fluid/electrolyte imbalances.

**Diagnosis:** Labs (CBC, BMP, liver panel, Hep B &C), abdominal ultrasound or CT/MRI, EGD, Hemodynamic measurement of the hepatic venous pressure gradient (HVPG)

**Treatment** includes:

- Restricted sodium intake & use diuretics as needed
- Endoscopic treatment of obstruction
- Portal vein shunting redirecting blood from the portal vein to the vena cava
- Liver transplant in severe cases
- These patients are at high risk for esophageal varices, which, if they rupture, can cause instantaneous hemorrhage and death

## Esophageal Varices

Esophageal varices are torturous, dilated veins in the submucosa of the esophagus (usually the distal portion). They are a complication of cirrhosis of the liver, in which obstruction of the portal vein causes an increase in collateral vessels and resulting decrease in circulation to the liver, increasing the pressure in the collateral vessels. This causes the vessels to dilate. Because they tend to be fragile and inelastic, they tear easily, causing sudden, massive esophageal hemorrhage.

**Signs/Symptoms:** Usually asymptomatic until rupture; projectile vomiting bright red blood, dark stools, and shock.

**Diagnosis:** EGD, capsule endoscopy, CT, and MRI.

**Treatment** (in the case of rupture) includes:

- Emergent fluid and blood replacement
- IV vasopressin, somatostatin, and octreotide to decrease venous pressure and provide vasoconstriction/clotting
- Endoscopic injection with sclerosing agents and band ligation
- Esophagogastric balloon tamponade using Sengstaken-Blakemore and Minnesota tubes (Note: always inflate gastric balloon first, keep scissors nearby in case of balloon migration, do not use longer than 24 hrs as there is increased risk of ulceration from pressure.)
- Transjugular intrahepatic portosystemic shunting (TIPS) creates a channel between systemic and portal venous systems to reduce portal hypertension

## Hepatic Coma

Hepatic coma or hepatic encephalopathy occurs when the liver's inability to remove ammonia and other toxins from the bloodstream causes a decrease in neurologic function. Hepatic encephalopathy often occurs in patients with severe liver disease, most commonly in patients diagnosed with cirrhosis of the liver. The fibrous tissue that forms in cirrhosis affects the liver structure and impedes the blood flow to the liver, ultimately causing the liver to fail. There are four stages of hepatic encephalopathy ranging from grade 0 to grade 4. Grade 4 encephalopathy is defined as hepatic coma. Neurologic alterations may progress slowly and if left untreated may result in irreversible neurologic damage.

**Signs and symptoms**: Altered mental status, personality or mood changes, poor judgment, and poor concentration. As symptoms progress, patients may experience agitation, disorientation, drowsiness, increasing confusion, lethargy, slurred speech, tremors, and seizures. In grade 4 encephalopathy, patients become unresponsive and ultimately comatose.

**Diagnosis**: Physical assessment, lab tests including a complete blood count, liver function tests, serum ammonia levels, BUN, creatinine and electrolyte levels, CT or MRI of the brain, and electroencephalogram may be used to diagnose hepatic encephalopathy.

**Treatment**: Address precipitating factors such as infection, gastrointestinal bleeding, dehydration, hypotension, or alcohol use. Other treatment options may include limiting protein intake, administration of lactulose to prevent the absorption of ammonia, and the administration of an antibiotic such as neomycin, rifaximin, or Flagyl to reduce the serum ammonia level.

## Acute Pancreatitis

Acute pancreatitis is related to chronic alcoholism or cholelithiasis in 90% of patients, but may have unknown etiology. It may also be triggered by a variety of drugs (tetracycline, thiazides, acetaminophen, and oral contraceptives). Complications may include shock, acute respiratory distress syndrome, and MODs.

**Signs/Symptoms:** acute pain (mid-epigastric, LUQ, or generalized), nausea and vomiting, Abdominal distension.

**Diagnosis:** Serum lipase (>2x normal), amylase (less accurate), CT with contrast, abdominal U/S, MRI cholangiopancreatography, ERCP.

**Treatment** (supportive) includes:

- **Medications**: IV fluids, antiemetics, antibiotics (if necrosis is secondary to infection), and analgesia. NOTE: do not give morphine, can cause spasms in sphincter of Oddi, making pain worse.
- **TPN, NPO, or restricted to clear liquids** may help manage vomiting, ileus, and aspiration.
- **Surgical**: may remove gallbladder and biliary duct obstructions if cause of recurrent pancreatitis.

**Prevention**: Avoid smoking and alcohol consumption; limit fat intake and increase fresh fruits/vegetables and water.

## Hernias

Hernias are protrusions into or through the abdominal wall and may occur in children and adults. Hernias may contain fat, tissue, or bowel. There are a number of **types:**

- **Direct inguinal hernias** occur primarily in adults and rarely incarcerate.
- **Indirect inguinal hernias** related to congenital defect is most common on the right in males and can incarcerate, especially during the first year and in females.
- **Femoral hernias** occur primarily in women and may incarcerate.
- **Umbilical hernias** occur in children, especially those of African-American descent, and rarely incarcerate. They may also occur in adults, primarily women, and may incarcerate.
- **Incisional hernias** are usually related to obesity or wound infections, and may incarcerate.

Hernias are evident on clinical examination.

**Symptoms** of incarceration include:

- Severe pain
- Nausea and vomiting
- Soft mass at hernia site
- Tachycardia
- Temperature

**Treatment** for hernias includes:

- Reduction if incarceration is very recent with patient in Trendelenburg position and gentle compression
- Surgical excision and fixation
- Broad-spectrum antibiotics

## Biliary Atresia

Biliary atresia is a rare life-threatening condition that occurs in infancy of unknown cause. Bile ducts are tubes that transport bile from the liver to the gallbladder (where it is stored) and the small intestine (where it aids in digestion). Biliary atresia occurs when the bile ducts (either inside or outside of the liver) become inflamed, causing damage to the ducts and an impedance of bile flow. Without treatment, the trapped bile causes damage to the liver eventually causing it to fail. The life expectancy for infants with untreated biliary atresia is approximately 2 years.

**Signs and symptoms**: Early identification is key in successfully treating biliary atresia. Signs and symptoms include dark urine, gray or white stools, slow weight gain and delayed growth, jaundice, abdominal swelling, and itching.

**Diagnosis**: Physical assessment, abdominal films, ultrasound, lab tests including bilirubin levels, and liver biopsy.

**Treatment**: The only treatment options for biliary atresia are liver transplant or the Kasai procedure. Named after the surgeon who invented it, the Kasai procedure involves using a loop of intestine to act as a new bile duct and removing the damaged ducts. Flow of bile is then restored to the small intestine. The Kasai procedure is most successful when performed on younger infants (less than 3 months old).

## Malnutrition and Malabsorption in Critically Ill Patients

**Malabsorption** occurs when an abnormality or alteration in the gastrointestinal tract affects the absorption of nutrients through the small intestine. It can also occur with damage to the small intestine due to infection, trauma, surgery, or radiation therapy; patients in ICU's are at an increased risk due to multiple illnesses, intubation/prolonged NPO status, vasopressors decreasing blood flow to the bowel, and other factors that make receiving adequate nutrition difficult. Malabsorption often leads to **malnutrition**. Hospitalized malnourished patients are at a higher risk for infection, respiratory failure, heart failure, arrhythmias and delayed or decreased wound healing.

**Signs and symptoms**: Bloating, cramping, gas, chronic diarrhea, failure to thrive, muscle wasting, weight loss, steatorrhea, anemia, electrolyte imbalance and vitamin/mineral deficiencies.

**Diagnosis**: Serum electrolytes, complete blood count, ferritin, vitamin B12, folate, albumin, and protein. Stool fat testing may be performed to assess for the presence of fat in the stool that occurs in certain disorders that affect fat absorption. Endoscopy may be used to diagnose an abnormality in the mucosa lining of the bowel.

**Treatment**: Replacement of nutrients that have been lost as a result of malabsorption as well as treatment for the cause of the malabsorption. Supplemental treatment with enzymes found to be deficient may also be incorporated into the treatment plan.

**Prevention**: Ensure patients with prolonged "NPO" status have alternative means of nutrition (TPN, tube feeds, etc.).

## NG Tubes, Sump Tubes, and Levin Tubes

Nasogastric **(NG) tubes** are plastic or vinyl tubes inserted through the nose, down the esophagus, and into the stomach. **Sump tubes** are radiopaque with a vent lumen to prevent a vacuum from forming with high suction. **Levin tubes** have no vent lumen and are used only with low suction. NG tubes drain gastric secretions, allow sampling of secretions, or provide access to the stomach and upper GI tract. They are used for lavage after medication overdose, for decompression, and for instillation of medications or fluids. NG tubes are contraindicated with obstruction proximal to the stomach or gastric pathology, such as hemorrhage.

*Tube-insertion length is estimated: earlobe to xiphoid + earlobe to nose tip + 15 cm.*

The tube is inserted through the naris with the patient upright, if possible, and swallowing sips of water. Vasoconstrictors and topical anesthetic reduce gag reflex. Placement is checked with insufflation of air or aspiration of stomach contents and verified by x-ray. The NG is secured and drainage bag provided. Tubes attached to continuous low or intermittent high suction must be monitored frequently.

**Levin Tube**

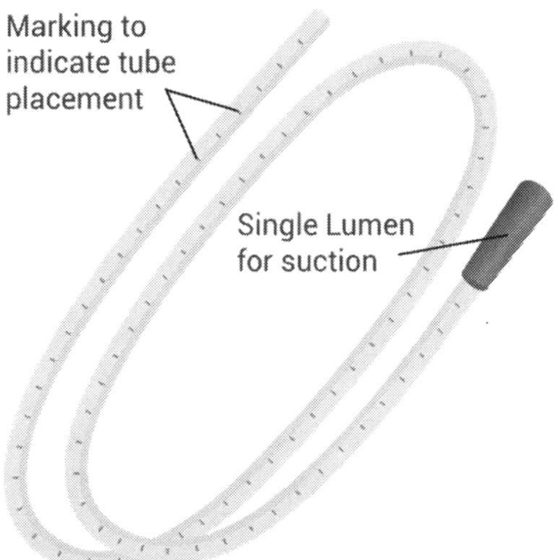


## PEG Tube

**Percutaneous endoscopic gastrostomy** (PEG), used for tube feedings, involves intubation of the esophagus with the endoscope and insertion of a sheathed needle with a guidewire through the abdomen and stomach wall so that a catheter can be fed down the esophagus, snared, and pulled out through the opening where the needle was inserted and secured. The PEG tube should not be secured to the abdomen until the PEG is fully healed, which usually takes 2 to 4 weeks, because tension caused by taping the tube against the abdomen may cause the tract to change shape and direction. The tract should be straight to facilitate insertion and removal of catheters. Once the tract has healed, the original PEG tube can generally be replaced with a balloon gastrostomy tube. External stabilizing devices can be applied to the skin to hold the tube in place but should be placed 1 to 2 cm above the skin surface to prevent excessive tension that may result in buried bumper syndrome (BBS) in which the internal fixation device becomes lodged in the mucosal lining of the gastric wall, resulting in ulceration.

## Drains

The following are different types of drains a patient may have, including pertinent nursing considerations:

- **Simple drains** are latex or vinyl tubes of varying sizes/lengths. They are usually placed through a stab wound near the area of involvement.
- **Penrose drains** are flat, soft rubber/latex tubes placed in surgical wounds to drain fluid by gravity and capillary action.

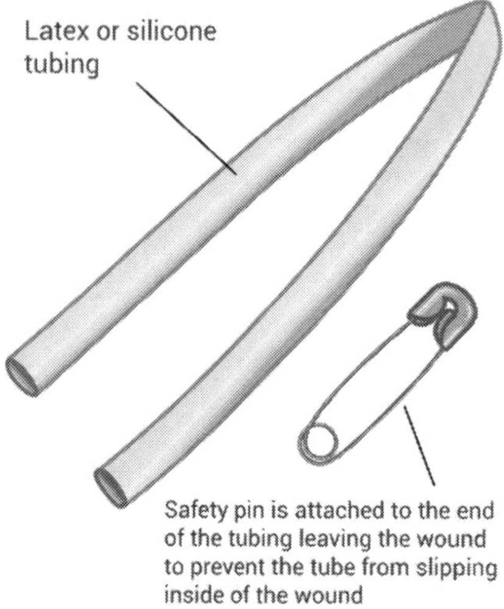


- **Sump drains** are double-lumen or tri-lumen tubes (with a third lumen for infusions). The multiple lumens produce venting when air enters the inflow lumen and forces drainage out of the large lumen.
- **A percutaneous drainage catheter** is inserted into the wound to provide continuous drainage for infection/fluid collection. Irrigation of the catheter may be required to maintain patency. Skin barriers and pouching systems may also be necessary.

SAFE PERCUTANEOUS DRAINAGE KIT

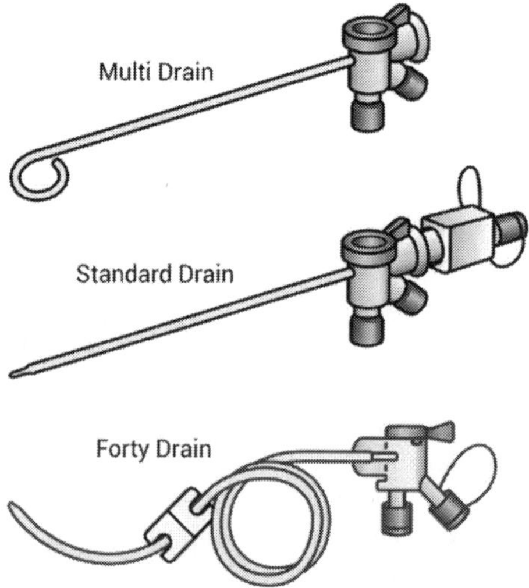

- **Closed drainage systems** use low-pressure suction to provide continuous gravity drainage of wounds. Drains are attached to collapsible suction reservoirs that provide negative pressure. The nurse must remember to always re-establish negative pressure after emptying these drains. There are two types in frequent use:
  - *Jackson-Pratt is* a bulb-type drain that is about the size of a lemon. A thin plastic drain from the wound extends to a squeeze bulb that can hold about 100 mL of drainage.

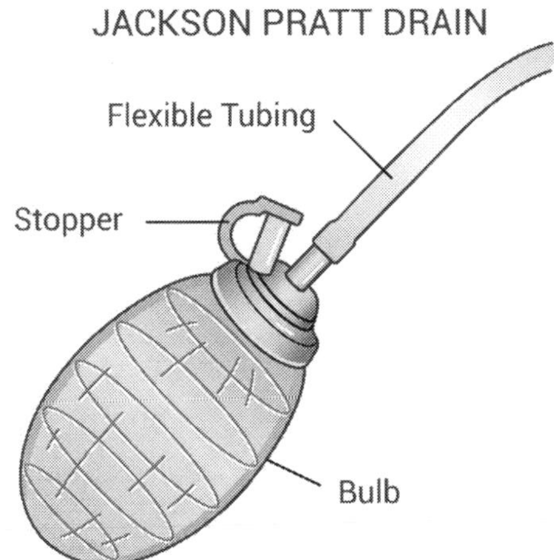


  - *Hemovac* is a round drain with coiled springs inside that are compressed after emptying to create suction. The device can hold up to 500 mL of drainage.

## Determining the Caloric Requirements of Critically Ill Patients

When an individual requires hospitalization for a critical illness, his or her **caloric requirements** must be determined so that normal body function is maintained, and so that recovery is as quick as possible. There are many factors that must be considered when attempting to determine the requirements of an ill patient. First, the **age** of the patient is important. If the patient is a growing child or adolescent, he or she will have very different nutritional requirements than an elderly individual would have. Also, to be considered is the **physical and nutritional status** of the patient, independent of the illness. A patient who is normally very active would have different requirements than an overweight, sedentary individual. Along the same lines, **comorbidities**, such as diabetes and atherosclerosis, need to be considered, as well as overall **stress levels** of the patient.

## Enteral Support and Parenteral Support

**Enteral nutrition** is a method of providing nutrition to a patient through a tube; the tube may be placed in either the nose (a nasogastric tube), the stomach (a percutaneous endoscopic gastrostomy [PEG] tube), or the small bowel (a percutaneous endoscopic jejunal [J] tube). When the tube has been placed, nutrition can be administered through the tube and absorbed by the patient's digestive system. Various **enteric formulas** exist, and the choice is dependent on the nutritional requirements of the patient.

**Parenteral nutrition** (also called total parenteral nutrition [**TPN**]) is a method of providing nutrition that completely bypasses the digestive system by administering nutrition through an intravenous line. Enteral support is the preferred method of providing nutrition, although in patients suffering from some compromise of the gastrointestinal tract, parenteral nutrition is the only option.

## Trouble-Shooting Problems Related to Enteral Feedings

**Feeding tubes** are commonly found in the critical care setting, as many patients are intubated and unable to take oral nutrition or medication. General maintenance involves checking placement before flushing anything into the tube (prevents aspiration), flushing the tubes with at least 30 mL of water before and after use, and every 4 hours. Never crush enteric-coated medications, and keep the HOB inclined at least 30° at all times during feeding. **Complications** include:

- **Vomiting/aspiration:** Caused by incorrect placement, gastric emptying, and/or formula intolerance.
    - Treatment: Confirm placement by checking pH (preferred to air bolus); delay feeding one hour and check residual volume before resuming. Refrigerate formula, check expiration, and use only for 24 hours.
- **Diarrhea:** Caused by rapid feeding, antibiotics/medications, intolerance of formula or hypertonic formula, and/or tube migration.
    - Treatment: Reduce rate of feeding, evaluate medications, avoid hanging feedings longer than 8 hours, and add fiber or decrease sodium in the feed.
- **Displacement of tube:**
    - Treatment: For NG tube, replace using the other nostril, only if not surgically placed. For G-tube or J-tube, cover the site and notify the physician.
    - Prevention: secure all tubes with the appropriate device and mark placement to identify migration.
- **Tube occlusion:**
    - Treatment: Check for kinks and obvious problems. Aspirate fluid, instill warm water, and aspirate to loosen occlusion. The physician may order an enzyme or sodium bicarb solution.

## TPN

**Total parenteral nutrition** (TPN) is an intravenous hypertonic solution containing glucose, fat emulsion, protein, minerals, and vitamins. TPN is generally given through a central line (PICC if short-term), and used only when other methods of nutrition are not feasible.

**Nursing considerations:**

- **Infection prevention**: Use aseptic technique for feedings and dressing changes; change solution, filter, and tubing every 24 hours, discard cloudy solutions, and monitor the site for signs of infection.
- **Risk of embolus/contamination**: Use micropore filter (TPN without fat emulsion) or 1.2-micron filter (TPN with fat emulsion); heparin can be added to the solution. Never infuse any medication or product in the same line as the TPN; blood cannot be drawn from this line either.
- **Malnutrition and electrolytes**: Check daily weight and check BMP and CBC 3x a week until stable, then weekly. Check the label and ingredients before administration and watch for signs of fluid overload. A cloudy blood specimen could indicate hyperlipidemia. Patients on TPN are also at risk for hyperammonemia (demonstrated by asterixis and altered mental status) and azotemia (demonstrated by dehydration and elevated BUN).
- **Hyper/hypoglycemia**: Initiate slowly, increasing rate over 24-48 hours. NEVER try to "catch-up" at a higher rate if there is a delay/pause in feeding; only administer with a pump and do not change the rate without order. If the bag runs out, hang a bag of D10W until a new bag can be obtained. Monitor BG every 4-6 hours; sliding scale insulin may be used.

## Gastrointestinal Surgery

### *Whipple*

The Whipple (pancreaticoduodenectomy) procedure is used to surgically remove the head of the pancreas, the gallbladder, part of the bile duct, the duodenum, and sometimes the distal portion of the stomach. After excision, the remaining pancreas, bile duct, and intestinal stump are sutured to the intestine so that secretions empty into the intestine. The Whipple procedure may be done as an open procedure or laparoscopically. This procedure is used primarily for malignant or benign tumors of the head of the pancreas but can also be used for chronic pancreatitis, duodenal cancer, cancer of the ampulla, and cholangiocarcinoma. Whipple is recommended only if the cancer has not spread beyond the pancreas and has not invaded major vessels.

Usually, the pancreas is still able to produce adequate insulin, but the production of pancreatic enzymes may be impaired. A pylorus-preserving variation preserves the stomach and part of the pylorus to decrease nutritional deficiencies and weight loss associated with the standard Whipple.

Post-op treatment includes monitoring fluid/electrolyte balance and monitoring drains. These patients have a very high risk of developing numerous complications, including peritonitis, bowel obstruction, sepsis, and acute abdomen, along with others.

### *Esophagectomy and Esophagogastrectomy*

**Esophageal cancer** starts in the inner layer of the esophagus and spreads. It may develop after long-term reflux because of cell changes brought about by gastric acid. Symptoms include throat or epigastric discomfort, increasing dysphagia and inability to swallow solids, unexplained weight loss, hoarseness, hiccups, hematemesis, and the feeling of something in the throat. *Treatment* for esophageal cancer involves surgical removal of the affected portion of the esophagus. Two common procedures include:

- **Esophagectomy** is the removal of all or part of the esophagus with the distal end resutured to the stomach or an intestinal graft used to replace the excised portion of the esophagus.
- **Esophagogastrectomy** is the removal of the distal portion of the esophagus, lymph nodes, and the upper portion of the stomach, after which the remaining esophagus and stomach are reattached.

#### Postoperative Management

Postoperative management for esophagectomy/gastrectomy includes the following:

- Monitor intubation and ventilation (increased risk for ARDS), encourage pulmonary hygiene, and monitor chest tubes (change in color or sudden increase in drainage could indicate leak; notify physician).
- Subcutaneous emphysema in the chest/neck could indicate a leak in the anastomosis and should be reported immediately.
- Manage pain, which is often severe; a PCA or epidural may be used initially.
- Hemodynamics: IV fluids, 100-200 mL/hr, bolus PRN; however, be cautious as there is an increased risk of pulmonary edema.
- Monitor the NG tube; **NEVER replace or irrigate the NG tube**, as it could damage the anastomosis. Notify MD if complications arise.
- Maintain NPO for 5-7 days; nutrition should be provided via J-tube or TPN.
- Drains: Penrose, Jackson-Pratt, possible drainage collection bag at the base of the cervical incision for saliva if >250 mL in 8 hr.
  *NOTE*: Patients often have history of alcohol abuse; observe for signs of DTs/withdrawal.
- Prior to initiating oral intake, a fluoroscopic examination with water-soluble contrast will be done to check for leaks. If no leaks, patients begin with clear liquids and progress to 6 to 8 small meals per day.

### *Bariatric Gastrointestinal Surgery*

Bariatric surgery is used to promote weight loss in the morbidly obese (100 pounds over normal weight or BMI of 35-40). Surgery is done to restrict intake and/or prevent the absorption of calories. Procedures are open surgical or laparoscopic and include:

- **Banding** places a band around the upper portion of the stomach, creating a small pouch with a small distal opening to slow gastric emptying.
- **Sleeve gastrectomy** removes about 2/3 of the stomach, and a distal part of the small intestine is attached, bypassing part of the small intestine, reducing absorption.

- **Roux-en-Y** uses staples and a vertical band to decrease the size of the stomach, creating a small pouch. Then, a section of the small intestine is attached to the pouch, bypassing the first and second segments of the intestine to reduce absorption.
- **Gastric ballooning** places a balloon in the stomach and fills it with liquid to decrease stomach capacity; this is used primarily in Europe.

**Nursing considerations:** Use extreme caution with post-bariatric NG/PEG tubes – generally do not check placement/irrigate with normal amounts (risk of rupturing stomach); ensure patient maintains strict NPO. There is an increased risk of respiratory complications post-surgery.

## Monitoring Devices for Abdominal Compartment Syndrome

Measurement of **intra-abdominal pressure** is obtained by attaching a pressure transducer or water-column manometer to a Foley catheter in the bladder, because bladder pressure correlates with abdominal pressure. The patient should be in the supine position if possible. The bladder must be empty for accurate measurement. The catheter should be clamped and transducer zeroed at the iliac crest along the midaxillary line. Then, 2-25 mL (usually about 10 mL for critically ill) of fluid is injected into the bladder and left in place for 30-60 seconds before the reading pressure following a patient expiration. Compartment pressures should be <30 mmHg and the difference between diastolic BP and compartment pressure should be >30 mmHg. Intraabdominal pressure may also be checked with an indwelling NG tube. If the risk for compartment syndrome exists, the wound should not be closed. Sudden release of pressure and reperfusion may cause acidosis, vasodilation, and cardiac arrest, so the patient should be given crystalloid solutions before decompression.

## Indwelling Fecal Management Systems

Indwelling fecal management systems are used for incontinent clients with loose or watery stools in order to prevent skin breakdown, discomfort, odor, and contamination of wounds, and to control the spread of organisms, such as *Clostridium difficile,* in bedridden or immobile clients. A number of different devices, such as the Flexi-Seal FMS, are available and work similarly. A typical management system includes:

- A silicone catheter
- A silicone retention balloon at end of the catheter
- A 45-mL syringe
- Charcoal filter collection bags

The application of the fecal management system is relatively simple: The catheter is inserted into the rectum and the balloon is inflated with water or saline (using the 45-mL syringe) to hold it in place and to block fecal leakage. Some systems, such as Flexi-Seal FMS, have a pop-up button to indicate when the balloon is adequately filled for the size of the rectum. The catheter contains an irrigation port so that irrigating fluid can be instilled if necessary. The charcoal filter collection bag is attached to the end of the silicone catheter to contain fecal material.

## Histamine Receptor Antagonists

Histamine (H) receptor antagonists (actually reverse agonists) are used to treat conditions in which excessive stomach acid causes heartburn and GERD. They block histamine 2 ($H_2$) (parietal) cell receptors in the stomach, thereby decreasing acid production. These drugs are used less commonly now than proton-pump inhibitors. **Common $H_2$ antagonists** include:

- **Cimetidine (Tagamet)**: The first $H_2$ antagonist, it is used less frequently than others because of inhibition of enzymes that results in drug interactions, especially with contraceptive agents and estrogen.
- **Famotidine (Pepcid)**: This may be combined with an antacid to increase the speed of effects as it has a slow onset. It may be used pre-surgically to reduce post-operative nausea.

- **Nizatidine**: The last $H_2$ antagonist developed, it is used to treat ulcers and GERD. It is about equal in potency and action to ranitidine, which was discontinued due to the presence of NDMA, a cancer-causing contaminant, when stored in high temperatures.

## Antacids

Antacids are medications used to reduce stomach acids by raising the pH and neutralizing the acids present. They are commonly used to treat heartburn or indigestion. Adverse reactions are relatively rare unless taken to excess or with renal impairment. Drugs include:

- **Aluminum hydroxide** (Amphojel) may cause constipation and with renal impairment, hypophosphatemia and osteomalacia.
- **Magnesium hydroxide** (Milk of Magnesia) may cause diarrhea and with renal impairment can cause hypermagnesemia.
- **Aluminum hydroxide with magnesium hydroxide** (Maalox, Mylanta) may cause nausea, vomiting and diarrhea, yeast infection (thrush), or hypophosphatemia.
- **Calcium carbonate** (TUMS, Rolaids, Titralac) may cause gastric distention. Excess calcium intake may cause toxic reactions, including kidney stones and renal failure, so excess intake should be avoided.
- **Alka-Seltzer** combines sodium bicarbonate with aspirin and citric acid so this compound may cause gastric irritation, nausea and vomiting, and tarry stools.
- **Bismuth subsalicylate** (Pepto-Bismol). Pepto-Bismol may react with sulfur in the body to create a black tongue and black stools, but this is temporary. Pepto-Bismol has been associated with Reye's syndrome in children with influenza or chickenpox.

## Proton Pump Inhibitors

Proton pump inhibitors (PPIs) are now used more frequently than histamine receptor antagonists. PPIs interfere with an acid-producing enzyme in the stomach wall, reducing stomach acid. PPIs are used to treat GERD, stomach ulcers, and *H. pylori* (with antibiotics). PPIs are similar in action and include:

- Esomeprazole (Nexium)
- Lansoprazole (Prevacid)
- Omeprazole (Prilosec)
- Pantoprazole (Protonix)
- Rabeprazole (Aciphex)
- Omeprazole/sodium bicarbonate (Zegerid) (Long-acting form of omeprazole)

Common side effects include gastrointestinal upset (nausea, diarrhea, and constipation), headache, and rash. In rare instances, PPIs may cause severe muscle pain; however, they are usually well-tolerated with few adverse effects. PPIs may interfere with the absorption of some drugs, such as those that are affected by stomach acid. Absorption of ketoconazole is impaired, and absorption of digoxin is increased, sometimes leading to toxicity. Omeprazole impacts the hepatic breakdown of drugs more than other PPIs and may cause increased levels of diazepam, phenytoin, and warfarin.

## ANTI-LIPIDS

Anti-lipid medications are frequently used to **lower cholesterol levels** if dietary modifications are unsuccessful in order to decrease coronary artery disease. Four primary **types** of medications include the following:

- **Statins** (3-hydroxy-3-methylglutaryl coenzyme A reductase inhibitors), such as atorvastatin (Lipitor), rosuvastatin (Crestor), fluvastatin (Lescol), lovastatin (Altoprev), pravastatin (Pravachol), and simvastatin (Zocor), inhibit the liver enzyme that produces cholesterol, but different statins vary in the ability to reduce cholesterol and in drug/other interactions (protease inhibitors, erythromycin, grapefruit juice, niacin, and fibric acids). Adverse effects include rhabdomyolysis (which causes severe muscle pain and weakness), headache, rash, weakness, and gastrointestinal disorders.
- **Nicotinic acid** (Niacor, Niaspan) decreases synthesis of lipoprotein, lowers low-density lipoprotein (LDL) and triglycerides, and increases high-density lipoprotein (HDL). It is used for low elevations of cholesterol and may be combined with statins. Adverse effects include flushing, hyperglycemia, gout, upper gastrointestinal disorders, and hepatotoxicity. Liver function must be monitored.
- **Bile acid sequestrants,** such as cholestyramine (Questran, Prevalite), colesevelam (WelChol), and colestipol HCL (Colestid), decrease LDL, increase HDL, and do not affect triglyceride levels. They bind to bile acids in the intestines so that more are excreted in the stool rather than returned to the liver, so the liver has to produce bile acids by converting cholesterol. Adverse effects include gastrointestinal disorders and decrease in absorption of other drugs.

## SEROTONIN ANTAGONISTS

Serotonin antagonists block 5-$HT_2$ receptors of serotonin in the central and peripheral nervous systems and gastrointestinal system. An open channel can result in agitation, nausea, and vomiting, but antagonists close the channel and reduce these symptoms. Serotonin antagonists are frequently used to prevent and treat nausea associated with chemotherapy and anesthesia. Medications include:

- **Metoclopramide** (Reglan) is used to reduce nausea and vomiting from a wide range of causes. It is also a prokinetic drug that increases gastrointestinal contractions and promotes faster gastric emptying, so it is used for heartburn, GERD, and diabetic gastroparesis.
- **Ondansetron** (Zofran) reduces vagal stimulation of the medulla oblongata (vomiting center) and is used for nausea related to chemotherapy.
- **Granisetron** (Sancuso) is used to reduce nausea related to chemotherapy, surgery, and radiation.

Serotonin antagonists have fewer side effects than other antiemetics, but they may cause muscle cramping, agitation, diarrhea/constipation, dizziness, and headache.

## LAXATIVES

The following are different types of laxatives:

- **Bulk formers** have high fiber content and both soften stool and create more formed stools. These include products such as Metamucil, Citrucel, and FiberCon, which are usually added to liquids because without adequate fluids, they can increase constipation.
- **Lubricants** include both oral mineral oil and glycerin suppositories. They coat the stool, preventing fluid absorption and keeping the stool soft. Mineral oil absorbs fat soluble vitamins and should be used only temporarily
- **Saline**, such as Milk of Magnesia and Epsom Salt, contain ions, such as magnesium phosphate, magnesium hydroxide, and citrate, which are not absorbed through the intestines and draw more fluid into the stool. The magnesium in the preparations also stimulates the bowel. People with impairment of kidney function should avoid magnesium products, and saline laxatives should be used infrequently to avoid dependence. Epsom Salt often has a purging effect and is rarely used.

- **Stool softeners** (emollients, such as Colace, and Philip's Liqui-Gels) use wetting agents, such as docusate sodium, to increase liquid in the stool, thereby softening it. They should not be used with mineral oil because of increased absorption of the oil through the intestines.
- **Hyperosmotics** (available by prescription) contain materials that are not digestible and serve to retain fluid in the stool. Products, such as Kristalose and MiraLAX soften the stool but may result in increased Abdominal distension and flatus, especially initially. There are three types of hyperosmolar laxatives: lactulose, polymer, and saline. Lactulose types use a form of sugar and work similarly to saline laxatives, but more slowly, and may be used for long-term treatment. The salines empty the bowels quickly and are used short-term. The polymers contain polyethylene glycol, which retains fluid in the stool and is used short-term.
- **Combinations** use two or more types, such as stool softener with stimulant, and should be used only short-term.

## STIMULANTS

Stimulants increase intestinal motility, moving the stool through the bowel faster and reducing the absorption of fluids so that the stool remains softer. Common ingredients include cascara in Castor oil and senna in Senokot. Stimulants work quickly and are effective but can result in electrolyte imbalance, Abdominal distension, and cramping. Chronic use may cause a cycle of constipation and diarrhea. Stimulant suppositories, such as Dulcolax, are also available.

**Review Video: Gastroenterological Drugs**
Visit mometrix.com/academy and enter code: 455152

# Genitourinary

## Assessment of Kidneys and Urinary Tract

Assessment of kidneys and urinary tract includes:

- Assess the health history for family urinary system disease and risk factors, such as previous urinary disease, increased age, immobility, hypertension, diabetes, chemical exposure, chronic disease, radiation to the pelvis, STDs, alcohol or drug use, and complications of pregnancy and delivery.
- Determine daily fluid intake.
- Question symptoms such as flank or abdominal pain, hesitancy, urgency, difficulty or straining with voiding, difficulty emptying the bladder, urinary incontinence, fatigue, SOB, exercise intolerance from anemia, fever, chills, blood in the urine, and GI symptoms.

**Physical assessment** includes vital signs, kidney and bladder palpation, and percussion over the bladder after urination:

- Palpate for ascites and edema.
- Measure the DTRs and check gait and ability to walk heel-to-toe.
- Examine the genitalia and check the urethra and vagina for herniation, irritation, or tears.

Urine specimen is obtained via clean catch midstream technique for analysis and culture if indicated. Blood is taken for a CBC, and in males, prostate-specific antigen (PSA) levels will also be measured via blood specimen.

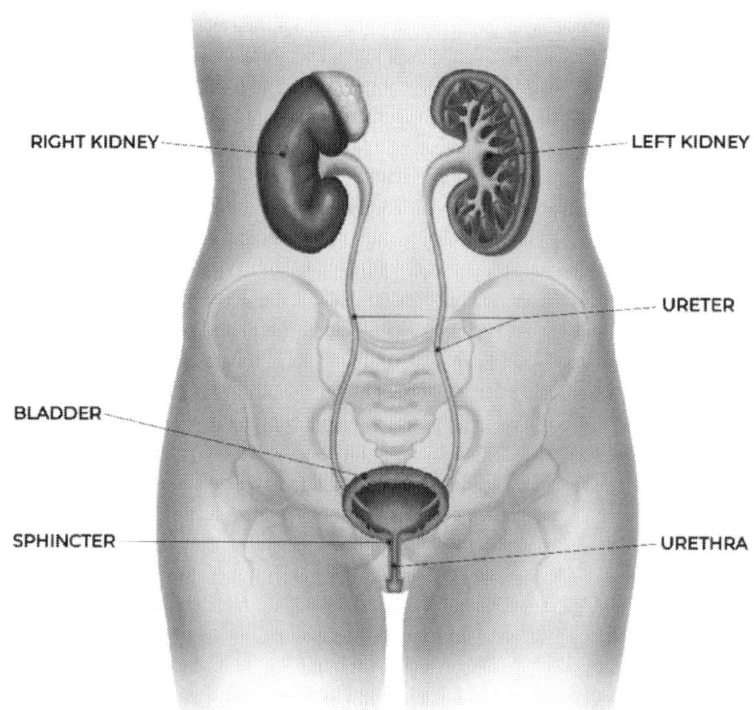


**Review Video: Urinary System**
Visit mometrix.com/academy and enter code: 601053

## Kidney Regulatory Functions Regarding Fluid Balance

Kidney regulatory functions include maintaining **fluid balance**. Fluid excretion balances intake with output, so increased intake results in a large output and vice versa:

- **Osmolality** (the number of electrolytes and other molecules per kg/urine) measures the concentration or dilution. With dehydration, osmolality increases; with fluid retention, osmolality decreases. With kidney disease, urine is dilute and the osmolality is fixed.
- **Specific gravity** compares the weight of urine (weight of particles) to distilled water (1.000). Normal urine is 1.010-1.025 with normal intake. High intake lowers the specific gravity, and low intake raises it. In kidney disease, it often does not vary.
- **Antidiuretic hormone** (ADH/vasopressin) regulates the excretion of water and urine concentration in the renal tubule by varying water reabsorption. When fluid intake decreases, blood osmolality rises, and this stimulates the release of ADH, which increases reabsorption of fluid to return osmolality to normal levels. ADH is suppressed with increased fluid intake, so less fluid is reabsorbed.

## Assessing Sexual Health and Preferences

Bringing up the topic of sex gives a patient permission to ask questions and openly discuss **sexual concerns**:

- Ask for permission to ask questions about sexual health and preferences during the gynecological/urological portion of the health history.
- If the patient refuses, go on with the rest of the health history, otherwise continue.
- Ask first if the person has sex with men, women, or both.
- Be nonjudgmental and do not assume that those who are elderly or disabled do not have sex. Use layman terms according to the patient's age and education level.
- Ask if the person is having any problems with relationships or sexual intercourse.
- Ask if the person has ever been forced to have sex or if is afraid of anyone close to them.
- End by asking if there are any questions about expression of sexual feelings, contraception, safe sex practices, or risky behavior.
- Refer those with problems to their doctor, or a gynecologist, urologist, or sex therapist.

## Renal Function Studies

Renal function studies are described below:

- **Osmolality (urine):** Normal: 350-900 mOsm/kg/day. Shows early changes when the kidney has difficulty concentrating urine.
- **Osmolality (serum):** Normal: 275-295 mOsm/kg. Gives a picture of the amount of solute in the blood.
- **Uric acid:** Normal: 3.0-7.2 mg/dL. Increases with renal failure.
- **Creatinine clearance (24-hour):** Normal: 75-125 mL/min. Evaluates the amount of blood cleared of creatinine in 1 minute. Approximates the GFR.
- **Serum creatinine:** Normal: 0.6-1.2 mg/dL. Increase with decreased renal function, urinary tract obstruction, and nephritis.
- **Urine creatinine:** Normal: 11-26 mg/kg/day. Product of muscle breakdown. Increase with decreased renal function.
- **Blood urea nitrogen (BUN):** Normal: 7-8 mg/dL (8-20 mg/dL if age >60). An increase indicates impaired renal function, as urea is the end product of protein metabolism.
- **BUN/creatinine ratio:** Normal: 10:1. Increases with hypovolemia. With intrinsic kidney disease, the ratio is increased.
- **Urinalysis:** Tests various qualities of a urine sample that are reflective of kidney function and other disease processes.

### *URINALYSIS*

Urinalysis components and normal findings are described below:

- **Color:** Pale yellow/amber and darkens when urine is concentrated or other substances (such as blood or bile) are present.
- **Appearance:** Clear but may be slightly cloudy.
- **Odor:** Slight. Bacteria may give urine a foul smell, depending upon the organism. Some foods, such as asparagus, change the odor.
- **Specific gravity:** Normal: 1.005-1.025. May increase if protein levels increase or if there is fever, vomiting, or dehydration.
- **pH:** Usually ranges from 4.5-8 with an average of 5-6.
- **Sediment:** Red cell casts from acute infections, broad casts from kidney disorders, and white cell casts from pyelonephritis. Leukocytes >10 per $mL^3$ are present with urinary tract infections.
- **Glucose, ketones, protein, blood, bilirubin, and nitrate:** Negative. Urine glucose may increase with infection (with normal blood glucose). Frank blood may be caused by some parasites and diseases but also by drugs, smoking, excessive exercise, and menstrual fluids. Increased red blood cells may result from lower urinary tract infections.
- **Urobilinogen:** 0.1-1.0 units.

## IVP AND RADIONUCLEOTIDE RENAL SCAN

**Intravenous pyelogram (IVP)** is done to identify structural defects and tumors and to observe urinary structures. The patient is administered an IV contrast medium and may be administered antihistamine or corticosteroid before the test to minimize allergic response. Serum creatinine and BUN are done prior to the IVP to ensure that the contrast medium can be excreted. During the procedure, radiographs are taken once every minute for five minutes and then again after 15 minutes (giving the contrast medium time to pass into the bladder). A post-voiding radiograph shows how efficiently the bladder is able to empty. Fluid intake should be increased post-procedure to flush contrast.

**Radionucleotide renal scan** with dimercaptosuccinic acid (DMSA) requires IV administration of a radioactive element followed by a series of CT scans taken over 20 minutes to 4 hours. The scan is used to assess function and perfusion of the kidney and can detect lesions, atrophy, and scars and differentiate among different causes for hydronephrosis. The patient must be well-hydrated and may need to be catheterized to measure the output of urine.

## RENAL BIOPSY

Renal biopsy to remove a small segment of cortical tissue helps to identify the extent of **kidney disease** with acute renal failure, transplant rejection, glomerulopathies, and persistent hematuria or proteinuria. Preoperative coagulation studies determine the risk of bleeding. The biopsy is done percutaneously per needle biopsy (guided by fluoroscopy or ultrasound) or surgically through a small flank incision. A urine specimen must be obtained so it can be compared with a post-procedure specimen. **Post-procedure**:

- Maintain the patient in a supine position immediately after the procedure for 4-6 hours and on bed rest overnight.
- Monitor urine for hematuria and compare it with the preop specimen.
- Monitor VS every 5-15 minutes for the first hour and then less frequently. To minimize bleeding, maintain blood pressure <140/90.
- Note anorexia, vomiting, and abdominal discomfort that may suggest bleeding.
- Note pain: Severe colicky pain may indicate a clot in the ureter.
- Monitor urinalysis and CBC post-procedure.
- Maintain fluid intake at 3,000 mL/day in absence of renal insufficiency.
- Provide blood component therapy and surgical repair if bleeding occurs.

## Renal Ultrasound

Renal ultrasound is a non-invasive method of viewing the **urinary structures**. Most patients that present with kidney disease of unknown origin should undergo a renal ultrasound to assess for possible obstruction. An ultrasound uses ultrasonic sound waves transmitted by a transducer, which picks up reflected sound waves that a computer converts to electronic images. An ultrasound can show fluid accumulation, the movement of blood through the kidney, masses, malformations (congenital abnormalities), changes in size of the kidney or other structures, and obstructions, such as renal calculi. An ultrasound is usually done before a renal biopsy, and may be done with a needle biopsy to guide the placement of the needle. Patient preparation includes drinking two 8-ounce glasses of water one hour before the examination to ensure that the bladder is full. The patient should be reminded not to urinate before the ultrasound. The patient usually remains in a supine position throughout the procedure but may be asked to turn to the side. No special precautions are necessary post-procedure.

## Urinary Incontinence

Urinary incontinence occurs more commonly in women than men and can range from an intermittent leaking of urine to a full loss of bladder control. Causes of urinary incontinence may include neurologic injury (including cerebral vascular accidents), infections, weakness of the muscles of the bladder, and certain medications, including diuretics, antihistamines, and antidepressants. **Stress incontinence** is defined as an involuntary leakage of urine with sneezing, coughing, laughing, lifting, or exercising. **Urge incontinence** is defined as an uncontrollable need to urinate on a frequent basis. **Total incontinence** is the full loss of bladder control.

**Signs and symptoms**: Urinary frequency and urgency may accompany the inability to control urine. If urinary incontinence is severe, incontinence-associated dermatitis may occur, predisposing the patient to skin breakdown and the development of pressure ulcers.

**Diagnosis**: Physical assessment and presence of symptoms. Ultrasound, urinalysis, urodynamic testing, and cystoscopy may be used to determine the underlying cause.

**Treatment**: Treatment options are dependent on the type of urinary incontinence and the severity. Bladder training and pelvic muscle exercises may be utilized to strengthen muscles to control leakage of urine. In female patients with stress incontinence, a vaginal pessary may be inserted into the vagina to help support the bladder. Suburethral slings may also be surgically implanted to support the urethra. Anticholinergics, antispasmodics, and tricyclic antidepressants may also be used in the treatment of urinary incontinence.

## Hydronephrosis

Hydronephrosis is a symptom of a disease involving swelling of the kidney pelvises and calyces because of an obstruction that causes urine to be retained in the kidney. In chronic conditions, symptoms may be delayed until severe kidney damage has occurred. Over time, the kidney begins to atrophy. The primary conditions that predispose to hydronephrosis include:

- Vesicoureteral reflux
- Obstruction at the ureteropelvic junction
- Renal edema (non-obstructive)
- Any condition that impairs drainage of the ureters can cause backup of the urine

**Symptoms** vary widely depending upon cause and whether the condition is acute or chronic.

- Acute episodes are usually characterized by flank pain, abnormal creatinine and electrolyte levels, and increased pH.
- The enlarged kidney may be palpable as a soft mass.

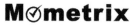

**Treatment** includes:

- Identifying the cause of obstruction and correcting it to ensure adequate drainage.
- A nephrostomy tube, ureteral stent or pyeloplasty may be done surgically in some cases.
- A urinary catheter may be inserted if there is outflow obstruction from the bladder.

## Acute Tubular Necrosis

Acute tubular necrosis (ATN) occurs when a hypoxic condition causes renal ischemia that damages tubular cells of the glomeruli so they are unable to adequately filter the urine, leading to acute renal failure. Causes include hypotension, hyperbilirubinemia, sepsis, surgery (especially cardiac or vascular), and birth complications. ATN may result from nephrotoxic injury related to obstruction or drugs, such as chemotherapy, acyclovir, and antibiotics, such as sulfonamides and streptomycin. Symptoms may be non-specific initially and can include life-threatening complications.

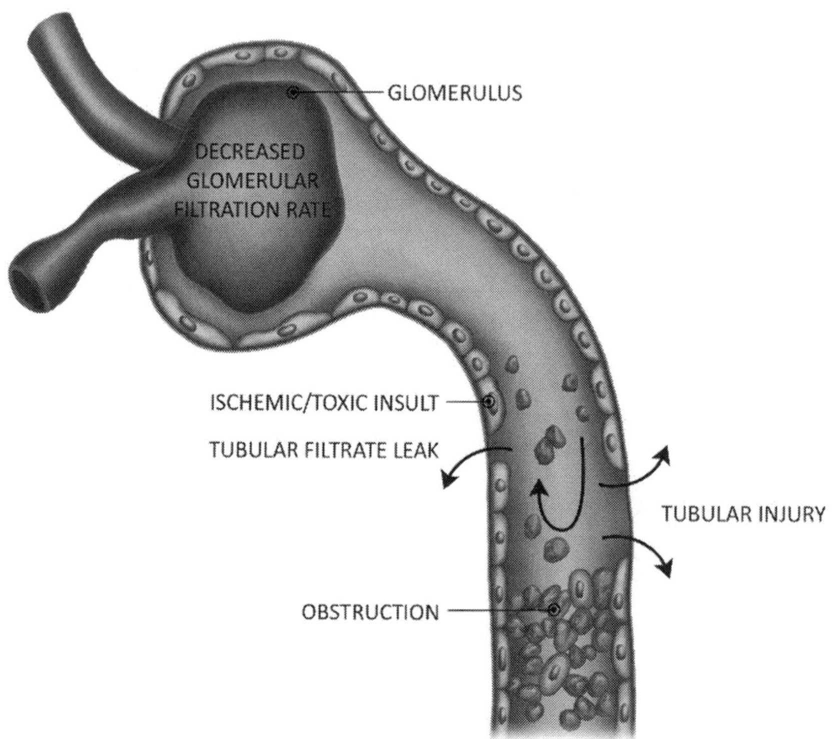


**Symptoms** include:

- Lethargy
- Nausea and vomiting
- Hypovolemia with low cardiac output and generalized vasodilation
- Fluid and electrolyte imbalance leading to hypertension, CNS abnormalities, metabolic acidosis, arrhythmias, edema, and congestive heart failure
- Uremia leading to destruction of platelets and bleeding, neurological deficits, and disseminated intravascular coagulopathy (DIC)
- Infections, including pericarditis and sepsis

**Treatment** includes:

- Identifying and treating underlying cause, discontinuing nephrotoxic agents
- Supportive care
- Loop diuretics (in some cases), such as Lasix
- Antibiotics for infection (can include pericarditis and sepsis)
- Kidney dialysis

## Acute Kidney Injury

Acute kidney injury (AKI), previously known as acute renal failure, is an acute disruption of kidney function that results in decreased renal perfusion, a decrease in glomerular filtration rate and a buildup of metabolic waste products (azotemia). Azotemia is the accumulation of urea, creatinine and other nitrogen containing end products into the bloodstream. The regulation of fluid volume, electrolyte balance and acid base balance is also affected. The causes of acute kidney injury are divided into pre-renal (caused by a decrease in perfusion), intrarenal or intrinsic (occurring within the kidney) and post-renal (caused by the inadequate drainage of urine). Acute kidney injury is common in hospitalized patients and even more common in critically ill patients, carrying a mortality rate of 50-80%. Risk factors for acute kidney injury include advanced age, the presence of co-morbid conditions, pre-existing kidney disease and a diagnosis of sepsis.

**Signs and symptoms**: Malaise, fatigue, lethargy, confusion, weakness, change in urine color, change in urine volume, and flank pain.

**Diagnosis**: Urinalysis, serum BUN and creatinine levels, renal ultrasound, CT or MRI and renal biopsy.

**Treatment**: The treatment of acute kidney injury is based on the underlying cause. Treatment options may include fluid and electrolyte replacement, diuretic therapy, fluid restriction, renal diet, and low dose dopamine to increase renal perfusion. Hemodialysis may also be necessary in patients with acute kidney injury.

## Renal and Ureteral Calculi

Renal and urinary calculi occur frequently, more commonly in males, and can relate to diseases (hyperparathyroidism, renal tubular acidosis, gout) and lifestyle factors, such as sedentary work. Calculi can form at any age, most composed of calcium, and can range in size from very tiny to larger than 6 mm. Those smaller than 4 mm can usually pass in the urine easily.

**Diagnostic** studies include clinical findings, UA, pregnancy test to rule out ectopic pregnancy, BUN and creatinine if indicated, ultrasound (for pregnant women and children), IV urography. Helical CT (non-contrast) is diagnostic.

**Symptoms** occur with obstruction and are usually of sudden onset and acute:

- Severe flank pain radiating to abdomen and ipsilateral testicle or labium majus, abdominal or pelvic pain (young children)
- Nausea and vomiting
- Diaphoresis
- Hematuria

**Treatment** includes:

- Instructions and equipment for straining urine
- Antibiotics if concurrent infection
- Extracorporeal shock-wave lithotripsy
- Surgical removal: percutaneous/standard nephrolithotomy
- Analgesia: opiates and NSAIDs

## CHRONIC KIDNEY DISEASE

Chronic kidney disease (CKD) occurs when the kidneys are unable to filter and excrete wastes, concentrate urine, and maintain electrolyte balance because of hypoxic conditions, kidney disease, or obstruction in the urinary tract. It results first in azotemia (increase in nitrogenous waste in the blood) and then in uremia (nitrogenous wastes cause toxic symptoms). When >50% of the functional renal capacity is destroyed, the kidneys can no longer carry out necessary functions, and progressive deterioration begins over months or years. Symptoms are often non-specific in the beginning, with loss of appetite and energy.

**Symptoms and complications** are as follows:

- Weight loss
- Headaches, muscle cramping, general malaise
- Increased bruising and dry or itchy skin
- Increased BUN and creatinine
- Sodium and fluid retention with edema
- Hyperkalemia
- Metabolic acidosis
- Calcium and phosphorus depletion, resulting in altered bone metabolism, pain, and retarded growth
- Anemia with decreased production on RBCs. Increased risk of infection
- Uremic syndrome

**Treatment** includes:

- Supportive/symptomatic therapy
- Dialysis and transplantation
- Diet control: low protein, salt, potassium, and phosphorus
- Fluid limitations
- Calcium and vitamin supplementation
- Phosphate binders

## UREMIC SYNDROME

Uremic syndrome is a number of disorders that can occur with end-stage renal disease and renal failure, usually after multiple metabolic failures and decrease in creatinine clearance to <10 mL/min. There is compromise of all normal functions of the kidney: fluid balance, electrolyte balance, acid-base homeostasis, hormone production, and elimination of wastes. Metabolic abnormalities related to uremia include:

- **Decreased RBC production**: The kidney is unable to produce adequate erythropoietin in the peritubular cells, resulting in anemia, which is usually normocytic and normochromic. Parathyroid hormone levels may increase, causing calcification of the bone marrow, causing hypoproliferative anemia as RBC production is suppressed.
- **Platelet abnormalities**: Decreased platelet count, increased turnover, and reduced adhesion leads to bleeding disorders.
- **Metabolic acidosis**: The tubular cells are unable to regulate acid-base metabolism, and phosphate, sulfuric, hippuric, and lactic acids increase, leading to congestive heart failure and weakness.
- **Hyperkalemia**: The nephrons cannot excrete adequate amounts of potassium. Some drugs, such as diuretics that spare potassium may aggravate the condition.
- **Renal bone disease**: Decreased calcium, elevated phosphate, elevated parathyroid hormone, decreased utilization of vitamin D lead to demineralization. In some cases, calcium and phosphate are deposited in other tissues (metastatic calcification).

- **Multiple endocrine disorders**: Thyroid hormone production is decreased and abnormalities in reproductive hormones may result in infertility/impotence. Males have decreased testosterone but elevated estrogen and LH. Females experience irregular cycles, lack of ovulation and menses. Insulin production may increase but with decreased clearance, resulting in episodes of hypoglycemia or decreased hyperglycemia in those who are diabetic.
- **Cardiovascular disorders**: Left ventricular hypertrophy is most common, but fluid retention may cause congestive heart failure and electrolyte imbalances, dysrhythmias. Pericarditis, exacerbation of valvular disorders, and pericardial effusions may occur.
- **Anorexia and malnutrition**: Nausea and poor appetite contribute to hypoalbuminemia, sometimes exacerbated by restrictive diets.

## Pyelonephritis

Pyelonephritis is a potentially organ-damaging bacterial infection of the parenchyma of the kidney. Pyelonephritis can result in abscess formation, sepsis, and kidney failure. Pyelonephritis is especially dangerous for those who are immunocompromised, pregnant, or diabetic. Most infections are caused by *Escherichia coli*. **Diagnostic studies** include urinalysis, blood and urine cultures. Patients may require hospitalization or careful follow-up.

**Symptoms** vary widely but can include:

- Dysuria and frequency, hematuria, flank and/or low back pain
- Fever and chills
- Costovertebral angle tenderness
- Change in feeding habits (infants)
- Change in mental status (geriatric)
- Young women often exhibit symptoms more associated with lower urinary infection, so the condition may be overlooked.

**Treatment** includes:

- Analgesia
- Antipyretics
- Intravenous fluids
- Antibiotics: started but may be changed based on cultures
    - IV ceftriaxone with fluoroquinolone orally for 14 days
    - Monitor BUN. Normal 7-8 mg/dL (8-20 mg/dL >age 60). Increase indicates impaired renal function, as urea is end product of protein metabolism.

## Cystitis

Cystitis is a common and often-chronic low-grade kidney infection that develops over time, so observing for symptoms of urinary infections and treating promptly are very important.

Changes in **character of urine**:

- **Appearance**: The urine may become cloudy from mucus or purulent material. Hematuria may be present.
- **Color**: Urine usually becomes concentrated and may be dark yellow/orange or brownish in color.
- **Odor**: Urine may have a very strong or foul odor.
- **Output**: Urinary output may decrease markedly.

**Pain**: There may be lower back or flank pain from inflammation of the kidneys.

**Systemic**: Fever, chills, headache, and general malaise often accompany urine infections. Some people suffer a lack of appetite as well as nausea and vomiting. Fever usually indicates that the infection has affected the kidneys. Children may develop incontinence or loose stools and cry excessively.

**Treatment:**

- Increased fluid intake
- Antibiotics

## Nephrotoxic Agents

Medications are a common cause of renal damage, especially among older patients. The **nephrotoxic effects** may be reversible if the drug is discontinued before permanent damage occurs. Those at increased risk include patients who are older than 60, have a history of renal insufficiency, suffer from volume depletion, or have diabetes mellitus, sepsis, or heart failure. Initial signs may be quite subtle. Preventive measures include baseline renal function tests and monitoring of renal function and vital signs during treatment. The following are some common effects, and the drugs that may cause them:

- **Chronic interstitial nephritis**: Acetaminophen, lithium, carmustine, cisplatin, cyclosporine.
- **Acute interstitial nephritis**: NSAIDs, acyclovir, beta-lactams, rifampin, quinolones, sulfonamides, vancomycin, indinavir, loop/thiazide diuretics, lansoprazole, allopurinol, phenytoin.
- **Rhabdomyolysis**: Amitriptyline, diphenhydramine, doxylamine, benzodiazepines, haloperidol, lithium, ketamine, methadone, methamphetamine, statins.
- **Crystal nephropathy**: Acyclovir, foscarnet, ganciclovir, quinolones, sulfonamides, indinavir, methotrexate, triamterene.
- **Tubular cell toxicity**: Aminoglycosides, amphotericin B, pentamidine, adefovir, tenofovir, contrast dye, zoledronate.
- **Thrombotic microangiopathy**: Cyclosporine, clopidogrel, mitomycin-C, quinine.
- **Impaired intraglomerular hemodynamics**: NSAIDs, cyclosporine, tacrolimus, ACE inhibitors.
- **Glomerulonephritis**: NSAIDs, lithium, beta-lactams, interferon-alpha, gold therapy, pamidronate.

## Phimosis and Paraphimosis

Phimosis and paraphimosis are both restrictive disorders of the penis that occur in males who are uncircumcised or incorrectly circumcised. **Phimosis** is the inability to retract the foreskin proximal to the glans penis, sometimes resulting in urinary retention or hematuria. **Treatments** include:

- Dilating the foreskin with a hemostat (temporary solution)
- Circumcision
- Application of topical steroids (triamcinolone 0.025% twice daily) from end of foreskin to glans corona for 4-6 weeks

**Paraphimosis** occurs when the foreskin tightens above the glans penis and cannot be extended to normal positioning. This results in edema of the foreskin and circulatory impairment of the glans penis, sometimes progressing to gangrene, so immediate treatment is critical. Symptoms include pain, swelling, and inability to urinate. **Treatments** include:

- Compression of the glans to reduce edema (wrapping tightly with 2-inch elastic bandage for 5 minutes)
- Reducing edema by making several puncture wounds with 22- to 25-gauge needle
- Local anesthetic and dorsal incision to relieve pressure

## Testicular Torsion

Testicular torsion is a twisting of the spermatic cord within or below the inguinal canal, causing constriction of blood supply to the testis. Testicular torsion is most common at puberty but can occur at any age, sometimes precipitated by strenuous athletic participation or trauma, but it can also occur during sleep.

**Symptoms** include acute onset of severe testicular pain and edema, although children may present with nonspecific abdominal discomfort initially.

**Diagnosis** is based on clinical examination that demonstrates a firm scrotal mass. Color-flow duplex Doppler ultrasound may be helpful if diagnosis is not clear.

**Treatment** includes:

- **Manual detorsion** (usually 1.5 rotations) with elective surgical repair. Right testicle is usually rotated counterclockwise and left, clockwise. Reduction of pain should occur. If pain increases with rotation, then rotation should be done in the opposite direction.
- **Emergency surgical repair** (if manual detorsion not successful)

## Epididymitis and Orchitis

**Epididymitis**, infection of the epididymis, is often associated with infection in a testis (epididymo-orchitis). In children, infection may be related to congenital anomalies that allow reflux of urine. In sexually active males 35 years or younger, it is usually related to STDs. In men older than 40, it is often related to urinary infections or benign prostatic hypertrophy with urethral obstruction.

**Symptoms** include progressive pain in lower abdomen, scrotum, and/or testicle. Late symptoms include large tender scrotal mass.

**Diagnosis** includes: Clinical examination. Pyuria. Urethral culture for STDs. Sonography.

**Orchitis** alone is rare but occurs with mumps, other viral infections, and epididymitis. Ultrasound may be needed to rule out testicular torsion.

**Treatment** for both conditions depends upon the cause, but epididymitis usually resolves with antibiotics:

- Younger than 40, associated with STDs:
  - Ceftriaxone 250 mg IM and doxycycline 100 mg twice daily for 10 days
- Older than 35, associated with other bacteria:
  - Ciprofloxacin 500 mg twice daily for 10-14 days
  - Levofloxacin 250 mg daily for 10-14 days
  - TMP/SMS DS twice daily for 10-14 days

## Prostatitis

Prostatitis is an acute infection of the prostate gland, commonly caused by *Escherichia coli, Pseudomonas aeruginosa, Staphylococcus aureus,* or other bacteria. *Symptoms* include fever, chills, lower back pain, urinary frequency, dysuria, painful ejaculation, and perineal discomfort. PSA will often be elevated in this patient population, unrelated to prostate cancer. *Diagnosis* is based on clinical findings of perineal tenderness and spasm of rectal sphincter. *Treatments* include Ciprofloxacin 500 mg orally twice daily for 1 month **or** TMP/SMX DS twice daily for 1 month. Most patients also have a urethral culture to check for STDs. Patients with suspected bacteremia should be admitted for monitoring.

## Procedures for Insertion and Removal of Urinary Catheter

Procedure for inserting and removing a urinary catheter:

1. Gather supplies (included in a urinary catheter insertion kit), perform hand hygiene, place a waterproof pad under the patient, and ensure that the light source is adequate to view the urinary meatus.
2. Place females in supine position with knees flexed and males in supine position.
3. Apply gloves and wash the perineal area with facility provided cleanser (sometimes included in the outside of the urinary catheter kit) and allow to dry.
4. Remove gloves and wash hands.
5. Using aseptic technique, place the catheter kit between the patient's legs, open the kit touching only the corners of the drape that wraps around the kit.
6. Apply sterile gloves.
7. Apply sterile drapes to the patient.
8. Following the steps provided with the kit, place the lubricant into the appropriate section of tray, remove the catheter from its plastic and place the tip into the lubricant, and pour iodine over the three cleansing swabs (if they do not come impregnated with iodine already). Attach the 10-cc syringe (filled with sterile water) to the appropriate port of the catheter.
9. Cleanse the urethral meatus with the iodine impregnated swabs.
10. Using the nondominant hand, hold the penis or open the labia to observe the urethral meatus. This hand now becomes "dirty" and cannot be used to touch the catheter.
11. Using the dominant hand, insert catheter with the drainage end attached to the collection bag. Insert until urine flows freely, advancing a little further after that point.
12. Inflate the balloon using the 10-cc sterile water syringe, and ensure the catheter is secure.
13. Secure the catheter to the patient's leg and hang the collection bag below the level of the patient. Secure any tubing to the bed and ensure no kinking is present.

**Removal**: Straight catheter—remove by pulling out slowly. To remove indwelling catheter, deflate the balloon using the appropriate port and gently pull the catheter out.

## Reducing Infection Risks Associated with Urinary Catheters

Strategies for reducing infection risks associated with urinary catheters include:

- Using **aseptic technique** for both the straight and indwelling catheter insertion
- **Limiting catheter use** by establishing protocols for use, duration, and removal; training staff; issuing reminders to physicians; using straight catheterizations rather than indwelling; using ultrasound to scan the bladder; and using condom catheters
- Utilizing **closed-drainage systems** for indwelling catheters
- **Avoiding irrigation** unless required for diagnosis or treatment
- Using **sampling port** for specimens rather than disconnecting catheter and tubing
- Maintaining **proper urinary flow** by proper positioning, securing of tubing and drainage bag, and keeping the drainage bag below the level of the bladder
- **Changing catheters** only when medically needed
- **Cleansing external meatal area** gently each day, manipulating the catheter as little as possible
- Avoiding placing catheterized patients adjacent to those infected or colonized with antibiotic-resistant bacteria to reduce **cross-contamination**

## Renal Dialysis

### Peritoneal Dialysis

**Renal dialysis** is used primarily for those who have progressed from renal insufficiency to uremia with end-stage renal disease (ESRD). It may also be temporarily for acute conditions. People can be maintained on dialysis, but there are many complications associated with dialysis, so many people are considered for renal transplantation. There are a number of different approaches to **peritoneal dialysis:**

- **Peritoneal dialysis:** An indwelling catheter is inserted surgically into the peritoneal cavity with a subcutaneous tunnel and a Dacron cuff to prevent infection. Sterile dialysate solution is slowly instilled through gravity, remains for a prescribed length of time, and is then drained and discarded.
- **Continuous ambulatory peritoneal dialysis:** a series of exchange cycles is repeated 24 hours a day.
- **Continuous cyclic peritoneal dialysis:** a prolonged period of retaining fluid occurs during the day with drainage at night.

Peritoneal dialysis may be used for those who want to be more independent, don't live near a dialysis center, or want fewer dietary restrictions.

### Hemodialysis

Hemodialysis, the most common type of dialysis, is used for both short-term dialysis and long-term for those with ESRD. Treatments are usually done three times weekly for 3-4 hours or daily dialysis with treatment either during the night or in short daily periods. **Hemodialysis** is often done for those who can't manage peritoneal dialysis or who live near a dialysis center, but it does interfere with work or school attendance and requires strict dietary and fluid restrictions between treatments. Short daily dialysis allows more independence, and increased costs may be offset by lower morbidity. A vascular access device, such as a catheter, fistula, or graft, must be established for hemodialysis, and heparin is used to prevent clotting. With hemodialysis, blood is circulated outside of the body through a dialyzer (a synthetic semipermeable membrane), which filters the blood. There are many different types of dialyzers. High flux dialyzers use a highly permeable membrane that shortens the duration of treatment and decreases the need for heparin.

### Dialysis Complications

There are many complications associated with dialysis, especially when used for long-term treatment:

- **Hemodialysis**: Long-term use promotes atherosclerosis and cardiovascular disease. Anemia and fatigue are common, as are infections related to access devices or contamination of equipment. Some experience hypotension and muscle cramping during treatment. Dysrhythmias may occur. Some may exhibit dialysis disequilibrium from cerebral fluid shifts, causing headaches, nausea and vomiting, and alterations of consciousness.
- **Peritoneal dialysis:** Most complications are minor, but it can lead to peritonitis, which requires removal of the catheter if antibiotic therapy is not successful in clearing the infection within 4 days. There may be leakage of the dialysate around the catheter. Bleeding may occur, especially in females who are menstruating as blood is pulled from the uterus through the fallopian tubes. Abdominal hernias may occur with long use. Some may have anorexia from the feeling of fullness or a sweet taste in the mouth from the absorption of glucose.

### Continuous Renal Replacement Therapy

Continuous renal replacement therapy (CRRT) circulates the blood by hydrostatic pressure through a semipermeable membrane. It is used in critical care and can be instituted quickly:

- **Continuous arteriovenous hemofiltration** (CAVH) circulates blood from an artery (usually the femoral) to a hemofilter using only arterial pressure and not a blood pump. The filtered blood is then returned to the patient's venous system, often with added fluids to offset those lost. Only the fluid is filtered.

- **Continuous arteriovenous hemodialysis** (CAVHD) is similar to CAVH except that dialysate circulates on one side of the semipermeable membrane to increase the clearance of urea.
- **Continuous venovenous hemofiltration** (CVVH) pumps blood through a double-lumen venous catheter to a hemofilter, which returns the blood to the patient in the same catheter. It provides continuous slow removal of fluid, is better tolerated with unstable patients, and doesn't require arterial access.
- **Continuous venovenous hemodialysis** is similar to CVVH but uses a dialysate to increase the clearance of uremic toxins.

# Obstetric and Gynecologic

## ABRUPTIO PLACENTAE

Abruptio placenta occurs when the placenta separates prematurely from the wall of the uterus. **Symptoms** include:

- Vaginal bleeding
- Tender uterus with increased resting tone
- Uterine contractions (hypertonic or hyperactive)
- Nausea and vomiting (in some patients)
- Dizziness

Complications include fetal distress, hypotension, and disseminated intravascular coagulopathy (DIC), as well as fetal and/or maternal death. Fetal death is common with at least 50% separation.

**Diagnosis** includes:

- Ultrasound
- Blood work: CBC, type and crossmatch, coagulation studies (50% have coagulopathy)

**Treatment** includes:

- Gynecological consultation
- Crystalloids to increase blood volume
- Fresh frozen plasma for coagulopathy

## PLACENTA PREVIA

Placenta previa occurs when the placenta implants over the cervical opening. Implantation may be complete (covering the entire opening), partial, or marginal (to the edge of the cervical opening). Symptoms include painless bleeding after the 20th week of gestation.

**Diagnosis** is per ultrasound. Vaginal examination with digit or speculum should be avoided. The condition may correct itself as the uterus expands, but bed rest may be needed. Emergency cesarean section is done for uncontrolled bleeding.

## ECTOPIC PREGNANCY

Ectopic pregnancy occurs when the fertilized ovum implants outside the uterus in an ovary, fallopian tube (the most common site), peritoneal cavity, or cervix.

- **Early symptoms** may include: Indications of pregnancy such as amenorrhea, breast tenderness, nausea, and vomiting. Positive Chadwick's sign (blue discoloration of cervix). Positive Hegar's sign (softening of isthmus). Bleeding may be the first indication as hormones fluctuate. Hormone hCG present in blood and urine.
- **Symptoms of rupture** include: One-sided or generalized abdominal pain. Decreased hemoglobin and hematocrit. Hypotension with hemorrhage. Right shoulder pain because of irritation of the subdiaphragmatic phrenic nerve.
- **Diagnostic studies** include: Vaginal exam. Pregnancy test. Transvaginal sonography (TVS) to rule out intrauterine pregnancy. hCG titers (increase more slowly with ectopic pregnancy) Progesterone level greater than 22 helps rule out ectopic pregnancy.

**Treatments** include:

- Methotrexate IM or IV if unruptured and 3.5 cm or less in size to inhibit growth and allow body to expel
- Laparoscopic linear salpingostomy or salpingectomy

## Nausea and Vomiting and Hyperemesis Gravidarum Related to Pregnancy

About 60-80% of pregnant woman suffer from nausea and vomiting (NV), especially during the first trimester, but only about 2% suffer severe (sometimes intractable) nausea and vomiting, known as **hyperemesis gravidarum (HG)**, associated with weight loss, dehydration, hypokalemia, or ketonemia. Nausea and vomiting may be associated with numerous disorders, including cholelithiasis, pancreatitis, hepatitis, and ectopic pregnancy, especially when accompanied by abdominal pain. **Diagnosis** includes:

- Physical examination to rule out other disorders
- CBC with serum electrolytes, BUN, creatinine, and urinalysis
- Ketonuria is an indication of inadequate nutrition

**Treatment** includes:

- IV fluids with glucose 5% in normal saline or Ringer's lactate
- Oral fluids after nausea and vomiting controlled
- Antiemetic drugs
- Acute treatment for NV and HG: promethazine, prochlorperazine, or chlorpromazine
- Maintenance for NV: Doxylamine with pyridoxine, diphenhydramine, or cisapride
- Maintenance for HG: Metoclopramide, trimethobenzamide, or ondansetron

## Hypertensive Disorders of Pregnancy During the Second Half of Pregnancy

Hypertensive disorders of pregnancy comprise a continuum ranging from mild to severe:

- **Hypertension**: BP increased to at least 140/90, or 20 mmHg increase in systolic or 10 mmHg diastolic. May be chronic or transient without signs of preeclampsia or eclampsia.
- **Preeclampsia**: Hypertension associated with proteinuria (300 mg per 24 hours) and edema (peripheral or generalized) or increase of at least 5 pounds of weight in 1 week after 20th week of gestation. Severe preeclampsia is BP at least 160/110. Symptoms include headache, abdominal pain, and visual disturbances.
- **Eclampsia**: Preeclampsia with seizures occurring at 20th week of gestation to 1 month after delivery.
- **HELLP syndrome**: Hemolysis, elevated liver enzymes [AST and ALT], and low platelets [less than 100,000]. Usually accompanied by epigastric or right upper quadrant pain.

**Treatments** include:

- **Chronic hypertension**: Methyldopa beginning with 250 mg every 6 hours.
- **Preeclampsia, eclampsia, HELLP:** Delivery of fetus (may be delayed with mild preeclampsia if fewer than 37 weeks gestation). Magnesium sulfate 4-6 g IV over 15 minutes initially and then 1-2 g/hr. Antihypertensive drugs.

## Vaginal Bleeding and Types of Abortion

Vaginal bleeding during the first trimester of pregnancy may indicate spontaneous abortion, ectopic pregnancy, gestational trophoblastic disease, or infection. All women of childbearing age with an intact uterus presenting with abdominal pain or vaginal bleeding should be assessed for pregnancy.

Abortion **classifications**:

- **Threatened**: Vaginal bleeding during first half of pregnancy without cervical dilatation
- **Inevitable**: Vaginal bleeding with cervical dilatation
- **Incomplete**: Incomplete loss of products of conception, usually at 6-14 weeks
- **Complete**: Complete loss of products of conception, before 20 weeks
- **Missed**: Death of fetus before 20 weeks without loss of products of conception within 4 weeks
- **Septic**: Infection with abortion

**Diagnostic** tests include:

- Pelvic examination. CBC, Rh factor, antibody screen, urinalysis, quantitative serum beta-hCG level
- Ultrasound to rule out ectopic pregnancy

**Treatment** includes:

- Suctioning of vaginal vault with Yankauer suction tip with pathologic examination of tissue
- Evacuation of uterus for incomplete abortion
- RhoGAM (50-150 mcg) for bleeding in unsensitized Rh-negative women

## Emergency Delivery

### *Prolapsed Umbilical Cord*

Prolapsed umbilical cord occurs when the umbilical cord precedes the presenting fetal part or, in some cases, presents at the same time, so that pressure is applied to the cord, decreasing circulation to the fetus. Decelerations in fetal pulse less than 110 may indicate prolapse. Pulsations may be felt in the cord or may be absent, but relieving pressure on the cord by holding back the presenting part is critical for fetal survival. Oxygen should be administered and fetal heart rate monitored. Infusing the bladder with 350-500 mL of fluid (warm normal saline) while pressure is held against the presenting part may lift the fetal head and relieve pressure on the cord. Other methods include placing the woman in the Trendelenburg position or with knees to chest as medical personnel apply continued pressure to the presenting part while awaiting Cesarean section for delivery.

### *Breech Presentation*

Emergency delivery may occur when there are complications of pregnancy or a woman is in advanced labor with birth imminent. The delivery may proceed normally, but complications may require immediate intervention. **Breech presentation** (common in premature births) is when the buttocks or lower extremities are the presenting part during delivery. Types include:

- **Complete**: knees and hips both flexed with buttocks and feet presenting
- **Frank**: hips flexed and knees extended with buttocks presenting
- **Footling** or **incomplete**: hips and legs extended and one or both feet presenting (In some incomplete cases, the knees may present.)

Complete and frank breech presentations may often be delivered vaginally as enough pressure is applied to adequately dilate the vagina, but the delivery should be spontaneous with medical staff keeping hands off until the umbilicus presents, then assisting with delivery of the legs and rotating the fetus to the sacrum anterior position and then gently turning to deliver the arms. Incomplete or footling presentations require Cesarean sections.

### *PROM*

**Preterm or premature labor** occurs between weeks 20 and 37. PROM occurs when the membranes rupture before the onset of labor, and may lead to premature labor. There are numerous causes for PROM, including infections and digital pelvic exams. When a woman presents in labor, the estimated date of delivery should be obtained by questioning the date of the last menstrual period (LMP) and using a gestation calculator wheel or estimating with **Naegele's rule**:

*First day LMP minus 3 months plus 7 days = estimated date of delivery*

Fetal viability is very low before 23 weeks of gestation but by 25 weeks, delaying delivery for 2 days can increase survival rates by 10%. Tocolytic drugs, which have many negative side effects, may be used to delay delivery in order to administer glucocorticoids, such as betamethasone or dexamethasone, to improve fetal lung maturity between weeks 24 and 36. **Tocolytics** include:

- Beta-adrenergic agonists
- Magnesium sulfates
- Calcium channel blockers
- Prostaglandin synthetase inhibitors

### *PRETERM INFANTS*

Emergency delivery often involves **preterm infants**, whose gestational age may not be clear upon delivery, so initial resuscitative efforts should be carried out until viability is determined. The infant should be dried and warmed immediately, such as by placing in a double-walled heated incubator or under a Plexiglas heat shield in a single-walled incubator to prevent heat loss. Radiant warmers and plastic wrap over the infant may also be used. The head and neck must be well supported to prevent blockage of the trachea. A small roll should be placed under the shoulders and the head slightly elevated if child is in supine position, but the prone position splints the chest and decreases respiratory effort. Gentle nasopharyngeal suctioning may be needed to clear secretions. The infant should be evaluated with the Apgar scale and transferred to the neonatal ICU as necessary for further interventions. Apgar score below 4 requires resuscitations (8 to 10 is normal range).

## POSTPARTUM HEMORRHAGE

Most postpartum hemorrhage is excessive vaginal bleeding (greater than 500 mL for vaginal and greater than 1,000 mL for Cesarean section) occurring within 24 hours of delivery, related to uterine atony caused by failure of the uterus to contract adequately, uterine rupture or inversion, lacerations, or coagulopathies. It is more common after Cesarean section than vaginal delivery. Hemorrhage may be delayed in some cases, related to retained products of conception, uterine polyps, or coagulopathies. Careful history and examination to determine the cause of bleeding is necessary. **Symptoms** include:

- Excessive bleeding
- Hypotension and tachycardia
- Decreased hematocrit
- Pain and/or edema in vagina/perineum

**Treatment** includes:

- Stabilizing patient
- Two IV lines (large bore) inserted
- Laboratory testing for CBC, clotting, and type and crossmatch
- Vaginal exam with speculum to identify and repair lacerations
- Oxytocin or methylergonovine maleate for uterine atony
- Ultrasound to check for retained products of conception
- Obstetric consultation for uterine inversion (observed as mass in vagina)
- Fresh frozen plasma for coagulopathies

## Trauma During Pregnancy

Trauma during pregnancy is one of the leading causes of death and injury to pregnant women. Automobile accidents, falls, and assault (often related to domestic abuse) can all result in death of the fetus. Complications of trauma may be uterine rupture, abruption, or uterine irritability, and the onset of premature labor. Fetal-maternal hemorrhage may also occur. Direct injury to the fetus is common only in the late stages of pregnancy when blunt abdominal trauma with pelvic fracture may cause fetal skull fracture or with gunshot wounds. Because fetal survival depends on maternal survival, initial resuscitation efforts are for the mother. After the airway is secured and IV (large bore) access is obtained, volume replacement is provided and any bleeding controlled. When the mother is stabilized, the gestational age of the fetus should be estimated and pelvic exam done. Radiologic exams should be done as indicated. All unsensitized Rh-negative (D-negative) women should receive **RhoGAM**. Tetanus prophylaxis should be given. Fetal assessment should include ultrasound and monitoring of fetal heart rate.

## Minimum Neonatal Resuscitation Equipment

The minimal equipment that should be present for neonatal resuscitation includes the following:

- **Temperature**: Thermometer, warmed drying towels, warmed swaddling blankets, radiant warmer, phototherapy equipment.
- **Respiration**: Oxygen tank and hood, flow meter, humidifier, heater, tubing, nasal prongs. Bag and mask set-up (assorted sizes). Laryngoscope with size 0 and 1 blades. Endotracheal tubes, sizes 2.5-4. Bulb syringe, suction catheters (sizes 6, 8, and 10 Fr.), suction canister. Cardiorespiratory monitor, oxygen analyzer.
- **Fluids**: IV needles and tubing, infusion pump, umbilical catheters (sizes 2.5 and 5 Fr.). Blood pressure monitor, pulse oximeter. Isotonic saline, D10W, sodium bicarbonate. If transfusions are done here, blood drainage system, volume expander, and blood warmer.
- **Drugs**: Epinephrine, Naloxone.
- **Procedures**: Various sterile surgical packs, dressings, chest tubes, scalpels, hemostat. Arterial blood gas equipment and portable x-ray machine.

## ABCs of Neonatal Resuscitation

The ABCs of resuscitation are a device to help remember in what order to do the steps of the resuscitation process. In this device, the letters stand for the following:

- **Airway**: An airway should be established as the very first thing to tend to. If there is no airway, air cannot be moved during resuscitation attempts. This step includes clearing the mouth and nose of secretions and properly positioning the infant in the "sniff" position.
- **Breathing**: This step involves initiating breathing after the airway has been established. This can be done with stimulation, supplemental oxygen, or through artificial ventilation. Oxygen should be initiated at 21% (up to 30% in preterm neonates) and titrated as needed.
- **Circulation**: Once an airway is open and breathing has been established, then circulation is considered. Chest compressions or the administration of volume expanders may be indicated. Epinephrine is only indicated if the heart rate remains <60 despite warming, ventilation, and chest compressions.

## Establishing Airway and Stimulating Respirations

To **establish an airway**, the infant is placed supine with the head slightly extended in the "sniffing" position. A small neck roll may be placed under the shoulders to maintain this position in a very small premature infant. Once the proper position is established, the mouth and nose are suctioned (mouth first, to prevent reflex aspiration of secretions when the nose is suctioned) with a bulb syringe or catheter if necessary. The infant's head can be turned momentarily to the side to allow secretions to pool in the cheek where they can be more easily suctioned and removed to establish the airway. **Stimulating** the newborn is often all that is needed to initiate spontaneous respirations. This tactile stimulation can be accomplished by gently rubbing the infant's back or trunk. Another technique used to provide stimulation is flicking or rubbing the soles of the feet. Slapping neonates as stimulation is no longer practiced and should NOT be used.

## Administration of Free-Flow Oxygen

If an infant remains cyanotic in the chest area (central cyanosis) after the initial steps of resuscitation have taken place, administering **free-flow oxygen** is the next step to take. Free-flow oxygen is administered to the neonate by the use of either a mask hooked up to an oxygen source or by the use of the oxygen tubing itself. If the tubing alone is used, the nurse can hold the tube with a cupped hand to help direct and concentrate the oxygen at the infant's airway. Free flow oxygen should be administered at a rate of 5 L/minute, initiated at 21% (up to 30% in preterm neonates). If the infant starts to turn pink, the oxygen can be carefully and slowly removed while continuing to closely monitor the infant for returning cyanosis. If the infant remains centrally cyanotic after the administration of free-flow oxygen, bag and mask ventilation must be considered as the next step.

## Bag and Mask Ventilation

Ventilation using a bag and mask is indicated when one or more of the following occurs and has not responded to other resuscitation attempts:

- Apnea that does not respond to tactile stimulation such as rubbing the chest or back or flicking the soles of the feet
- Gasping respirations
- Heart rate of <100 bpm, determined by auscultation at the apex of the heart or palpation of the base of the umbilical cord
- Central cyanosis that persists after administering free-flow oxygen (Acrocyanosis alone is NOT an indication for the need for further oxygenation or ventilation.)

The flowmeter is set at 5-10 L/min, and opening breath pressures of 30-40 $cmH_2O$ are used for full term infants and 20-25 $cmH_2O$ for preterm. Ventilation is done at 40-60 breaths/min with pressure of 15-20 $cmH_2O$ for normal lungs and 20-50 $cmH_2O$ for immature or compromised lungs.

### *Flow-Inflating Bag and Mask Ventilation*

Bag and mask ventilation is indicated for persistent apnea or gasping respirations, bradycardia (<100 bpm), and persistent cyanosis unrelieved by free-flowing oxygen.

**Flow-inflating bag and mask** (connected to oxygen flow, which inflates bag) equipment includes:

- Oxygen inlet
- Flow control valve
- Pressure manometer attachment
- Patient outlet for mask attachment

**Advantages**: Flow-inflating bag and mask ventilation has the ability to deliver anywhere from 21% (room air) to 100% oxygen; any pressure desired can be set. This type of bag and mask also has the ability to maintain positive end-expiratory pressure (PEEP) and CPAP.

**Disadvantages**: Because this bag must be connected to a gas (oxygen) source to inflate, it can only be used where a gas supply exists. It requires some experience to deliver the desired quantity of air with each breath. The high pressures possible with this type of equipment make overinflation of the lungs possible, resulting in pneumothorax. A complete seal is necessary to deliver a tidal volume.

### *Self-Inflating Bag and Mask Ventilation*

Self-inflating bag and mask (does not require gas source) equipment includes:

- Air inlet
- Oxygen inlet
- Patient outlet for mask attachment
- Valve assembly
- Oxygen reservoir
- Pop-off valve
- Pressure manometer attachment

**Advantages**: Self-inflating bag and mask ventilation is simple to use and does not require much practice or experience to operate. It can be operated anywhere, even if no oxygen source is near, and can easily deliver a tidal volume.

**Disadvantages**: These bags usually have a pop-off valve that will open at a pressure set by the manufacturer to prevent over inflation of the lungs. This valve popping off can prevent the ability to deliver enough pressure to ventilate very noncompliant lungs. Another disadvantage is that if 90% or higher oxygen delivery is desired, this equipment must have a reservoir attached to deliver this concentration. The inability to deliver PEEP is also a disadvantage to the self-inflating bag and mask.

## Gastric Suctioning Following Neonatal Resuscitation

When an infant is resuscitated using a bag and mask, air is inadvertently pumped into the stomach as it is being pumped into the lungs, so **gastric suctioning** is necessary. Once respirations have been stabilized, either spontaneously or with mechanical ventilation, the stomach should be aspirated to remove any air pumped into it. If the air is left in the abdomen, it remains distended, causing an upward pressure on the lungs; this compromises lung capacity and breathing effort. Use this procedure:

1. Select an orogastric catheter or size 8 Fr. feeding tube.
2. Measure the distance from the nose to the earlobe, then to the xiphoid.
3. Mark the tube at this distance.
4. Advance the tube to the mark.
5. Attach a 20 mL syringe to the tube.
6. Aspirate the contents of the stomach.
7. Leave the tube in place, open to air, and taped to the infant's cheek to keep the stomach decompressed.

## Chest Compressions

If **chest compressions** are indicated for resuscitation, these steps should be followed.

1. Position the neonate in the "sniffing" position with the neck slightly extended.
2. Make sure there is firm support for the infant's back.
3. Using a two-finger technique, proceed with the compressions on the lower third of the sternum with a depth of one third of the anterior-posterior diameter of the chest. The compression rate is 90 compressions per minute and 30 breaths per minute, equaling 120 "events" per minute. Essentially, one cycle is 3 compressions and 1 breath every 2 seconds.
4. When performing the compressions, the hands should be placed in a circle around the chest to provide support to the infant's back. The ratio of compressions to breaths should be 3:1.
5. Check the heart rate again after 30 seconds of compressions—about 45 compressions total.
6. If the heart rate is less than 60 beats per minute, continue with another round of compressions, but if the rate is 60 beats per minute or higher, stop compressions.

During chest compressions, oxygen should be delivered at a concentration of 100%.

## Indications for Stopping or Not Providing Resuscitation to Newborn

The decision to **discontinue or not perform resuscitative efforts** in the newborn (DNR) is very difficult to make. Whenever possible, the decision to withhold or stop resuscitative efforts in the newborn should be made by the attending physician with parental input, especially in situations with variable degrees of morbidity and mortality. Infants born under these conditions associated with certain death should not be resuscitated:

- Extreme prematurity (less than 23 weeks gestation)
- Extremely low birth weight (less than 400 grams)
- Congenital anomalies that are incompatible with life (anencephaly, trisomy 13 or 18)

Discontinue resuscitation of the infant who has not responded to appropriate resuscitation for 10 minutes and shows no signs of life (no heart rate or respiratory effort).

## Resuscitation Medications

### *Epinephrine*

**Epinephrine** is a naturally-occurring hormone produced by the adrenal glands. Epinephrine is used to resuscitate both adults and children. It is a sympathomimetic that supports the circulatory system by:

- Increasing heart rate
- Increasing contraction strength
- Vasoconstricting vessels in the skin, mucosa, and circulation of the gastrointestinal tract, causing a rise in blood pressure

If positive pressure ventilation and chest compressions have not caused the neonate's heart rate to rise above 60 beats per minute during resuscitation, then epinephrine is indicated. The recommended IV dose is 0.01-0.03 mg/kg. The usual concentration of epinephrine is 1:10,000 or 0.1 mg/mL. Endotracheal administration is not widely recommended, but may be used if no IV access is available. Higher doses are required for endotracheal administration (0.05-0.1 mg/kg).

### *Volume Expanders*

**Volume expanders** used in neonatal resuscitation include:

- Normal saline
- Ringer's Lactate
- O- blood, or blood that has been crossmatched with the mother

Prepare 40 mL in a syringe or IV. Give 10 mL/kg over 5-10 minutes. Repeat if necessary. Rapid infusion of a large volume causes intraventricular hemorrhage. (5% albumin in saline is no longer the solution of choice.) Consider volume expanders in instances where neonatal blood loss is suspected and/or the neonate is showing signs of shock that is not responding to other resuscitative efforts. Blood loss occurs due to trauma of the placenta or umbilical cord, or with neonatal hemolysis. Shock is inadequate perfusion in tissues and organs. Signs and symptoms of shock are pallor, cold extremities, neurological depression, and weak pulse.

### *Naloxone Hydrochloride*

**Naloxone hydrochloride**, an opiate antagonist, is not used in the routine resuscitation of an infant but is used in one very specific situation following birth. Naloxone is considered the antidote for narcotics administered to the mother of the infant within 4 hours of birth if the infant shows signs of serious respiratory depression from secondary absorption. If the mother of the infant has narcotics in her system as a result of an addiction to narcotics rather than as treatment for labor pain, however, naloxone cannot be given to this infant. If naloxone is given to an infant born to a narcotic-addicted mother, the drug will cause a severe abstinence reaction in the newborn that can result in seizure.

## NEONATAL TRANSPORT

An infant that is severely compromised at birth or <32 weeks gestation often requires **transport** to specialized neonatal care units, usually because of respiratory distress, preterm birth, congenital anomalies, and suspected cardiac abnormalities. The infant should be resuscitated and stabilized prior to transport. Communication with the regional center should be immediate and detailed. The **STABLE program** (**s**ugar, **t**emperature, **a**rtificial breathing, **b**lood pressure, **l**ab work, and **e**motional support) can guide efforts to stabilize the infant. The transport team must take copies of all records and lab reports. Transport teams may include NICU nurses, NNPs, physicians, and respiratory therapists. Adequate supplies (similar to those needed for resuscitation) must be available as well as oxygen, air-blended mixtures, monitors, and transport incubators. The incubator must control temperature while allowing access. Insulating material may be needed for very cold environments.

# Mental Health Emergencies

## Psychosocial Assessment

### Elements of the Psychosocial Assessment

A psychosocial assessment should provide additional information to the physical assessment to guide the patient's plan of care and should include:

- Previous hospitalizations and experience with healthcare
- Psychiatric history: Suicidal ideation, psychiatric disorders, family psychiatric history, history of violence and/or self-mutilation
- Chief complaint: Patient's perception
- Complementary therapies: Acupuncture, visualization, and meditation
- Occupational and educational background: Employment, retirement, and special skills
- Social patterns: Family and friends, living situation, typical activities, support system
- Sexual patterns: Orientation, problems, and sex practices
- Interests/abilities: Hobbies and sports
- Current or past substance abuse: Type, frequency, drinking pattern, use of recreational drugs, and overuse of prescription drugs
- Ability to cope: Stress reduction techniques
- Physical, sexual, emotional, and financial abuse: Older adults are especially vulnerable to abuse and may be reluctant to disclose out of shame or fear
- Spiritual/Cultural assessment: Religious/Spiritual importance, practices, restrictions (such as blood products or foods), and impact on health/health decisions

### Cognitive Assessment

Individuals with evidence of dementia, delirium, or short-term memory loss should have cognition assessed. The **mini-mental state exam (MMSE)** or the **mini-cog test** are both commonly used. These tests require the individual to carry out specified tasks and are used as a baseline to determine change in mental status.

**MMSE:**

- Remembering and later repeating the names of 3 common objects
- Counting backward from 100 by 7s or spelling "world" backward
- Naming items as the examiner points to them
- Providing the location of the examiner's office, including city, state, and street address
- Repeating common phrases
- Copying a picture of interlocking shapes
- Following simple 3-part instructions, such as picking up a piece of paper, folding it in half, and placing it on the floor

*A score of ≥24/30 is considered a normal functioning level.*

**Mini-cog:**

- Remembering and later repeating the names of 3 common objects
- Drawing the face of a clock, including all 12 numbers and the hands, and indicating the time specified by the examiner

*A score of 3-5 (out of 5) indicates a lower chance of dementia but does not rule it out.*

## Confusion Assessment Method

The Confusion Assessment Method is an assessment tool intended to be used by those without psychiatric training in order to assess the progression of delirium in patients. The tool covers 9 factors, some factors have a range of possibilities, and others are rated only as to whether the characteristic is present, not present, uncertain, or not applicable. The tool also provides room to describe abnormal behavior. Factors indicative of delirium include:

- **Onset**: Acute change in mental status
- **Attention**: Inattentive, stable, or fluctuating
- **Thinking**: Disorganized, rambling conversation, switching topics, illogical
- **Level of consciousness**: Altered, ranging from alert to coma
- **Orientation**: Disoriented (person, place, and time)
- **Memory**: Impaired
- **Perceptual disturbances**: Hallucinations, illusions
- **Psychomotor abnormalities**: Agitation (tapping, picking, moving) or retardation (staring, not moving)
- **Sleep-wake cycle**: Awake at night and sleepy in the daytime

**The Confusion Assessment Method indicates delirium if there is an acute onset, fluctuating inattention, and disorganized thinking OR altered level of consciousness.*

## Hamilton Anxiety Scale

The Hamilton Anxiety Scale (HAS or HAMA) is utilized to evaluate the anxiety related symptomatology that may be present in adults as well as children. It provides an evaluation of overall **anxiety** and its degree of severity. This includes **somatic anxiety** (physical complaints) and **psychic anxiety** (mental agitation and distress). This scale consists of 14 items based on anxiety produced symptoms. Each item is ranked 0-4 with 0 indicating no symptoms present and 4 indicating severe symptoms present. This scale is frequently utilized in psychotropic drug evaluations. If performed before a particular medication has been started and then again at later visits, the HAS can be helpful in adjusting medication dosages based in part on the individual's score. It is often utilized as an outcome measure in clinical trials.

## Beck Depression Inventory

The Beck Depression Inventory (BDI) is a widely utilized, self-reported, multiple-choice questionnaire consisting of 21 items, which measures the **degree of depression**. This tool is designed for use in adults ages 17-80. It evaluates physical symptoms such as weight loss, loss of sleep, loss of interest in sex, fatigue, and attitudinal symptoms such as irritability, guilt, and hopelessness. The items rank in four possible answer choices based on an increasing severity of symptoms. The test is scored with the answers ranging in value from 0 to 3. The total score is utilized to determine the degree of depression. The usual ranges include: 0-9 no signs of depression, 10-18 mild depression, 19-29 moderate depression, and 30-63 severe depression.

## Evaluation for Suicidal or Homicidal Thoughts

During a risk assessment two of the most important areas to evaluate are the patient's **risk for self-harm or harm to others**. The staff member performing the assessment should very closely evaluate for any descriptions or thoughts the patient may have concerning these risks. Direct questioning on these subjects should be performed and documented. Close evaluation of any delusional thoughts the patient may be having should be carefully evaluated. Does the patient believe he or she is being instructed by others to perform either of these acts? Safety of the patient and others needs to be a top priority and carefully documented. If the patient indicates that they are having these thoughts or ideas, they must be placed in either suicidal or assault precautions with close monitoring per facility protocol.

### Suicide Risk Assessment

A suicide risk assessment should be completed and documented upon admission, with each shift change, at discharge, or any time suicidal ideations are suggested by the patient. This risk assessment should evaluate some of the following criteria:

- Would the patient sign a contract for safety?
- Is there a suicide plan? How lethal is the plan?
- What is the elopement risk?
- How often are the suicidal thoughts, and have they attempted suicide before?

Any associated symptoms of hopelessness, guilt, anger, helplessness, impulsive behaviors, nightmares, obsessions with death, or altered judgment should also be assessed and documented. The higher the score the higher the risk for suicide.

### Alcohol Use Assessment

The **Clinical Instrument for Withdrawal for Alcohol (CIWA)** is a tool used to assess the severity of alcohol withdraw. Each category is scored 0-7 points based on the severity of symptoms, except #10, which is scored 0-4. A score <5 indicates mild withdrawal without need for medications; for scores ranging 5-15, benzodiazepines are indicated to manage symptoms. A score >15 indicates severe withdrawal and the need for admission to the unit.

1. Nausea/Vomiting
2. Tremor
3. Paroxysmal Sweats
4. Anxiety
5. Agitation
6. Tactile Disturbances
7. Auditory Disturbances
8. Visual Disturbances
9. Headache
10. Disorientation or Clouding of Sensorium

The **CAGE** tool is used as a quick assessment to identify problem drinkers. Moderate drinking, (1-2 drinks daily or one drink a day for older adults) is usually not harmful to people in the absence of other medical conditions. However, drinking more can lead to serious psychosocial and physical problems. One drink is defined as 12 ounces of beer/wine cooler, 5 ounces of wine, or 1.5 ounces of liquor.

- **C** - *Cutting Down*: "Do you think about trying to cut down on drinking?"
- **A** - *Annoyed at Criticism*: "Are people starting to criticize your drinking?"
- **G** - *Guilty feeling*: "Do you feel guilty or try to hide your drinking?"
- **E** - *Eye opener*: "Do you increasingly need a drink earlier in the day?"

"Yes" on one question suggests the possibility of a drinking problem. "Yes" on ≥2 indicates a drinking problem

### Screening for Risk-Taking Behavior

The ability to assess outcomes and respond appropriately to risks are part of the decision-making process. Decision making can be impaired in patients with mental health disorders such as depression, anxiety, bipolar disorder, and personality disorders, as well as in patients who have experienced a brain injury or have a dependence on drugs or alcohol. Health care providers should screen patients for the presence of high-risk behaviors. This may be accomplished through a self-administered questionnaire or through a patient interview with a trained clinician. Examples of **high-risk behaviors** include substance use/abuse, high risk sexual behaviors, high risk driving behaviors such as drinking and driving, speeding or riding with a drunk driver, and violence related behaviors. Patients with an increased response to risk taking may exhibit signs of impulsivity and sensation seeking. Conversely, other patients may exhibit abnormally cautious behavior.

## Assessment of Unique Needs of Veterans

Assessment of **veterans** must include not only the standard assessments appropriate for the patient's age and gender but also assessment of combat-associated injuries and illnesses:

- Shrapnel and/or gunshot injuries: Associated physical limitations, pain
- Amputations: Mobility and prosthesis issues; body image issues
- PTSD: Extent, frequency of attacks, limiting factors, triggers
- Depression, suicidal ideation
- Substance abuse: Type and extent

Because a large number of veterans are among the homeless population, the veteran's living arrangements should be explored and appropriate referrals made if the patient is in need of housing. Veterans may be unaware of programs offered through the US Department of Veterans Affairs and should be provided information about these programs as appropriate for the patient's needs.

# Psychosocial Pathophysiology

## Developmental Delays and Intellectual Disability

Developmental delays occur when a patient does not progress mentally at the same rate as the general population. Intellectual disability is a condition in which individuals may have difficulty adapting to changing environments, need guidance in decision-making, and have self-care or communication deficits. Behaviors range from shy and passive to hyperactive and aggressive. Intellectual disability may be inherited (Tay-Sachs), toxin-related (maternal alcohol consumption), perinatal (hypoxia), environmental (lack of stimulation/neglect), or acquired (encephalitis, brain injury). **Diagnosis** involves performance results from standardized tests with behavior analysis. Intellectual disability classifications are based on IQ:

- **55-69 (mild, 85% of cases):** Educable to about 6th grade level. May not be diagnosed until adolescence. Usually able to learn skills and be self-supporting but may need assistance and supervision.
- **40-54 (moderate, 10% of cases):** Trainable and may be able to work and live in sheltered environments or with supervision.
- **25-39 (severe, 3-4% of cases):** Language usually delayed and can learn only basic academic skills and perform simple tasks.
- **≤25 (profound, 1-2% of cases):** Usually associated with neurological disorder with sensorimotor dysfunction. Require constant care and supervision.

**Nursing considerations:** Always treat patients according to their developmental level, not their physical age. This is especially important when considering education and consent. People with developmental delays are at increased risk for injury and abuse.

## Personality Disorder

A personality disorder is a fixed and enduring set pattern or traits of behavior that **deviate from expected behaviors within a culture**. These disorders inhibit the individual's ability to have meaningful interpersonal relationships, to be fulfilled, or to enjoy life. Onset usually occurs during adolescence or early adulthood. A personality disorder is an attitude directed toward the whole world including one's own self. This attitude is expressed through thoughts, feelings, and behaviors. Many times, the behaviors will become less extreme as the person gets older.

### *DSM Classification Groupings*

The DSM-5 lists 10 personality disorders grouped into three clusters: A, B, and C.

- **Cluster A** includes disorders that are characterized by odd or eccentric behaviors and a tendency for social awkwardness and withdrawal.
- **Cluster B** includes disorders that are characterized by erratic, highly emotional, dramatic, or impulsive behaviors.
- **Cluster C** includes disorders that are characterized predominantly by fearful or anxious symptoms.

#### Specific Diagnoses Included in Cluster A for Personality Disorders

**Cluster A:** The classification of Cluster A for personality disorders includes the diagnoses of paranoid, schizoid, and schizotypal personality disorders.

- The **paranoid** individual is very distrustful and suspicious of others. They believe that other people are up to no good, are keeping secrets, and may intend to harm them. There is usually no basis or evidence to support this belief.

- The **schizoid** individual exhibits a consistent social detachment. Many of their behaviors indicate a restricted emotional response and can include appearing cold and indifferent, having no desire for close personal relationships, having no desire for intimacy, choosing solidarity over socializing, and usually having no close friends or relatives.
- Like the schizoid individual, the **schizotypal** individual tends to lack intimate relationships, but this is due to social ineptitude and fear rather than a lack of interest in relationship. They also experience cognitive and perceptual distortions, seeing or hearing things that are not there, and hold odd or superstitious beliefs.

#### Specific Diagnoses Included in Cluster B for Personality Disorders

**Cluster B:** The classification of Cluster B for personality disorders includes the diagnoses of antisocial, borderline, histrionic, and narcissistic personality disorders.

- The **antisocial** individual exhibits a blatant disregard for other people. They frequently lie, manipulate, exploit, and commit illegal acts.
- The **borderline** individual has a markedly unstable self-image. They are very impulsive, self-destructive, have unstable and intense interpersonal relationships, mood instability, inappropriate and intense anger, and may have recurrent suicidal or self-mutilating behaviors.
- The **histrionic** individual is extremely emotional and desires to be the center of attention. They often perform attention-seeking behaviors and have frequent, intense, and short-lived relationships.
- The **narcissistic** individual has a great sense of self-importance and is often arrogant. They lack empathy for others and can be exploitative and manipulative, and they tend to react violently if they perceive disrespect or opposition.

#### Specific Diagnoses Included in Cluster C for Personality Disorders

**Cluster C***:* The classification of Cluster C for personality disorders includes the diagnoses of avoidant, dependent, and obsessive-compulsive personality disorders.

- The **avoidant** individual is socially inhibited and consequently avoids interaction with others. They are very sensitive to criticism or rejection and often have feelings of inadequacy.
- The **dependent** individual has very low self-esteem and will be submissive and dependent in behaviors and relationships, making them susceptible to being taken advantage of. If they lose their primary supportive relationship, they will quickly seek to establish another one.
- The **obsessive-compulsive** individual will have an extreme preoccupation with minute details, and will possess an inflexible perfectionism and desire for control. They also exhibit cold, unfeeling, and superior attitudes towards others.

### Bipolar Disorder

Bipolar disorder causes severe mood swings between hyperactive states and depression, accompanied by impaired judgment because of distorted thoughts. The hypomanic stage may allow for creativity and good functioning in some people, but it can develop into more severe mania, which may be associated with psychosis and hallucinations with rapid speech and bizarre behavior, and then into periods of profound depression. While most cases are diagnosed in late adolescence, there is increasing evidence that some children present with symptoms earlier; especially at risk are children with a bipolar parent. Bipolar disorder is associated with high rates of suicide, so early diagnosis and treatment is critical.

**Symptoms** may be relatively mild or involve severe rapid cycling between mania and depression.

**Treatment** includes both medications (usually given continually) to prevent cycling and control depression and psychosocial therapy, such as cognitive therapy, to help control disordered thought patterns and behavior. Psychiatric referral should be made.

## Obsessive-Compulsive Disorder

Anxiety disorders also include the diagnosis of obsessive-compulsive disorder (OCD). OCD involves either **obsessions** or **compulsions** that are persistent impulses or thoughts that are uncontrollable by the person. These thoughts lead to an **abnormally elevated anxiety response**. Some examples of obsessions can include fear of dirt, germs, robbery, contracting a medical disease, unintentional discarding of important information, having images of a sexual nature, or things not being symmetrical or completed. Compulsions are when the individual is driven to perform certain repetitive behaviors in ritualistic order with the outcome being resolution of the anxiety caused by the obsession.

Some examples of **compulsive repetitive behaviors** can include hand washing, checking locks, counting objects found routinely within their normal day, hoarding, ordering or arranging items, or saying words silently.

### *Comorbidities*

When an individual has two or more disorders occurring at the same time, these disorders are considered to share **comorbidity**. Obsessive-compulsive disorder (OCD) is often found sharing comorbidity with other psychological disorders. Many times, individuals with OCD also have Tourette's syndrome, depression, panic attacks, mood disorders, social and specific phobias, eating disorders, or personality disorders. It has been found that Tourette's syndrome and OCD actually cause similar brain dysfunctions. Depression is commonly seen in patient's suffering from OCD due to the isolating effects it can have upon their lifestyle. It is also common for these individuals to have substance abuse problems due to trying to self-medicate to solve their struggles with OCD.

## Depression

Depression is a mood disorder characterized by profound feelings of sadness and withdrawal. It may be acute (such as after a death) or chronic with recurring episodes over a lifetime. The cause appears to be a combination of genetic, biological, and environmental factors. A major depressive episode is a depressed mood, profound and constant sense of hopelessness and despair, or loss of interest in all or almost all activities for a period of at least two weeks. Some drugs may precipitate depression: diuretics, Parkinson's drugs, estrogen, corticosteroids, cimetidine, hydralazine, propranolol, digitalis, and indomethacin. Depression is associated with neurotransmitter dysregulation, especially serotonin and norepinephrine. Major depression can be mild, moderate, or severe.

**Symptoms** include changes in mood, sadness, loss of interest in usual activities, increased fatigue, changes in appetite and fluctuations in weight, anxiety, and sleep disturbance.

**Treatment** includes tricyclic antidepressants (TCAS) and SSRIs, but SSRIs have fewer side effects and are less likely to cause death with an overdose. Counseling, undergoing cognitive behavioral therapy, treating underlying cause, and instituting an exercise program may help reduce depression.

### *Anxiety and Depression Due to Intensive Care Stays*

Anxiety and depression affect over half of patients who are treated in intensive care not only during the stay but also after discharge, especially if care is long-term or if their needs for moderate or high care continue. Additionally, studies have shown that those who suffer depression during and after ICU stays have increased risk of mortality over the next two years. Patients with anxiety may appear restless (thrashing about the bed), have difficulty concentrating, exhibit tachycardia and tachypnea, experience insomnia and feelings of dread, and complain of various ailments, such as stomach ache and headache. Symptoms of depression may overlap (and patients may have both anxiety and depression) and may also include fatigue, insomnia, withdrawal, appetite change, irritability, pessimistic outlooks, feelings of worthlessness, sadness, and suicidal ideation. Brief screening tools for anxiety and depression should be used with all ICU patients and interventions per psychological referral made as needed.

## Anxiety Disorders

Anxiety is a human emotion and experience that everyone has at some point during their life. Feelings of uncertainty, helplessness, isolation, alienation, and insecurity can all be experienced during an **anxiety response**. Many times, anxiety occurs without a specific known object or source. It can occur because of the unknown. Anxiety occurs throughout the life cycle, and therefore anxiety disorders can affect people of all ages. Populations that are most commonly affected include women, smokers, people under the age of 45, individuals that are separated or divorced, victims of abuse, and people in the lower socioeconomic groups. An individual can have one single anxiety disorder, experience more than one anxiety disorder, or have other mental health disorders all occurring at the same time.

### *Generalized Anxiety Disorder*

Generalized anxiety disorder can be very insidious and occurs when an individual consistently experiences **excessive anxiety and worry**. This anxiety and worry will be present almost every day and lasts for a period of at least six months. The worry and anxiety will be uncontrollable, intrusive, and not related to any medical disease process. It will pertain to real-life events, situations, or circumstances and may occur along with mild depression symptoms. The individual will also experience three or more of the following symptoms: fatigue, inability to concentrate, irritability, insomnia, restlessness, loosing thought processes or going blank, and muscle tension. The continued anxiety and worry will eventually affect daily functioning and cause social and occupational disturbances.

#### Comorbidities

Individuals with generalized anxiety disorder (GAD) will often have **other mental health disorders**. When a person has more than one psychological disorder occurring at the same time, these disorders are considered to be **comorbid**. Most patients suffering from GAD will have at least one more psychiatric diagnosis. The most common comorbid disorders can include major depressive disorder, social or specific phobias, panic disorder, and dysthymic disorder. It is also common for these individuals to have substance abuse problems, and they may look to alcohol or barbiturates to help control their symptoms of anxiety.

### *Levels of Anxiety*

There are four main levels of anxiety that were named by Peplau. They are as follows:

1. **Mild anxiety** is associated with normal tensions of everyday life. It can increase awareness and motivate learning and creativity.
2. **Moderate anxiety** occurs when the individual narrows their field of perception and focuses on the immediate problem. This level decreases the perceptual field; however, the person can tend to other tasks if directed.
3. **Severe anxiety** leads to a markedly reduced field of perception and the person focuses only on the details of the problem. All energy is directed at relieving the anxiety and the person can only perform other tasks under significant persuasion.
4. **Panic** is the most extreme level of anxiety and associated with feelings of dread and terror. The individual is unable to perform any other tasks no matter how strongly they are persuaded to do so. This level can be life-threatening with complete disorganization of thought occurring.

### *Physical Symptoms*

Anxiety produces a very physical response and effects the largest body systems, such as cardiovascular, respiratory, GI, neuromuscular, urinary tract, and skin. Symptoms vary and can increase upon a continuum depending upon the level of anxiety the person is experiencing.

- **Cardiovascular symptoms** can include palpitation, tachycardia, hypertension, feeling faint or actually fainting, hypotension, or bradycardia.
- **Respiratory symptoms** can include tachypnea, shortness of breath, chest pressure, shallow respirations, or choking sensation.
- **GI symptoms** can include revulsion toward food, nausea, diarrhea, and abdominal pain or discomfort.

Even though anxiety occurs psychologically, it can produce extreme **physical responses** from the neuromuscular system, urinary tract, and skin. These symptoms can range from mild to severe depending upon the degree of anxiety the person is experiencing.

- **Neuromuscular symptoms** can include hyperreflexia, being easily startled, eyelid twitching, inability to sleep, shaking, fidgeting, pacing, wobbly legs, or clumsy movements.
- **Urinary tract symptoms** can include increased frequency and sensation of need to urinate.
- **Skin symptoms** can include flushed face, sweaty palms, itching, sensations of being hot and/or cold, pale facial coloring, or diaphoresis.

### *Behavioral and Affective Responses*

Behavioral and affective symptoms along with a multitude of physical symptoms are observable in anxious patients. The effects of these responses can affect the person experiencing the anxiety along with their relationships with others.

- Some **behavioral responses** can include restlessness and physical tension, hypervigilance, rapid speech, social or relationship withdrawal, decreased coordination, avoidance, or flight.
- **Affective responses** are the patient's emotional reactions and can be described subjectively by the individual. Patients may describe symptoms such as edginess, impatience, tension, nervousness, fear, frustration, jitteriness, or helplessness.

### *Cognitive Responses*

Anxiety not only produces physical and emotional symptoms, but it can also greatly affect the individual's intellectual abilities. **Cognitive responses** to anxiety occur in three main categories. These include sensory-perceptual, thought difficulties, and conceptualization. Responses that affect the patient's **sensory-perceptual fields** can include feeling that their mind is unclear or clouded, seeing objects indistinctly, perceiving a surreal environment, increased self-consciousness, or hypervigilance. **Thinking difficulties** can include the inability to remember important information, confusion, inability to focus thoughts or attention, easily distracted, blocking thoughts, difficulty with reasoning, tunnel vision, or loss of objectivity. **Conceptual difficulties** can include the fear of loss of control, inability to cope, potential physical injury, developing a mental disorder, or receiving a negative evaluation. The patient may have cognitive distortion, protruding scary visual images, or uncontrollable repetition of fearful thoughts.

## Panic Attacks

Panic attacks are short episodes (peaking in 5-10 minutes) of intense anxiety that can result in a wide variety of **symptoms** that include:

- Dyspnea
- Palpitations
- Hyperventilation
- Nausea and vomiting

- Intense fear or anxiety
- Pain and pressure in the chest
- Dizziness and fainting
- Tremors

Panic attacks may be associated with agoraphobia, depression, or intimate partner violence and abuse (IPVA), so a careful history is important. Typically, patients believe they are dying or having a heart attack and require reassurance and treatment, such as diazepam or lorazepam, in the ED for the acute episode. In severe cases, ASA may be given and EKG done to rule out cardiac abnormalities. Patients should be referred for psychiatric evaluation for ongoing medications such as SSRIs (sertraline, paroxetine, fluoxetine) to prevent recurrence. Panic attacks become chronic panic disorders if they are recurrent, with each attack each followed by at least a month of fear of another attack.

## PTSD

Patients that experience a traumatic event may re-experience the trauma through distressing thoughts and recollections of the event. In addition, psychological effects of the trauma may include difficulty sleeping, emotional lability and problems with memory and concentration. Patients may also wish to avoid places or activities that remind them of their trauma. These are all characteristics of **post-traumatic stress disorder (PTSD)** and may cause patients extreme distress and significantly impact their quality of life.

**Signs and symptoms**: Nightmares, flashbacks, insomnia, symptoms of hyperarousal including irritability and anxiety, avoidance, and negative thoughts and feelings about oneself and others.

**Diagnosis**: PTSD is diagnosed through psychological assessment and criteria defined in the Diagnostic and Statistical Manual of Mental Disorders, Fifth Edition (DSM-5).

**Treatment**: Pharmacologic therapy may be utilized to help control the symptoms of PTSD. Non-pharmacologic therapy options include group and individual/family therapy, cognitive behavioral therapy, and anxiety management/relaxation techniques. Hypnosis may also be utilized.

## Stress

### *Relationship Between Stress and Disease*

Stress causes a number of physical and psychological changes within the body:

- Cortisol levels increase
- Digestion is hindered and the colon stimulated
- Heart rate increases
- Perspiration increases
- Anxiety and depression occur and can result in insomnia, anorexia or weight gain, and suicide
- Immune response decreases, making the person more vulnerable to infections
- Autoimmune reaction may increase, leading to autoimmune diseases

The body's **compensatory mechanisms** try to restore homeostasis. When these mechanisms are overwhelmed, pathophysiological injury to the cells of the body result. When this injury begins to interfere with the function of the organs or systems in the body, symptoms of dysfunction will occur. If the conditions are not corrected, the body changes the structure or function of the affected organs or systems.

### *Adaptation of Cells to Stress*

The most common stressors to cells include the lack of oxygen, presence of toxins or chemicals, and infection. **Cells react to stress** by making the following changes:

- **Hypertrophy**: Cells swell, leading to an overall increase in the size of the affected organ.
- **Atrophy**: Cells shrivel and the overall organ size decreases in size.
- **Hyperplasia**: The cells divide and overgrowth and thickening of the tissue results.
- **Dysplasia**: The cells are changed in appearance as a result of irritation over an extended period of time, sometimes leading to malignancy.
- **Metaplasia**: Cells change type as a result of stress.

If the stress that caused the cells to change continues, the cells become injured and die. When enough cells die, organ and systemic failure occur.

### *Psychological Response to Stress*

When stress is encountered, a person **responds** according to the threat perceived to compensate. The threat is evaluated as to the amount of harm or loss that has occurred or is possible. If the stress is benign (such as with marriage), then a challenge is present that demands change. Once the threat or challenge is defined, the person can gather information, resources, and support to make the changes needed to resolve the stress to the greatest degree possible. Immediate psychological response to stress may include shock, anger, fear, or excitement. Over time, people may develop chronic anxiety, depression, flashbacks, thought disturbances, and sleep disturbances. Changes may occur in emotions and thinking, in behavior, or in the person's environment. People may be more able to adapt to stress if they have many varied experiences, a good self-esteem, and a support network to help as needed. A healthy lifestyle and philosophical beliefs, including religion, may give a person more reserve to cope with stress.

### *Impact of Different Kinds of Stress*

Everyone encounters **stress** in life and it **impacts** each person differently. There are the small daily "hassles," major traumatic events, and the periodic stressful events of marriage, birth, divorce, and death. Compounded stress experienced on a daily basis can impact health status over time. Stressors that occur suddenly are the hardest to overcome and result in the greatest tension. The length of time that a stressor is present affects the impact with long-term, relentless stress, such as that generated by poverty or disability, resulting in disease more often. If there is **ineffective coping**, a person will suffer greater changes resulting in even more stress. The nurse can help patients to recognize those things that induce stress in their lives, find ways to reduce stress when possible, and teach effective coping skills and problem-management.

## Violence and Aggression

Violence and aggression are sometimes seen in critical care settings. The nurse must be aware of signs of impending violence or aggression in order to intervene and prevent injury to self or staff.

- **Violence** is a physical act perpetrated against an inanimate object, animal, or other person with the intent to cause harm. Violence often results from anger, frustration, or fear. It often occurs because the perpetrator believes that he is threatened in some way. Violence may occur suddenly without warning or following an escalating pattern of aggressive behavior.
- **Aggression** is the communication of a threat or intended act of violence that often occurs before the act of violence is carried out. This communication can occur verbally or nonverbally. Gestures, shouting, increasing volume of speech, invasion of personal space, and prolonged eye contact are all examples of aggression. The nurse should promptly recognize all forms of aggression and redirect or remove the patient from the situation to avoid an act of violence.

### MANAGEMENT OF PATIENTS WITH VIOLENT BEHAVIOR

Patients may exhibit **violent behavior** for a number of reasons, including metabolic disorders (hypoglycemia), neurological disorders (brain tumor), psychiatric disorders (schizophrenia), or substance abuse (drugs and alcohol). Patients who make threats or have a history of violent behavior should be approached with caution.

**Diagnosis** includes history, physical exam, CBC and chemistry panel, toxicology screening, ECG, and, in some cases, CT scans or lumbar punctures. Violent behavior tends to escalate from anxiety to defensiveness to aggression, so identifying these signs and providing support through information, setting limits, using restraints, and seclusion can avoid injuries. Handcuffs should not be removed in the ED, and patients who are so violent they must be restrained should not be allowed to leave the ED against medical advice.

**Pharmacologic treatment** includes:

- **Antipsychotic drugs**: Haloperidol 5 mg IM (1-2 mg for elderly patients)
- **Benzodiazepines**: Lorazepam 2-4 mg IM/IV (often in conjunction with antipsychotic drugs)
- **Hypnotics**: Droperidol 2.5 mg IM/IV

## HOMICIDAL IDEATION

Homicidal ideation, the intention to kill another person, can occur for a variety of reasons:

- **Sociopathy/psychopathy**: These patients usually appear quite normal and may even seem charming, but they can be very dangerous because they lack empathy for others. Some are involved in gangs in which violent behavior is expected and valued.
- **Psychosis**: Uncontrolled schizophrenia and paranoia may result in a patient behaving in a homicidal manner. In some cases, these changes may be brought about by pathology, such as TBI or brain tumor.
- **Medications**: Medications such as antidepressants, SSRIs, and antipsychotics as well as interferon have been associated with homicidal ideation in some patients. Patients on multiple medications may experience an involuntary intoxication that results in rage reactions and sometimes even the death of others.

Indications of homicidal ideation may include verbal threats, use of weapons, and violent behavior. Patients who express homicidal ideation or have attempted homicide require immediate psychiatric referral and may require restraint. The nurse should conduct a complete review of medications and notify security personnel if the patient poses a danger.

## PSYCHOSIS

Psychosis is a severe reaction to stressors (psychological, physical) that results in alterations in affect and impaired psychomotor and behavioral functions, including the onset of hallucinations and/or delusions. Psychosis is not a diagnosis but is a symptom that may be caused by a mental disorder (such as schizophrenia or bipolar disease) or a physical disorder (such as a brain tumor or Alzheimer's disease). Psychosis may also be induced by some prescription drugs (muscle relaxants, antihistamines, anticonvulsants, corticosteroids, antiparkinson drugs), illicit drugs (cocaine, PCP, amphetamines, cannabis, LSD), and alcohol. Treatment depends on identifying the underlying cause of the psychosis and initiating treatment. For example, if caused by schizophrenia, then antipsychotic drugs and hospitalization in a mental health facility may be indicated. In most cases of drug-induced psychosis, stopping the drug alleviates the symptoms although some may benefit from the addition of a benzodiazepine or antipsychotic drug until symptoms subside.

## SUICIDAL IDEATION

Patients may attempt suicide for many reasons, including severe depression, social isolation, situational crisis, bereavement, or psychotic disorder.

**Suicidal indications** are as follows:

- Depression or dysphoria
- Hostility to others
- Problems with peer relationships, and lack of close friends
- Post-crisis stress (divorce, death in family, graduation, college)
- Withdrawn personality; quiet or lonely appearance or behavior
- Change in behavior (dropping grades, unkempt appearance, change in sleeping patterns)
- A sudden increase in positive mood may indicate patient has a plan
- Co-morbid psychiatric problems (bipolar, schizophrenia)
- Substance abuse

The following are indicators of **high risk for repeated suicide attempt**:

- Violent suicide attempt (knives, gunshots)
- Suicide attempt with low chance of rescue
- Ongoing psychosis or disordered thinking
- Ongoing severe depression and feeling of helplessness
- History of previous suicide attempts
- Lack of social support system

**Nursing considerations:** Take all suicidal ideations seriously; do not minimize them. Suicidal patients should be watched continuously, given plastic utensils, break-away wall rails/shower heads, no cords/sharp instruments.

## SUBSTANCE ABUSE

Substance abuse is the abuse of drugs, medicines, or alcohol that causes mental and physical problems for the abuser and family. Abusers use substances out of boredom, to hide negative self-esteem, to dampen emotional pain, and to cope with daily stress. As the abuse continues, abusers become unable to take care of daily needs and duties. They lack effective coping mechanisms and the ability to make healthy choices. They can't identify and prioritize stress or choose positive behavior to resolve the stress in a healthy way. Some family members may act as codependents because of their desire to feel needed by the abuser, to control the person, and to stay with him or her. The nurse can help the family to confront an individual with their concerns about the person and their proposals for treatment. Family members can enforce consequences if treatment is not sought. Family members may also need counseling to learn new behaviors to stop enabling the abuser to continue substance abuse.

### *PATHOPHYSIOLOGY OF ADDICTION*

Genetic, social, and personality factors may all play a role in the development of **addictive tendencies**. However, the main factor of the development of substance addiction is the pharmacological activation of the **reward system** located in the central nervous system (CNS). This reward systems pathway involves **dopaminergic neurons**. Dopamine is found in the CNS and is one of many neurotransmitters that play a role in an individual's mood. The mesolimbic pathway seems to play a primary role in the reward and motivational process involved with addiction. This pathway begins in the ventral tegmental area of the brain (VTA) and then moves forward into the nucleus accumbens located in the middle forebrain bundle (MFB). Some drugs enhance mesolimbic dopamine activity, therefore producing very potent effects on mood and behavior.

### *Indicators of Substance Abuse*

Many people with substance abuse (alcohol or drugs) are reluctant to disclose this information, but there are a number of **indicators** that are suggestive of substance abuse:

**Physical signs** include:

- Burns on fingers or lips
- Pupils abnormally dilated or constricted, eyes watery
- Slurring of speech, slow speech
- Lack of coordination, instability of gait, tremors
- Sniffing repeatedly, nasal irritation, persistent cough
- Weight loss
- Dysrhythmias
- Pallor, puffiness of face
- Needle tracks on arms or legs
- Odor of alcohol/marijuana on clothing or breath

**Behavioral signs** include:

- Labile emotions, including mood swings, agitation, and anger
- Inappropriate, impulsive, or risky behavior
- Lying
- Missing appointments
- Difficulty concentrating, short term memory loss, blackouts
- Insomnia or excessive sleeping; disoriented, confused
- Lack of personal hygiene

### *Alcohol Withdrawal*

Chronic abuse of ethanol (alcoholism) can lead to physical dependency. Sudden cessation of drinking, which often happens in the inpatient setting, is associated with **alcohol withdrawal syndrome.** It may be precipitated by trauma or infection and has a high mortality rate, 5-15% with treatment and 35% without treatment.

**Signs/Symptoms:** Anxiety, tachycardia, headache, diaphoresis, progressing to severe agitation, hallucinations, auditory/tactile disturbances, and psychotic behavior (delirium tremens).

**Diagnosis:** Physical assessment, blood alcohol levels (on admission).

**Treatment** includes:

- Medication: IV benzodiazepines to manage symptoms; electrolyte and nutritional replacement, especially magnesium and thiamine.
- Use the CIWA scale to measure symptoms of withdrawal; treat as indicated.
- Provide an environment with minimal sensory stimulus (lower lights, close blinds) & implement fall and seizure precautions.
- Prevention: Screen all patients for alcohol/substance abuse, using CAGE or other assessment tool. Remember to express support and comfort to patient; wait until withdrawal symptoms are subsiding to educate about alcohol use and moderation.

## EATING DISORDERS

### *ANOREXIA NERVOSA*

Eating disorders are a profound health risk and can lead to death, especially for adolescent girls, although boys also have eating disorders, often presenting as excessive exercise. Anorexia nervosa is characterized by profound fear of weight gain and severe restriction of food intake, often accompanied by abuse of diuretics and laxatives, which can cause electrolyte imbalances, kidney and bowel disorders, and delay or cessation of menses.

- **Symptoms** include growth retardation, amenorrhea (missing 3 consecutive periods), unexplained and sometimes precipitous weight loss (at least 15% below normal weight), dehydration, loss of appetite, hypoglycemia, hypercholesterolemia, or carotenemia with yellowing of skin, emaciated appearance, osteoporosis, bradycardia, and food obsessions and rituals.
- **Diagnosis** includes complete history, physical, and psychological exam with CBC and chemical panels to rule out other disorders.
- **Treatment** includes volume and electrolyte replacement initially with referral to psychiatric care for long-term management of the disorder and nutritional plans.

### *BULIMIA NERVOSA*

Bulimia nervosa includes binge eating followed by vomiting (at least 2 times monthly for at least 3 months), often along with diuretics, enemas, and laxatives. Some may engage in periods of fasting or excessive exercise rather than vomiting to offset the effects of binging. Gastric acids from purging can damage the throat and teeth. While bulimics may maintain a normal weight, they are at risk for severe electrolyte imbalances that can be life-threatening. Binge eating affects 2% to 5% of females and includes grossly overeating, often resulting in obesity, depression, and shame. Symptoms include hypokalemia, metabolic acidosis, fluctuations of weight, dental caries and loss of enamel, knuckle scars (from contact with teeth while inducing vomiting), parotid and submandibular gland enlargement, and insulin-dependent diabetes. Diagnosis includes complete history, physical, and psychological exam with CBC and chemical panels to rule out other disorders. Treatment includes volume and electrolyte replacement initially with referral to psychiatric care for long-term management of the disorder and nutritional plans, as well as SSRIs, naltrexone, and ondansetron.

# Psychosocial Interventions

## TRAUMA-INFORMED CARE

Trauma-informed care acts on the premise that many individuals have experienced some sort of trauma, and therefore every patient should be approached with sensitivity and care. Traumatic events are deeply individualized, and what may have been traumatic to one individual, may not be to the next. Withholding judgment of what qualifies as trauma is imperative for the psychiatric-mental health nurse.

The five elements of **trauma-informed care** include the following:

- **Safety**: Ensuring that the patient feels emotionally and physically safe must be the first priority in order to create a conducive environment for treatment.
- **Choice**: Treatment cannot be forced and must honor the individual's right to choose.
- **Collaboration**: The patient and the nurse must work collaboratively through shared decision-making.
- **Trustworthiness**: The patient must trust the nurse in order for treatment to be effective. Trustworthiness can be established by communicating what is happening and what will happen next to the patient.
- **Empowerment**: Empower the patient with tools to cope on their own so that their recovery extends outside the walls of treatment.

## PSYCHIATRIC AND MENTAL HEALTH PROGRAMS

A variety of psychiatric and mental health programs are available and should be evaluated, according to the needs of the individual patient.

- **Inpatient programs** provide a secure environment and comprehensive care, often with psychologists, psychiatrists, occupational therapists, social workers, and other allied health personnel. Programs may be tailored to one specific type of patient (e.g., criminally insane, substance abusers) or to a general population. They may offer short-term or long-term care.
- **Outpatient programs** provide assessment and treatment, such as group therapy, cognitive-behavioral therapy, and family therapy. Programs may be community-based, targeting specific groups of people, such as alcoholics or the homeless.
- **Partial/day hospitalization programs** provide daily inpatient care during prescribed hours (e.g., 8 a.m. to 3 p.m.) as well as outpatient services. The stay is usually short-term (1–2 weeks) and may serve as a transition from inpatient to outpatient care.

## NONVIOLENT CRISIS INTERVENTION AND DE-ESCALATION TECHNIQUES

Nonviolent crisis intervention and de-escalation techniques begin with self-awareness because the normal response to aggression is a stress response (freezing, fight/flight, fear). The nurse must control these responses in order to deal with the situation. The nurse should recognize signs of impending conflict (clenched fists, and sudden change in tone of voice or body stance, and change in eye contact). Steps include:

- Maintain social distance (≥12 feet) if possible and stay at the same level as the person (sitting or standing).
- Speak in a quiet calm tone of voice, limiting eye contact and avoiding changes in voice tone, facial expression, and gestures (especially avoid pointing or waving a finger at the person).
- Ask the person's name (if necessary) and use the name when addressing the person.
- Validate the person by acknowledging their issue: "I can see that you are angry about the changes in your treatment."
- Show empathy without being judgmental: "I'm sorry you are upset."
- Ignore questions that are challenging and avoid arguing.

- Practice active listening by paraphrasing and clarifying.
- Assist the person to explore options and the results of those options: "What is it that you would like to do?"

## Physical Restraints

Restraints are used to restrict movement and activity when other methods of controlling patient behavior have failed and there is a risk of harm to the patient or others. There are two primary types of **physical restraints**: violent (behavioral) and non-violent (clinical). Violent restraints are more commonly used in the psychiatric unit or when individuals exhibit aggressive behavior. More commonly, non-violent restraints are used to ensure that the individual does not interfere with safe care. Non-violent restraints are commonly used in the confused elderly or intubated patient to prevent pulling out lines/removing equipment. The federal government and the Joint Commission have issued strict **guidelines** for temporary restraints or those not part of standard care (such as post-surgical restraint):

- Each facility must have a written policy and restraints are only used when ordered by a physician (usually require written/signed order every 24hrs and within 4 hours of restraint initiation).
- An assessment must be completed frequently, including circulation, toileting, and nutritional needs (generally every 1-2 hours).
- All alternative methods should be tried before applying a restraint and the least restrictive effective restraint should be used.
- A nurse must remove the restraint, assess, and document findings at least every 2 hours, every hour for violent restraints.

*Key: Least restrictive option for the least amount of time.*

## Chemical Restraints

Chemical restraints involve the use of pharmacological sedatives to manage an individual's behavior problems. This type of restraint is indicated only when severe agitation/violence puts the patient at risk for injury to themselves or others. **Chemical restraints** inhibit the individuals' physical movements, making their behavior more manageable. It is important to realize that medication used on an ongoing basis as part of treatment is not legally considered a chemical restraint, even though the medications may be the same. There is little consensus about the use of chemical restraints, although benzodiazepines and antipsychotics are frequently used to control severe agitation (haloperidol, lorazepam, etc.). Oral medications should be tried first before injections, as oral medication is less coercive. It is important for the nurse to realize that chemical restraints are used as a last resort when other measures (such as de-escalation and environmental modification) have failed and there is an immediate risk of harm to the patient or others.

# Psychosocial Pharmacology

## ANTIPSYCHOTIC MEDICATIONS

### *FIRST-GENERATION*

There are a variety of first-generation antipsychotics available, though their use is becoming less prominent now that atypical antipsychotic agents are available. Some **first-generation antipsychotics** include:

- Chlorpromazine (Thorazine)
- Thioridazine hydrochloride (Mellaril)
- Haloperidol (Haldol)
- Pimozide (Orap)
- Fluphenazine hydrochloride (Prolixin)
- Molindone hydrochloride (Moban)
- Trifluoperazine hydrochloride (Stelazine)

**Possible side effects** include photosensitivity, sexual dysfunction, dry mouth, dry eyes, nasal congestion, blurred vision, constipation, urinary retention, exacerbation of narrow-angle glaucoma, various cardiac effects, extrapyramidal effects, dyskinesia, sedation, cognitive dulling, amenorrhea, menstrual irregularities, hyperglycemia or hypoglycemia, increased appetite, and weight gain. The most common extrapyramidal symptom caused by antipsychotic agents is tardive dyskinesia, in which clients are unable to control their movements, such as tics, lip-smacking, and eye blinking. The extrapyramidal system is a group of neural connections outside of the medulla that control movement. **Extrapyramidal effects** are the result of drug influence on the extrapyramidal system and include:

- Akinesia (inability to start movement)
- Akathisia (inability to stop movement)
- Dystonia (extreme and uncontrolled muscle contraction, torticollis, flexing, and twisting)

### *SECOND-GENERATION*

Second-generation antipsychotics (SGAs), also called atypical antipsychotics, are used for bipolar disorders, schizophrenia, and psychosis, and include aripiprazole (Abilify), clozapine (Clozaril), olanzapine (Zyprexa), quetiapine (Seroquel), risperidone (Risperdal), and ziprasidone (Geodon). Females report more side effects than males, but the recommended doses for males and females are identical. Women were underrepresented when SGAs were clinically tested, because researchers feared teratogenic effects on fetuses:

- Side effects include constipation, increased appetite, weight gain, urinary retention, various sexual side effects, increased prolactin, menstrual irregularities, increased risk of diabetes mellitus, decreased blood pressure, dizziness, agranulocytosis, and leucopenia.
- Atypical antipsychotics may interact with fluvoxamine, phenytoin, carbamazepine, barbiturates, nicotine, ketoconazole, phenytoin, rifampin, and glucocorticoids.
- The use of atypical antipsychotic agents correlates with significant weight gain. Overweight and obese clients are likely to develop insulin resistance and glucose intolerance, which may lead to diabetes mellitus. Data show clozapine and olanzapine as the greatest offenders. Ziprasidone seems to present the lowest risk.

**Review Video: Anti-Psychotic Drugs: Clozapine, Haloperidol, Etc.**
Visit mometrix.com/academy and enter code: 369601

## Antidepressants

### *Indications for Treatment with Antidepressant*

The main **indicator** for use of an antidepressant is simply **depression**. This can be further expanded to include major depression, atypical depression, and anxiety disorders. Depression-type symptoms commonly include loss of interest in usual or pleasurable activities, decreased levels of energy, having a depressed mood, decreased ability to concentrate, loss of appetite, or suicidal thoughts. Antidepressants are also commonly used to treat **anxiety disorders** that include panic attacks, obsessive-compulsive disorder (OCD), social phobias, and post-traumatic stress disorder. They may also be beneficial in treating chronic pain syndromes, premenstrual syndrome, insomnia, attention deficit hyperactivity disorder, or bed-wetting.

### *SSRIs*

Selective serotonin reuptake inhibitors (SSRIs) prevent the reuptake of serotonin at the presynaptic membrane. This increases the amount of serotonin in the synapse for neurotransmission. This class of antidepressants has been shown to reduce depression and anxiety symptoms. Common side effects are usually short in duration and include headache, GI upset, and sexual dysfunction. They do not cause significant anticholinergic, cardiovascular, or significant patient sedation side effects. Examples of SSRIs include citalopram (Celexa), escitalopram (Lexapro), fluoxetine (Prozac), Fluvoxamine (Luvox), paroxetine (Paxil), and sertraline (Zoloft). These drugs are not highly lethal in overdose.

#### Monitoring

SSRI monitoring includes the following:

- Monitor for increased depression and suicidal ideation, especially in adolescents.
- Inform patients of the following:
  - Smoking decreases effectiveness.
  - Fatal reactions may occur with monoamine oxidase inhibitors.
  - Taking SSRIs with benzodiazepines or alcohol has an additive effect.
  - Some drugs, such as citalopram, may increase the effects of β-blockers and warfarin.
- Avoid cimetidine, which is prescribed for ulcers and gastroesophageal reflux disease, and St. John's wort.
- Inform patients of possible decreased libido and sexual functioning.
- Monitor for insomnia and gastrointestinal upset.

### *Tricyclic Antidepressants*

Tricyclic antidepressants not only block the reuptake of serotonin and norepinephrine, they also act to block muscarinic cholinergic receptors, histamine H1 receptors, and alpha1 noradrenergic receptors. These receptors do not affect depression symptoms, but their blockade is implicated in some of the side effects associated with tricyclics. The blockade of the muscarinic receptors produces anticholinergic side effects such as dry mouth, blurred vision, constipation, urinary retention, and tachycardia. The blockade of the histamine receptors is associated with drowsiness, low blood pressure, and weight gain. The alpha1 noradrenergic receptor blocking action produces the side effects associated with orthostatic hypotension, vertigo, and some memory disturbances.

#### Mechanism of Action and Necessary Evaluations

Most of the tricyclic antidepressants have very similar mechanisms of action and side effects. Although their exact **mechanism of action** is unknown, they are believed to act to inhibit the reuptake of both serotonin and norepinephrine. These drugs have a high **first-pass rate of metabolism** and are excreted by the kidneys. A complete **physical and history** should be obtained before starting a patient on tricyclic drugs. Because this class of antidepressants can cause death with an overdose, an initial **suicide risk assessment** must be obtained, and continued assessments for this risk are necessary. This class of drug can cause a prolongation in the electrical conduction of the heart. Therefore, a **baseline ECG** should be performed in children, young teenagers, anyone with cardiac electrical conduction problems, and adults over age 40.

#### MONITORING

Tricyclics monitoring includes the following:

- Observe for toxicity.
- Inform patients not to take with monoamine oxidase inhibitors.
- Observe for decreased therapeutic response to hypertensives (e.g., clonidine, guanethidine).
- Monitor other medications; the patient should avoid other central nervous system depressants, including alcohol. Some medications potentiate the effects of tricyclics, including bupropion, cimetidine, haloperidol, selective serotonin reuptake inhibitors, and valproic acid.
- Inform the patient to avoid prolonged exposure to sunlight or sunlamps.
- Administer major dosage of the drug at bedtime if the patient experiences drowsiness.
- Monitor for sedation, cardiac arrhythmias, insomnia, gastrointestinal upset, and weight gain.

### *MAOIs*

The **mechanism of action** for monoamine oxidase inhibitors (MAOIs) is exactly what their name indicates. These drugs act to inhibit the enzyme **monoamine oxidase (MAO)**. There are actually two of these enzymes, **MAO-A** and **MAO-B**, and this class of medication inhibits both. These enzymes act to metabolize serotonin and norepinephrine. By inhibiting the production of these enzymes, there are increased levels of **serotonin** and **norepinephrine** available for neurotransmission. Medications that selectively inhibit MAO-B have no antidepressant effects and can be used to treat disease processes such as Parkinson's.

#### SIDE EFFECTS

Side effects associated with the use of monoamine oxidase inhibitors (MAOIs) are similar to antipsychotic medications. They can include symptoms such as GI upset, vertigo, headaches, sleep disturbances, sexual dysfunction, dry mouth, visual disturbances, constipation, peripheral edema, urinary hesitancy, weakness, increased weight, or orthostatic hypotension. The elderly population is at greatest risk for problems with **orthostatic hypotension** and should have lying, sitting, and standing blood pressure checks to monitor for this side effect. Orthostatic hypotension can lead to injuries related to falls, such as fractures. The most dangerous side effect can be an extreme **elevation in blood pressure** or **hypertensive crisis**. Hypertension can develop due to the presence of increased levels of **tyramine**. These levels increase because **monoamine oxidase**, which normally metabolizes tyramine, is inhibited. Increased levels of tyramine produce a vasoconstrictive response by the body that leads to increased blood pressure. Symptoms associated with hypertensive crisis can include severe occipital headache, palpitations, chest pain, diaphoresis, nausea and vomiting, flushed face, or dilated pupils. Complications associated with hypertensive crisis include hemorrhagic stroke, severe headache, or death. It is vital that patients receive in-depth education about the symptoms of hypertension, the need for close monitoring of blood pressure, and methods for sustaining a low-tyramine diet.

#### DIET RESTRICTIONS

Monoamine oxidase inhibitors can lead to increased levels of **tyramine** in the nerve cell. These increased levels can lead to a dangerous and possibly fatal increase in **blood pressure**. Certain **foods that contain tyramine** should be avoided to help prevent hypertensive episodes. Foods high in tyramine include strong or aged cheeses, cured meats, smoked or processed meats, pickled or fermented foods, sauces, such as soy or teriyaki sauce, soybeans, snow peas or broad beans, dried or overripe fruits, meat tenderizers, products containing monosodium glutamate, yeast-extract spreads, alcoholic beverages, and improperly stored foods or spoiled foods.

## Anti-Anxiety Medications

### *Benzodiazepines*

Benzodiazepines are the most commonly prescribed medications for **anxiety**. Some of the more commonly prescribed include chlordiazepoxide, lorazepam, diazepam, flurazepam, and triazolam. Benzodiazepines act to enhance the neurotransmitter **GABA**. This neurotransmitter inhibits the firing rate of neurons and therefore leads to a decline in anxiety symptoms. Indications for their use can include anxiety, insomnia disorders, alcohol withdrawal, seizure control, skeletal muscle spasticity, or agitation. They can also be utilized to reduce the anxiety symptoms preoperatively or before any other type of medical procedure such as cardiac catheterization or colonoscopy. This class of drug is also the treatment of choice for alcohol withdrawal.

#### Side Effects

There are several common side effects associated with the use of benzodiazepines. One of the most common is the effect of **drowsiness**. Patients should be advised to use caution when operating motor vehicles or machinery. Activity will help decrease this effect. Other side effects include feelings of detachment, irritability, emotional lability, GI upset, dependency, or development of tolerance. The elderly population is at high risk for the development of **dizziness** or **cognitive impairment**, which places them at high risk for falls with associated injuries. When discontinuing a benzodiazepine after long-term use, the drug should be weaned off to prevent withdrawal side effects.

#### Treatment of Insomnia

Benzodiazepines are used to treat **insomnia** because of their **sedative-hypnotic effects**. There are three different types of insomnia, which include the inability to fall asleep, inability to stay asleep, or the combination of both. Many times, insomnia can be helped by a change in habits or talking about worries or stress the patient may be experiencing. When using a sedative-hypnotic to treat sleep disturbances, the medication should have rapid onset and allow the patient to wake up feeling refreshed instead of tired and groggy. When administered at bedtime, most benzodiazepines will produce a sleep-inducing effect and should be used on a short-term basis.

### *Use of Buspirone for Treatment of Anxiety*

Due to the addictive potential of benzodiazepines, the use of **nonbenzodiazepines** to treat anxiety has increased. One of the most commonly used nonbenzodiazepine medications is the drug **buspirone**. This medication is highly effective in treating anxiety and its associated symptoms such as insomnia, poor concentration, tension, restlessness, irritability, and fatigue. Buspirone has no addiction potential, is not useful in alcohol withdrawal and seizures, and is not known to interact with other CNS depressants. Because it may take several weeks of continual use for the effects of this drug to be realized by the patient, it cannot be used on an as-needed basis. Buspirone does not increase depression symptoms and therefore is useful in treating anxiety associated with depression. Side effects associated with medication can include GI upset, dizziness, sleepiness, excitement, or headache.

# Medical Emergencies

## Hematologic Disorders

### Red Blood Cells

Red blood cells (RBCs or erythrocytes) are biconcave disks that contain **hemoglobin** (95% of mass), which carries oxygen throughout the body. The heme portion of the cell contains **iron**, which binds to the oxygen. RBCs live about 120 days, after which they are destroyed and their hemoglobin is recycled or excreted. Normal values of **red blood cell count** vary by gender:

- Males >18 years: 4.7-6.1 million per $mm^3$
- Females >18 years: 4.2-5.4 million per $mm^3$

The most common **disorders of RBCs** are those that interfere with production, leading to various types of **anemia**:

- Blood loss
- Hemolysis
- Bone marrow failure

The **morphology** of RBCs may vary depending upon the type of anemia:

- Size: Normocytes, microcytes, macrocytes
- Shape: Spherocytes (round), poikilocytes (irregular), drepanocytes (sickled)
- Color (reflecting concentration of hemoglobin): Normochromic, hypochromic

#### *Laboratory Tests*

A number of different tests are used to evaluate the condition and production of red blood cells in addition to the red blood cell count.

**Hemoglobin**: Carries oxygen and is decreased in anemia and increased in polycythemia. Normal values:

- Males >18 years: 14.0-17.46 g/dL
- Females >18 years: 12.0-16.0 g/dL

**Hematocrit**: Indicates the proportion of RBCs in a liter of blood (usually about 3 times the hemoglobin number). Normal values:

- Males >18 years: 40-50%
- Females >18 years: 35-45%

**Mean corpuscular volume (MCV)**: Indicates the size of RBCs and can differentiate types of anemia. For adults, <80 is microcytic and >100 is macrocytic. Normal values:

- Males >18 years: 84-96 $\mu m^3$
- Females >18 years: 76-96 $\mu m^3$

**Reticulocyte count**: Measures marrow production and should rise with anemia. Normal values: 0.5-1.5% of total RBCs.

## WBC Count and Differential

**White blood cell (leukocyte) count** is used as an indicator of bacterial and viral infection. WBC count is reported as the total number of all white blood cells.

- Normal WBC for adults: 4,800-10,000
- Acute infection: 10,000+; 30,000 indicates a severe infection
- Viral infection: 4,000 and below

The **differential** provides the percentage of each different type of leukocyte. An increase in the white blood cell count is usually related to an increase in one type, and often an increase in immature neutrophils (bands), referred to as a "shift to the left," is an indication of an infectious process:

- Normal immature neutrophils (bands): 1-3%, increases with infection
- Normal segmented neutrophils (segs) for adults: 50-62%, increases with acute, localized, or systemic bacterial infections
- Normal eosinophils: 0-3%, decreases with stress and acute infection
- Normal basophils: 0-1%, decreases during acute stage of infection
- Normal lymphocytes: 25-40%, increases in some viral and bacterial infections
- Normal monocytes: 3-7%, increases during recovery stage of acute infection

## C-Reactive Protein and Erythrocyte Sedimentation Rate

**C-reactive protein** is an acute-phase reactant produced by the liver in response to an inflammatory response that causes neutrophils, granulocytes, and macrophages to secrete cytokines. Thus, levels of C-reactive protein rise when there is inflammation or infection. It is helpful to measure the response to treatment for pyoderma gangrenosum ulcers:

- Normal values: 2.6-7.6 μg/dL

**Erythrocyte sedimentation rate (sed rate)** measures the distance erythrocytes fall in a vertical tube of anticoagulated blood in one hour. Because fibrinogen, which increases in response to infection, also increases the rate of the fall, the sed rate can be used as a non-specific test for inflammation when infection is suspected. The sed rate is sensitive to osteomyelitis and may be used to monitor treatment response. Values vary according to gender and age:

- <50: Males 0-15 mm/hr; females 0-20 mm/hr
- >50: Males 0-20 mm/hr; females 0-30 mm/hr

## ELEMENTS OF THE COAGULATION PROFILE

The coagulation profile measures clotting mechanisms, identifies clotting disorders, screens preoperative patients, and diagnoses excessive bruising and bleeding. Values vary depending on lab:

- **Prothrombin time (PT)**: 10-14 seconds
  - Increases with anticoagulation therapy, vitamin K deficiency, decreased prothrombin, DIC, liver disease, and malignant neoplasm. Some drugs may shorten PT.
- **Partial thromboplastin time (PTT)**: 25-35 seconds
  - Increases with hemophilia A and B, von Willebrand disease, vitamin deficiency, lupus, DIC, and liver disease.
- **Activated partial thromboplastin time (aPTT)**: 21-35 seconds
  - Similar to PTT, but decreases in extensive cancer, early DIC, and after acute hemorrhage. Used to monitor heparin dosage.
- **Thrombin clotting time (TCT) or Thrombin time (TT)**: 7-12 seconds
  - Used most often to determine the dosage of heparin. Prolonged with multiple myeloma, abnormal fibrinogen, uremia, and liver disease.
- **Bleeding time**: 2-9.5 minutes
  - (Using the IVY method on the forearm) Increases with DIC, leukemia, renal failure, aplastic anemia, von Willebrand disease, some drugs, and alcohol.
- **Platelet count**: 150,000-400,000 per μL
  - Increased bleeding <50,000 (transfusion required) and increased clotting >750,000.

## ANEMIA

Anemia occurs when there is an insufficient number of red blood cells to sufficiently oxygenate the body. As a result of the decreased level of oxygen being supplied to the organs, the body will attempt to compensate by increasing cardiac output and redistributing blood to the brain and heart. In return, the blood supply to the skin, abdominal organs, and kidneys is decreased. Anemia can occur from blood loss, increased destruction of red blood cells (hemolytic anemia), or as a result of a decreased production in red blood cells.

**Signs and symptoms**: Pallor, fatigue, hypotension, weakness, and mental status changes. As perfusion decreases and the body attempts to compensate for the lack of oxygenation, tachycardia, chest pain, and shortness of breath may occur. In hemolytic anemias, jaundice and splenomegaly may occur as the result of the breakdown of red blood cells and the excretion of bilirubin.

**Diagnosis**: A complete blood count, reticulocyte count, and iron studies may be used to diagnose anemia.

**Treatment**: The treatment of anemia is focused on treating the underlying cause. Parenteral iron may be given for patients with iron deficiency anemias caused from chronic blood loss, or inadequate iron intake or absorption. Blood transfusions are used to treat patients with active bleeding as well as those patients who are displaying significant clinical symptoms. Erythropoietin stimulating proteins may also be utilized to decrease the need for a transfusion.

## SICKLE CELL DISEASE

Sickle cell disease is a recessive genetic disorder of chromosome 11, causing hemoglobin to be defective so that red blood cells (RBCs) are sickle-shaped and inflexible, resulting in their accumulating in small vessels and causing painful blockage. While normal RBCs survive 120 days, sickled cells may survive only 10-20 days, stressing the bone marrow that cannot produce fast enough and resulting in severe anemia. There are 5 variations of sickle cell disease, with sickle cell anemia the most severe. Different types of crises occur (aplastic, hemolytic, vaso-occlusive, and sequestrating), which can cause infarctions in organs, severe pain, damage to organs, and rapid enlargement of liver and spleen. Complications include anemia, acute chest syndrome, congestive heart failure, strokes, delayed growth, infections, pulmonary hypertension, liver and kidney disorders, retinopathy, seizures, and osteonecrosis. Sickle cell disease occurs almost exclusively in African Americans in the United States, with 8-10% carriers.

**Review Video: What is Sickle Cell Disease?**
Visit mometrix.com/academy and enter code: 603869

### *TREATMENT*

Treatment for sickle cell disease includes:

- **Prophylactic penicillin** for children from 2 months to 5 years to prevent pneumonia
- **IV fluids** to prevent dehydration
- **Analgesics** (morphine) during painful crises
- **Folic acid** for anemia
- **Oxygen** for congestive heart failure or pulmonary disease
- **Blood transfusions** with chelation therapy to remove excess iron OR erythropheresis, in which red cells are removed and replaced with healthy cells, either autologous or from a donor
- **Hematopoietic stem cells transplantation** is the only curative treatment, but immunosuppressive drugs must be used and success rates are only about 85%, so the procedure is only used on those at high risk. It requires ablation of bone marrow, placing the patient at increased risk.
- **Partial chimerism** uses a mixture of the donor and the recipient's bone marrow stem cells and does not require ablation of bone marrow. It is showing good success.

## POLYCYTHEMIA VERA

Polycythemia vera is a condition in which there is abnormal production of blood cells in the bone marrow. Erythrocytes (red blood cells) are primarily affected. The disease is more common in men older than 40 years. Polycythemia may be primary or secondary, related to conditions causing hypoxia. The blood increases in viscosity, resulting in a number of **symptoms**:

- Dizziness, headache, weakness, and fatigue
- Dyspnea, especially when supine
- Flushing of skin, blue-tinged skin discoloration, and red lesions
- Itching after warm bath
- Left upper abdominal fullness and splenomegaly
- Phlebitis from blood clots
- Vision disturbances
- Complications include stroke, hemorrhage, and heart failure

**Diagnosis** includes CBC with differential, chemistry panel, bone marrow biopsy, and Vitamin $B_{12}$ level. Red cell mass will be more than 25% above normal.

**Treatment** includes:

- **Phlebotomy** to remove 500 mL (lesser amounts for children) of blood to decrease blood viscosity, repeated weekly until hematocrit stable (less than 45%)
- Referral for **chemotherapy** (hydroxyurea) to suppress marrow production
- **Interferon** to decrease need for phlebotomy

## Von Willebrand Disease

Von Willebrand disease is a group of congenital bleeding disorders (inherited from either parent) affecting 1-2% of the population, associated with deficiency or lack of von Willebrand factor (vWF), a glycoprotein that is synthesized, stored, and secreted by vascular endothelial cells. This protein interacts with thrombocytes to create a clot and prevent hemorrhage; however, with von Willebrand disease, this clotting mechanism is impaired. There are three types:

- **Type I**: Low levels of vWF and also sometimes factor VIII (dominant inheritance)
- **Type II**: Abnormal vWF (subtypes a, b) may increase or decrease clotting (dominant inheritance)
- **Type III**: Absence of vWF and less than 10% factor VIII (recessive inheritance)

**Symptoms** vary in severity and include bruising, menorrhagia, recurrent epistaxis, and hemorrhage.

**Treatment** includes:

- **Desmopressin acetate** parenterally or nasally to stimulate production of clotting factor (mild cases)
- **Severe bleeding**: factor VIII concentrates with vWF, such as Humate-P

## Hemophilia

Hemophilia is an inherited disorder in which the person lacks adequate clotting factors. There are three types:

- **Type A**: lack of clotting factor VIII (90% of cases)
- **Type B**: lack of clotting factor IX
- **Type C**: lack of clotting factor XI (affects both sexes, rarely occurs in the United States)

Both Type A and B are usually X-linked disorders, affecting only males. The severity of the disease depends on the amount of clotting factor in the blood.

**Symptoms**:

- Bleeding with severe trauma or stress (mild cases)
- Unexplained bruises, bleeding, swelling, joint pain
- Spontaneous hemorrhage (severe cases), often in the joints but can be anywhere in the body
- Epistaxis, mucosal bleeding
- First symptoms often occur during infancy when the child becomes active, resulting in frequent bruises

**Treatment**:

- Desmopressin acetate parenterally or nasally to stimulate production of clotting factor (mild cases)
- Infusions of clotting factor from donated blood or recombinant clotting factors (genetically engineered), utilizing guidelines for dosing
- Infusions of plasma (Type C)

## Disseminated Intravascular Coagulation

### *Pathology*

Disseminated intravascular coagulation (DIC) (consumption coagulopathy) is a secondary disorder that is triggered by another disorder such as trauma, congenital heart disease, necrotizing enterocolitis, sepsis, and severe viral infections. DIC triggers both coagulation and hemorrhage through a complex series of events. Trauma causes tissue factor (transmembrane glycoprotein) to enter the circulation and bind with coagulation factors, triggering the coagulation cascade. This stimulates thrombin to convert fibrinogen to fibrin, causing aggregation and destruction of platelets and forming clots that can be disseminated throughout the intravascular system. These clots increase in size as platelets adhere to the clots, causing blockage of both the microvascular systems and larger vessels, which can result in ischemia and necrosis. Clot formation triggers fibrinolysis and plasmin to breakdown fibrin and fibrinogen, causing the destruction of clotting factors and resulting in hemorrhage. Both processes, clotting and hemorrhage, continue at the same time, placing the patient at high risk for death, even with treatment.

### *Symptoms and Treatment*

The onset of symptoms of DIC may be very rapid or be a slower chronic progression from a disease. Those who develop the chronic manifestation of the disease usually have fewer acute symptoms and may slowly develop ecchymosis or bleeding wounds.

**Symptoms** include:

- Bleeding from surgical or venous puncture sites
- Evidence of GI bleeding with distention, bloody diarrhea
- Hypotension and acute symptoms of shock
- Petechiae and purpura with extensive bleeding into the tissues
- Laboratory abnormalities:
  - Prolonged prothrombin and partial prothrombin times
  - Decreased platelet counts and fragmented RBCs
  - Decreased fibrinogen

**Treatment** includes:

- Identifying and treating underlying cause
- Massive blood transfusion protocol; replacement of blood products, such as platelets and fresh frozen plasma
- Anticoagulation therapy (heparin) to increase clotting time
- Cryoprecipitate to increase fibrinogen levels
- Coagulation inhibitors and coagulation factors

## Thrombocytopenia

Thrombocytopenia is a deficiency of circulating platelets in the blood. It can be caused by a decrease in the production of platelets from the bone marrow or an increase in destruction of platelets. Thrombocytopenia may also be caused from the use of heparin. Heparin induced thrombocytopenia can occur after heparin therapy (average 4-14 days post therapy) and is characterized by a decrease in platelet count to less than 50% of baseline or the occurrence of an unexplained thrombolytic event. A decreased production of platelets within the bone marrow can occur as a result of malignancy, bone marrow failure, infection, alcohol abuse, or a nutritional deficiency. An increase in the destruction of platelets may occur in disseminated intravascular coagulation, vasculitis, thrombotic thrombocytopenic purpura, sepsis, or idiopathic thrombocytopenic purpura.

**Signs and symptoms**: Signs and symptoms may include petechiae, ecchymosis, bleeding from the mouth or gums, epistaxis, pallor, weakness, fatigue, splenomegaly, blood in the urine or stool, and jaundice.

**Diagnosis**: Physical exam and lab studies including complete blood count, partial thromboplastin time and prothrombin time may be used to diagnosis thrombocytopenia. A bone marrow biopsy may be indicated to determine the cause of the decreased production of platelets.

**Treatment**: Treatment of thrombocytopenia involves identifying and treating the underlying cause. Medications that decrease the platelet count should be held. Platelet transfusions may be administered to patients with extremely low counts (less than 50,000) or if spontaneous bleeding occurs. Platelet transfusions are contraindicated in patients with thrombotic thrombocytopenia purpura.

## ITP

The autoimmune disorder **idiopathic thrombocytopenic purpura (ITP)** causes an immune response to platelets, resulting in decreased platelet counts. ITP affects primarily children and young women although it can occur at any age. The acute form primarily occurs in children, but the chronic form affects primarily adults. Platelet counts are usually 150,000–400,000 per mcL. With ITP, platelet levels are less than 100,000. Maintaining a platelet count of at least 30,000 is necessary to prevent intracranial hemorrhage, the primary concern. The cause of ITP is unclear and may be precipitated by viral infection, sulfa drugs, and conditions, such as lupus erythematosus. ITP is usually not life threatening and can be controlled. **Symptoms** include:

- Bruising and petechiae with hematoma in some cases
- Epistaxis
- Increased menstrual flow in post-puberty females

**Treatment** includes:

- Corticosteroids to depress immune response and increase platelet count
- Splenectomy may be indicated for chronic conditions
- Platelet transfusions
- Avoiding aspirin, ibuprofen, or other NSAIDs

## HITTS

**Heparin-induced thrombocytopenia and thrombosis syndrome** (HITTS) occurs in patients receiving heparin for anticoagulation. There are two types:

- **Type I** is a transient condition occurring within a few days and causing depletion of platelets (<100,000 $mm^3$), but heparin may be continued as the condition usually resolves without intervention.
- **Type II** is an autoimmune reaction to heparin that occurs in 3–5% of those receiving unfractionated heparin and also occurs with low-molecular-weight heparin. It is characterized by low platelets (<50,000 $mm^3$) that are ≥50% below baseline. Onset is 5–14 days but can occur within hours of heparinization. Death rates are <30%. Heparin-antibody complexes form and release platelet factor 4 (PF4), which attracts heparin molecules and adheres to platelets and endothelial lining, stimulating thrombin and platelet clumping. This puts the patient at risk for thrombosis and vessel occlusion rather than hemorrhage, causing stroke, myocardial infarction, and limb ischemia with symptoms associated with the site of thrombosis. Treatment includes:
    - Discontinuation of heparin
    - Direct thrombin inhibitors (lepirudin, argatroban)
    - Monitor for signs/symptoms of thrombus/embolus

## Transfusion Components

**Blood components** that are commonly used for transfusions include:

- **Packed red blood cells:** RBCs (250-300 mL per unit) should be warmed >30 °C (optimal 37 °C) before administration to prevent hypothermia and may be reconstituted in 50-100 mL of normal saline to facilitate administration. RBCs are necessary if blood loss is about 30% (1,500-2,000 mL lost; Hgb ≤7). Above 30% blood loss, whole blood may be more effective. RBCs are most frequently used for transfusions.
- **Platelet concentrates:** Transfusions of platelets are used if the platelet count is <50,000 cells/mm³. One unit increases the platelet count by 5,000-10,000 cells/mm³. Platelet concentrates pose a risk for sensitization reactions and infectious diseases. Platelet concentrate is stored at a higher temperature (20-24 °C) than RBCs. This contributes to bacterial growth, so it is more prone to bacterial contamination than other blood products and may cause sepsis. Temperature increase within 6 hours should be considered an indication of possible sepsis. ABO compatibility should be observed but is not required.
- **Fresh frozen plasma** (FFP) (obtained from a unit of whole blood frozen ≤6 hours after collection) includes all clotting factors and plasma proteins, so each unit administered increases clotting factors by 2-3%. FFP may be used for deficiencies of isolated factors, excess warfarin therapy, and liver-disease-related coagulopathy. It may be used for patients who have received extensive blood transfusions but continue to hemorrhage. It is also helpful for those with antithrombin III deficiency. FFP should be warmed to 37 °C prior to administration to avoid hypothermia. ABO compatibility should be observed if possible, but it is not required. Some patients may become sensitized to plasma proteins.
- **Cryoprecipitate** is the precipitate that forms when FFP is thawed. It contains fibrinogen, factor VIII, von Willebrand, and factor XIII. This component may be used to treat hemophilia A and hypofibrinogenemia.

## Transfusion Administration

Prior to the transfusion of any blood component, the nurse should obtain the patient's transfusion history along with a consent form. A type and crossmatch must be completed on the patient's blood and an IV in place for administration. An 18-gauge catheter is standard, but 22-gauge can also be used at a slower rate. Baseline vital signs need to be taken prior to starting the infusion, and then the patient should be under direct observation for at least the first 15 minutes. Vital signs should be monitored at 5 minutes, 15 minutes, and then at least every 30 minutes during the transfusion and one hour post-transfusion.

## Transfusion-Related Complications

There are a number of transfusion-related complications, which is the reason that transfusions are given only when necessary. Complications include:

- **Infection**: Bacterial contamination of blood, especially platelets, can result in severe sepsis. A number of infective agents (viral, bacterial, and parasitic) can be transmitted, although increased testing of blood has decreased rates of infection markedly. Infective agents include HIV, hepatitis C and B, human T-cell lymphotropic virus, CMV, WNV, malaria, Chagas' disease, and variant Creutzfeldt-Jacob disease (from contact with mad cow disease).
- **Transfusion-related acute lung injury (TRALI):** This respiratory distress syndrome occurs ≤6 hours after transfusion. The cause is believed to be antileukocytic or anti-HLA antibodies in the transfusion. It is characterized by non-cardiogenic pulmonary edema (high protein level) with severe dyspnea and arterial hypoxemia. Transfusion must be stopped immediately and the blood bank notified. TRALI may result in fatality but usually resolves in 12-48 hours with supportive care.
- **Graft vs. host disease:** Lymphocytes cause an immune response in immunocompromised individuals. Lymphocytes may be inactivated by irradiation, as leukocyte filters are not reliable.

- **Post-transfusion purpura:** Platelet antibodies develop and destroy the patient's platelets, so the platelet count decreases about 1 week after transfusion.
- **Transfusion-related immunosuppression:** Cell-mediated immunity is suppressed, so the patient is at increased risk of infection, and in cancer patients, transfusions may correlate with tumor recurrence. This condition relates to transfusions that include leukocytes. RBCs cause a less pronounced immunosuppression, suggesting a causative agent is in the plasma. Leukoreduction is becoming more common to reduce transmission of leukocyte-related viruses.
- **Hypothermia**: This may occur if blood products are not heated. Oxygen utilization is halved for each 10 °C decrease in normal body temperature.

## AUTOTRANSFUSION

Autotransfusion (autologous blood transfusion) is collecting of the patient's blood and re-infusing it. This is life-saving if another donor's blood is not available. Blood in trauma cases is usually collected from a body cavity, such as pleural (hemothorax with ≥1,500 mL blood) or peritoneal space (rare). **Autotransfusion** is contraindicated if malignant lesions are present in the area of blood loss, contamination of pooled blood, or wounds more than 4-6 hours old. Commercial collection/transfusion kits (Pleur-Evac, Thora-Klex) are available, but blood can be collected through the chest tube into a sterile bottle, which is then disconnected and connected to IV tubing for infusion, or the blood in the bottle may be transferred to a blood collection bag for use. Commercial kits use either a chest tube or suction tube to withdraw blood and provide specific procedures. Blood is filtered. Heparin is not routinely used, but citrate phosphate dextrose (CPD) (25-70 mL per 500 mL blood) is often added to the aspirant to prevent clotting. Complications from autotransfusion are rare.

## PLASMAPHERESIS

With plasmapheresis, whole blood is removed from the body, anticoagulant is added, cellular components are separated from the plasma (which is removed), and cellular components are suspended in saline, albumin (most common), or another substitute for plasma. This is reinfused into the patient. The purpose is to remove harmful antibodies found in plasma. ACE inhibitors increase risk of hypotension and should be withheld for 24 hours before the procedure. Machine settings may vary. Typically, the patient's height and weight are entered into the automated system to aid in calculating the plasma volume. The patient must be carefully monitored during the procedure for signs of hypocalcemia (perioral/fingertip tingling, alterations in mental status, VT), which requires the administration of calcium; hypomagnesemia (confusion, headaches, dizziness, twitching), which requires administration of magnesium; and hypotension, which requires saline bolus. If the patient shows indications of transfusion reaction, the infusion must be discontinued and medications (diphenhydramine, corticosteroids) administered. The patient should be kept warm to avoid hypothermia. Post-procedure, the patient may experience thrombocytopenia and hypofibrinogenemia, so the patient must be observed for signs of bleeding.

## EXCHANGE TRANSFUSION

Exchange transfusions replace a person's blood with donor blood to remove sickled blood for sickle cell anemia or to remove toxins. The exchange may be complete or partial. An automated machine is generally used, and the time on the machine ranges from 1-4 hours. (If done manually, removal and replacement are done in cycles with blood first removed followed by replacement.) A catheter is inserted (usually in the arm) to drain the blood and another, usually in the femoral area (under local or moderate sedation), to administer donor blood, plasma, or another substitute for plasma. During the exchange, the patient's VS must be carefully monitored. If the patient exhibits signs of hypocalcemia (perioral/finger tingling) then calcium is administered. Some may receive calcium routinely during administration. Blood may be taken from the femoral line for testing after the exchange. When the femoral catheter is removed, pressure must be applied to the area for at least 5 minutes and the patient instructed to lie flat for at least 30 minutes to prevent bleeding.

## LEUKOCYTE DEPLETION

Red blood cell and platelet transfusions typically contain some leukocytes, which are recognized as foreign by the immune system of a patient receiving the transfusion. This can lead to adverse reactions, especially in patients who are immunocompromised. **Leukocyte depletion** is carried out by various processes, including filtration. One disadvantage to leukodepletion of RBCs is that the process results in the loss of about 10% of the RBCs, and some hemolysis may occur. Leukocyte depleted RBCs are given in volumes of 200-250 mL within a 4-hour time period.

## BLOOD CONSERVATION

Blood conservation includes methods to:

- **Minimize the loss of blood during surgical procedures**: May include regional anesthesia instead of general, positioning to reduce blood loss, cell salvage, autotransfusion, non-invasive monitoring (BP, pulse oximetry), limited blood draws, normovolemic hemodilution, and medications to reduce bleeding (vitamin K, tranexamic acid, desmopressin, somatostatin, vasopressin, recombinant factor VIIa).
- **Lower the threshold for receiving transfusions**: Transfusion threshold lowered from 10 g/dL to 7 g/dL.
- **Maintain the hematocrit at acceptable levels**: Administration of oral or parenteral iron therapy to increase tolerance for blood loss. Erythropoietin alpha may also be administered perioperatively to stimulate the production of RBCs.
- **Ensure optimal oxygenation of tissue**: Hyperoxic ventilation during surgery, crystalloid/colloid volume replacement, and utilizing techniques to minimize consumption of oxygen.

Blood conservation includes a commitment to bloodless surgery as much as possible, especially through the utilization of minimally-invasive procedures.

## MASSIVE TRANSFUSION PROTOCOL

A massive transfusion protocol (MTP) is a proactive standardized protocol used during an uncontrolled hemorrhage, designed to ensure effective management of massive blood loss and to improve patient outcome.

Indications for activation of **massive transfusion protocol** (MTP) include:

- Uncontrolled hemorrhage.
- Actual/anticipated use of ≥4 units of RBCs in less than 4 hours or ≥10 units in 24 hours (some may need up to 30 units in 8 hours).
- Hemodynamic instability despite initial management of bleeding and resuscitation efforts that should include avoiding hypothermia and the use of excessive crystalloid.
- Allowing permissive hypotension to 80-100 systolic BP to help control bleeding. Autotransfusion may be used when appropriate.

Protocols may vary somewhat:

- MTPs are activated by a clinician in response to massive bleeding, generally after transfusion of 4-10 units.
- Obtain baseline laboratory tests (CBC, coagulation screen, blood gases, and chemistry panel) and repeat CBC, blood gases, coagulation screen, and ionized calcium test hourly.
- MTP packs have a predetermined ratio (e.g., 1:1:1 or 2:1:1 ratio) of RBCs, FFPs, and platelet units for transfusion, prepared by the blood bank for rapid and timely delivery.
- Targets of resuscitation include:
  - Mean arterial pressure (MAP) around 60 mmHg
  - Core temperature >35 °C

- Hemoglobin 7–9 g/dL
- pH 7.35–7.45
- Lactate <4 mmol/L
- Calcium >1.1 mmol/L
- Platelets >50,000
- PT/aPTT <1.5 times normal
- INR ≤1.5
- Fibrinogen >1.5–2.0 g/L

## ANTICOAGULANTS

Common anticoagulants used at home and in the hospital setting are discussed below, including possible complications and the antidotes for each:

- **Antithrombin activators**: Heparin (unfractionated) and derivatives, LWM (Dalteparin, Enoxaparin, tinzaparin), and Fondaparinux.
  - Possible complications: Thrombocytopenia, bleeding/hemorrhage, osteopenia, hypersensitivity.
  - Antidote: Protamine sulfate 1% solution—dosage varies according to drug and drug's dosage. (1 mg protamine neutralizes 100 units of heparin or 1 mg of enoxaparin.)
- **Direct thrombin inhibitors**: Hirudin analogs (bivalirudin, desirudin, lepirudin). Others: Apixaban, Argatroban, and dabigatran.
  - Possible complications: Bleeding/hemorrhage, GI upset, backpain, hypertension, headache.
  - No antidote is available.
- **Direct Xa inhibitor**: Rivaroxaban
  - Possible complications: Bleeding/hemorrhage.
  - No antidote is available.
- **Antithrombin (AT)**: Recombinant human AT, Plasma-derived AT
  - Possible complications: Bleeding/hemorrhage, hypersensitivity.
  - No antidote is available.
- **Warfarin**
  - Possible complications: Bleeding/hemorrhage. Drug interactions may cause thrombosis or increased risk of bleeding.
  - Antidote: Vitamin $K_1$ usually at 2.5 mg PO or 0.5–1.0 mg IV. If ineffective, FFP or fresh whole blood may be administered.

### *HEPARIN*

#### PHARMACOLOGY

**Heparin** is an **anticoagulant** derived from the intestinal mucosa of the pig and the lung of the pig. The mechanism of action of heparin is to bind to the surface of the endothelial cell membrane. The activity of heparin depends upon plasma protease inhibitor antithrombin III. Antithrombin III inhibits thrombin and other anti-clotting proteases. In addition, heparin binding causes a change in antithrombin III inhibitor form, resulting in increased antithrombin-protease complex formation activity. After antithrombin-protease complex formation, heparin is subsequently released and is available to bind to more antithrombin molecules.

#### RISK FACTORS

The major risk factor of heparin use is hemorrhage. Predisposing factors for hemorrhage include advanced age and renal failure. Prolonged use of heparin can result in osteoporosis and fractures. Other risk factors of heparin use include transient thrombocytopenia, severe thrombocytopenia, paradoxical thromboembolism, and heparin-induced aggregation of platelets. These risks can be reduced by careful selection of patients who receive heparin therapy, careful control of the dosage of heparin, and meticulous monitoring of the partial thromboplastin time, or PTT. It is important to remember that thrombocytopenia or the development of a thrombus may be due to heparin itself.

#### CONTRAINDICATIONS

There are numerous contraindications to the use of heparin, including: hypersensitivity to heparin; diseases of the hematologic system (hemophilia, purpura, or thrombocytopenia); uncontrolled hypertension; intracranial bleed; infectious endocarditis; active tuberculosis; gastrointestinal ulcers; cancer of the gastrointestinal visceral organs; severe liver dysfunction; severe kidney dysfunction; and threatened miscarriage or abortion. Heparin is contraindicated in the following medical procedures: following brain surgery; following spinal cord surgery; following eye surgery; after a lumbar puncture; and after regional anesthesia blocks. The effects of heparin may be reversed by stopping heparin or by the use of a specific antagonist (protamine sulfate).

**Review Video: Heparin**
Visit mometrix.com/academy and enter code: 127426

### *WARFARIN*

#### PHARMACOLOGY

**Warfarin** causes a deficiency in prothrombin in the plasma and is used as an **anti-thrombotic agent** and to decrease the risk of embolism in humans. This agent causes the liver to manufacture less of the proteins necessary for blood coagulation. Since it is 99% bound to albumin in the plasma, warfarin has a high bio-availability. The mechanism of action of warfarin involves prothrombin, factor VII, factor IX, factor X, and protein C. Warfarin inhibits the g-carboxylation of the glutamate residues in the aforementioned factors. The mechanism of action of warfarin also involves vitamin K. Warfarin has a slow onset of action, usually 24 hours, and a typical duration of 2 to 5 days. Using increased dosages of warfarin as loading dosages will serve to speed up the onset of anti-coagulation. Patients on warfarin must discontinue this medication five days before planned surgery due to its longer duration.

#### DRUG-DRUG INTERACTIONS

Warfarin has many drug-drug interactions, the most serious of which increases the risk of bleeding. Sulfinpyrazone and phenylbutazone interact with warfarin to cause enhanced decrease in prothrombin, increased inhibition of platelets, and increased risk of peptic ulcer. The following drugs can have adverse effects when co-administered with warfarin: antibiotics such as metronidazole, azithromycin, clarithromycin, dirithromycin, erythromycin, roxithromycin, and telithromycin; broad-spectrum antibiotics such as amoxicillin, imipenem, levofloxacin; antifungal agents such as fluconazole, miconazole, and ketoconazole; barbiturates; and trimethoprim-sulfamethoxazole, amiodarone, cimetidine, and disulfiram. Aspirin inhibits metabolism of the warfarin and nonsteroidal anti-inflammatory drugs (NSAIDs) inhibit the clotting of platelets. The third-generation cephalosporins increase the risk of bleeding with warfarin because these drugs destroy the intestinal bacteria that produce vitamin K. Always check on possible drug-drug interactions when administering warfarin and monitor patients who might be at risk.

**Review Video: Warfarin**
Visit mometrix.com/academy and enter code: 844117

## THROMBOLYTICS

Thrombolytics are drugs used to dissolve clots in myocardial infarction, ischemic stroke, DVT, and pulmonary embolism. **Thrombolytics** may be given in combination with heparin or low-weight heparin to increase anticoagulation effect. Thrombolytics should be administered within 90 minutes but may be given up to 6 hours after an event. They may increase the danger of hemorrhage and are contraindicated with hemorrhagic strokes, recent surgery, or bleeding. Thrombolytics include:

- **Alteplase tissue-type plasminogen activator** (t-PA) (Activase) is an enzyme that converts plasminogen to plasmin, which is a fibrinolytic enzyme. t-PA is used for ischemic stroke, MI, and pulmonary embolism and must be given IV within 3–4.5 hours or by catheter directly to the site of occlusion within 6 hours.
- **Anistreplase** (Eminase) is used for treatment of acute MI and is given intravenously in a 30-unit dose over 2–5 minutes.
- **Reteplase** (Retavase) is a plasminogen activator used after MI to prevent CHF (contraindicated for ischemic strokes). It is given in 2 doses, a 10-unit bolus over 2 minutes and then repeated in 30 minutes.
- **Streptokinase** (Streptase) is used for pulmonary emboli, acute MI, intracoronary thrombi, DVT, and arterial thromboembolism. It should be given within 4 hours but can be given after up to 24 hours. Intravenous infusion is usually 1,500,000 units in 60 minutes. Intracoronary infusion is done with an initial 20,000-unit bolus and then 2000 units per minute for 60 minutes.
- **Tenecteplase** (TNKase) is used to treat acute MI with large ST elevation. It is administered in a one-time bolus over 5 seconds and should be administered within 30 minutes of the event.

**Contraindications** to thrombolytic therapy include:

- Evidence of cerebral or subarachnoid hemorrhage or other internal bleeding or history of intracranial hemorrhage, recent stroke, head trauma, or surgery (ruled out by CT scan before administration for ischemic stroke)
- Uncontrolled hypertension, seizures
- Intracranial AVM, neoplasm, or aneurysm
- Current anticoagulation therapy
- Low platelet count (<100,000 $mm^3$)

# Electrolyte and Fluid Imbalance

## *Sodium*

Sodium (**Na**) regulates fluid volume, osmolality, acid-base balance, and activity in the muscles, nerves, and myocardium. It is the primary **cation** (positive ion) in extracellular fluid (ECF), necessary to maintain ECF levels that are needed for tissue perfusion:

- Normal range: 135-145 mEq/L
- Hyponatremia: <135 mEq/L
- Hypernatremia: >145 mEq/L

**Hyponatremia** may result from inadequate sodium intake, excess sodium loss through diarrhea, vomiting, or NG suctioning, or illness, such as severe burns, fever, SIADH, and ketoacidosis.

- **Symptoms**: Irritability to lethargy and alterations in consciousness, cerebral edema with seizures and coma, dyspnea to respiratory failure.
- **Treatment**: Identify and treat the underlying cause and provide Na replacement.

**Hypernatremia** may result from renal disease, diabetes insipidus, and fluid depletion.

- **Symptoms**: Irritability to lethargy to confusion to coma; seizures; flushing; muscle weakness and spasms; thirst.
- **Treatment**: Identify and treat the underlying cause, monitor Na levels carefully, and give IV fluid replacement.

## *Potassium*

Potassium (**K**) is the primary **electrolyte** in intracellular fluid (ICF), with about 98% inside cells and only 2% in ECF, although this small amount is important for neuromuscular activity. Potassium influences activity of the skeletal and cardiac muscles. Its level is dependent upon adequate renal functioning because 80% is excreted through the kidneys and 20% through the bowels and sweat:

- Normal range: 3.5-5.5 mEq/L
- Hypokalemia: <3.5 mEq/L. Critical value: <2.5 mEq/L
- Hyperkalemia: >5.5 mEq/L. Critical value: >6.5 mEq/L

A healthy NPO patient will need about 40 mEq of K per day to maintain serum K levels. Expect alterations in renal disease and other disease processes.

**Hypokalemia** is caused by alkalosis, decreased intake associated with starvation, nephritis, and loss of potassium through diarrhea, vomiting, gastric suction, and diuresis.

- **Symptoms**: Lethargy and weakness; nausea and vomiting; paresthesia and tetany; muscle cramps with hyporeflexia; hypotension; dysrhythmias with EKG changes: PVCs or flattened T-waves.
- **Treatment**: Treatment involves identifying and treating the underlying cause and replacing K. When possible, oral replacement is preferable to IV, as it allows slower adjustment of K levels. When given IV, K should be given no faster than 20 mEq/hour via central line if possible. If given peripherally, 10 mEq/hour is preferable for patient comfort.

**Hyperkalemia** is caused by renal disease, adrenal insufficiency, metabolic acidosis, severe dehydration, burns, hemolysis, and trauma. It rarely occurs without renal disease but may be induced by treatment (such as NSAIDs and potassium-sparing diuretics). Untreated renal failure results in reduced excretion. Those with Addison's disease and deficient adrenal hormones suffer sodium loss that results in potassium retention.

- **Symptoms**: The primary symptoms relate to the effect on the cardiac muscle: ventricular arrhythmias with increasing changes in EKG lead to cardiac and respiratory arrest, weakness with ascending paralysis and hyperreflexia, diarrhea, and increasing confusion.
- **Treatment**: Treatment includes identifying the underlying cause and discontinuing sources of increased K. Calcium gluconate to decrease cardiac effects. Sodium bicarbonate, insulin, and hypertonic dextrose shift K into the cells temporarily. Cation exchange resin (Kayexalate) to decrease K. Peritoneal dialysis or hemodialysis to remove excess K.

*Note*: When a tourniquet is on, a patient opening and closing their hand can lead to falsely elevated K levels.

### CALCIUM

More than 99% of calcium (**Ca**) is in the skeletal system with 1% in serum, but it is important for transmitting nerve impulses and regulating muscle contraction and relaxation, including the myocardium. Calcium activates enzymes that stimulate chemical reactions and has a role in the coagulation of blood:

- Normal range: 8.2-10.2 mg/dL
- Hypocalcemia: <8.2. Critical value: <7 mg/dL
- Hypercalcemia: >10.2 mg/dL. Critical value: >12 mg/dL

**Hypercalcemia** may be caused by acidosis, kidney disease, hyperparathyroidism, prolonged immobilization, and malignancies. Crisis carries a 50% mortality rate.

- **Symptoms**: Increasing muscle weakness with hypotonicity; anorexia; nausea and vomiting; constipation; bradycardia and cardiac arrest.
- **Treatment**: Identify and treat underlying cause, loop diuretics, IV fluids, phosphate.

**Hypocalcemia** may be caused by damage to the parathyroid resulting in hypoparathyroidism (directly decreasing calcium production), vitamin D resistance or inadequacy, or liver/kidney disease.

- **Symptoms**: Muscle cramping or spasms; seizures; numbness or tingling of the feet, hands, or lips; tetany if severe.
- **Treatment**: Identify and treat underlying cause, replace calcium by administering IV calcium gluconate in acute circumstances or increasing oral Vitamin D and calcium in chronic cases.

### PHOSPHORUS

Phosphorus, or phosphate, (**$PO_4$**) is necessary for neuromuscular and red blood cell function, the maintenance of acid-base balance, and provides structure for teeth and bones. About 85% is in the bones, 14% in soft tissue, and <1% in ECF.

- Normal range: 2.4-4.5 mEq/L
- Hypophosphatemia: <2.4mEq/L
- Hyperphosphatemia: >4.5 mEq/L

**Hypophosphatemia** occurs with severe protein-calorie malnutrition, hyperventilation, severe burns, diabetic ketoacidosis, and excess antacids with magnesium, calcium, or aluminum.

- **Symptoms**: Irritability, tremors, seizures to coma; hemolytic anemia; decreased myocardial function; respiratory failure.
- **Treatment**: Identify and treat underlying cause and replace phosphorus.

**Hyperphosphatemia** occurs with renal failure, hypoparathyroidism, excessive intake, neoplastic disease, diabetic ketoacidosis, muscle necrosis, and chemotherapy.

- **Symptoms**: Tachycardia; muscle cramping; hyperreflexia and tetany; nausea and diarrhea.
- **Treatment**: Identify and treat underlying cause, correct hypocalcemia, and provide antacids and dialysis.

### *Magnesium*

Magnesium (**Mg**) is the second most common intracellular electrolyte (after potassium) and activates many intracellular enzyme systems. Mg is important for carbohydrate and protein metabolism, neuromuscular function, and cardiovascular function, producing vasodilation and directly affecting the peripheral arterial system:

- Normal range: 1.7-2.2 mg/dL
- Hypomagnesemia critical value: <1.2 mg/dL
- Hypermagnesemia critical value: >4.9 mg/dL

**Hypomagnesemia** occurs with chronic diarrhea, chronic renal disease, chronic pancreatitis, excess diuretic or laxative use, hyperthyroidism, hypoparathyroidism, severe burns, and diaphoresis.

- **Symptoms**: Neuromuscular excitability or tetany; confusion, headaches, dizziness; seizure and coma; tachycardia with ventricular arrhythmias; respiratory depression.
- **Treatment**: Identify and treat underlying cause, provide magnesium replacement. IV magnesium is a vasodilator, 2 g over 60 mins.

**Hypermagnesemia** occurs with renal failure or inadequate renal function, diabetic ketoacidosis, hypothyroidism, and Addison's disease.

- **Symptoms**: Muscle weakness, seizures, and dysphagia with decreased gag reflex; tachycardia with hypotension.
- **Treatment**: Identify and treat underlying cause, IV hydration with calcium, and dialysis.

**Review Video: Fluid and Electrolytes**
Visit mometrix.com/academy and enter code: 384389

# Acid Base Imbalances

## Invasive Blood Gas Monitoring

Invasive blood gas monitoring options include the following:

- **Arterial blood gas (ABG)** is the most informative measurement of blood gas status. If an arterial catheter is in place, it is easily obtained by aspirating 1-2 mL of blood.
- **Venous blood gas (VBG)** is easier to obtain if an arterial catheter is not in place. In order to compare the values in the VBG with an ABG, make the following calculations:
  - Add 0.05 to the pH of the VBG.
  - Subtract 5-10 mmHg from the $PCO_2$ of the VBG.
- **Capillary blood gas (CBG)** can be obtained with a heel stick, without a venous or arterial line, but the values obtained in a CBG are the least accurate and are rarely useful. This is used most often in neonates.

### *Components of a Blood Gas Reading*

The following are components of a blood gas reading:

- **pH** measures the circulating acid and base levels. Neutral pH for humans is 7.4. A value below 7.35 indicates acidosis and a value greater than 7.45 indicates alkalosis.
- **$pCO_2$** is the partial pressure of carbon dioxide and it determines the respiratory component of pH. An elevated $pCO_2$ lowers the pH. A low $pCO_2$ raises the pH. The $pCO_2$ value is dependent on adequate pulmonary ventilation and respiration. Changes in respiratory status quickly alter this value. Normal value range for $pCO_2$ is 35-45 mmHg.
- **$pO_2$** is the partial pressure of oxygen, which indicates how well the individual is transporting oxygen from the lungs into the bloodstream. Normal value is 75-100 mmHg.
- **$HCO_3^-$** is bicarbonate, the metabolic component of pH. This value may slowly change in response to abnormal pH, or a disease process may cause an elevation or depression. Low values decrease the pH and high values raise the pH. Normal value for bicarbonate is 22-26 mEq/L.

## Metabolic and Respiratory Acidosis

### *Pathophysiology*

- Metabolic acidosis
  - Increase in fixed acid and inability to excrete acid, or loss of base, with compensatory increase of $CO_2$ excretion by lungs
- Respiratory acidosis
  - Hypoventilation and $CO_2$ retention with renal compensatory retention of bicarbonate ($HCO_3$) and increased excretion of hydrogen

### *Laboratory*

- Metabolic acidosis
  - Decreased serum pH (<7.35) and $PCO_2$ normal if uncompensated and decreased if compensated
  - Decreased $HCO_3$
- Respiratory acidosis
  - Decreased serum pH (< 7.35) and increased $PCO_2$
  - Increased $HCO_3$ if compensated and normal if uncompensated

### *CAUSES*

- Metabolic acidosis
    - DKA, lactic acidosis, diarrhea, starvation, renal failure, shock, renal tubular acidosis, starvation
- Respiratory acidosis
    - COPD, overdose of sedative or barbiturate (leading to hypoventilation), obesity, severe pneumonia/atelectasis, muscle weakness (Guillain-Barré), mechanical hypoventilation

### *SYMPTOMS*

- Metabolic acidosis
    - Neuro/muscular: Drowsiness, confusion, headache, coma
    - Cardiac: Decreased BP, arrhythmias, flushed skin
    - GI: Nausea, vomiting, abdominal pain, diarrhea
    - Respiratory: Deep inspired tachypnea
- Respiratory acidosis
    - Neuro/muscular: Drowsiness, dizziness, headache, coma, disorientation, seizures
    - Cardiac: Flushed skin, VF, ↓BP
    - GI: Absent
    - Respiratory: Hypoventilation with hypoxia

## METABOLIC AND RESPIRATORY ALKALOSIS

### *PATHOPHYSIOLOGY*

- Metabolic alkalosis
    - Decreased strong acid or increased base with possible compensatory $CO_2$ retention by lungs
- Respiratory alkalosis
    - Hyperventilation and increased excretion of $CO_2$ with compensatory $HCO_3$ excretion by kidneys

### *LABORATORY*

- Metabolic alkalosis
    - Increased serum pH (>7.45)
    - $PCO_2$ normal if uncompensated and increased if compensated
    - Increased $HCO_3$
- Respiratory alkalosis
    - Increased serum pH (>7.45)
    - Decreased $PCO_2$
    - $HCO_3$ normal if uncompensated and decreased if compensated

### *CAUSES*

- Metabolic alkalosis
    - Excessive vomiting, gastric suctioning, diuretics, potassium deficit, excessive mineralocorticoids and $NaHCO_3$ intake
- Respiratory alkalosis
    - Hyperventilation associated with hypoxia, pulmonary embolus, exercise, anxiety, pain, and fever
    - Encephalopathy, septicemia, brain injury, salicylate overdose, and mechanical hyperventilation

### Symptoms

- Metabolic alkalosis
  - Neuromuscular: Dizziness, confusion, nervousness, anxiety, tremors, muscle cramping, tetany, tingling, seizures
  - Cardiac: Tachycardia and arrhythmias
  - GI: Nausea, vomiting, anorexia
  - Respiratory: Compensatory hypoventilation
- Respiratory alkalosis
  - Neuro/muscular: Light-headedness, confusion, lethargy
  - Cardiac: Tachycardia and arrhythmias
  - GI: Epigastric pain, nausea, and vomiting
  - Respiratory: Hyperventilation

# Endocrine Disorders

## Assessing for Endocrine Disorders

The **endocrine system** comprises organs that produce hormones that are critical to growth, sexual development, and metabolism, so changes in these areas are suggestive of endocrine disorders. While symptoms may vary widely, there are often generalized symptoms that can be associated with most endocrine disorders. One should question the patient about fatigue and ability to perform ADLs, heat or cold intolerance, changes in sexual libido, sexual functioning, and secondary sexual characteristics, weight fluctuation, sleep problems, decreased concentration and memory, and mood changes. During the physical exam, one should assess the patient for edema, "moon" face or "buffalo hump," exophthalmos, hair loss, female facial hair, enlarged trunk with thin extremities, and enlarged hands and feet. Vital signs should be assessed for hypo or hypertension, and one should assess for changes in skin appearance and vision.

## Thyroid Imaging

Thyroid imaging plays a critical role in assessment of many thyroid diseases. This test may be used to determine the uptake characteristics of the thyroid gland in addition to the size and shape of the gland. In addition, **thyroid imaging** may determine how much iodine-131 is needed in order to safely ablate the gland when necessary. The radioactive iodine uptake scan (RAIU) is basically administration of iodine-123 with imaging performed 8 and 24 hours later:

Uptake of radioactive iodine is increased in disorders such as Graves' disease, "hot" nodules of various etiologies (including toxic multinodular goiter), TSH-secreting pituitary tumor, and iodine deficiency.

Uptake of radioactive iodine is decreased in the setting of thyroiditis and iodine excess.

**Ultrasound imaging** is used in thyroid disease to determine the size and structure of a thyroid nodule, such as to determine uniformity of shape, irregular contour, solid/cystic structure, and depth.

## Glucose Laboratory Test

Glucose is manufactured by the liver from ingested carbohydrates and is stored as glycogen for use by the cells. If intake is inadequate, glucose can be produced from muscle and fat tissue, leading to increased wasting. High levels of glucose are indicative of diabetes mellitus, which predisposes people to skin injuries, slow healing, and infection. **Fasting blood glucose levels** are used to diagnose and monitor this condition:

- Normal values: 70–99 mg/dL
- Impaired: 100–125 mg/dL
- Diabetes: ≥126 mg/dL

There are a number of different conditions that can increase glucose levels, including stress, renal failure, Cushing syndrome, hyperthyroidism, and pancreatic disorders. Medications, such as steroids, estrogens, lithium, phenytoin, diuretics, tricyclic antidepressants, may increase glucose levels. Other conditions, such as adrenal insufficiency, liver disease, hypothyroidism, and starvation can decrease glucose levels.

## Hemoglobin A1c Laboratory Test

Hemoglobin A1c comprises hemoglobin A with a glucose molecule because hemoglobin holds onto excess blood glucose, so it shows the average blood glucose levels over a 3-month period and is used primarily to monitor long-term diabetic therapy:

- Normal value: <6%
- Elevation: >7%

## Basic Thyroid Function Testing and Antibody Testing

**Thyroid stimulating hormone (TSH)** is produced by the pituitary as a result of thyrotropin releasing hormone (TRH) from the hypothalamus. TSH stimulates the thyroid to produce T4 (mostly) and T3. T4 is deiodinated to T3 (active hormone), and the free hormone is active while the majority is bound to albumin and thyroxine-binding globulin. The best testing of thyroid function is the free T4 (unbound). Free T4 and TSH testing allows appropriate screening for thyroid disease.

Additionally, certain antibodies are used to screen for thyroid disease. Thyroglobulin antibodies are found in 50% of patients with Graves' disease and about 90% of those with Hashimoto's thyroiditis. Thyroid peroxidase antibodies are detected in >90% of those with Hashimoto's thyroiditis. TSH receptor antibodies (TSHR) may be either thyroid stimulating immunoglobulin (TSI) which stimulate the receptor to produce thyroid hormone (found in Graves' disease), or TSHR-blocking antibodies, which may inhibit production of thyroid hormone.

Lab values to consider include:

- **Thyroid stimulating hormone (TSH)** (0.4-6.15 mIU/L). Increase in TSH indicates hypothyroidism and decrease indicates hyperthyroidism.
- **Free thyroxine**: (FT4) (0.9-2.4 ng/dL). FT4 is used to confirm TSH abnormalities. Serum T3 (80-180 ng/dL) and T4 (4.5-11.5 mcg/dL). These usually increase together, but T3 more accurately diagnoses hyperthyroidism. T3 resin uptake (25-35%). Increases with hyperthyroidism and decreases with hypothyroidism.

## Additional Endocrine Function Studies

There is a wide range of endocrine function studies:

- **Pituitary:** Serum levels of pituitary hormones and hormones of target organs, dependent on stimulation by pituitary hormones, are measured to determine abnormalities.
- **Parathyroid:** Parathyroid hormone (PTH) level (10-65 ng/L) and serum calcium levels (8.5-10.2 mg/dL) both increase with hyperparathyroidism. Calcium levels decrease with hypoparathyroidism, and phosphate levels (2.5-4.5 mg/dL) increase.
- **Adrenal**: Catecholamine (urine and serum) levels: Epinephrine (<75 ng/L) and norepinephrine (<100-550 ng/mL) elevate with pheochromocytoma. Electrolyte and glucose levels.
- **ACTH** and **serum cortisol levels** and **ACTH stimulation test** to evaluate for Addison's. Dexamethasone suppression test for Cushing's disease.

## Diabetes Mellitus Types 1 and 2

Diabetes mellitus is the most common metabolic disorder. Over 6% of adults have diabetes, but only 4% of adults are diagnosed. Insulin resistance tends to increase in older adults, so there is less ability to handle glucose. Type II is more common in older adults, with incidence increasing with age.

- **Type I:** Immune-mediated form with insufficient insulin production because of the destruction of pancreatic beta cells
    - **Symptoms** include pronounced polyuria and polydipsia, short onset, obesity or recent weight loss, and ketoacidosis present on diagnosis.
    - **Treatment** includes insulin as needed to control blood sugar, glucose monitoring 1–4 times daily, diet with carbohydrate control, and exercise.
- **Type II:** Insulin resistant form with defect in insulin secretion

- **Symptoms** include long onset, obesity with no weight loss or significant weight loss, mild or absent polyuria and polydipsia, ketoacidosis or glycosuria without ketonuria, androgen-mediated problems such as hirsutism and acne (adolescents), and hypertension.
- **Treatment** includes diet and exercise, glucose monitoring, and oral medications.

**Review Video: Diabetes Mellitus: Diet, Exercise, & Medications**
Visit mometrix.com/academy and enter code: 774388

**Review Video: Diabetes: Complications**
Visit mometrix.com/academy and enter code: 996788

## Diabetic Ketoacidosis

Diabetic ketoacidosis is a complication of type 1 diabetes mellitus, usually related to noncompliance with treatment, stress, illness, or lack of awareness of having diabetes (this event often being the first time that diabetes is diagnosed). Inadequate production of insulin results in glucose being unavailable for metabolism, so lipolysis (breakdown of fat) produces free fatty acids (FFAs) as an alternate fuel source. Glycerol is converted to ketone bodies which are used for cellular metabolism less efficiently than glucose. Excess ketone bodies are excreted in the urine (ketonuria) or exhalations. Acidosis of any type causes potassium in cells to shift to the serum. The ketone bodies lower serum pH, leading to ketoacidosis.

**Symptoms** include:

- Kussmaul respirations: "Ketone breath," or fruity smelling breath; progresses to CNS depression with loss of airway
- Fluid imbalance, including loss of potassium and other electrolytes from cellular death resulting in dehydration and diuresis with excess thirst
- Dangerous cardiac arrhythmias, related to potassium loss; hypotension, chest pain, tachycardia
- GI: Nausea/vomiting, abdominal pain, loss of appetite
- Neurological: malaise, confusion/lethargy progressing to coma

**Diagnosis** is based on:

- Labs: Blood glucose >250 mg/dL, lower Na and elevated K (switches after treatment), elevated beta-hydroxybutyrate (byproduct of ketones)
- ABG: pH <7.3, $HCO_3$ <18 mEq/L
- Urine: + glucose, ketones

### *Treatment and Potential Complications*

**Treatment** of DKA:

- **Fluids**: Priority is fluid resuscitation with 1-2 liters of isotonic fluids given in the first hour, up to 8 liters in the first 24 hours. Potassium will be added to the fluids when levels begin to fall.
- **Insulin**: Continuous drip IV, with/without loading dose. Will usually begin at 0.1 unit/kg/ hour (5-7 units an hour generally), with a goal of decreasing blood glucose 50–75 mg/dL an hour. Blood glucose is checked every hour, and when levels are < 200 mg/dL, add dextrose to IV fluids to prevent rebound hypoglycemia.
- **Potassium**: Watch carefully, as fluids and insulin will cause rapid fall in serum levels. When K <5 mEq/L, it should be added to the IV fluids (Per liter: 20 mEq for K 4-5, 40 mEq for K 3–4). If potassium falls below 3, stop insulin drip and give 10–20 an hour until >3.5.

- **Sodium and Magnesium**: Na has an inverse relationship with potassium, and will increase as potassium falls. If sodium levels rise above 150 mEq, switch fluids to 0.45 NS. Low magnesium levels prevent potassium uptake, so replace as necessary.
- **Electrolytes**: Continue to monitor electrolytes and anion gap during ICU stay. When ABG and electrolytes normalized, transition to SQ insulin.

**Potential complications** include:

- Sudden electrolyte shifts (potassium) leading to catastrophic arrythmias, cerebral edema, and other complications
- Vomiting and decreased LOC leading to aspiration/ARDS
- Mechanical ventilation stops respiratory alkalosis and increases acidosis

## HHNK

Hyperglycemic hyperosmolar nonketotic syndrome (HHNK) occurs in people without history of diabetes or with mild type 2 diabetes, resulting in persistent hyperglycemia leading to osmotic diuresis. Fluid shifts from intracellular to extracellular spaces to maintain osmotic equilibrium, but the increased glucosuria and dehydration results in hypernatremia and increased osmolarity. This condition is most common in those 50–70 years old and often is precipitated by an acute illness, such as a stroke, medications (thiazides), or dialysis treatments. HHNK differs from ketoacidosis because, while the insulin level is not adequate, it is high enough to prevent the breakdown of fat. Onset of symptoms often occurs over a few days. Glucose levels are often higher than those in DKA due to the gradual increase over time (often greater than 600), and the body living in a state of hyperglycemia, therefore the individual is not symptomatic until the blood glucose level is at an extreme high.

**Symptoms:** Polyuria, dehydration, hypotension, tachycardia, changes in mental status, seizures, hemiparesis.

**Diagnosis:** Increased glucose, Na, osmolality (urine and serum), BUN/Creatinine.

**Treatment** is similar to that for ketoacidosis:

- Insulin drip with frequent (hourly) blood sugar monitoring.
- Intravenous fluids and electrolytes.
- Correct blood glucose and other labs.

## Acute Hypoglycemia

Acute hypoglycemia (hyperinsulinism) may result from pancreatic islet tumors or hyperplasia, increasing insulin production, or from the use of insulin to control diabetes mellitus. Hyperinsulinism can cause damage to the central nervous and cardiopulmonary systems, interfering with functioning of the brain and causing neurological impairment. Other causes may include: genetic defects (chromosome 11: short arm), severe infections, and toxic ingestion of alcohol or drugs (salicylates).

**Symptoms** include:

- Blood glucose <50-60 mg/dL
- Central nervous system: seizures, altered consciousness, lethargy, and poor feeding with vomiting, myoclonus, respiratory distress, diaphoresis, hypothermia, and cyanosis
- Adrenergic system: diaphoresis, tremor, tachycardia, palpitation, hunger, and anxiety

**Diagnosis:** Blood work, patient history, presentation.

**Treatment** depends on underlying cause:

- Glucose/Glucagon administration to elevate blood glucose levels
- Diazoxide (Hyperstat) to inhibit release of insulin
- Somatostatin (Sandostatin) to suppress insulin production
- Careful monitoring

### Diabetes Insipidus

Diabetes insipidus (DI) is caused by a deficiency of the antidiuretic hormone (ADH), or vasopressin. DI may develop secondary to head trauma, primary brain tumor, meningitis, encephalitis, or surgical ablation or irradiation of the pituitary gland, or metastatic tumors. This is different from congenital nephrogenic diabetes insipidus, in which production of ADH is normal but the renal tubules do not respond.

**Symptoms:**

- Polydipsia—enormous quantities of fluid may be ingested (3-30 L/day)
- Polyuria—large volumes of very dilute urine is excreted (3-30 L/day); nocturia almost always occurs
- Dehydration and hypovolemia can develop quickly if urinary losses are not continuously replaced

**Diagnosis:** A water deprivation test is the most reliable diagnostic test, but should only be done while the patient is under constant supervision. The test measures urine production, blood electrolyte levels, and weight over about 12 hours, during which the person is not allowed to drink. At the end of the 12 hours, vasopressin is given and a diagnosis of DI is confirmed if the person's excessive urination stops, BP rises to normal, and HR is normal.

**Treatment** includes:

- **Hormonal drugs**—Desmopressin, a synthetic analog of vasopressin, has prolonged antidiuretic activity, lasting 12 to 24 hours in most patients, and may be given intranasally, SQ, IV, or orally. Overdosage can lead to water intoxication, so monitor neurological status.
- **Nonhormonal drugs**—Three groups of nonhormonal drugs can reduce polyuria:
  - Diuretics, primarily thiazides (hydrochlorothiazide)
  - Vasopressin-releasing drugs (chlorpropamide or carbamazepine)
  - Prostaglandin inhibitors (indomethacin)

## SIADH

Syndrome of inappropriate secretion of antidiuretic hormone (SIADH) is related to hypersecretion of the posterior pituitary gland. This causes the kidneys to reabsorb fluids, resulting in fluid retention, and triggers a decrease in sodium levels (dilutional hyponatremia), resulting in production of only concentrated urine. This syndrome may result from central nervous system disorders, such as brain trauma, surgery, or tumors. It may also be triggered by other disorders, such as tumors of various organs, pneumothorax, acute pneumonia, and other lung disorders. Some medications (vincristine, phenothiazines, tricyclic antidepressants, and thiazide diuretics) may also trigger SIADH.

**Symptoms:** Edema, dyspnea, crackles on auscultation, anorexia with nausea and vomiting, irritability, stomach cramps, alterations of personality, stupor, and seizures (related to progressive sodium depletion).

**Diagnosis:** Increased urine specific gravity, decreased Na and serum osmolality.

**Treatment** includes: (treat underlying cause)

- Correct fluid volume excess and electrolytes.
- Monitor urine output continuously: <0.5-1 mL/kg/hour is cause for concern.

- Seizure precautions.
- With SIADH expect low serum sodium and serum osmolality with high urine osmolality.

## CHRONIC ADRENAL INSUFFICIENCY (ADDISON'S DISEASE)

Adrenal/Adrenocortical insufficiency (Addison's disease) is caused by damage to the adrenal cortex related to a variety of causes, such as autoimmune disease or genetic disorders, but it may relate to destructive lesions or neoplasms. Without treatment the condition is life threatening.

**Symptoms** may be vague and the condition undiagnosed until 80–90% of the adrenal cortex has been destroyed:

- Chronic weakness and fatigue
- Abdominal distress with nausea and vomiting
- Salt or licorice craving as a result of aldosterone deficiency
- Pigmentary changes in skin and mucous membranes, hyperpigmentation
- Hypotension
- Hypoglycemia
- Recurrent seizures (more common in children)

**Treatment** includes hormone replacement therapy with glucocorticoids (cortisol) and mineralocorticoids (aldosterone), which may be taken orally or by monthly parenteral injections. Androgen replacement is sometimes recommended for women.

**Note:** During times of stress or illness, the demand for glucocorticoids may increase, and dosages up to 3 times the normal dosage may be needed to prevent an acute crisis.

## ACUTE ADRENAL INSUFFICIENCY (ADRENAL CRISIS)

Acute adrenal insufficiency (adrenal crisis) is a sudden, life-threatening condition resulting from an exacerbation of primary chronic adrenal insufficiency (Addison's disease), often precipitated by sepsis, surgical stress, adrenal hemorrhage related to septicemia, anticoagulation complications, and cortisone withdrawal related to a decreased or inadequate dose to compensate for stress. Acute adrenal insufficiency may occur in those who do not have Addison's disease, such as those who have received cortisone for various reasons, usually a minimum of 20 mg daily for at least 5 days.

**Symptoms**:

- Fever
- Nausea and vomiting
- Abdominal pain
- Weakness and general fatigue
- Disorientation, confusion
- Hypotensive shock
- Dehydration
- Electrolyte imbalance with hyperkalemia, hypercalcemia, hypoglycemia, and hyponatremia

**Treatment**:

- IV fluids in large volume
- Glucocorticoid
- 50% dextrose if indicated (hypoglycemia)
- Mineralocorticoid may be needed after intravenous solutions
- The precipitating cause must be identified and treated as well

## HYPERTHYROIDISM

Hyperthyroidism (thyrotoxicosis) usually results from excess production of thyroid hormones (Graves' disease) from immunoglobulins providing abnormal stimulation of the thyroid gland. Other causes include thyroiditis and excess thyroid medications.

**Symptoms** vary and may be non-specific, especially in the elderly:

- Hyperexcitability
- Tachycardia (100-160) and atrial fibrillation
- Increased systolic (but not diastolic) BP
- Poor heat tolerance, skin flushed and diaphoretic
- Dry skin and pruritis (especially in the elderly)
- Hand tremor, progressive muscular weakness
- Exophthalmos (bulging eyes)
- Increased appetite and intake but weight loss

**Treatment** includes:

- Radioactive iodine to destroy the thyroid gland. Propranolol may be used to prevent thyroid storm. Thyroid hormones are given for resultant hypothyroidism.
- Antithyroid medications, such as Propacil or Tapazole to block conversion of T4 to T3.
- Surgical removal of thyroid is used if patients cannot tolerate other treatments or in special circumstances, such as large goiter. Usually one-sixth of the thyroid is left in place and antithyroid medications are given before surgery.

**Review Video: 7 Symptoms of Hyperthyroidism**
Visit mometrix.com/academy and enter code: 923159

**Review Video: Graves' Disease**
Visit mometrix.com/academy and enter code: 516655

**Review Video: Thyroid and Antithyroid**
Visit mometrix.com/academy and enter code: 666133

## THYROTOXIC STORM

Thyrotoxic storm is a severe type of hyperthyroidism with sudden onset, precipitated by stress such as injury or surgery, in those un-treated or inadequately treated for hyperthyroidism. If not promptly diagnosed and treated, it is fatal. Incidence has decreased with the use of antithyroid medications but can still occur with medical emergencies or pregnancy. Diagnostic findings are similar to hyperthyroidism and include increased T3 uptake and decreased TSH.

**Symptoms**:

- Increase in symptoms of hyperthyroidism
- Increased temperature >38.5 °C
- Tachycardia >130 with atrial fibrillation and heart failure
- Gastrointestinal disorders such as nausea, vomiting, diarrhea, and abdominal discomfort
- Altered mental status with delirium progressing to coma

**Treatment**:

- Controlling production of thyroid hormone through antithyroid medications such as propylthiouracil and methimazole
- Inhibiting release of thyroid hormone with iodine therapy (or lithium)
- Controlling peripheral activity of thyroid hormone with propranolol
- Fluid and electrolyte replacement
- Glucocorticoids, such as dexamethasone
- Cooling blankets
- Treatment of arrhythmias as needed with antiarrhythmics and anticoagulation

## HYPOTHYROIDISM

Hypothyroidism occurs when the thyroid produces inadequate levels of thyroid hormones. Conditions may range from mild to severe myxedema. There are a number of **causes**:

- Chronic lymphocytic thyroiditis (Hashimoto's thyroiditis)
- Excessive treatment for hyperthyroidism
- Atrophy of thyroid
- Medications such as lithium and iodine compounds
- Radiation to the area of the thyroid
- Diseases that affect the thyroid such as scleroderma
- Iodine imbalances

**Symptoms** may include chronic fatigue, menstrual disturbances, hoarseness, subnormal temperature, low pulse rate, weight gain, thinning hair, thickening skin. Some dementia may occur with advanced conditions. Clinical findings may include increased cholesterol with associated atherosclerosis and coronary artery disease. Myxedema may be characterized by changes in respiration with hypoventilation and $CO_2$ retention resulting in coma.

**Treatment** involves hormone replacement with synthetic levothyroxine (Synthroid) based on TSH levels, but this increases the oxygen demand of the body, so careful monitoring of cardiac status must be done during early treatment to avoid myocardial infarction while reaching euthyroid (normal) level.

## HYPERPARATHYROIDISM

Hyperparathyroidism occurs when there is **overproduction of parathyroid hormone (PTH)**. Normal range is 10-55 pg/mL. This occurs more often in women and those over 50 years old. Hypercalcemia (total $Ca^{++}$ >10.4 mg/dL) is the most common finding in hyperparathyroidism. Patients may complain signs of hypercalcemia which can be easily remembered with *bones, stones, groans, and moans.* This includes **bone pain** due to demineralization, **kidney stones**, **abdominal groans** (nausea, vomiting, constipation, loss of appetite), and **psychiatric moans** (nervous system issues: muscle weakness, fatigue, lethargy, depression, confusion). Polyuria can occur with renal failure. Cardiac arrhythmias, hypertension, and even coma can occur. $Ca^{++}$ levels >12 mg/dL may be due to cancer, and therefore cancer must be ruled out, especially if $Ca^{++}$ levels rise rapidly. Hyperparathyroidism is treated with parathyroidectomy of affected glands.

## HYPOPARATHYROIDISM

Hypoparathyroidism is the **deficiency of PTH**. This is more common in women and is usually due to accidental damage during thyroid/neck surgery, radioactive iodine treatment for hyperthyroidism, radiation, or due to autoimmune causes. As $Ca^{++}$ levels drop, patients may complain of paresthesia of the fingers, toes, and perioral area. Patients will show other signs of neuromuscular irritability with muscle aches, hyperreflexia, carpopedal spasm (tetany), laryngospasm, and facial grimacing. A positive Chvostek sign (unilateral spasm of the facial muscles when the facial nerve is tapped) and a positive Trousseau sign (carpal spasm when upper arm is compressed with a blood pressure cuff) may be present. Irritability, confusion, fatigue, seizures, brittle hair and nails, and personality changes may occur. Diagnose with an ionized $Ca^{++}$ level (<4.7 mg/dL), reduced PTH, and elevated phosphate. Treat with $Ca^{++}$ and vitamin D supplements. Patients with renal failure must also reduce the amount of phosphate in their diet. Patients with tetany are treated with IV calcium gluconate.

### Cushing Syndrome and Cushing's Disease

Cushing syndrome results when **cortisol levels** are increased. Most commonly, this is due to steroid treatment with **prednisone**. Endogenous causes include a pituitary adenoma producing excess amounts of adrenocorticotropic hormone (ACTH) which leads to elevated cortisol (termed **Cushing's disease**) or a primary tumor of the adrenal gland causing increased cortisol secretion. Forms of cancer (e.g., lung, carcinoid) can present with ectopic sources of ACTH secretion. Patients will develop proximal muscle weakness, muscular atrophy, truncal obesity with thin arms and legs, round facies, buffalo hump, and purple striae usually across the abdomen. Patients may bruise easily, have non-healing sores, and women may be affected with hirsutism and oligomenorrhea/amenorrhea. Osteoporosis can occur as can glucose intolerance. For diagnosis a patient should be screened with one of the following: 24-hour urine free cortisol x3, low dose (1 mg) dexamethasone suppression test, midnight serum or salivary cortisol. Once Cushing syndrome is established, determine the cause using an ACTH and simultaneous cortisol measurement (elevated = adrenal adenoma or carcinoma) or a high-dose (8 mg overnight, or 2-day) dexamethasone suppression test (differentiates between pituitary cause and ectopic ACTH cause). Patients should be weaned off prednisone if possible. Removal of a pituitary adenoma can decrease ACTH production. Removal of an adrenal adenoma or other ectopic source of hormone secretion can decrease cortisol levels. Complications include hypertension, CV disease, DM, osteoporosis, risk of adrenal crisis, and psychosis.

### Hyperaldosteronism

Hyperaldosteronism leads to hypokalemia and hypernatremia (and often resulting hypertension). In fact, patients with untreated hypertension and potassium <2.8meq/dL often have primary hyperaldosteronism:

- **Aldosterone-producing adenoma** (Conn's syndrome) accounts for most primary hyperaldosteronism and affects women more often than men.
- **Idiopathic hyperaldosteronism** accounts for about 30% of primary hyperaldosteronism and has no identifiable changes on imaging.
- **Glucocorticoid suppressible hyperaldosteronism** is familial and rare.
- **Aldosterone-producing adrenocortical carcinoma** is another rare cause and presents with hyperandrogenism.

**Diagnosis** of hyperaldosteronism requires diastolic hypertension without edema, low renin levels that do not respond to volume depletion, and high aldosterone levels that fail to drop with saline boluses. An adrenal CT scan is performed to distinguish between Conn's syndrome and idiopathic hyperaldosteronism. **Treatment** includes spironolactone or eplerenone to block the mineralocorticoid receptor, normalizing potassium and improving blood pressure. Adrenalectomy is indicated for unilateral hyperplasia or Conn's syndrome.

## Pheochromocytoma

Pheochromocytoma is a rare tumor of chromaffin tissue. Ninety percent of these occur in the adrenal medulla, 10% are bilateral, and 10% are malignant. These tumors produce epinephrine and norepinephrine, leading to episodic symptoms of headaches, chest pain, palpitations, diaphoresis, tremor, nausea, vomiting, weight loss, and constipation. Initial diagnosis requires a 24-hour urine test to check for metanephrine, VMA, and catecholamines. These are always elevated with pheochromocytoma. If associated with a multiple endocrine neoplasia (MEN) syndrome, then one must check serum free metanephrine. Then one should begin imaging with CT or MRI scanning of the adrenals. If the adrenals appear normal, a radiolabeled iodine (called MIBG-metaiodobenzylguanidine scintigraphy) scan can localize extra-adrenal pheochromocytoma tissue or metastases. This scan uses a compound that concentrates in the adrenals to highlight the pheochromocytoma tissue. **Treatment** is surgical. But first, phenoxybenzamines are used to block the catecholamines, and then beta-blockers are used to control heart rate. Surgery has a 90% cure rate. Urinary catecholamines should be followed for at least 10 years.

## Paget's Disease

Paget's disease is a disease of high bone turnover and disorganized osteoid formation. It is most prevalent in patients in the northeast US or of European descent and in older patients. The disease is usually asymptomatic, being detected on radiographs. However, it may present with bone pain, fractures, and bony deformities. Commonly involved bones include the skull, femur, tibia, pelvis, and humerus. Specifically, with skull involvement, the patient may note frequent headaches and increasing hat size, sometimes associated with deafness. Examination findings include frontal bossing, bowed legs, and superficial erythema and warmth, due to the increased vascularity of the bones. This disease is **diagnosed** with increased alkaline phosphatase, and elevated urinary hydroxyproline. Calcium and phosphorous are often normal. Imaging reveals hyperdense and enlarged bones in some regions and erosions in others. Bone scanning reveals increased uptake in certain areas. **Treatment** includes bisphosphonate and management of complications, including CHF, spinal cord compression, or nerve entrapment.

## Oral Hypoglycemic Agents

Oral hypoglycemic agents are **anti-diabetic treatments** generally used in the treatment of Type II Diabetes. There are five classic categories of oral hypoglycemic agents: sulfonylureas, biguanides, meglitinides, competitive inhibitors of alpha-glucosidases (located in the intestinal brush border), and thiazolidinediones. More recently, two additional novel classes of oral hypoglycemics, DPP-4 inhibitors and SGLT2 inhibitors, were introduced with proven effectiveness when used in conjunction with changes in diet and exercise. Some examples of sulfonylurea oral hypoglycemic agents include the first-generation agents tolbutamide, tolazamide, chlorpropamide, and acetohexamide; and second-generation agents glyburide, glimepiride, and glipizide. The biguanide oral hypoglycemic agent is metformin. Metformin has the distinct advantage of not causing weight gain or hypoglycemic reactions. The meglitinide agent is repaglinide. Examples of alpha-glucosidase inhibitors are acarbose and miglitol. Alpha-glucosidase inhibitors bind tightly to intestinal alpha-glucosidases and decrease the postprandial rise in glucose levels. The only available thiazolidinedione oral hypoglycemic agent is currently pioglitazone; troglitazone was removed from US market in 2000, and rosiglitazone was removed from US market in 2011. Examples of DPP-4 inhibitors include linagliptin, vildagliptin, sitagliptin, and saxagliptin. Examples of SGLT2 inhibitors include canagliflozin, dapagliflozin, and empagliflozin.

## INSULIN USED TO TREAT GLYCEMIC DISORDERS

There are a number of different types of **insulin** with varying action times. Insulin is used to metabolize **glucose** for those whose pancreas does not produce insulin. People may need to take a combination of insulins (short- and long-acting) to maintain glucose control. Duration of action may vary according to the individual's metabolism, intake, and level of activity:

- **Humalog** (Lispro H) is a fast-acting, short-acting insulin with onset in 5–15 minutes, peaking at 45–90 minutes and lasting 3–4 hours.
- **Regular** (R) is a relatively fast-acting insulin with onset in 30 minutes, peaks in 2–5 hours, and lasts 5–8 hours.
- **NPH** (N) insulin is intermediate-acting with onset in 1–3 hours, peaking at 6–12 hours, and lasting for 16–24 hours.
- **Insulin Glargine** (Lantus) is a long-acting insulin with onset in 3–6 hours, no peak, and lasting for 24 hours.
- **Combined NPH/Regular** (70/30 or 50/50) has an onset of 30 minutes, peaks at 7–12 hours, and lasts 16–24 hours.

# Immunocompromise

## Immune Deficiencies

There are multiple disorders that fall into the category of **primary immunodeficiency diseases.** These disorders are genetic or inherited disorders in which the body's immune system does not function properly. These disorders may involve low levels of antibodies, defects in the antibodies, or defects in cells that make up the immune system (T-cells, B-cells). Common variable immune deficiency is a common immune deficiency diagnosed in adulthood. This disorder is characterized by low levels of serum immunoglobins and antibodies, which substantially increases the risk of infection.

- **Signs and symptoms**: Recurrent infections are the hallmark sign of immune deficiency disorders. Recurrent infections most often involve the ears, sinuses, bronchi, and lungs. Lymphadenopathy may occur as well as splenomegaly. GI symptoms may include abdominal pain, nausea, vomiting, diarrhea, and weight loss. Some patients may experience polyarthritis. Granulomas are also common and may occur in the lungs, lymph nodes, liver, and skin.
- **Diagnosis**: A physical assessment and patient history are used to diagnose immune deficiency disorders. Since immune deficiency disorders are genetic or inherited, family history should also be evaluated. Lab tests such as serum antibodies, serum immunoglobin levels and a complete blood count may also be used to assist in the diagnosis of immune deficiency disorders.
- **Treatment**: Patients with immune deficiency disorders often receive immunoglobulin replacement. Long term antibiotics may also be administered for recurrent infections. Educate patients to frequently wash hands, cook foods thoroughly, avoid large crowds, and other infection prevention techniques.

### *Congenital Immunodeficiencies*

Congenital immunodeficiencies include:

- **Common variable immunodeficiency** is primarily an IgG deficiency due to absent plasma cells and B cell differentiation. These patients have increased susceptibility to encapsulated organisms and are more likely to develop bronchiectasis from the recurrent damage. They are also at higher risk for B cell neoplasms, GI malignancy, and autoimmune disease. Test is with functional antibody response and treatment with IVIG.
- **Congenital Agammaglobulinemia** (Bruton's, x-linked) usually leads to a susceptibility to recurrent pyogenic infections and low IgG and no IgA, IgM, IgE, IgD, or B cells.
- **Selective IgA deficiency** is the most common Ig deficiency and leads to recurrent sinopulmonary infections. It has association with recurrent giardiasis, GI malignancy, and autoimmune disorders, including celiac sprue. One should withhold IVIG due to possible anaphylactic reaction to IgA.
- **Wiskott-Aldrich syndrome** is the combination of thrombocytopenia, eczema, and immunodeficiency. It has associated low IgM and elevated IgA and IgE. BMT treats this successfully.

### *Complement Deficiencies*

There are deficiencies of all parts of the complement pathway, including the following:

- **Classical deficiency** may include C1 (q, r, s), C2, and C4. This leads to immune complex syndromes and pyogenic infection, such as recurrent sinopulmonary infections with encapsulated bacteria. There is an association with SLE and other rheumatoid diseases. C2 is the most common deficiency in Caucasians in the US.
- **C3 and alternative complement deficiency** may lead to immune complex syndromes and recurrent infections, such as severe pyogenic infections. It may also be associated with HUS.
- **Membrane attack complex (MAC) deficiency** is also known as terminal complement deficiency. This is associated with recurrent Neisseria infections (which can cause meningitis and sepsis) and immune complex diseases. The CH50 assay must be checked to determine the activity of the classical pathway. CH50 may also be used to follow disease activity in SLE.

## Autoimmune System Disorders

**Allergic interstitial/tubulointerstitial nephritis** is inflammation and edema of the interstitial areas of the kidneys. Up to 92% of cases caused by allergic reaction to medications, such as antibiotics (B-lactams, fluoroquinolones, macrolides, and anti-tuberculin drugs), antivirals, NSAIDs, PPIs, antiepileptics, diuretics, chemotherapy, and allopurinol. **Symptoms** include fever, rash, and renal enlargement as well as fatigue, nausea, vomiting, and weight loss. **Diagnosis** is by renal biopsy. Urine tests may show eosinophils, blood, RBC casts and sterile pyuria. Increased protein may be seen in response to NSAIDs. **Treatment** is primarily supportive but requires stopping the triggering medication.

**Eosinophilic esophagitis** is the accumulation of eosinophils in the esophagus, resulting in chronic inflammation. Damage from proteins produced in esophageal tissue causes scarring and narrowing, resulting in dysphagia, vomiting, choking, GERD, upper abdominal pain, heartburn, and regurgitation. **Causes** include allergic reaction to pollens or foods. **Risk factors** include cold/dry climate, male gender, family history, allergies, and asthma. **Diagnosis** is per endoscopy with biopsy. Blood tests may help confirm allergic reactions. **Treatment** may include dietary limitations, PPIs, and topical steroids. Some may require dilation of the esophagus.

**Churg-Strauss syndrome** (AKA **eosinophilic granulomatosis with polyangiitis**) is an idiopathic form of pulmonary vasculitis that can affect multiple systems (skin and lungs most often) as well as affecting small- and medium-sized arteries in those with asthma. **Symptoms** include dyspnea, chest pain, skin rash, myopathy, arthropathy, rhinitis, sinusitis, abdominal pain, blood in stools, and paresthesia (from the involvement of nerves). The syndrome is characterized by eosinophilia >1500 cells/mcL or >10% of peripheral total WBC count. X-rays or CTs may show transient opacities or multiple nodules. Tissue biopsies typically show allergic granulomas. **Treatment** usually begins with corticosteroids but other immunosuppressive drugs (cyclophosphamide, methotrexate, azathioprine) may be used, especially if critical organs are involved. The goal of treatment is remission, but patients usually need to take drugs at least 2 years before they are tapered off of the drugs. Up to 50% of patients have relapses.

### Neutropenia

Neutropenia is identified as a **polymorphonuclear neutrophil count** equal to or less than 500/mL. **Chronic neutropenia** is a sustained condition of minimal neutrophils lasting 3 or more months. Neutropenia may occur from a decreased production of **white blood cells** (e.g., from chemotherapy or radiation therapy). It may also occur from a loss of white blood cells from autoimmune disease processes. Neutropenia is silent but dangerous. It leaves essentially no neutrophils to fight any threat of infection. Neutrophils make up as much as 70% of the white blood cells circulating in the blood. Neutropenia can be the cause of a septic situation, which can be life-threatening. Up to 70% of patients experiencing a fever while in a neutropenic state will die within 48 hours if not treated aggressively.

### Leukopenia

Leukopenia is defined as a decrease in white blood cells. Neutropenia is defined as a low number of neutrophils and is often used interchangeably with the term leukopenia. With a decrease in the number of circulating white blood cells, the patient is at an increased risk for the development of an infection. Leukopenia and neutropenia can occur from either a decrease in the production of white blood cells or an increase in their destruction. Infections, malignancy, autoimmune disorders, medications (including chemotherapy) and a history of radiation therapy may contribute to the development of leukopenia/neutropenia.

**Signs and symptoms**: Malaise, fever, chills, night sweats, shortness of breath, headache, cough, abdominal pain, tachycardia, and hypotension. A patient with neutropenia/leukopenia is at risk for the development of infections including pneumonia, skin infections, urinary tract infections and gastrointestinal infections. In addition, the patient is at an increased risk for sepsis.

**Diagnosis**: Complete blood count including an absolute neutrophil count. In addition, a bone marrow biopsy may be performed to determine the cause of the decrease in neutrophils.

**Treatment**: Supportive therapy is used in the treatment of leukopenia including the aggressive treatment of infections that may develop. Precautions should be taken to protect the patient from additional infections, including strict adherence to sterile technique and infection control procedures. Hematopoietic growth factors may also be given to stimulate the production of neutrophils.

### LYMPHEDEMA

Lymphedema results from untreated or incurable **edema**. It is a chronic condition marked by swelling and accumulated fluids within the tissue. This accumulation is a result of lymphatic drainage failure, inadequate lymph transport capacity, an increased lymph production, or a combination of these. Primary disease is a result of **inadequately developed lymphatic pathways**, while the secondary disease process is due to **damage outside of the pathways**. The process is worsened and complicated as **macrophages** are released to control inflammation caused by the increased release of fibroblasts and keratinocytes. There is a gradual increase in adipose tissue and leakage of lymph through the skin. The skin and tissues gradually thicken and change in color, texture, tone, and temperature. It begins to blister and produce hyperkeratosis, warts, papillomatosis, and elephantiasis. There is an ever-increasing risk of infection and further complications.

## HIV/AIDS

**AIDS** is a progression of infection with **human immunodeficiency virus** (HIV). AIDS is diagnosed when the following criteria are met:

- HIV infection
- CD4 count less than 200 cells/mm$^3$
- AIDS defining condition, such as opportunistic infections (cytomegalovirus, tuberculosis), wasting syndrome, neoplasms (Kaposi sarcoma), or AIDS dementia complex

Because there is such a wide range of AIDS defining conditions, the patient may present with many types of **symptoms**, depending upon the diagnosis, but more than half of AIDS patients exhibit:

- Fever
- Lymphadenopathy
- Pharyngitis
- Rash
- Myalgia/arthralgia
- It is important to review the following:
  - CD4 counts to determine immune status
  - WBC and differential for signs of infection
  - Cultures to help identify any infective agents
  - CBC to evaluate for signs of bleeding or thrombocytopenia

Treatment aims to cure or manage opportunistic conditions and control underlying HIV infection through highly active anti-retroviral therapy (HAART), 3 or more drugs used concurrently.

### LUNG CANCER

#### *SCLC*

Small cell lung cancer (SCLC) is a rapidly-growing variant of lung cancer found in about 15% of new cases. Its origin is in the bronchi and this type of lung cancer occurs predominantly in smokers. At the time of diagnosis, the disease is usually symptomatic and metastases have generally already occurred. There are 3 subtypes of SCLC: oat cell or small-cell carcinoma, intermediate cell, and small cell combined with squamous cell carcinoma or adenocarcinoma. Differential diagnosis includes tests to distinguish it from slower-growing non-small cell lung cancer, lymphoma, sarcoidosis, metastases due to other primary tumors, or infectious processes. In addition to routine procedures like history, physical examination, and laboratory tests, SCLC is generally staged using imaging tests. In particular, a CT scan with contrast is done to assess the involvement in the lung and other sites, and an MRI of the brain and/or a bone scan may also be done to look for metastases. A bone marrow biopsy may also be indicated.

### NSCLC

Non-small cell lung cancer (NSCLC) is a blanket term for several histological types of lung cancer not classified as SCLC. The major histological variants are adenocarcinoma, squamous cell carcinoma, and large cell. The large cell type is anaplastic, which means the cells are relatively undifferentiated. Diagnosis of NSCLCs includes exclusion of small cell lung carcinoma, metastatic lung lesions from other primary sources, sarcoidosis, and infections. The clinician generally stages the disease through use of history, physical examination, and laboratory tests. Imaging studies usually include not only CT scans but also positron emission tomography (PET) and, if metastases are suspected, a brain MRI and possibly a bone scan. Mediastinal node biopsies are generally performed if the PET scan indicates later stage disease; various types of incisions can be made, such as those into the sternum or mediastinum.

## Breast Cancer

### Staging

The American Joint Committee on Cancer **TNM Staging** has recently developed a complex staging classification for breast cancer. In general, however, early invasive breast cancer would be Stage I or II (IIA or IIB). In these stages, there is either no lymph node involvement or only same-side axillary region lymph node involvement with no distant metastases. Nevertheless, diagnostic tests should include bilateral mammography (and possibly other imaging techniques), blood profiles, hepatic and renal function tests, serum alkaline phosphatase levels, and lymph node biopsy or mapping. Assays for prognostic factors like high levels of HER2 or hormone receptors may also be done. Management is surgery that either conserves the breast or a modified radical mastectomy in which the pectoral muscles are not removed. If there is nodal involvement or other factors exist (such as positive hormone receptors or large tumor size), adjuvant chemotherapy or endocrine treatment is added.

### Locally Advanced or Recurrent Breast Cancer or Distant Metastases

Locally advanced stage III breast cancer is a comprehensive term for a highly heterogeneous grouping. All Stage III patients have either some sort of nodal involvement and/or their tumor has extended into the chest wall or skin. They do not have distant metastases. Once the disease has reached this stage, multiple treatment strategies are needed, including chemotherapy (and endocrine therapy in receptor-positive women), surgery, and radiation. Locally recurrent breast cancer, on the other hand, is generally due to insufficient removal of the primary lesion (such as with breast conservation surgery); it can often be managed with further surgery, although other modalities may be needed if there has been nodal or metastatic spread. Once there is metastatic involvement, therapies are merely palliative and the prognosis is poor.

## Prostate Cancer

At present, about one out of nine men will develop **prostate cancer** at some point, and approximately 2-3% of those will die of the disease. There are familial groupings of prostate cancer; for example, mutations in the RNASEL and MSR1 loci coding for host response to infection appear to predispose a man to prostate cancer. Diet affects susceptibility to prostate cancer; in particular, consumption of red meat cooked at high temperature to release aromatic compounds is highly correlated to development of the cancer. Ethnicity may play a role, as African Americans in the U. S. have an especially high rate of prostate cancer, but this may be due in part to diet.

### *Mechanisms That Contribute to Development of Prostate Cancer*

Germline mutations in the RNASEL and MSR1 genes have been associated with an increased risk of developing prostate cancer. There is some evidence that inflammation and infection may play a role in the progression of the disease, and development of lesions termed proliferate inflammatory atrophy (PIA) may predispose a man to later prostate intraepithelial neoplasia and prostate cancer. Molecular changes have also been closely associated with disease progression. These include somatic inactivation of the GSTP1 gene, which fosters susceptibility to oxidant and electron-accepting carcinogens and depression of various functions caused by gene mutations, such as the PTEN tumor-suppressor gene, NKA3.1, and CDKN1B. As discussed previously, screening tests include serum prostate-specific antigen (PSA) levels and digital rectal examination. Diagnosis is generally confirmed by core needle biopsy.

### *Staging and Grading*

There are two **staging systems** that are commonly used for prostate cancer.

- The **TNM system**, which is adapted to many types of cancer, defines the primary tumor (T) when observable as T1 (identified only by histology or needle biopsy), T2 (limited to the prostate), T3 (reaches through the prostate capsule) or T4 (invasion of adjacent structures). The TMN system also expresses regional lymph node involvement from N1 to N3 and distant metastases as M1 if present. An *X* after the T, N, or M indicates inability to assess and a zero means no evidence of presence.
- The **American Urological Association or AUA staging system** classifies prostate cancer in four stages. These stages are fairly similar to the primary tumor staging of the TMN program. Basically, Stage A is disease that is not clinically observable. Stage B is a tumor confined within the prostate gland. Stage C involves malignancy that extends outside the prostate capsule but remains within the area. Stage D is malignancy with metastatic involvement. A Gleason score is a combined measurement of histological grading of the two most prevalent differentiation patterns; a lower score reflects a higher amount of differentiation and each component can be graded from 1 to 5.

## Colon Cancer

The factor most closely associated with development of **colon cancer** is age, with about 9 out 10 cases identified after age 50. The vast majority of cases have not been correlated to any heritable gene mutation. However, there is a several-fold increase in risk of development of the disease when a close relative is affected, and there are several familial syndromes related to colon cancer (most notably familial adenomatous polyposis or FAP and HNPCC or hereditary nonpolyposis colon cancer). Risk of colon cancer has been associated with certain dietary practices, including high intake of low fiber and high fat foods. It has also been associated with environmental influences, such as exposure to tobacco. The disease often develops through mutations attributable to either chromosomal instability or to a lesser extent microsatellite (repetitive DNA sequence) instability. The genetic change most often found in patients with both precursor adenomatous polyps or actual colon cancer is a defective APC tumor suppressor locus.

### *Procedures for Prevention, Diagnosis, and Staging of Colon Cancer*

Identification of individuals with familial syndromes or known genetic changes associated with colon cancer is theoretically a means of preventing colon cancer. Realistically, at present this is rarely done. COX-2 inhibitors, which are basically anti-inflammatory agents, are sometimes used as chemo preventive drugs. Patients usually present with symptoms like anemia, fatigue, weight loss, or changes in bowel habits. A small portion of them have other cancers and up to 40% have polyps in addition to the primary tumor. Colonoscopy is suggested as a diagnostic procedure every 10 years beginning at age 50, and it involves inspection of the entire large intestine using a flexible fiberoptic endoscope. Benign polyps, possible cancer precursors, can be immediately excised. Other diagnostic probes include sigmoidoscopy and virtual colonoscopy. Staging is usually done utilizing imaging techniques like CT scans, MRIs, or PET scans. Liver metastases, common in conjunction with colorectal cancers, can be best visualized using intraoperative ultrasound.

### *Staging*

There are several classification systems for **staging** colorectal cancers. The most common scheme utilized is the Astler-Coller modified Duke's system. The emphasis of this classification scheme is the depth of tumor invasion into the colon wall. The modified Astler-Coller (MAC), the traditional Duke, and the American Joint Committee on Cancer or AJCC (based on TMN) classification schemes are interrelated. According to Astler-Coller, MAC A is comprised of lesions limited to the mucosa or sub mucosa; MAC B1 and B2 involve extension into or through the muscularis propria; MAC C1, 2, or 3 imply nodal involvement along with extension into or through the bowel wall; MAC D means evidence of distant metastases. These correspond roughly to Duke's A, B, C and D. The AJCC or TMN classification defines stages 0 (carcinoma in situ) through IV.

## Skin Cancer

### *Melanomas*

The severity of melanoma is primarily related to the thickness of the primary lesion and to the presence of histologic ulceration. The American Joint Commission on Cancer's Stage Grouping for melanoma reflects these parameters. The T or tumor size component for identifiable melanomas is up to 1.0 mm thick for T1, 1.01 to 2.0 mm for T2, 2.01 to 4.0 mm for T3, and greater than 4.0 mm thick for T4. Within each of these groups for cases of melanoma in situ, an *a* is added for no ulceration and a *b* is added to indicate ulceration. Regional lymph node involvement is described by an N followed by a 1, 2 or 3 (for 1, 2-3, or 4 or more involved lymph nodes) and an *a* or *b* to indicate either micro- or macrometastases. Distant metastases, if present, are classified as M1a, b, or c, depending on the site. As with other schemes, an *X* after the letter indicates inability to assess, and a zero means no evidence. Staging is from 0 (in situ) to stage IV (distant metastases). Stages I and II have no nodal or metastatic involvement, and stage III means regional lymph node presence. Within each stage (I, II, and III) there are various subgroups, and the presence of ulceration can put a thinner melanoma in the same stage with a thicker but non-ulcerated lesion.

### *Basic Features of Nonmelanoma Skin Cancers*

About four out of every five cases of nonmelanoma skin cancer are **basal cell carcinoma** (BCC), which usually presents as either a reddish ulcerated bump on the skin or as a lighter hardened plaque. Most other nonmelanoma skin cancers are **squamous cell carcinomas** (SCC), which usually appear as raised areas that are either red or skin-toned and have ulcerations and patchy areas of hard horny tissue called keratoses.

Organ transplant patients are prone to develop SCC. Patients with SCC are more likely to develop metastases than those with BCC, although the latter can reoccur at the primary site. Lack of differentiation in either type can portend a more clinically aggressive tumor. There are other generally rare and often more aggressive malignancies that can emulate BCC or SCC that should be excluded via differential diagnosis such as sebaceous gland carcinoma and Merkel cell carcinoma.

## Leukemia

Leukemia is a condition in which the proliferating cells compete with normal cells for nutrition. Leukemia affects all cells because the abnormal cells in the bone marrow depress the formation of all elements, resulting in several consequences, regardless of the type of leukemia:

- Decrease in production of **erythrocytes** (RBCs), resulting in anemia
- Decrease in **neutrophils**, resulting in increased risk of infection
- Decrease in **platelets**, with subsequent decrease in clotting factors and increased bleeding
- Increased risk of **physiological fractures** because of invasion of bone marrow that weakens the periosteum
- Infiltration of **liver, spleen, and lymph glands**, resulting in enlargement and fibrosis

- Infiltration of the **CNS**, resulting in increased intracranial pressure, ventricular dilation, and meningeal irritation with headaches, vomiting, papilledema, nuchal rigidity, and coma progressing to death
- **Hypermetabolism** that deprives cells of nutrients, resulting in anorexia, weight loss, muscle atrophy, and fatigue

**Review Video: Leukemia**
Visit mometrix.com/academy and enter code: 940024

### *Relationship of Leukocytosis to Leukemia*

Leukemia occurs when one type of WBC proliferates with immature cells, with the defect occurring in the hematopoietic stem cell, either lymphoid or myeloid. Usually, leukemias classified as blast cell or stem cell refer to lymphoid defects. With acute leukemia, WBC count remains low because the cells are halted at the blast stage and the disease progresses rapidly. Chronic leukemia progresses more slowly and most cells are mature.

## Tumor Lysis Syndrome

Tumor lysis syndrome occurs when intracellular contents are released from tumor cells, leading to electrolyte imbalances (hyperkalemia, hyperphosphatemia, hypocalcemia, and hyperuricemia) when the kidneys are unable to excrete the large volume of metabolites. **Tumor lysis syndrome** is most common after treatment of hematologic malignancies but can occur due to any type of tumor that is sensitive to chemotherapy. The primary goals of therapy for tumor lysis syndrome are to increase urine production through IV hydration in order to prevent renal failure and to decrease uric acid concentration, usually with administration of allopurinol. The urine pH should be maintained at 7 or higher. Electrolyte levels should be closely monitored, as hyperkalemia is a risk. Patients at moderate risk (intermediate grade lymphomas, acute leukemias) should begin prophylactic allopurinol before chemotherapy, and those at higher risk (high grade lymphomas or acute leukemias with WBC count >50,000) should begin rasburicase.

## Cancer-Specific Treatment

### *Leukemia Treatment*

Leukemia treatment depends upon the protocol established for each type of leukemia. Combined drugs are usually more effective than any single drug. Chemotherapy usually includes three stages:

- **Induction therapy**: The purpose is to induce remission to the point that the bone marrow is clear of disease and blood cell counts are normal. Chemotherapy is usually given for about 4-6 weeks, followed by transplantation or the next stage of chemotherapy. The chemotherapy is potent and suppresses blood elements, leaving the body at risk for serious infections and hemorrhage, so supportive care is critical.
- **Consolidation therapy**: The goal is to kill any cells that may have escaped the induction stage. This stage lasts 4-8 months. Intrathecal chemotherapy may be co-administered as a prophylaxis to prevent CNS involvement.
- **Maintenance therapy**: Treatment may continue for another 2-3 years, but with less intense chemotherapy to maintain remission. Weekly blood cell counts monitor progress and side effects.

Sometimes after the three stages of chemotherapy are completed, the patient will relapse and leukemic cells return. In that case, **reinduction** is carried out, usually using a different arsenal of drugs. Many drugs in use now, especially for relapses, are those in clinical trials. Clinical trials are ongoing for many chemotherapeutic agents to determine the best combination of drugs and duration of treatment. Other treatments may be instituted, depending on the severity of the disease:

- **Intrathecal chemotherapy** is administered into the spinal fluid for treatment of infiltration of the CNS.
- **Radiation** to the brain may be indicated in addition to intrathecal chemotherapy with severe disease but poses danger to brain development.
- **Bone marrow or cord blood transplant**, also known as hematopoietic stem cell transplantation (HCST), may be done if chemotherapy fails or after the first remission for AML, which has a lower cure rate.

### *Lung Cancer Treatment*

Since SCLC is an aggressive disease, surgical procedures are not useful and not generally performed. If the cancer is relatively limited, chemotherapy and irradiation of both the chest and brain (to prevent brain metastases) are done. Otherwise, several cycles of combination or multi-agent chemotherapy are tried but the prognosis is poor.

For NSCLC, surgical resection is usually effective for the early stages I and II. For stages IIIA and IIIB, indicating metastatic involvement, chemotherapy possibly combined with radiation is generally used either before surgery (IIIA) or as the treatment modality. If the latter patients also have a malignant pleural effusion, they are treated as stage IV. Stage IV patients are given combination chemotherapy, mainly to improve their quality of life. Individuals with recurrent NSCLC are also treated with combination chemotherapy.

### *Management of Localized Versus Advanced Prostate Cancer*

**Localized prostate cancer** would be defined as falling into the TMN categories of T1 or T2. Usually, these individuals also have serum PSA levels of ≤10 ng/mL and a Gleason score in the range of 2 to 6. Patients falling into these categories are often just watched carefully, but a radical retropubic prostatectomy may be performed or radiation (either external beam or brachytherapy) may be used. Androgen deprivation has also been used as an adjunct to external beam radiation treatment. Radiation therapy can be utilized after prostatectomy if the disease recurs, usually monitored by looking for rising PSA levels. More **advanced stages of prostate cancer** are generally managed primarily through suppression of androgens by luteinizing hormone-releasing (LHRH) agonists and possibly antiandrogens. However, if the disease progresses (usually indicated by rising PSA levels) systemic chemotherapy may be initiated. Other modalities are under investigation as well. Any of these approaches can produce side effects related to sexual function or pleasure or urinary function, and the androgen deprivation can lead to loss of muscle mass or bone density.

### *Colon Cancer Treatment*

Standard **treatment** for colorectal cancer is radical surgical resection followed by anastomosis of the remaining colon, including elimination of lymphatic drainage portals. The bowel must be cleared of fecal matter through liquid diet, hydration, and the use of salt solutions and lavage before the surgery. The most suitable surgical option for management of obstructive colon cancers is a subtotal colectomy. After surgery, recommendations for surveillance are physical examination every three months for two years tapering to twice yearly, quarterly monitoring by CEA levels and CT scans, and colonoscopy a year later with follow-up every three to five years. Most cases of recurrence happen within the first few years and many can be successfully surgically removed. Systemic chemotherapy (such as 5-fluorouracil combined with leucovorin) is also administered to most patients in an attempt to eliminate possible micrometastases. Similar chemotherapeutic regimens, possibly in conjunction with additional agents, are used to manage metastatic disease. The liver is the most common site of disease spread.

### *Procedures for Primary or Salvage Therapy of Melanomas*

Primary melanomas are surgically excised. The margin around the site required is ascertained by the thickness of the melanoma and the area where it is located. A thicker lesion requires a larger excision margin, and some sites such as the fingers, toes, soles of the foot or ears may necessitate other surgical procedures in conjunction. Sentinel nodes are often biopsied if regional lymph node involvement is not clinically evident. If regional nodes are metastatic, they are dissected. Patients who have large primary lesions or nodal involvement are generally also given interferon alpha or dacarbazine (DTIC), the only currently approved agents, or they may be enrolled in other clinical trials. These systemic adjuvants mainly alleviate symptoms. Once metastatic disease becomes systemic, patient survival is typically only about six to nine months.

#### *Treatment of Nonmelanoma Skin Cancers*

Primary basal cell or squamous cell carcinomas are generally surgically excised. A procedure called Mohs surgery is used in more aggressive or indistinct cases. Other approaches include radiation treatment, obliteration of the lesion by physical means, and administration of interferons or their activators. Once metastasis has occurred, treatment is generally multimodal, including surgery, radiation, and chemotherapy. Most people with nonmelanoma skin cancers have a much better chance of survival than those who present with melanoma. The prognosis for patients with either BCC or SCC is usually excellent, but if metastases develop in SCC cases, the individual has a less than 50% chance of surviving 5 years. The rarer skin cancers are associated with greater severity. Most skin cancers are associated with exposure to ultraviolet radiation, and there are available potential chemopreventive agents such as retinoids and COX-2 inhibitors.

### Immunosuppressant Drugs

| Drugs | Actions | Side effects |
|---|---|---|
| **Corticosteroids** | Depress cell-mediated immune response, humoral immune response, and inflammation, reducing proliferation of T cells and B cells. Used with transplantations and to prevent GVHD disease. | Weight gain, edema, Cushing syndrome, hyperglycemia, bruising, and osteoporosis. Abruptly stopping drugs may trigger Addisonian crisis. |
| **Ciclosporin** | Inhibit activation of T cells. Used to prevent transplantation rejection and to treat autoimmune diseases and nephrotic syndrome. | Tremor, excessive facial hair, gingivitis, bone marrow suppression with increased risk of infection and cancer, especially skin cancer. |
| **Intravenous immuno-globulin G (IVIG)** | Used to combat immunosuppression by increasing antibodies to prevent infection or treat acute infection, such as Guillain-Barre. Used off-label for many different disorders and infections. | Dermatitis, headache, renal failure, and venous thrombosis. Infections can occur because IVIG is extracted from pooled plasma. |

**Review Video: Immunomodulators and Immunosuppressors**
Visit mometrix.com/academy and enter code: 666131

### Chemotherapy

Chemotherapy may be offered during palliative care to enhance patient comfort, wellbeing, and symptom control for **enhanced quality of life**. It is understood that the treatment is not expected to provide a cure and should not be given as a means to maintain a sense of false hope within the patient or family. It should be clear that the expectation of treatment is **prolonged survival** and **control of cancer-related symptoms**. Not all patients will benefit from palliative chemotherapy. The decision to provide chemotherapy is based on the clinical indicators and the patient's wishes. The benefit and cost ratios of treatment need to be considered. Tumor response to treatment, metastasis, and other disease specific factors will help define chemotherapy's usefulness for an individual patient. Patients also need to be aware that chemotherapy involves a commitment to repeated travel, hospitalizations, invasive procedures, and assessments in order to make an informed decision.

### CHEMOTHERAPEUTIC AGENTS

The major chemotherapy agents are alkylating agents, antimetabolites, plant alkaloids, antitumor antibiotics, and steroid hormones.

- **Alkylating agents** work directly by attacking the DNA of cancers such as chronic leukemias, Hodgkin's disease, lymphomas, and lung, breast, prostate, and ovary cancers.
- **Nitrosoureas** inhibit repair in damaged DNA. They are able to cross the blood-brain barrier and are frequently used to treat brain tumors, lymphomas, multiple myeloma, and malignant melanoma.
- **Antimetabolites** block cell growth. This class of chemotherapeutic drugs is used to treat leukemias, choriocarcinoma, and gastrointestinal, breast, and ovary cancers.
- **Antitumor antibiotics** are a broad category of agents that bind to DNA and prevent RNA synthesis and are used with a wide variety of cancers.
- **Plant (vinca) alkaloids** are extracted from plants and block cell division. These are used to treat acute lymphoblastic leukemia, Hodgkin and non-Hodgkin lymphomas, neuroblastomas, Wilms tumor, and lung, breast, and testes cancers.
- **Steroid hormones** have an unclear action but may be useful in treating hormone-dependent cancers such as ovary and breast cancer.

### ROUTES OF DELIVERY

Chemotherapy treatments may be provided orally, intramuscularly, intravenously, intra-arterially, intralesionally (directly into the tumor), intraperitoneally, intrathecally, or topically. **Oral chemotherapy** is the easiest and often used in the home. **Intravenous delivery** is the most common chemotherapy route but **intramuscular delivery** may have more lasting effects. The goal of **intra-arterial chemotherapy** is to introduce the agent directly into the blood supply feeding the tumor or affected organ. Ovarian cancer with tumors greater than 2 cm in diameter may be treated with **intraperitoneal therapy**. Acute lymphocytic leukemia is primarily treated with **intrathecal administration**. **Intralesional treatments** are used for melanoma and Kaposi sarcoma. **Topical treatment** is most common with skin cancers.

### SIDE EFFECTS

Not every patient will experience every symptom, or in the same degree. **Side effects** can vary greatly; some can be easily controlled with additional medications. Many side effects are due to the effects of the chemotherapy on **cells**, such as bone marrow, hair, and gastrointestinal cells, which have a rapid mitotic rate and rapid turnover. Common side effects can include bone marrow suppression, hair loss (alopecia), mouth ulcers, sore throat and gums, heartburn, nausea, vomiting, loss of appetite, weight loss, anorexia and cachexia, anemia, nerve and muscle problems, dry or discolored skin, kidney and bladder irritation, fatigue, and increased bruising, bleeding, and infection. The patient's sexual function can also be affected, including possible infertility.

### RISKS

**Infection** is a common concern of chemotherapy because of the decreased number of **neutrophils** in the patient's system. **Neutropenia** is silent but dangerous, leaving no neutrophils to fight the threat of infections. Neutropenia can cause a septic situation, which can be life-threatening. Severe **anemia** may result in the need for blood transfusions. **Neurological damage** may include mild alterations in taste or smell, peripheral neuropathy, mental status changes, or seizures. Some anticancer drugs can cause **heart damage** if not monitored closely. Many anticancer drugs cause **kidney damage**, as well as increasing the risk of drug toxicity from decreased renal function. Anticancer drugs can also cause **cataracts** and **retina damage**.

## PALLIATIVE SEDATION

Palliative sedation is a treatment method focused on controlling and easing symptoms that have proven otherwise refractory or unendurable in nature. This process was originally named **terminal sedation**. It was changed to palliative sedation to emphasize the differences between symptom management and euthanasia.

The purpose of palliative sedation is **symptom control**; it does not hasten or cause death. Through the monitored use of medications such as midazolam or propofol, relief can be provided through varying levels of unconsciousness. Among terminally ill patients, palliative sedation is most often used to calm persistent agitation and restlessness. The second most frequent need is for pain control, followed by confusion, shortness of breath, muscle twitching or seizures, and anguish.

# Sepsis and Shock

## Range of Severe Infection

There are a number of terms used to refer to severe infections which are often used interchangeably. It is important to know these terms to properly perform the continuum of care.

- **Bacteremia** is the presence of bacteria in the blood without systemic infection.
- **Septicemia** is a systemic infection caused by pathogens (usually bacteria or fungi) present in the blood.
- **Systemic inflammatory response syndrome** (SIRS) is a generalized inflammatory response affecting many organ systems. It may be caused by infectious or non-infectious agents, such as trauma, burns, adrenal insufficiency, pulmonary embolism, and drug overdose. If an infectious agent is identified or suspected, SIRS is an aspect of sepsis. Infective agents include a wide range of bacteria and fungi, including *Streptococcus pneumoniae* and *Staphylococcus aureus.* SIRS includes 2 of the following:
  - Elevated (>38 °C) or subnormal rectal temperature (<36 °C)
  - Tachypnea or $PaCO_2$ <32 mmHg
  - Tachycardia
  - Leukocytosis (>12,000) or leukopenia (<4000)
- **Sepsis** is the presence of infection either locally or systemically in which there is a generalized life-threatening inflammatory response (SIRS). It includes all the indications for SIRS as well as one of the following:
  - Changes in mental status
  - Hypoxemia without preexisting pulmonary disease
  - Elevation in plasma lactate
  - Decreased urinary output <5 mL/kg/hr for ≥1 hour
- **Severe sepsis** includes both indications of SIRS and sepsis as well as indications of increasing organ dysfunction with inadequate perfusion and/or hypotension.
- **Septic shock** is a progression from severe sepsis in which refractory hypotension occurs despite treatment. There may be indications of lactic acidosis.
- **Multi-organ dysfunction syndrome** (MODS) is the most common cause of sepsis-related death. Cardiac function becomes depressed, acute respiratory distress syndrome (ARDS) may develop, and renal failure may follow acute tubular necrosis or cortical necrosis. Thrombocytopenia appears in about 30% of those affected and may result in disseminated intravascular coagulation (DIC). Liver damage and bowel necrosis may occur.

## Shock

There are a number of different types of shock, but there are general characteristics that they have in common. In all types of shock, there is a marked decrease in tissue perfusion related to hypotension, so that there is insufficient oxygen delivered to the tissues and inadequate removal of cellular waste products, causing injury to tissue:

- Hypotension (systolic below 90 mmHg); this may be somewhat higher (110 mmHg) in those who are initially hypertensive
- Decreased urinary output (<0.5 mL/kg/hr), especially marked in hypovolemic shock
- Metabolic acidosis
- Peripheral/cutaneous vasoconstriction/vasodilation resulting in cool, clammy skin
- Alterations in level of consciousness

**Types of shock** are as follows:

- **Distributive:** Preload decreased, CO increased, SVR decreased
- **Cardiogenic:** Preload increased, CO decreased, SVR increased
- **Hypovolemic:** Preload decreased, CO decreased, SVR increased

## Septic Shock

Septic shock is caused by toxins produced by bacteria and cytokines that the body produces in response to severe infection, resulting in a complex syndrome of disorders. **Symptoms** are wide-ranging:

- **Initial**: Hyper- or hypothermia, increased temperature (>38 °C) with chills, tachycardia with increased pulse pressure, tachypnea, alterations in mental status (dullness), hypotension, hyperventilation with respiratory alkalosis ($PaCO_2$ ≤30 mmHg), increased lactic acid, unstable BP, and dehydration with increased urinary output
- **Cardiovascular**: Myocardial depression and dysrhythmias
- **Respiratory**: Acute respiratory distress syndrome (ARDS)
- **Renal**: Acute kidney injury (AKI) with decreased urinary output and increased BUN
- **Hepatic**: Jaundice and liver dysfunction with an increase in transaminase, alkaline phosphatase, and bilirubin
- **Hematologic**: Mild or severe blood loss (from mucosal ulcerations), neutropenia or neutrophilia, decreased platelets, and DIC
- **Endocrine**: Hyperglycemia, hypoglycemia (rare)
- **Skin**: Cellulitis, erysipelas, and fasciitis, acrocyanotic and necrotic peripheral lesions

### *Diagnosis and Treatment*

Septic shock is most common in newborns, those >50, and those who are immunocompromised. There is no specific test to confirm a diagnosis of septic shock, so **diagnosis** is based on clinical findings and tests that evaluate hematologic, infectious, and metabolic states: Lactic acid, CBC, DIC panel, electrolytes, liver function tests, BUN, creatinine, blood glucose, ABGs, urinalysis, ECG, radiographs, blood and urine cultures.

**Treatment** must be aggressive and includes:

- Oxygen and endotracheal intubation as necessary
- IV access with 2-large bore catheters and central venous line
- Rapid fluid administration at 0.5L NS or isotonic crystalloid every 5-10 minutes as needed (to 4-6 L)
- Monitoring urinary output to optimal >30 mL/hr (>0.5-1 mL/kg/hr)
- Inotropic or vasoconstrictive agents (dopamine, dobutamine, norepinephrine) if no response to fluids or fluid overload
- Empiric IV antibiotic therapy (usually with 2 broad spectrum antibiotics for both gram-positive and gram-negative bacteria) until cultures return and antibiotics may be changed
- Hemodynamic and laboratory monitoring
- Removing source of infection (abscess, catheter)

## Distributive Shock

Distributive shock occurs with adequate blood volume but inadequate intravascular volume because of arterial/venous dilation that results in decreased vascular tone and hypoperfusion of internal organs. Cardiac output may be normal or blood may pool, decreasing cardiac output. **Distributive shock** may result from anaphylactic shock, septic shock, neurogenic shock, and drug ingestions.

**Symptoms** include:

- Hypotension (systolic <90 mmHg or <40 mmHg below normal), tachypnea, tachycardia (>90) (may be lower if patient receiving β-blockers)
- Hypoxemia
- Skin initially warm, later hypoperfused
- Hyper- or hypothermia (>38 °C or <36 °C)
- Alterations in mentation
- Decreased urinary output
- Symptoms related to underlying cause

**Treatment** includes:

- Treating underlying cause while stabilizing hemodynamics
- Oxygen with endotracheal intubation if necessary
- Rapid fluid administration at 0.25-0.5 L NS or isotonic crystalloid every 5-10 minutes as needed to 2-3 L
- Vasoconstrictive and inotropic agents (dopamine, dobutamine, norepinephrine) if necessary, for patients with profound hypotension

## Neurogenic Shock

Neurogenic shock is a type of distributive shock that occurs when injury to the CNS from trauma resulting in acute spinal cord injury (from both blunt and penetrating injuries), neurological diseases, drugs, or anesthesia, impairs the autonomic nervous system that controls the cardiovascular system. The degree of symptoms relates to the level of injury with injuries above T1 capable of causing disruption of the entire sympathetic nervous system and lower injuries causing various degrees of disruption. Even incomplete spinal cord injury can cause neurogenic shock.

**Symptoms** include:

- Hypotension and warm dry skin related to lack of vascular tone that results in hypothermia from loss of cutaneous heat
- Bradycardia (common but not universal)

**Treatment** includes:

- ABCDE (airway, breathing, circulation, disability evaluation, exposure)
- Rapid fluid administration with crystalloid to keep mean arterial pressure at 85-90 mmHg
- Placement of pulmonary artery catheter to monitor fluid overload
- Inotropic agents (dopamine, dobutamine) if fluids don't correct hypotension
- Atropine for persistent bradycardia

## Hypovolemic Shock/Volume Deficit

Hypovolemic shock occurs when there is inadequate intravascular fluid. The loss may be *absolute* because of an internal shifting of fluid or an external loss of fluid, as occurs with massive hemorrhage, thermal injuries, severe vomiting or diarrhea, and internal injuries (such as ruptured spleen or dissecting arteries) that interfere with intravascular integrity. Hypovolemia may also be *relative* and related to vasodilation, increased capillary membrane permeability from sepsis or injuries, and decreased colloidal osmotic pressure that may occur with loss of sodium and some disorders, such as hypopituitarism and cirrhosis.

Hypovolemic shock is **classified** according to the degree of fluid loss:

- **Class I:** <750 mL or ≤15% of total circulating volume (TCV)
- **Class II:** 750-1500 mL or 15-30% of TCV
- **Class III:** 1500-2000 mL or 30-40% of TCV
- **Class IV:** >2000 mL or >40% of TCV

### *Symptoms and Treatment*

Hypovolemic shock occurs when the total circulating volume of fluid decreases, leading to a fall in venous return that in turn causes a decrease in ventricular filling and preload, indicated by ↓ in right atrial pressure (RAP) and pulmonary artery occlusion pressure (PAOP). This results in a decrease in stroke volume and cardiac output. This in turn causes generalized arterial vasoconstriction, increasing afterload (↑ systemic vascular resistance), causing decreased tissue perfusion.

**Symptoms**: Anxiety, pallor, cool and clammy skin, delayed capillary refill, cyanosis, hypotension, increasing respirations, weak, thready pulse.

**Treatment** is aimed at identifying and treating the cause:

- Administration of blood, blood products, autotransfusion, colloids (such as plasma protein fraction), and/or crystalloids (such as normal saline)
- Oxygen—intubation and ventilation may be necessary
- Medications may include vasopressors, such as dopamine. **Note: Fluids must be given before starting vasopressors**!

## Anaphylactic Shock

Anaphylactic reaction or anaphylactic shock may present with a few symptoms or a wide range of potentially lethal effects.

**Symptoms** may recur after the initial treatment (biphasic anaphylaxis), so careful monitoring is essential:

- Sudden onset of weakness, dizziness, confusion
- Severe generalized edema and angioedema; lips and tongue may swell
- Urticaria
- Increased permeability of vascular system and loss of vascular tone leading to severe hypotension and shock
- Laryngospasm/bronchospasm with obstruction of airway causing dyspnea and wheezing
- Nausea, vomiting, and diarrhea
- Seizures, coma, and death

**Treatments**:

- Establish patent airway and intubate if necessary, for ventilation
- Provide oxygen at 100% high flow
- Monitor VS
- Administer epinephrine (Epi-pen or solution)
- Albuterol per nebulizer for bronchospasm
- Intravenous fluids to provide bolus of fluids for hypotension
- Diphenhydramine if shock persists
- Methylprednisolone if no response to other drugs

# Multisystem Procedures and Interventions

## Multisystem Trauma-Treatment Prioritization Guidelines

In order to give the trauma patient the best chance at survival, treatment must be appropriately **prioritized** and managed. Immediate priority should be given to maintaining the airway and ensuring adequate ventilation. Pre-hospital management should also include control of bleeding, prevention of shock, spine immobilization, and neurological assessment. Upon arrival to the closest trauma center, the primary survey conducted by the healthcare trauma team is centered on determining which injuries are potentially life-threatening. The airway is the number one priority, followed by an assessment of hemodynamic status (assess for hypovolemia) and core body temperature (assess for hypothermia). Baseline data is also collected, including laboratory studies, EKG, and radiologic testing. Treatment may include fluid resuscitation, the administration of blood products, and surgical intervention (if indicated). Complications of multisystem trauma include disseminated intravascular coagulopathy, acute respiratory distress syndrome, renal failure, infection, compartment syndrome, dysrhythmias, and sepsis.

## Thermoregulation in Critically Ill Patients

The hypothalamus, limbic system, lower brainstem, reticular formation, spinal cord, and sympathetic ganglia all play a role in the regulation of core temperature. The normal core body temperature of 35.5-37.5 °C is a narrow range which is frequently disrupted in the critically ill patient. **Impaired thermoregulation** can occur in patients with sepsis, brain or spinal cord trauma, stroke, and tumors of the central nervous system. Mild hypothermia is common during deep sedation. Hypothermia (core temperature of <35 °C) is associated with an increased risk of postoperative wound infections, blood loss, and adverse cardiovascular events. Hypothermia may occur in trauma patients, patients with sepsis, postoperative patients, and patients with severe burns. Hyperthermia (core temperature of >38 °C) may occur in systemic inflammatory response syndrome, malignant hyperthermia, heatstroke, neuroleptic malignant syndrome, and serotonin syndrome. Hyperpyrexia occurs when the core temperature exceeds 40 °C. Core temperatures exceeding 41.5 °C may be life-threatening.

## Targeted Temperature Management

Targeted temperature management (previously referred to as therapeutic hypothermia) is used to reduce ischemic tissue damage associated with cardiac arrest, ischemic stroke, traumatic brain/spinal cord injury, neurogenic fever, and subsequent coma (3 on Glasgow scale). Reducing the body's temperature to below normal range has a neuroprotective effect by making cell membranes less permeable, thus reducing neurologic edema and damage. Hypothermia should be initiated immediately after an ischemic event if possible, but some benefit remains up to 6 hours. Hypothermia to 33 °C may be induced by cooled saline through a femoral catheter, reducing temperature 1.5-2.0 °C/hr by an electronic control unit. Hypothermic water blankets covering ≥80% of the body's surface can also lower body temperature. In some cases, both a femoral cooling catheter and a water blanket are used for rapid reduction of temperature. Rectal probes are used to measure core temperature, but Foley temperature catheters are more common. Desflurane or meperidine is given to reduce the shivering response. Hypothermia increases risk of bleeding (decreased clotting time), infection (due to impairing leukocyte function and introducing catheters), arrhythmias, hyperglycemia, and DVT. Rewarming is done slowly at 0.5-1.0 °C/hr. through warmed intravenous fluids, warm humidified air, and/or warming blanket. The warming process is a critical time, as it causes potassium to be moved from extracellular to intracellular spaces and the patient's electrolyte levels must be monitored regularly.

## Continuous Temperature Monitoring

Continuous temperature monitoring may be carried out through various means:

- Pulmonary artery catheter (most accurate but generally not recommended because of invasiveness and potential for complications)
- Rectal or Foley temperature probes
- Skin probes

- Wearable Bluetooth monitors (patch applied to the skin), which transmit information to an external monitor or the patient's electronic health record. (For external temperature monitoring, the device must be applied properly and for the correct duration of time [e.g., the TempTraQ wearable patch is applied in the underarm area and measures temperature for 72 hours].)

**Indications** for continuous temperature monitoring include:

- Skin flap transplantation—to assess perfusion
- Brain injury—to assess thermoregulation
- Therapeutic hypothermia—for cardiac arrest or post-cardiac surgery
- Malignant hyperthermia
- Immunocompromised patients—to assess for signs of infection
- Critically ill patients—at risk for temperature dysregulation

## PERMISSIVE HYPOTENSION

Permissive hypotension procedures allow the systolic blood pressure to fall low enough to prevent or control hemorrhage while still high enough to maintain perfusion. With trauma patients, this means restricting fluid resuscitation when active bleeding is occurring. While protocols vary, permissive hypotension usually includes systolic blood pressure no higher than 80 mmHg, although this may vary. For example, permissive hypotension with systolic blood pressure maintained at 80-100 mmHg may be indicated when massive transfusion protocols are activated. Permissive hypotension helps decrease some of the adverse effects associated with rapid and high-dose fluid resuscitation (emboli, coagulopathy, and hypothermia). However, the patient does remain at risk of hypoperfusion and must be monitored carefully. Permissive hypotension is generally contraindicated with brain or spinal cord injury, although studies are ongoing (and mostly conducted with animals) and some controversy remains about the use of permissive hypotension.

## SEDATION

### *MINIMAL SEDATION*

Minimal sedation includes local/topical anesthesia, peripheral nerve blocks, administration of <50% nitrogen oxide in oxygen by itself, or administration of one sedative or analgesic medication in a dosage that does not typically require supervision. The patient should be fully aware, able to respond appropriately to verbal and tactile stimulation, and able to maintain an airway independently, as these medications should not have cardiovascular or respiratory effects. The purpose of minimal sedation is to decrease perception of pain, relax the patient, and reduce fear. The patient's level of consciousness, sedation, and pain should be monitored throughout the procedure to ensure the dosage is adequate and the patient is not excessively sedated. Medications may include benzodiazepines (diazepam, lorazepam) and opioids (fentanyl, morphine, meperidine). Reversal agents (flumazenil, naloxone) should be available. Minimal sedation is often used during labor and delivery and for minor procedures, such as skin biopsies and removal of skin lesions.

### *CONTINUOUS VS. INTERMITTENT SEDATION*

Sedation for critically ill patients may include:

- **Intermittent sedation** is that administered through IV push, so the expected duration is relatively short. Typical agents include benzodiazepines and opioids. Intermittent sedation is most often used for endoscopic procedures but is also sometimes used for patients who are on mechanical ventilation, especially if they have regular trials of weaning. Also, intermittent sedation is less likely to result in oversedation.
- **Continuous sedation** is that administered through a steady intravenous infusion to ensure longer-lasting sedation. Typical agents include opioids, midazolam, and propofol. Continuous sedation is more commonly used for patients on mechanical ventilation because it requires less intervention and maintains a steady blood level. Daily interruptions of continuous sedation may be carried out as a trial for weaning patients on mechanical ventilation.

With both intermittent sedation and continuous sedation, the patient's vital signs, respiratory status, temperature, and oxygen saturation should be monitored. Arousal scales (Richmond or Riker Agitation/Sedation Scales) should be utilized to assess arousal and to adjust sedation dosages.

### *Neuromuscular Blockade Agents*

Neuromuscular blocker agents are used for induced paralysis of those who have not responded adequately to sedation, especially for intubation and mechanical ventilation. NMBAs do not produce unconsciousness, amnesia, or analgesia, therefore it is critical that they are administered *after* the patient has been adequately sedated. NMBAs include:

- **Depolarizing agents**: Succinylcholine. Risk for severe hyperkalemia after denervation injury persists for 7-10 days. Post-operative myalgia is common, and succinylcholine may trigger malignant hyperthermia and severe anaphylactic/anaphylactoid reactions.
- **Non-depolarizing agents**: Short-acting (mivacurium, rapacuronium), intermediate-acting (rocuronium, vecuronium, atracurium, cisatracurium), and long-acting (pancuronium, doxacurium, pipecuronium). Should be given for ≤2 days for those on ventilators because they may develop persistent quadriparesis. Most are not associated with malignant hyperthermia.

Eye lubricant should be applied every 2 hours and the eyes kept closed. Range of motion exercises should not extend beyond normal range because of the potential to damage joints. The patient must be repositioned frequently while paralyzed and on an adequate support surface. Pupil reactivity should be assessed every 1-4 hours to evaluate neurological status. Temperature should be monitored hourly if <36 °C or if placed under a cooling blanket because heat production is depressed. After cessation, the patient should be closely monitored to ensure that muscle function has returned to normal.

**Review Video: Muscle Relaxants**
Visit mometrix.com/academy and enter code: 862193

### *Moderate (Conscious) Sedation*

The ASA sedation guidelines (2018) are intended for **moderate (conscious) sedation** used for procedures, such as colonoscopy. Steps include:

- **Pre-procedure evaluation**: Includes review of health records, physical examination and laboratory testing as indicated a few days or weeks prior to the procedure, and re-evaluating the patient again before the procedure.
- **Patient preparation**: Consult with a specialist if indicated, ensure the patient has informed consent and has been compliant with pre-procedure fasting, and insert intravenous line.
- **Patient monitoring**: LOC (every 5 minutes), oxygenation/ventilation (capnography, pulse oximetry), and hemodynamic with a designated person responsible for monitoring and recording.
- **Supplemental oxygen:** Use unless contraindicated by condition.
- **Emergency interventions**: Resuscitative equipment and reversal agents for opioids (naloxone) and benzodiazepines (Romazicon) must be present with a person trained in assessment and use available.
- **Sedatives**: Analgesics (opioids) and combinations of drugs as appropriate may be used (benzodiazepines and dexmedetomidine).
- **Sedative (propofol, ketamine, etomidate) and analgesics (local anesthetics, NSAIDs, and opioids) intended for general anesthesia**: Care must be consistent with that of general anesthesia and IV medications administered incrementally.
- **Recovery care**: Monitor oxygenation, ventilation, and circulation every 5-15 minutes.

### *Sedation Using Propofol*

Sedation used for a drug-induced coma often includes **propofol**. Propofol is an IV non-opioid hypnotic anesthetic, the most common used for induction. It is also used for maintenance and postoperative sedation.

Onset of action is rapid because of high lipid solubility, and propofol has a short distribution half-life and rapid clearance, so recovery is also fast. Propofol is metabolized by the liver, as well as through the lungs. Propofol decreases cerebral blood flow, metabolic rate of oxygen consumption, and ICP. Propofol causes vasodilation with resultant hypotension, but with bradycardia rather than tachycardia. Propofol is a respiratory depressant, resulting in apnea after induction and decreased tidal volume, respiratory rate, and hypoxic drive during maintenance. Propofol has antiemetic properties as well but does not produce analgesia.

### *Delayed Emergence*

Delayed emergence (failure to emerge for 30-60 minutes after anesthesia ends) is more common in the elderly because of slowed metabolism of anesthetic agents but may have a variety of causes, such as drug overdose during surgery, overdose related to preinduction use of drugs or alcohol that potentiates intraoperative drugs. In this case, naloxone or flumazenil may be indicated if opioids or benzodiazepines are implicated. Physostigmine may also be used to reverse effects of some anesthetic agents. Hypothermia may also cause delay in emergence, especially core temperatures <33 °C, and may require forced-air warming blankets to increase the temperature. Other metabolic conditions, such as hypoglycemia or hyperglycemia, may also affect emergence. Patients suffering from delayed emergence must be evaluated for perioperative stroke, especially after neurological, cardiovascular, or cerebrovascular surgery. Metabolic disturbance may also delay emergence.

## Postanesthetic Respiratory Complications

Postoperative respiratory complications are most common in the postanesthesia period, so monitoring of oxygen levels is critical to preventing hypoxemia:

- **Airway obstruction** may be partial or total. Partial obstruction is indicated by sonorous or wheezing respirations, and total by absence of breath sounds. Treatment includes supplemental oxygen, airway insertion, repositioning (jaw thrust), or succinylcholine and positive-pressure ventilation for laryngospasm. If edema of the glottis is causing obstruction, IV corticosteroids may be used.
- **Hypoventilation** ($PaCO_2$ >45 mmHg) is often mild but may cause respiratory acidosis. It is usually related to depression caused by anesthetic agents. A number of factors may slow emergence (hypothermia, overdose, metabolism) and cause hypoventilation. It may also be related to splinting because of pain, requiring additional pain management.
- **Hypoxemia** (mild is $PaO_2$ 50-60 mmHg) is usually related to hypoventilation and/or increased right to left shunting and is usually treated with supplementary oxygen (30-60%) with or without positive airway pressure.

## Postanesthetic Cardiovascular Complications

Cardiovascular complications after surgery are sometimes related to respiratory complications, which may need to be addressed as well. Complications include:

- **Hypotension** is most often mild and requires no specific treatment. It is most commonly caused by hypovolemia and is significant if BP falls 20-30% below the normal baseline. A bolus (100-250 mL IV colloid) is used to confirm hypovolemia. If severe, then medications such as vasopressors may be indicated. Hypotension may occur with pneumothorax, so careful respiratory assessment must be done.
- **Hypertension** usually occurs ≤30 minutes after surgery and is common in those with a history of hypertension. It may be secondary to hypoxemia or metabolic acidosis. Mild increases usually don't require treatment but medications may be used for moderate (β-adrenergic blockers) or severe (nitroprusside) increases.
- **Arrhythmias** usually relate to respiratory complications or effects of anesthetic agents. Bradycardia may relate to cholinesterase inhibitors, opioids, or propranolol. Tachycardia may relate to anticholinergics, β-agonists, and vagolytic drugs. Hypokalemia and hypomagnesemia may cause premature atrial and ventricular beats.

# Musculoskeletal and Wound Emergencies

## Musculoskeletal Assessment

### Assessing Risk of Falling

Many factors must be examined and combined to determine the **fall risk** status of a patient. They include age, sensory deficits, mobility problems, neurological disorders, past history of falling, cognitive impairment, and depression. Some medications, such as those associated with postural hypotension and psychotropic medications, may increase the danger of falls. The presence of dizziness, acute or chronic illness, poor physical status, elimination requirements, medications, and environmental concerns contribute to the risk for falls.

Multiple factors increase risk, so careful history and physical exam are necessary as part of assessment. When the presence of risk factors shows a risk for falls, this information should be communicated to other caregivers by wristband, colored markers on doors, care plans, or other effective means. The factors are then modified as much as possible. The patient should be re-evaluated as their condition changes or after a fall to determine the cause.

**Review Video: Muscular System**
Visit mometrix.com/academy and enter code: 967216

**Review Video: Skeletal System**
Visit mometrix.com/academy and enter code: 256447

### Assessing Patients with Disabilities

A patient with **disabilities** may find it very difficult to obtain screening for health problems due to inaccessibility:

- Work with the patient to resolve barriers to obtain weight, mammography, bone density tests, and pap/pelvic exams on a regular basis.
- Ask how to best assist the patient during the assessment.
- Observe the patient carefully for nonverbal communication, such as grimacing.
- If sensation is affected, warn the patient before touching any part of the body.
- Always address all areas of the patient's history, including sexual history.
- Use an interpreter that is not a family member if needed.
- Give the patient extra time to respond to questions when there is aphasia or other communication problems.
- Address the impact of the disability on the ability to perform ADLs, health status in general, access to healthcare, financial status, emotional status, work, community roles, and family wellbeing.

### Assessment to Establish Mechanism of Injury

Assessment to establish the mechanism of injury for an injury to the musculoskeletal system includes:

- **Question/Listen**: Reports from the patient (if responsive and cognitively aware), family or friends, and first responders often can establish how, when, and where an injury occurred. Police reports may be available in some cases. The trauma nurse should ask questions to clarify any information provided.
- **Observation**: The patient's general appearance (clean, soiled, unkempt, well-dressed, sporting clothes/uniform), obvious injuries (bruises, swelling, and bleeding), and odor (fruity, alcohol, urine, feces) may provide clues as to the mechanism of injury or the patient's general health and living situation.

- **Physical examination**: The trauma nurse should look for typical patterns of injury associated with different mechanisms of injury. For example, a fall from a height may result in fractures of both feet and back injuries. Hip and wrist fractures are common with falls. Blistering, redness, and sloughing of tissue may suggest burns.

## FAST Assessment

**Focused abdominal sonography for trauma (FAST)** assessment is a non-invasive ultrasound procedure that is part of the ATLS protocol for assessment of trauma and is generally now used in place of peritoneal lavage to detect free fluid (generally blood). FAST is about 85% to 90% effective in diagnosing intraperitoneal bleeding (usually associated with hepatic or splenic injury) as well as pneumo- and hemothorax (can detect as small a volume as 20 mL, depending on the sonographer's skill), and pericardial effusion associated with blunt or penetrating cardiac trauma. FAST may help to prioritize treatment when a patient presents with multiple penetrating injuries (especially involving inferior chest and superior abdomen). However, FAST is less effective in identifying bowel injuries. In some cases where a patient's condition is not clear, observation and a series of FAST assessments may help to identify problems, such as a slow bleed.

# Musculoskeletal Pathophysiology

## Carpal Tunnel Syndrome

Carpal tunnel syndrome is a type of entrapment neuropathy in which the median nerve is compressed by thickening of the flexor tendon sheath, skeletal encroachment, or mass in the soft tissue. Carpal tunnel syndrome is often associated with repetitive hand activities, arthritis, hypothyroidism, diabetes, and pregnancy. Patients complain of pain in wrist, radiating to forearm, and numbness and tingling in the first 2 to 3 fingers, especially during the night.

**Diagnosis** is based on symptoms and tests such as:

- **Positive Tinel test**: Gentle percussion over medial nerve in inner aspect of wrist elicits numbness and pain.
- **Positive Phalen test**: The backs of the hands are pressed together and the wrists sharply flexed for 1 minute to elicit pain and numbness.

**Treatment** includes identifying and treating the underlying cause:

- Steroid injection may relieve symptoms
- Splint during the night or during repetitive activities
- Modification of activities
- Referral for decompression surgery in recalcitrant cases or those with severe loss of sensation

## Infectious Arthritis

Infectious arthritis may be bacterial, viral (rubella, parvovirus, and hepatitis B), parasitic, or fungal, with bacterial arthritis causing the most rapid destruction to the joint. *Neisseria gonorrhoeae* (most common), *Staphylococcus*, *Streptococcus*, and *Escherichia coli* are the most common bacterial agents. The infection may be bloodborne or spread from an infection near the joint or from direct implantation or postoperative contamination of the wound. Usually, the infection involves just one joint.

**Symptoms** include acute edema, erythema, and pain in a joint. Systemic reactions, such as fever and polyarthralgia, may occur, especially with gonorrhea.

**Diagnosis** requires a complete history and physical examination, arthrocentesis and synovial fluid culture, and WBC.

**Treatment** includes:

- Antibiotics as indicated by organism
- Arthrocentesis to drain fluid accumulation in joint (may need to be repeated)
- Analgesia

## Bursitis and Tendinitis

**Bursitis** is inflammation of the bursa, fluid-filled spaces or sacs that form in tissues to reduce friction, causing thickening of the lining of the bursal walls. This can be the result of infection, trauma, crystal deposits, or chronic friction from trauma.

**Tendinitis** is inflammation of the long, tubular tendons and tendon sheaths adjacent to the bursa. Causes of tendinitis are similar to bursitis but tendinitis may also be caused by quinolone antibiotics. Frequently, both bursa and tendons are inflamed. Common types of bursitis include shoulder, olecranon (elbow), trochanteric (hip), and prepatellar (front of knee). Common types of tendinitis include wrist, Achilles, patellar, and rotator cuff.

**Symptoms** include pain with movement, edema, dysfunction, and decreased range of motion.

**Diagnosis** is by clinical examination, although x-rays may rule out fractures. The bursa may be aspirated diagnostically to aid in ruling out other diagnosis, like gout or infection.

**Treatment** for bursitis and tendinitis includes:

- Rest and immobilization
- NSAIDs
- Application of cold packs to affected area
- Steroid injections

## Joint Effusion and Arthrocentesis

Joint effusion is the accumulation of fluid (clear, bloody, or purulent) within a joint capsule. Joint effusion can cause pressure on the joint and severe pain. Arthrocentesis relieves the pressure and the fluid aspirated can be examined to aid in diagnosis. Arthrocentesis is usually contraindicated in the presence of overlying infection, prosthetic joint, and coagulopathy without referral to an orthopedic specialist.

**Procedure**:

1. Patient is **positioned** according to joint to be aspirated and encouraged to relax muscles.
2. **Overlying area** is cleansed with povidone-iodine solution, air-dried a few minutes, and cleansed of iodine with alcohol wipe.
3. **Local anesthetic** is given to the area (but not into the joint) with 25- to 30-gauge needle (lidocaine 1-2%) or a regional nerve block for severe pain.
4. The joint is **aspirated** with insertion in a straight line, using a 30-60 mL syringe (depending upon expected amount of fluid) and an 18- to 22-gauge needle or IV catheter.
5. The joint is completely **drained** of fluid.
6. Observe for **complications**: bleeding, infection, or allergic reaction.

## Lumbosacral Pain

Lumbosacral (low back) pain may be related to strain, muscular weakness, osteoarthritis, spinal stenosis, herniated disks, vertebral fractures, bony metastasis, infection, or other musculoskeletal disorders. Disk herniation or other joint changes put pressure on nerves leaving the spinal cord, causing pain to radiate along the nerve. Pain may be acute or chronic (more than 3 months).

**Symptoms** include local or pain radiating down the leg (radiculopathy), impaired gait and reflexes, difference in leg lengths, decreased motor strength, and alteration of sensation, including numbness.

**Diagnosis** is by careful clinical examination and history as well as x-ray (fractures, scoliosis, dislocations), CT (identifies underlying problems), MRI (spinal pathology), and/or EMG and nerve conduction studies. Diagnostic studies may be deferred in many cases for 4-6 weeks as symptoms may resolve over time. **Treatments** for nonspecific back pain include:

- Analgesia: acetaminophen, NSAIDS, opiates
- Encourage activity to tolerance but not bed rest
- Muscle relaxants: diazepam 5-10 mg every 6-8 hours
- Cold and heat compresses

## Strains and Sprains

A **strain** is an overstretching of a part of the musculature ("pulled muscle") that causes microscopic tears in the muscle, usually resulting from excess stress or overuse of the muscle. Onset of pain is usually sudden with local tenderness on use of the muscle. A **sprain** is damage to a joint, with a partial rupture of the supporting ligaments, usually caused by wrenching or twisting that may occur with a fall. The rupture can damage blood vessels, resulting in edema, tenderness at the joint, and pain on movement with pain increasing over 2-3 hours after injury. An avulsion fracture (bone fragment pulled away by a ligament) may occur with strain, so x-rays rule out fractures.

**Treatment** for both strains and sprains includes:

- **RICE protocol**: rest, ice, compression, and elevation
- **Ice compresses** (wet or dry) applied 20-30 minutes intermittently for 48 hours and then intermittent heat 15-20 minutes 3-4 times daily
- Monitor **neurovascular status** (especially for sprain)
- **Immobilization** as indicated for sprains for 1-3 weeks

## High Energy Joint Injuries

Low energy injuries include those that occur as a result of a fall from standing position or less than one-meter height, but **high energy injuries** include those with greater impact, such as from an automobile accident, fall from greater height, and sports accidents (downhill skiing, ice hockey) as well as gunshot wounds, stab wounds, and blast injuries. High energy injuries are likely to be more severe and may include:

- Fractures, both open and closed
- Compression fractures
- Dislocations and fracture-dislocations
- Comminution
- Strains and sprains, injury to ligaments and tendons
- Lacerations, bleeding
- Soft tissue trauma, edema, and ecchymosis
- Shock

Patients typically have severe pain, and the affected joint may be very unstable with obvious misalignment if fractures or dislocations are present. Older adults are particularly at risk for fractures because of osteoporosis, and healing may be impaired because of chronic disease. With high energy injuries, patients also have greater risk of complications, such as fat embolism, hemorrhage, pulmonary embolism, compartment syndrome, infection, neurological damage, avascular necrosis, and mal-union, delayed union, or non-union.

## Fractures and Dislocations

### *Types of Fractures*

Fractures and dislocations usually occur as the result of trauma, such as from falls and auto accidents, but *pathologic* fractures can result from minor force to diseased bones such as those with osteoporosis or metastatic lesions. *Stress* fractures are caused by repetitive trauma, such as from forced marching. *Salter* fractures involve the cartilaginous epiphyseal plate near the ends of long bones in children who are growing. Damage to this area can impair bone growth. Orthopedic injuries that are of special concern include:

- **Open fractures** with soft tissue injury overlying the fracture, including puncture wounds from external forces or bone fragments, can result in osteomyelitis.
- **Subluxation, partial dislocation of a joint, and luxation** (complete dislocation) can cause neurovascular compromise, which can be permanent if reduction is delayed. Dislocation of the hip can result in avascular necrosis of the femoral head.

### *Diagnosis and Treatment*

Fractures and dislocations are commonly **diagnosed** by clinical examination, history, and radiographs. Careful inspection and observation of range of motion, palpation, and observation of abnormalities is important because pain may be referred. Neurovascular assessment should be done immediately to prevent vascular compromise. Radiographs should usually precede reduction of dislocations to ensure there are no fractures and follow reduction to ensure the dislocation is reduced.

**Treatment** includes:

- Analgesia and sedation as indicated
- Application of cold compresses and elevation of fractured area to reduce edema
- Reduction of fracture: steady and gradual longitudinal traction to realign bone
- Immobilization with brace, cast, sling, or splint indicated
- Reduction of dislocation: Varies according to area of dislocation
- Open fracture: Wound irrigation with NS
- Tetanus prophylaxis
- Antibiotic prophylaxis
- Referral to orthopedic specialist for open fractures, irreducible dislocations, and complications such as compartment syndrome or circulatory impairment

### *Pelvic Fractures*

Pelvic fractures may be fairly benign or seriously life threatening, depending on the degree and type of fracture. They most often result from high-speed trauma related to vehicular accidents or skiing accidents:

- **Open book**: Pelvis is pulled apart, usually from frontal injury (may cause severe hemorrhage)
- **Closed book**: Lateral compression occurs from side injury
- **Vertical shear**: Injury occurs from fall

Indications of pelvic fracture include localized edema, tenderness, obvious pelvic deformity, abnormal pelvic movement, and abdominal bruising. Associated intra-abdominal injuries and complications are common, including paralytic ileus, hemorrhage, urethral, colon, or bladder laceration. Patients may develop sepsis, peritonitis, fat embolism syndrome, or DVT. Displaced fractures may require open reduction and internal fixation. Treatment usually includes bedrest (up to 6 weeks) with care in handling to prevent further injury. Patients should be turned and moved in accordance with specific physician's orders. Ambulation using walker or crutches may be allowed for non-displaced fractures.

### *Acetabular Fractures*

Acetabular (hip-socket) fractures occur primarily in young adults with motor vehicle accidents or falls from a height, resulting in impact pressure from the head of the femur to the joint and frequently associated (up to 50% of cases) with other severe injuries, including dislocation (which can lead to avascular necrosis if not promptly reduced). Up to 20% of those with acetabular fractures also have pelvic fractures. The degree of displacement that occurs depends on the amount of force as well as the position of the femur during impact. Acetabular fracture may be classified as posterior-wall, posterior-column, anterior-column, or transverse. Acetabular fractures in children less than 12 years may result in growth arrest. Complications may include sepsis, chondrolysis, and injury to vessels and/or nerves. Post-traumatic arthritis of the joint may develop. **Diagnosis** is per examination, radiograph, and/or CT with Doppler ultrasound with suspected DVT. Treatment includes emergent closed reduction if necessary, longitudinal skeletal traction, and open reduction and internal fixation (ORIF) for displaced fractures and serious injury (usually delayed for 2-3 days because of initial bleeding).

### *Closed Fractures and Open Fractures*

**Closed fractures** are those in which the damage to the bone and tissue (bleeding, swelling) remains enclosed within intact skin and does not invade any internal cavity. The bone segments are more likely to be aligned, although some comminution may have occurred from splintering when the bone breaks. It may be difficult to differentiate a closed fracture from an open fracture if there are abrasions and lacerations over the area of the fractures, but it is closed if there is no continuity between the fracture and the external injury.

**Open fractures**, on the other hand, cause an external wound and may result from fragments of the fractured bone penetrating the skin or an external force penetrating the skin and bone. Open fractures may also appear closed on the surface but invade a body cavity. Open fractures carry a much higher risk of contamination and infection as well as severe bleeding. The external wounds associated with open fractures may vary in size, but even small wounds are considered emergent because of risk of infection.

### *Fat Embolism as Complication of Traumatic Fracture*

In instances of **traumatic fracture**, the possibility of **fat embolism** should be considered; this is especially true in fractures involving the long bones (femur, humerus). When the bone is fractured, this allows for some of the fatty marrow contained within the bone to escape. Because the fracture and subsequent trauma to the area surrounding the fracture results in broken vessels, it is possible that the fatty marrow can be introduced into the bloodstream. When this happens, the events are similar to that of a deep venous thrombosis; the fat embolus dislodges from the lumen of the vessel and travels to the lung. When the embolus enters the pulmonary circulation, it eventually blocks blood flow as the caliber of the vessel through which it travels decreases, keeping blood from flowing to the lung tissue. The disruption in blood flow results in inflammation and necrosis of the lung, and eventually pulmonary failure ensues.

## Osteomyelitis

**Musculoskeletal infections** encompass a variety of different disorders with differing pathologies. Osteomyelitis, cellulitis, and septic arthritis are examples of musculoskeletal infections that can be both serious and debilitating in nature.

**Osteomyelitis** is an infection of the bone that can occur from an open fracture or an infection that has occurred somewhere else in the body. Osteomyelitis can also be caused by wounds or soft tissue infections that have progressed and extended to the bone. Signs and symptoms of osteomyelitis include pain, swelling, erythema and possible drainage at the site. The patient may also experience fever and chills. Diagnosis includes lab work including a complete blood count, erythrocyte sedimentation rate (ESR), C-reactive protein (CRP), and blood cultures, as well as radiologic testing that may include CT, MRI, x-ray, bone scan, or a bone biopsy. Treatment includes the administration of IV antibiotics. A needle aspiration may be performed to determine the organism and drain the area. Surgical irrigation and debridement may also be indicated.

## Compartment Syndrome

Compartment syndrome occurs when there is an increase in the amount of pressure within a grouping of muscles, nerves, and blood vessels resulting in compromised blood flow to muscles and nerves. This is a medical emergency. If left untreated, tissue ischemia and eventual tissue death will occur. **Compartment syndrome** most often occurs after a fracture, particularly a long bone fracture, but can also occur with crushing syndrome and rhabdomyolysis. Risk factors include lower extremity trauma, massive tissue injury, venous obstruction, the use of certain medications (anticoagulants), burns and compressive dressings or casts. Compartment syndrome can affect the hand, forearm, upper arm, abdomen, and lower extremities. It can be acute or chronic in nature with acute compartment syndrome requiring immediate intervention.

**Signs and symptoms**: Intense pain, decreased sensation and paresthesia, firmness at the affected site, swelling and tightness at the affected site, pallor and pulselessness (late signs).

**Diagnosis**: Physical assessment and the measurement of intra-compartmental pressures.

**Treatment**: The goal of treatment in compartment syndrome is decompression and the restoration of perfusion to the affected area. Surgical fasciotomy is often indicated to relieve pressure and prevent tissue death. Fasciotomy involves the opening of the skin and muscle fascia to release the pressure within the compartment and restore blood flow to the area.

**Prevention**: Leave large abdominal wounds open to drain, delay casting on affected extremities, and use flexible casts. Watch circumferential burns closely and perform frequent neurovascular checks on those at risk.

## RHABDOMYOLYSIS

Rhabdomyolysis occurs when damage of the cells of the skeletal muscles causes the release of toxins from injured cells into the bloodstream. Rhabdomyolysis may be caused by trauma, tissue ischemia, infection, certain medications (statins, selective serotonin reuptake inhibitors, lithium, and antihistamines), sepsis, immobilization, extraordinary physical exertion, myopathies and cocaine or alcohol abuse. Additionally, rhabdomyolysis may occur with exposure to certain toxins such as snake/insect venoms or mushroom poisoning. In rare circumstances, the identifiable cause cannot be determined. The most serious complication of rhabdomyolysis is renal failure. Rhabdomyolysis may be life threatening. Early recognition and treatment are critical to avoid serious complications and for patients to make a full recovery.

**Signs and symptoms**: Electrolyte imbalance, muscle pain and weakness, fever, tachycardia, dehydration, fatigue, lethargy, hypotension, and metabolic acidosis. Dark, reddish-brown urine may occur due to the presence of myoglobin released from the muscles and excreted into the urine.

**Diagnosis**: Laboratory studies such as creatinine kinase (CK) level, metabolic panel, urinalysis, and blood gases.

**Treatment**: The treatment of rhabdomyolysis includes fluid administration to eliminate toxins and prevent renal failure. Bicarbonate may be administered to correct metabolic acidosis. Mannitol or dopamine may be administered to increase renal perfusion. Electrolyte replacement may also be indicated. In severe cases, emergency dialysis may be necessary.

# Musculoskeletal Procedures and Interventions

## Pelvic Stabilizer

Pelvic stabilizers are used to prevent excessive bleeding associated with pelvic fractures, to maintain the bones in the correct position, and to prevent further damage. Maintaining pressure and reducing the fracture often reduces bleeding. Various methods of stabilizing the pelvis may be employed, including the sheet wrap method in which a sheet is folded, center under the patient, wrapped tightly about the pelvis, and secured. The pneumatic anti-shock garment (PASG) is indicated for hypovolemic shock, and hypotension associated with and for stabilization of pelvic and bilateral femur fractures. PASG is contraindicated with respiratory distress, pulmonary edema, pregnancy (after the first trimester), heart failure, myocardial infarction, stroke, evisceration, abdominal or leg impalement, head injuries, and uncontrolled bleeding above the garment. Another device is the SAM pelvic sling, which has a wide band that fits under and about the pelvis and lateral hips and a belt anteriorly that allows adjustment.

## Immobilization Devices

Immobilization devices include:

- **Cervical collar**: Support the head to prevent spinal cord injury with suspected injury to cervical vertebrae.
- **Cervical extrication splints**: Short board used to immobilize and protect the head and neck during extrication.
- **Backboards**: Used to immobilize the spine to prevent further injury to spinal cord. Both long and short spine boards are available in a number of different shapes and sizes.
- **Full-body splints** (such as vacuum mattress splint): Provide cushioned support to maintain body alignment.
- **Various types of splints for extremities**: Include rigid (should be padded), non-rigid (moldable), traction, and air (pneumatic devices) as well as the use of blankets, rolled towels, sheets, and pillows to maintain position. Traction splints are used for fractured femurs to keep bones in position.
- **Pneumatic anti-shock garment** (PASG): Provides pressure on lower extremities and abdomen and is used to control hemorrhage and shock to prevent pooling of blood in extremities and return blood to general circulation. Often used for pelvic fractures, but may increase risk of internal hemorrhage.

## Spinal Immobilization

Spinal immobilization, once a standard for trauma patients, has been shown to have little effect and in some cases may cause harm. Because of these findings, spinal immobilization with backboard is now recommended only for patients with neurological complaints, such as numbness, tingling, weakness, paralysis, pain or tenderness in the spine, spinal deformity, blunt trauma associated with alterations of consciousness, and high energy injuries associated with drugs/alcohol, inability of the patient to communicate, and/or distracting injury. Cervical collars for cervical spine immobilization are to be utilized for trauma based on the NEXUS criteria or Canadian C-spine rules (CCR). According to **NEXUS criteria**, a patient who exhibits all of the following does not require a cervical collar:

- Alert and stable
- No intoxication
- No midline tenderness of the spine
- No distracting injury
- No neurological deficit

Spinal immobilization should be continued for the shortest time possible, so imaging, such as CT, should be carried out upon admission. Cervical collars are applied while the head is supported in neutral position, and the patient is logrolled onto a backboard and strapped in place.

### IMMOBILIZATION OF FRACTURES AND DISLOCATIONS

Immobilization techniques for fractures and dislocations include:

- **Cast**: Plaster and fiberglass casts are applied after reduction to ensure that the bone is correctly aligned. Cast should be placed over several layers of padding that extends slightly beyond the cast ends. Cast material, such as plaster, should NOT be immersed in hot water but water slightly above room temperature (70 °F).
- **Splint**: Plaster splints use 12 or more layers of plaster measured to the correct length and then several layers of padding (longer and wider than splint should be measured and cut). The plaster splint is submerged in water to saturate, removed, laid on a flat surface, and massaged to fuse the layers. The padding is laid on top, and the splint is positioned and wrapped with gauze to hold it in place. While setting the splint, position can be maintained by holding it in place with the palm of the hand (not the fingers). After setting, the splint may be wrapped by elastic compression bandages.

### TOURNIQUETS

Tourniquets are used to control hemorrhage in an extremity and should be applied immediately with arterial bleeds or if pressure does not stop bleeding. Commonly used **tourniquets** include adjustable bands that are tightened and secured and then include a windlass handle twisted until blood flow stops and the handle is secured. Another type is a wide elastic band that is stretched, wrapped about the extremity tightly a number of times and secured. Blood pressure cuffs may also be used to apply pressure if standard tourniquets are not available. Regardless of the type, the tourniquet should be placed as high on the extremity as possible (avoiding joints), and the date and time of placement should be documented (on the tourniquet if possible). Tourniquets may be contraindicated with DVT, Reynaud's disease, crushing injuries, sickle cell disease, severe peripheral arterial disease, and open lower extremity fractures. Risks include damage to muscles, nerves, and vessels as well as increased risk of amputation. However, the first priority is always to prevent exsanguination.

# Wound

## General Skin Assessment

**Skin color** varies according to ethnicity. Color changes should be assessed to determine if they are local or extend over the entire body, and if they are permanent or transient. Pallor may indicate stress, impaired oxygenation, and vasoconstriction. Erythema may indicate vasodilation, local inflammation, and blushing. Cyanosis indicates impaired oxygenation, and jaundice indicates increased bilirubin.

**Temperature** is typically assessed by touching the skin with the back of the hand. Skin should be warm and equal bilaterally. Hypothermia may indicate impaired circulation, intravenous infusion, and immobilized limb (such as in a cast). Hyperthermia may indicate fever, infection, and excessive exercise.

**Review Video: Skin Assessment**
Visit mometrix.com/academy and enter code: 794925

## Effects of Age on Skin

**Age** is an important consideration when evaluating the skin because the characteristics of the skin change as people age.

- An **infant's** skin is thinner than an adult's because, while the epidermis is developed, the dermis layer is only about 60% of that of an adult and continues to develop after birth. The skin of premature infants is especially friable, allowing for transepidermal water loss and evaporative heat loss.
- During **adolescence**, the hair follicles activate, the thickness of the dermis decreases about 20%, and epidermal turnover time increases, so healing slows.
- As people **continue to age**, Langerhans' cells decrease in number, making the skin more prone to cancer, and the inflammatory reactions decrease. The sweat glands, vascularity, and subcutaneous fat all decrease, interfering with thermoregulation and contributing to dryness and irritation of the skin. The epidermal-dermal junction flattens, resulting in skin that is prone to tearing. The elastin in the skin degrades with age and solar exposure. The thinning of the hypodermis can lead to pressure ulcers.

**Review Video: Integumentary System**
Visit mometrix.com/academy and enter code: 655980

## BRADEN SCALE

The Braden scale is a risk assessment tool that has been validated clinically as predictive of the risk of patient's developing pressure sores. It was developed in 1988 by Barbara Braden and Nancy Bergstrom and is in wide use. The scale scores six different areas with five areas scored 1-4 points, and one area 1-3 points. The lower the score, the greater the risk.

| Area | Score of 1 | Score of 2 | Score of 3 | Score of 4 |
|---|---|---|---|---|
| **Sensory perception** | Completely limited | Very limited | Slightly limited | No impairment |
| **Moisture** | Constantly moist | Very moist | Occasionally moist | Rarely moist |
| **Activity** | Bed | Chair | Occasional walk | Frequent walk |
| **Mobility** | Immobile | Limited | Slightly limited | No limitations |
| **Nutritional pattern** | Very poor | Inadequate | Adequate | Excellent |
| **Friction and shear** | Problem | Potential problem | No apparent problem | |

## EVALUATING WOUNDS FOR ETIOLOGY

Wounds should be evaluated for **etiology** during the initial assessment to ensure proper treatment. Wounds can arise from a number of different causes:

- **Pressure**: Wounds that occur over bony prominences, such as the heels and coccyx, may be related to pressure, shear, or friction. The skin should be carefully examined for discolorations or changes in texture that might indicate compromise.
- **Arterial**: Arterial insufficiency is associated with a decrease in pedal pulses, and cool atrophic (shiny, dry) skin. It may result in small punctate-type ulcers, frequently on the dorsum of foot.
- **Venous stasis**: A decrease in venous circulation often results in hemoglobin leaking into the tissues of the lower leg, giving a brown discoloration. Tissue is often edematous, and ulcers are most common near the medial malleolus.
- **Diabetic neuropathy/ischemia**: Neuropathy can result in a lack of sensation to pain so that injuries to the feet may go unnoticed. Diabetes may also cause damage to small vessels, resulting in ischemia that can lead to ulcerations.
- **Trauma**: Injuries resulting from accidents or other types of trauma may vary considerably with some resulting in extensive damage to bones, tissues, organs, and circulation. Additionally, the wounds may be contaminated. Each wound must be assessed individually for multiple factors.
- **Burns**: Burn wounds may be chemical or thermal and should be assessed according to the area, the percentage of the body burned, and the depth of the burn. First-degree burns are superficial and affect the epidermis only. Second-degree burns extend through the dermis. Third degree burns affect underlying tissue, including vasculature, muscles, and nerves.
- **Infection**: An infected surgical or wound site can result in pain, edema, cellulitis, drainage, erosion of the sutures and ulceration of the tissue. Surgical sites must be assessed carefully and laboratory findings reviewed.

## Elements of Wound Assessment

### Location and Size

**Wound location** should be described in terms of anatomic position using landmarks (such as sternal notch, umbilicus, lateral malleolus), correct medical terminology, and directional terms:

- Anterior (in front)
- Posterior (behind)
- Superior (above)
- Inferior (below)

**Wound size** should be carefully described through actual measurement rather than association (the size of a dime). Measurements should be done with a disposable ruler in millimeters or centimeters. The current standard for measurement:

$$\text{Length} \times \text{width} \times \text{depth} = \text{dimension}$$

However, a clear description requires more detail. The measurement should be done at the greatest width and greatest length. More than two measurements may be needed if the wound is very irregularly shaped. The depth of the wound should be measured by inserting a sterile applicator and grasping or marking the applicator at skin level and then measuring the length below. Ideally, the wound should be photographed as well, following protocols for photography.

### Wound Bed Tissue

Wound bed tissue should be described as completely as possible, including color and general appearance:

- **Granulation tissue** is slightly granular in appearance and deep pink to bright red and moist, bleeding easily if disturbed.
- **Clean non-granular tissue** is smooth and deep pink or red and is not healing.
- **Hypergranulation** is excessive, soft, flaccid granulating tissue that is raised above the level of the periwound tissue, preventing proper epithelization, and may reflect excess moisture in the wound.
- **Epithelization** should appear at wound edges first and then eventually cover the wound. It is dry and light pink or violet in color.
- **Slough** is necrotic tissue that is viscous, soft, and yellow-gray in appearance and adheres to the wound.
- **Eschar** is hard dark brown or black leathery necrotic tissue that accumulates with death of the tissue.

### Wound Margins

Wound margins and the tissue surrounding the wound should be described carefully and with correct terminology:

- **Color** should be described using color descriptions and such terms as blanched, erythematous (red), or ecchymosed (purple, green, yellow).
- **Skin texture** may be normal, indurated (hardened), or edematous (swollen). Note if there is cellulitis or maceration evident.
- **Wound edges** may be diffuse (without clear margins), well defined, or rolled. A healing ridge may be evident if granulation has begun. Note if the wound is closed (as with a surgical incision) or open (as with dehiscence or ulcerations). Note if wound edges are attached or unattached (indicating undermining or tunneling).
- **Tunneling or undermining** should be assessed by probing the wound margins with a moist sterile cotton applicator, using clock face locators (toward the head is 12 o'clock, for example). Tunneling may be described as extending from 3 o'clock to 4 o'clock. A large area is usually described as undermining. The size should be measured or estimated as closely as possible.

### *Distribution, Drainage, and Odor*

**Distribution** of lesions should be clearly delineated if there is more than one lesion over an area. The arrangement of the lesions can be helpful for diagnosis and treatments.

- Linear (in a line)
- Satellites (small lesions around a larger one)
- Diffuse (scattered freely over an area)

**Drainage** may vary considerably from nothing at all to copious outpourings of discharge.

- Serous drainage is usually clear to slightly yellow.
- Serosanguineous drainage is a combination of serous drainage and blood.
- Sanguineous drainage is bloody.
- Purulent discharge may be thick and milky, yellow, brownish, or green, depending upon the infective agent.

**Odor** requires more subjective assessment, but the odor and type of discharge together can provide useful information. Some infective agents, such as *Pseudomonas*, produce distinctive odors, which may be described in various ways: musty, foul, sweet.

## Assessment Characteristics of Arterial, Neuropathic, and Venous Ulcers

The assessment process is important in delineating between the arterial, neuropathic, or venous origin of the ulcer. Characteristics of each must be known and closely examined:

**Location**

- **Arterial**: Ends of toes, pressure points, traumatic nonhealing wounds
- **Neuropathic**: Plantar surface, metatarsal heads, toes, and sides of feet
- **Venous**: Between knees and ankles, medial malleolus

**Wound Bed**

- **Arterial**: Pale, necrotic
- **Neuropathic**: Red (or ischemic)
- **Venous**: Dark red, fibrinous slough

**Exudate**

- **Arterial**: Slight amount, infection common
- **Neuropathic**: Moderate to large amounts, infection common
- **Venous**: Moderate to large amounts

**Wound Perimeter**

- **Arterial**: Circular, well-defined
- **Neuropathic**: Circular, well-defined, often with callous formation
- **Venous**: Irregular, poorly-defined

**Pain**

- **Arterial**: Very painful
- **Neuropathic**: Pain often absent because of reduced sensation
- **Venous**: Pain varies

**Skin**

- **Arterial**: Pale, friable, shiny, and hairless, with dependent rubor and elevational pallor
- **Neuropathic**: Ischemic signs (as in arterial) may be evident with comorbidity
- **Venous**: Brownish discoloration of ankles and shin, edema common

**Pulses**

- **Arterial**: Weak or absent
- **Neuropathic**: Present and palpable, diminished in neuroischemic ulcers
- **Venous**: Present and palpable

## Cellulitis

Cellulitis occurs when an area of the skin becomes infected, usually following injury or trauma to the skin. Cellulitis is most likely to be caused by staphylococcus or streptococcus bacteria. Patients with peripheral vascular disease, diabetes mellitus, and immunosuppression are at a higher risk for the development of cellulitis. **Signs and symptoms** include pain, erythema, and warmth at the affected site that progresses rapidly. In addition, the patient may experience fever, chills, fatigue, and malaise. **Diagnosis** is made by physical exam. Labs include complete blood count, culture of the involved area and blood. **Treatment** for cellulitis is the administration of antibiotics. Surgical irrigation and debridement may be indicated in severe cases.

## Extravasation

Extravasation occurs when an intravenously infused vesicant medication or fluid leaks from the vein and into the subcutaneous space. Vesicant medications are those that cause tissue injury if extravasated and that may ultimately lead to tissue necrosis. Extravasation and infiltration are similar in nature, with infiltration occurring when the infusate is a non-vesicant solution or medication. Extravasation occurs more commonly in peripheral IVs; however, it can also occur with central venous catheters. Common vesicant agents include several chemotherapeutic agents, vancomycin, electrolytes, dobutamine, norepinephrine, phenytoin, promethazine, propofol, and vasopressin.

**Signs and symptoms**: Pain, burning, erythema, and edema at the site of the extravasation. Oftentimes, a blood return from the peripheral IV or central venous catheter is not present. Long term complications include complex regional pain syndrome, tissue necrosis, and nerve or tendon damage.

**Diagnosis**: Physical assessment and review of patient symptoms and medications/infusions administered.

**Treatment**: Early recognition is key to the successful treatment of an extravasation. When an extravasation is suspected, the IV infusion should be immediately stopped and the infusion site assessed. For some medications, antidotes may be available to minimize the damage caused by the extravasation. Heat or cold therapy may also be utilized depending on the medication. In cases of severe damage, debridement, skin grafting, and even amputation may result.

## Tissue Damage Related to Allergic Contact Dermatitis

**Contact dermatitis** is a localized response to contact with an allergen, resulting in a rash that may blister and itch. Common allergens include poison oak, poison ivy, latex, benzocaine, nickel, and preservatives, but there is a wide range of items, preparations, and products to which people may react.

**Treatment** includes:

- Identifying the causative agent through evaluating the area of the body affected, careful history, or skin patch testing to determine allergic responses
- Corticosteroids to control inflammation and itching

- Soothing oatmeal baths
- Pramoxine lotion to relieve itching
- Antihistamines to reduce allergic response
- Lesions should be gently cleansed and observed for signs of secondary infection
- Antibiotics are used only for secondary infections as indicated
- Rash is usually left open to dry
- Avoidance of allergen to prevent recurrence

## PRESSURE ULCERS

Pressure ulcers occur when pressure from the weight of the body causes a decrease in perfusion, affecting arterial and capillary blood flow and resulting in ischemia. Ulcers may then develop from pressure, shearing, and friction. Common pressure points include the occiput, scapula, sacrum, buttocks, ischium, and heels. Patients with a decreased level of consciousness, brain/spinal cord injuries, peripheral neuropathies, malnutrition, dehydration, PVD, or impaired mobility are at a higher risk for pressure ulcers. Critically ill patients are at an increased risk due to prolonged immobility, sedation, and often incontinence of urine and stool. In addition, patients on vasopressors are at a higher risk due to the constriction of the peripheral circulation.

**Signs and symptoms**: Early stages include redness, tenderness, and firmness at the site of the ulcer. Once the ulcer progresses to severe tissue injury, bone, muscle, or tendons may be exposed, and there may be a yellow or black wound base in addition to pain and drainage at the site.

**Diagnostics**: Skin and wound assessment, including staging of the ulcer.

**Treatment**: Wet-to-Dry dressings, Wound VAC therapy, and hyperbaric oxygen may be used; a wound care consult is often advised.

**Prevention**: Begins with a risk assessment; the Braden scale is a commonly used scale. A score of 16 or below indicates that the patient is at risk. At-risk patients or patients with active ulcers should be placed on a turning and positioning schedule or on a specialty bed to relieve pressure. Moisture barriers and skin protectants may also be utilized.

### *NATIONAL PRESSURE INJURY ADVISORY PANEL STAGING*

Pressure ulcers result from pressure or pressure with shear and/or friction over bony prominences. The **National Pressure Injury Advisory Panel (NPIAP) stages** include:

- **Suspected deep tissue injury**: Skin discolored, intact or blood blister
- **Stage I**: Intact skin with non-blanching reddened area
- **Stage II**: Abrasion or blistered area without slough but with partial-thickness skin loss
- **Stage III**: Deep ulcer with exposed subcutaneous tissue; tunneling or undermining may be evident with or without slough
- **Stage IV**: Deep ulcer, full thickness, with necrosis into muscle, bone, tendons, and/or joints
- **Unstageable**: Eschar and/or slough prevents staging prior to debridement

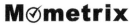

Patients should be placed on pressure-reducing support surfaces and turned at least every two hours, avoiding the area(s) with a pressure ulcer. Wound care depends on the stage of the wound and the amount of drainage but includes irrigation, debridement when necessary, antibiotics for infection, and appropriate dressing. Patients should be encouraged to have adequate protein and iron in their diets to promote healing and to maintain adequate hydration.

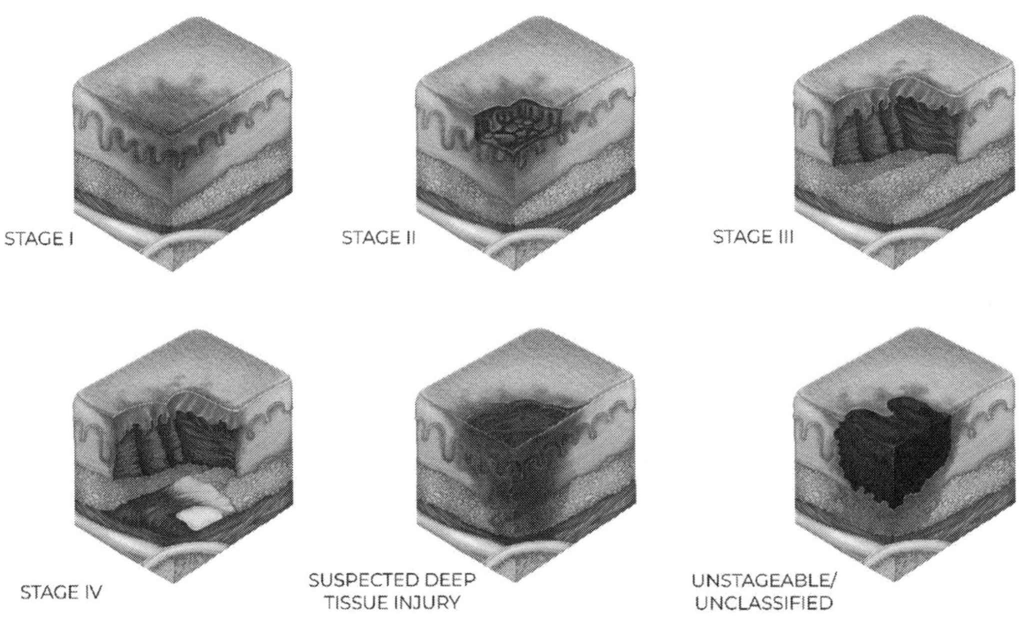


## Infectious Wounds

All types of wounds have the potential to become infected. Infectious wounds are commonly health care acquired. Wound infections increase a patient's risk of sepsis, multisystem organ failure and death. Trauma patients are at an increased risk of developing an infected wound due to exposure to various contaminants that they may have encountered during their injury (e.g., dirt from a motor vehicle accident).

**Signs and symptoms**: Erythema, edema, induration, drainage, increasing pain and tenderness, fever, leukocytosis, and lymphangitis.

**Diagnosis**: Wound infections are diagnosed by wound cultures (anaerobic and aerobic). Fluid or tissue biopsy may also be performed.

**Treatment**: Wound infections are treated with antibiotics and a wound care regimen that includes routine cleaning and dressing of the wound. Wound care treatment is based on the type and severity of the wound. Surgical irrigation and debridement may also be indicated. For deep, complex wounds, a wound-care consult is often indicated.

## Necrotizing Fasciitis

Necrotizing fasciitis is an infection that develops deep within the fascia, causing a rapidly developing tissue necrosis resulting in destruction and death of the soft tissue and nerves. Complications of necrotizing fasciitis may include the loss of the affected limb, sepsis, and death. Group A *Streptococcus*, *Klebsiella*, *Clostridium*, *Escherichia coli*, *Staphylococcus aureus*, and *Aeromonas hydrophila* are organisms that have the potential to cause necrotizing fasciitis.

**Signs and symptoms**: Edema, erythema, and pain at the affected site. Nausea, vomiting, fatigue, malaise, fever, and chills may also occur.

**Diagnosis**: Diagnosis is based on physical assessment and patient history. In addition, excisional deep skin biopsy and gram staining may be performed to determine the causative organism. CT/MRI may also be utilized to assess the extent of the infection.

**Treatment**: Treatment options for necrotizing fasciitis include antibiotics and fasciotomy with radical debridement. Hyperbaric oxygen therapy may also be utilized.

## Surgical Wounds

Surgical wounds or incisions are made during a surgical procedure in a sterile, controlled environment. The American College of Surgeons has defined four classes of surgical wound types. This classification can help to predict how the wound will heal and the risk of infection.

- **Class I** is defined as clean (e.g., laparoscopic surgeries and biopsies).
- **Class II** is defined as clean contaminated (e.g., GI and GU surgeries).
- **Class III** is defined as contaminated (e.g., traumatic wounds such as a gunshot wound).
- **Class IV** is defined as dirty (e.g., traumatic wound from a dirty source).

Surgical wounds should be assessed for signs and symptoms of infection including erythema, edema, fever, increasing pain, and drainage. Surgical drains are commonly placed near the surgical incision to promote drainage—inspect drains for patency, amount, and characteristics of drainage. Patients are often treated with antibiotics prophylactically to help prevent a surgical site infection. Wound vacuum assisted closure devices may also be utilized to remove blood or serous fluid from the surgical wound/incision site.

## Management of Inflammation Resulting from Tattoos and Piercing

Tattoos and piercing have both been implicated in **MRSA infections**. Tattooing uses needles that inject dye, sometimes resulting in local infection with erythema, edema, and purulent discharge. Body piercing for insertion of jewelry carries similar risks. Piercings of concern include the upper ear cartilage, nipples, navel, tongue, lip, penis, and nose. Some people who do piercings use reusable piercing equipment that is difficult to adequately clean and sterilize. Infections resulting from piercing in cartilage are often resistant to antibiotics because of lack of blood supply.

**Treatment** includes:

- **Cleansing wounds**. Jewelry may need to be removed in some cases.
- **Antibiotics**: Culture should be obtained, but medications for community-acquired MRSA should be started immediately:
  - **Mupirocin** may be used topically 3 times daily for 7-10 days with or without systemic antimicrobials.
  - **Trimethoprim-sulfamethoxazole DS** (TMP 160 mg/SMX 800 mg), 1-2 tablets twice daily. Children, dose based on TMP: 8-12 mg/kg/day in 2 doses.

## Tissue Damage

**Abrasion** is damage to superficial layers of skin, such as with road burn or ligature marks.

**Contusion** occurs when friction or pressure causes damage to underlying vessels, resulting in bruising. Contusions that are bright red/purple with clear margins have occurred within 48 hours and those with receding edges or yellow-brown discoloration are older than 48 hours.

**Laceration** is a tear in the skin resulting from blunt force, often from falls on protuberances, such as elbows, or other blunt trauma. Lacerations may be partial to full-thickness.

**Avulsion** is tissue that is separated from its base and lost or without adequate base for attachment.

**Treatments** include:

- Local anesthetic if needed
- Low pressure, high volume irrigation with 35-50 mL syringe of open wound with normal saline, water, or non-antiseptic nonionic surfactants, and mechanical scrubbing of surrounding tissue with disinfectant
- Topical antibiotics as indicated
- Prophylactic antibiotics or antibiotic irrigation if wound contaminated
- Suturing/debridement as needed
- Hydrocolloids, Steri-Strips, and transparent dressings to stabilize flaps

## TRAUMATIC WOUNDS

Traumatic wounds include cuts, punctures, lacerations, force trauma, gunshot wounds, bites, abrasions, crush injuries, degloving injuries, and contusions. Trauma wounds can vary in severity and may be associated with serious underlying injuries. Once the patient is stabilized, wound management is initiated and should include thorough wound cleansing and debridement with removal of any foreign objects or materials. Irrigation and debridement are critical steps in minimizing the risk of infection. **Signs and symptoms** include bleeding, pain, erythema, and edema. With severe traumatic injury patients may experience signs of hemorrhagic shock including heavy bleeding, loss of consciousness, tachypnea, tachycardia, hypotension, decreased urinary output, and pallor.

**Treatment** of traumatic wounds is dependent on the location and severity of the wound. Treatment options may include irrigation and debridement, foreign body removal, wound closure including sutures, staples or fibrin glue, antibiotics, prophylactic tetanus injection, and fasciotomy.

### *MECHANICAL TRAUMA*

Mechanical trauma may result in stripping of the epidermis and sometimes the dermis of the skin or lacerations. Mechanical trauma may occur from tape removal or blunt trauma, such as colliding with furniture. Skin tears are categorized with the **Payne-Martin Classification System**:

- Skin tear leaves avulsed skin adequate to cover wound; tears may be linear or flap-type
- Skin tear with loss of partial thickness, involving either scant (less than 25% of epidermal flap over tear is lost) to moderate-large (more than 25% of dermis in tear is lost)
- Skin tear with complete loss of tissue, involving a partial-thickness wound with no epidermal flap

**Treatment** includes:

- Recognizing fragile skin and treating carefully
- Applying emollients, skin sealants, and skin barriers as indicated
- Applying and removing tape appropriately
- Avoiding adhesives when possible
- Using hydrocolloids, Steri-Strips, and transparent dressings to stabilize flaps

## FOREIGN BODIES IN SUBCUTANEOUS TISSUE

Foreign bodies (FB) imbedded in subcutaneous tissue can include metal, glass, plastic, and wood.

**Symptoms** may include pain, infection, or inflammatory response, pseudotumor, sinus tracts, or osteomyelitis. Patients often sense presence of FB.

**Treatment** includes careful history and examination to determine if the trauma of removing the foreign object is worse than leaving the object in place. Inert objects, such as metal and sometimes plastic or glass may be left in place, but wood always causes infection and must be removed. **Diagnosis** includes:

- Radiographs of soft tissue (metal and glass)
- Ultrasound (wood or thorns)
- CT for dangerous FB only

**MRIs** are usually only done if the initial attempt to remove the FB was unsuccessful and infection has developed, but metal fragments may move during an MRI so it is contraindicated for intraorbital or intracranial FBs.

### *Removal of Foreign Bodies in Subcutaneous Tissue*

Treatment to remove a foreign body (FB) should not exceed 30 minutes in the ED. Open tissue should not be probed with a gloved finger to locate the FB because of the danger of tearing a glove:

- Palpate tissue and use **metal instrument** to search for glass fragments rather than gloved finger
- **Local anesthetic**: lidocaine with epinephrine
- Use **radiographs or ultrasound** for guidance, using metal markers or inserting 2 needles to isolate location
- **BP cuff or tourniquet** may be needed to slow arterial flow to extremity
- **Incise** tissue adequately and use hemostat to remove the FB
- **Irrigate** wound with normal saline
- Wound is usually left **opened and bandaged**; large wounds may be sutured closed in 3-5 days
- **Antibiotics** as indicated
- FBs under **nails** may require removing all or part of nail:
    - **Digital block**
    - Sterile **hypodermic needle** (straight or bent) slid under nail to capture the FB
    - **$CO_2$ laser vaporization** may be used to vaporize nail above foreign object

## High-Pressure Injection Injuries

High-pressure injection injuries involve injection of materials (such as nails) or substances (water, air, oil, paint) into the tissue under high pressure. The severity of the injury depends on the location of the injury, the material or substance, and the size or amount of the injection. High-pressure injection injuries may result in ischemia, tissue destruction, open wounds, and inflammatory response even though the external injury may appear small.

**Signs and symptoms** include pain and swelling. Crepitus may be present with air injection. Ischemia may occur. These injuries may result in fractures, contractures, amputations, fibrosis, and fistulae. Common substances involved in high-pressure injection injuries include grease (over half of injuries) and diesel fuel. Injuries often occur on fingers of the non-dominant hand.

**Diagnosis** includes clinical symptoms and may include CBC (as some substances may cause increase WBC count) and electrolytes (some substances cause imbalance).

**Treatment** depends on the extent of the injury and includes supportive care, tetanus prophylaxis, and broad-spectrum antibiotic. Surgical repair may be required.

## Management of Missile Injuries

Missile injuries include arrow, gunshot, paint gun, nail gun, and shrapnel wounds. These injuries are usually circular, oval, or triangular, and may have both an entry (with abrasion at periphery) and exit site. Other residue, such as gunpowder, may be evident at the entry. Careful documentation should be done and clothes retained for evidence in gunshot wounds. Puncture wounds are difficult to properly cleanse and become easily infected, even with treatment.

**Treatment** varies according to the site, type, and degree of injury and may include:

- Tetanus prophylaxis
- Irrigation of wound with NS if both entry and exit
- Incision over puncture wound to create a linear incision that can be irrigated and cleansed adequately
- Removal of foreign body if in place
- Antibiotics as indicated
- Follow-up care to check for infection

## Wound VACs

**Wound vacuum-assisted closure (wound VAC)** (AKA negative pressure wound therapy) uses subatmospheric (negative) pressure with a suction unit and a semi-occlusion vapor-permeable dressing. The suction reduces periwound and interstitial edema, decompressing vessels, improving circulation, stimulating production of new cells, and decreasing colonization of bacteria. Wound VAC also increases the rate of granulation and re-epithelialization to hasten healing. The wound must be debrided of necrotic tissue prior to treatment. Wound VAC is used for a variety of difficult-to-heal wounds, especially those that show less than 30% healing in 4 weeks of post-debridement treatment or those with excessive exudate, including chronic stage II and IV pressure ulcers, skin flaps, diabetic ulcer, acute wounds, burns, surgical wound, and those with dehiscence and nonresponsive arterial and venous ulcers. Contraindications include:

- Wound malignancy
- Untreated osteomyelitis
- Exposed blood vessels or organs
- Non-enteric, unexplored fistulas.

Nonadherent porous foam is cut to fit and cover the wound and is secured with occlusive transparent film with an opening cut to accommodate the drainage tube, which is attached to a suction canister in a closed system. The pressure should be set at 75-125 psi and the dressing changed 2-3 times weekly.

## Pressure Reduction Surfaces

Pressure reduction surfaces redistribute pressure to prevent pressure ulcers and reduce shear and friction. There are various types of support surfaces for beds, examining tables, operating tables, and chairs. Functions of pressure reduction surfaces include temperature control, moisture control, and friction/shear control. **General use guidelines** include:

- Pressure redistribution support surfaces should be used for patients with stage II, III, and IV ulcers, as well as for those that are at risk for developing pressure ulcers.
- Chairs should have gel or air support surfaces to redistribute pressure for chair-bound patients, critically ill patients, or those who cannot move independently.
- Support surface material should provide at least an inch of support under areas to be protected when in use to prevent bottoming out. (Check by placing hand palm-up under the overlay below the pressure point.)
- Static support surfaces are appropriate for patients who can change position without increasing pressure to an ulcer.
- Dynamic support surfaces are needed for those who need assistance to move or when static pressure devices provide less than an inch of support.

## Biological Wound Debridement with Maggots

**Medical maggots** are applied to the open wound; periwound tissue must be protected:

- A **wound pattern** is transferred onto a hydrocolloid pad, an opening is cut, and a pad is applied to the skin with the wound exposed. The pattern is used to cut an opening in a semi-permeable film for an outer dressing.
- Maggots are wiped from the container with a saline-dampened 2×2 **gauze** (about 5-10 maggots per $cm^2$ wound size). The gauze is loosely packed into the wound.
- A porous **mesh** (*Creature Comfort*) is placed over the wound and secured to the hydrocolloid with tape or glue, creating a maggot cage.
- **Transparent film** is placed over the hydrocolloid, making sure that the cutout area is over the cage so that the maggots have air and drainage can escape. Saline-dampened gauze is placed loosely over the cage.
- **Dry gauze** is used for the outer dressing and changed every 4-8 hours as needed.

Maggots are wiped from the wound after 48 hours and the wound is **irrigated** with normal saline.

## Pharmacologic Treatment of Wound Pain

### *Topical Anesthetics*

There are numerous different types of pain medications that may be used to control pain from wounds, including **topical anesthetics**:

- **Lidocaine 2-4%** is frequently used during debridement or dressing changes. Lidocaine is useful only superficially and may take 15-30 minutes before it is effective.
- **Eutectic Mixture of Local Anesthetics (EMLA Cream)** provides good pain control. The wound is first cleansed and then the cream is applied thickly (1/4 inch) extending about 1/2 inch past the wound to the periwound tissue. The wound is then covered with plastic wrap, which is secured and left in place for about 20 minutes. The wrapped time may be extended to 45-60 minutes if necessary, to completely numb the tissue. The tissue should remain numb for about 1 hour after the plastic wrap is removed, allowing time for the wound to be cleansed, debrided, and/or redressed.

### *Regional Anesthesia*

Regional anesthesia (injectable subcutaneous and perineural medications) is administered locally about the wound or as nerve blocks. Medications include lidocaine, bupivacaine, and tetracaine in solution. Epinephrine is sometimes added to increase vasoconstriction and reduce bleeding, although it is avoided in distal areas of the limbs (hands and feet) to prevent ischemia.

- **Field blockade** involves injecting the anesthetic into the periwound tissue or into the wound margins. The effect may be decreased by inflammation. The effects last for limited periods of time.
- **Regional nerve blocks** may involve single injections, the effects of which are limited in duration but can provide pain relief for treatments. Techniques that use continuous catheter infusions are longer lasting and can be controlled more precisely. Blocks may involve nerves proximal to affected areas, such as peripheral nerve blocks, or large nerve blocks near the spinal cord, such as percutaneous lumbar sympathetic blocks (LSB). Long-term blocks may use alcohol-based medications to permanently inactivate the nerves.

# Maxillofacial and Ocular Emergencies

## Maxillofacial

### Peritonsillar Abscess

Peritonsillar abscess (PTA), which usually derives from tonsillitis, progresses from cellulitis to abscess between the palatine tonsil and capsule. It is often polymicrobial. It usually occurs bilaterally between the ages of 20 and 30. Complications include obstruction of airway, rupture with aspiration of purulent material, septicemia, endocarditis, and epiglottitis. The infection is often polymicrobial. Symptoms include fever, pain, hoarseness, muffling of voice, dysphagia, tonsillar edema, erythema, exudate, and edema of palate with displacement of uvula.

**Diagnosis**:

- Aspiration of purulent material (usually diagnostic)
- CT with contrast, ultrasound
- On exam: Displacement of the uvula, with enlarged tonsils

**Treatments** include:

- Needle aspirations (often multiple) with needle penetrating 1 cm or less to avoid carotid artery
- Abscess incision and drainage if aspiration not successful
- IV volume replacement
- **Antibiotics**: IV ampicillin-sulbactam or clindamycin until culture results come back and in areas with high rates of CA-MRSA vancomycin may be added. Once the patient shows signs of clinical improvement, they may switch to oral antibiotics (needing 14 days total).

### Dental Avulsions

Dental avulsions are the complete displacement of a tooth from its socket. The tooth may be reimplanted if done within one to two hours after displacement, although only permanent teeth are reimplanted, not primary.

**Procedure**:

1. Tooth can be **transported** from accident site to the emergency department in Hank solution, saline, or milk.
2. **Cleanse** tooth with sterile NS or Hank solution, handling only the crown and avoiding any disruption of fibers.
3. If tooth has been dry for 20-60 minutes, **soak** tooth in Hank solution for 30 minutes before reimplantation.
4. If tooth has been dry for more than 60 minutes, **soak** tooth in citric acid for 5 minutes, stannous fluoride 2% for 5 minutes, and doxycycline solution for 5 minutes prior to reimplantation.
5. Remove **clot** in socket and gently irrigate with NS.
6. Place tooth into **socket** firmly, cover with gauze, and have patient bite firmly on gauze until splinting can be applied.
7. Apply **splinting material and mold packing** over implanted tooth and 2 adjacent teeth on both sides (encompasses 5 teeth).

## Dental Fractures

Dental fractures, most commonly of the maxillary teeth, may occur in association with other oral injuries and may be overlooked unless a careful dental examination is carried out. Fractures are classified according to severity of fracture with treatment to prevent further damage and necrosis.

- **Ellis I**: Chipping of enamel
  - Smoothen rough edges
- **Ellis II**: Fracture of enamel and dentin with pain on pressure and air sensitivity
  - Protect dentin with glass ionomer dental cement and refer to dentist within 24 hours
- **Ellis III**: Fracture of enamel, dentin, and pulp with pain on movement; air and temperature sensitivity; blood may be evident
  - Protect dentin with ionomer dental cement or calcium hydroxide base and refer to dentist for prompt treatment
  - Administer oral analgesics
- **Alveolar/root fracture:** Loose tooth and malocclusion, sensitivity to percussion
  - Prompt referral to dentist for splinting and/or root canal

**Review Video: Anatomical and Clinical Parts of Teeth**
Visit mometrix.com/academy and enter code: 683627

## Temporomandibular Fracture and/or Dislocation

Temporomandibular fracture and/or dislocation can occur as a result of trauma, such as a direct blow to the jaw, or chronic disorders. Dislocations may be anterior (most common and often after extreme mouth opening), posterior, lateral, or superior.

**Symptoms**:

- Acute pain
- Dysphagia
- Difficulty speaking
- Edema and rigidity of surrounding muscles
- Inability to open mouth

**Diagnosis** includes:

- Complete head, neck, ear, and dental examination
- Radiography, such as x-rays or CT, with significant trauma
- Tongue blade test: Patient bites hard on tongue blade while examiner twists blade, attempting to break it. If fracture, patient opens mouth to release blade

**Treatment** (dislocation) includes:

- Short-acting muscle relaxant
- Narcotic analgesia/conscious sedation
- Reduction: Patient on chair with head against hard surface
- Examiner in front of patient places gloved thumbs in patient's mouth, posteriorly over the surface of the mandibular molars
- Examiner applies pressure posteriorly and inferiorly
- Alternately, examiner stands behind recumbent patient and applies pressure posteriorly and inferiorly

## Nasal Fracture

Nasal fracture can result from any type of blunt trauma to the face. Fracture may be overlooked because of edema, so careful examination of the nose with facial injuries is important. Common causes include altercations and sporting injuries. Septal cartilage is often fractured as well as nasal bones.

**Symptoms** include:

- Edema
- Pain
- Crepitation
- Ecchymosis
- Deformity
- Nasal bleeding

**Diagnosis** is based on clinical examination and otoscope. Radiographic studies are not indicated unless other facial fractures are suspected. Clear nasal discharge following injury to the face may indicate leaking of cerebrospinal fluid from torn meninges resulting from fracture of cribriform plate. A drop of clear drainage should be placed on filter paper and examined for a clear area around a central stain of blood. If CSF drainage is suspected, the patient should be placed upright, and have a CT scan and neurological consult.

**Treatment** for fracture includes:

- Realignment if necessary
- Analgesia
- Nasal decongestant
- Protective covering
- Packing only for persistent epistaxis

## Maxillary Fractures

Maxillary fractures of the face often are associated with significant other trauma because of the degree of force necessary to fracture the maxilla. Three primary types include:

- **Le Fort I**: Horizontal (low downward force)
- **Le Fort II**: Pyramidal (low or mid maxilla force)
- **Le Fort III**: Transverse (force to bridge of nose or upper maxilla)

However, many injuries are a combination with more than one type of fracture.

**Symptoms** may include:

- Malocclusion and open bite
- Apparent lengthening of face
- CSF rhinorrhea (clear nasal discharge)
- Periorbital ecchymosis

**Diagnosis**: Grasping and moving the hard palate back and forth may shift the facial bones. Complete head, neck, ear, oral, and nasal examination with slit headlamp, suction as needed, nasal speculum, and otoscope. CT scans of face and brain.

**Treatment**:

- Stabilize patient and ensure patent airway
- Disimpaction of displaced fragments manually

- Obtain pre-injury photograph to guide surgical fixation
- Referral to surgeon for fixation

## Recurrent Epistaxis

Recurrent epistaxis is common in young children (2 to 10 years), especially boys, and is often related to nose picking, dry climate, or central heating in the winter. Incidence also increases between 50 and 80 years of age, and may be caused by NSAIDs and anticoagulants. Kiesselbach plexus in the anterior nares has plentiful vessels and bleeds easily. Bleeding in the posterior nares is more dangerous and can result in considerable blood loss. Bleeding from the anterior nares is usually confined to one nostril, but from the posterior nares, blood may flow through both nostrils or backward into the throat and the person may be observed swallowing. People abusing cocaine may suffer nosebleeds because of damage to the mucosa. Hematocrit and hemoglobin should be done to determine if blood loss is significant. Bleeding should stop within 20 minutes. Treatment:

- Upright position, leaning forward so blood does not flow down throat.
- Applying pressure below the nares or by pinching the nostrils firmly for 10 minutes.
- Severe bleeding: packing and/or topical vasoconstrictors.
- Humidifiers may decrease irritation.

## Bell's Palsy

Bell's palsy is caused by inflammation of cranial nerve VII, usually from a herpes simplex I or II infection, and generally affects only one side of the paired nerves. Onset is generally sudden, and symptoms peak by 48 hours with a wide range of presentation. **Symptoms** usually subside within two to six months but may persist one year:

- Mild weakness on one side of face to complete paralysis with distortion of features
- Drooping of eyelid and mouth
- Tearing in affected eye
- Taste impairment

**Diagnosis** includes:

- Neurological, eye, parotid gland, and ear exam to rule out other cranial nerve involvement or conditions.

**Treatment** includes:

- Artificial tears during daytime with lubricating ophthalmic ointment and patch at night to protect eye
- Prednisone 60 mg daily for 5 days with tapering over 5 days.
- For severe cases use prednisone AND acyclovir 400 mg 5 times daily for 7 days.

## Temporal Arteritis

Temporal arteritis (TA), also called giant cell arteritis, is inflammation of the blood vessels of the head, especially the temporal artery, and the thoracic aorta and branches. TA is commonly associated with polymyalgia rheumatica (30% or less of patients) but can occur with other systemic disorders such as lupus erythematous, Sjögren syndrome, and rheumatoid arthritis. TA is a progressive disorder that can result in blindness and is most common in those older than 50. **Symptoms** include:

- New onset of headaches
- Vision fluctuations, including decreased visual acuity and loss of vision
- Intermittent claudicating pain in jaw, tongue, and upper extremities
- Fever

**Diagnosis** includes:

- Temporal artery biopsy (definitive)
- ESR greater than 50 mm/hr (may be normal in about 20%)
- CRP greater than 2.45 mg/dL

**Treatment** should begin immediately if the diagnosis is suspected to prevent blindness:

- Prednisone 60 mg daily

## TRIGEMINAL NEURALGIA

Trigeminal neuralgia (tic douloureux) is a neurological condition in which blood vessels press on the trigeminal nerve as it leaves the brainstem causing severe pain on one side of the face or jaw. The shock-like pains may involve a small area or half the face and in rare cases both sides of the face at different times. The pain lasts from seconds to two minutes and is extremely debilitating and may be precipitated by movement, vibration, or contact with the face or mouth. Trigeminal neuralgia is most common in women older than 50. Patients may go through periods of remission and recurrences. Diagnosis is by history and neurological exam.

**Treatment** includes:

- **Carbamazepine** is the drug of choice and usually controls pain initially, but the effects may decrease over time.
- **Phenytoin or oxcarbazepine** may be used in place of carbamazepine.
- **Baclofen** (muscle relaxant) potentiates other drugs.
- **Surgical procedures** may be done if no response to medications.

## FOREIGN BODIES

### *FOREIGN BODIES IN THE EAR*

Foreign bodies in the ear (most often in children) can be organic or inorganic materials or insects. Careful history should be done to determine the type of foreign body before attempting removal. Children may require conscious sedation or general anesthesia for deep insertions. Irrigations should not be done if tympanic membrane is ruptured or cannot be visualized. Procedure:

1. Examine ear to determine if tympanic membrane is intact.
2. Drown insects with lidocaine 2% solution and then suction.
3. Irrigate small nonorganic particles with pulsatile flow aimed at wall of the canal.
4. Use cerumen loops, right-angle hooks, and/or alligator forceps to grasp and remove item.
5. Carefully examine the ear canal after removal of the item for lacerations or abrasions.
6. Topical antibiotic if extensive cutaneous abrasion or laceration or for organic material.

### *FOREIGN BODIES IN THE EYE*

Foreign bodies in the eye should be assessed carefully with slit lamp with corneal examination using optical sectioning before attempting removal of the foreign body. Foreign bodies that penetrate the cornea full-thickness should not be removed in the ED, but superficial foreign bodies can safely be removed. Procedure:

1. Apply topical anesthetic to both eyes (to suppress blinking in the unaffected eye).
2. Eye held open by hand or with wire eyelid speculum.
3. Foreign body is carefully removed with small gauge needle or moistened cotton swab.
4. Rust ring from metallic objects should be removed with ophthalmic burr (if not over pupil), and patient referred to ophthalmologist for further rust ring removal within 24 hours.
5. Eyelid everted and examined carefully for further foreign bodies.
6. Abrasions treated as indicated.

### *Foreign Bodies in the Nares*

Children may insert various organic and inorganic foreign bodies in the nose. In most cases, this is observed, but persistent unilateral obstruction of nose, foul discharge, or epistaxis is suggestive of foreign body. Small or uncooperative children may need to be restrained with conscious sedation or papoose board.

**Procedure**:

1. Vasoconstrictor/topical anesthetic applied: 1 mL of phenylephrine with 3 mL of lidocaine 4%.
2. Aerosolized racemic epinephrine may be used for decongestion, to loosen foreign body.
3. Examine nares with speculum.

**Removal techniques**:

- Positive pressure: Blowing nose on command. For small children, block opposite nares and have caregiver blow puff of air in mouth, forcing item out of nares.
- Suction with catheter.
- Use alligator or bayonet forceps to grasp item.
- Pass a curette behind item, rotate, and the use to pull item out.
- Pass Fogarty vascular catheter past item, inflate balloon, pull catheter back out.

## Ludwig Angina

Ludwig angina is cellulitis, usually caused by *Streptococcus* or *Staphylococcus,* of the submandibular spaces and lingual space that can result in obstruction of the airway as the swelling in the mouth floor pushes the tongue superior and posterior.

**Symptoms** include:

- Evidence of poor dental hygiene and odontogenic abscess (usually from lower third molars or surrounding gums) that has spread into soft tissue
- Dysphagia
- Odynophagia, trismus, edema of the upper neck (midline)
- Erythema, stridor, and cyanosis (late signs of obstruction)
- Changes in mental status

**Diagnosis** includes:

- Examination of the head and neck to observe for swelling of the upper neck, floor of mouth, and tongue
- CT scan
- Culture (treatment should, however, begin immediately)

**Treatments** include:

- Nasotracheal intubation (with fiberoptic tube if necessary) and ventilation if respiratory obstruction
- IV antibiotics, such as penicillin or clindamycin
- Referral to surgeon for incision and drainage as indicated

## Otitis Externa

Otitis externa is infection of the external ear canal, either bacterial or mycotic. Common pathogens include bacteria, *Pseudomonas aeruginosa, Staphylococcus aureus,* and fungi, *Aspergillus* and *Candida.* OE is often caused by chlorine in swimming pools killing normal flora and allowing other bacteria to multiply. Fungal infections may be associated with immune disorders, diabetes, and steroid use.

**Symptoms** include:

- Pain, swelling, and exudate
- Itching (pronounced with fungal infections)
- Red pustular lesions
- Black spots over tympanic membrane (fungus)

**Diagnosis**: On exam, tenderness when touched on tragus or when the auricle is pulled, erythema, and history.

**Treatment** includes:

- Irrigate ear with Burow's solution or saline to clean and remove debris or foreign objects.
- **Bacteria**: Antibiotic ear drops, such as ciprofloxacin and ofloxacin. If impetigo, flush with hydrogen peroxide 1:1 solution and apply mupirocin twice daily for 5-7 days. Lance pointed furuncles.
- **Fungus**: Solution of boric acid 5% in ethanol; clotrimazole-miconazole solution with/without steroid for 5-7 days.
- Analgesics as needed.

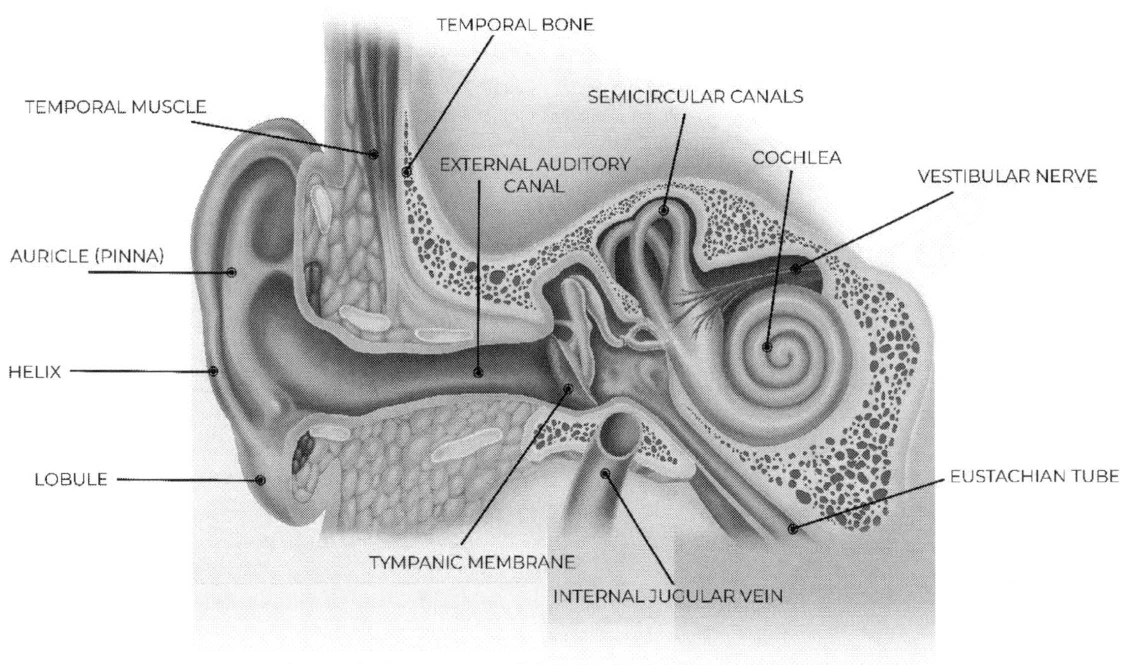


## Otitis Media

Otitis media, inflammation of the middle ear, usually follows upper respiratory tract infections or allergic rhinitis. The eustachian tube swells and prevents the passage of air. Fluid from the mucous membrane pools in the middle ear, causing infection. Common pathogens include *Streptococcus pneumoniae, Haemophilus influenzae,* and *Moraxella catarrhalis.* Some genetic conditions, such as trisomy 21 and cleft palate, may include abnormalities of the eustachian tube, increasing risk. There are four forms:

- **Acute**: 1-3 weeks with swelling, redness, and possible rupture of the tympanic membrane, fever, pain (ear pulling), and hearing loss.
- **Recurrent**: 3 episodes in 6 six months or 4-6 in 12 months.

- **Bullous**: Acute infection with ear popping pressure in middle ear, pain, hearing loss, and bullae between layers of tympanic membrane, causing bulging.
- **Chronic**: Persists at least 3 months with thick retracted tympanic membrane, hearing loss, and drainage.

**Diagnosis**: Distinguishing features on assessment of acute otitis media include a bulging or perforated tympanic membrane, signs of inflammation, or purulent fluid present.

**Treatment**: 75-90% resolve spontaneously, so antibiotics are **withheld** for 2-3 days. Amoxicillin for 7-10 days. Referral for **tympanostomy and pressure-equalizing tubes** (PET) for severe chronic or recurrent infections.

**Review Video: Otitis Media**
Visit mometrix.com/academy and enter code: 328778

## Mastoiditis

Mastoiditis usually results from extension of acute otitis media because the mucous membranes of the middle ear are continuous with the mastoid air cells in the temporal bone. All patients with otitis media should be considered at risk for mastoiditis. Patients with chronic otitis media also often develop chronic mastoiditis, which can result in formation of benign cholesteatoma. Signs and symptoms of mastoiditis include persistent fever, pain in or behind the ear (especially during the night), and hearing loss. Differential diagnoses may include Bell's palsy, otitis externa, and otitis media. **Diagnosis** is based on symptoms, CBC, audiometry, tympanocentesis or myringotomy with culture and sensitivities, and CT scan (definitive). Acute mastoiditis is treated with antibiotics, usually beginning with a 3rd generation cephalosporin or penicillin/aminoglycoside combination until culture and sensitivity results return. If spreading empyema or osteitis is present, then surgical mastoidectomy is required.

## Sinusitis

Sinusitis is inflammation of the nasal sinuses, of which there are two maxillary, two frontal, and one sphenoidal, as ethmoidal air cells. Inflammation causes obstruction of drainage with resultant discomfort.

**Symptoms** include:

- Frontal and maxillary presents with pain over sinuses
- Ethmoidal present with dull aching behind eye
- Tenderness to palpation and percussion of sinuses
- Mucosa of nasal cavity edematous and erythematous
- Purulent exudate

**Diagnosis** includes:

- Transillumination of sinus (diminished with inflammation)
- CT for those who are immunocompromised or if diagnosis is not clear
- Careful examination to rule out spreading infection, especially with signs of fever, altered mental status, or unstable vital signs

**Treatment** includes:

- Symptomatic relief with analgesia
- Topical decongestants and nasal irrigation
- Antimicrobial therapy if symptoms persist at least seven days or are severe (avoid routine use): Amoxicillin or TMP/SMX
- Steroid nasal spray twice daily

## Meniere's Disease

Meniere's disease occurs when a blockage in the endolymphatic duct of the inner ear causes dilation of the endolymphatic space and abnormal fluid balance, which causes pressure or rupture of the inner ear membrane.

**Symptoms** include:

- Progressive fluctuating sensorineural hearing loss
- Tinnitus
- Pressure in the ear
- Severe vertigo that lasts minutes to hours
- Diaphoresis
- Poor balance
- Nausea and vomiting

**Diagnosis** includes:

- Complete physical exam and evaluation of cranial nerves
- Tuning fork sounds may lateralize to unaffected ear
- Assessment of hearing loss

**Treatment**:

- Low sodium diet
- Vestibular suppressant (antihistamine): Meclizine
- Benzodiazepine or SSRI for anxiety
- Antiemetics, such as promethazine suppositories
- Diuretics, such as hydrochlorothiazide
- Referral for surgical repair for persistent vertigo, but this will not correct other symptoms

## Labyrinthitis

Labyrinthitis is a viral or bacterial inflammation of the inner ear, and it may occur secondary to bacterial otitis media. Viral labyrinthitis may be associated with mumps, rubella, rubeola, influenza, or other viral infections, such as upper respiratory tract infections. Because the labyrinth includes the vestibular system that is responsible for sensing head movement, labyrinthitis causes balance disorders. The condition often persists for 1 to 6 weeks with acute symptoms the first week and then decreasing symptoms. **Symptoms** include:

- Sudden onset of severe vertigo
- Hearing loss and sometimes tinnitus
- Nausea and vomiting
- Panic attacks from severe anxiety related to symptoms

**Treatment** includes:

- **Bacterial**: IV antibiotics
- **Viral**: Symptomatic as for bacterial (except for antibiotics)
- Volume replacement
- Antiemetics, such as promethazine suppositories
- Vestibular suppressant (antihistamine): Meclizine
- Benzodiazepine or SSRI for anxiety
- Referral to surgeon for I&D if necessary

## TMD

Temporomandibular disorder (TMD) is jaw pain caused by dysfunction of the temporomandibular joint (TMJ) and the supporting muscles and ligaments. It may be precipitated by injury, such as whiplash, or grinding or clenching of the teeth, stress, or arthritis.

**Symptoms** include:

- Clicking or popping noises on jaw movement
- Limited jaw movement or "locked" jaw
- Acute pain on chewing or moving jaw
- Headaches and dizziness
- Toothaches

**Diagnosis** includes:

- Complete dental exam with x-rays to rule out other disorders
- MRI or CT may be needed

**Treatment** usually begins conservatively:

- Ice pack to jaw area for 10 minutes followed by jaw stretching exercises and warm compress for 5 minutes 3-4 times daily
- Avoidance of heavy chewing by eating soft foods and avoiding hard foods, such as raw carrots and nuts
- NSAIDs to relieve pain and inflammation
- Night mouthguard
- Referral for dental treatments to improve bite as necessary

# Ocular

## Corneal Abrasions

Corneal abrasion results from direct scratching or scraping trauma to the eye, often involving contact lenses. This causes a defect in the epithelium of the cornea. Infection with corneal ulceration can occur with abrasions.

**Symptoms** include:

- Pain
- Intense photophobia
- Tearing

Determining the **cause and source** of the abrasion is important for treatment as organic sources pose the danger of fungal infection and soft contact lenses pose the danger of *Pseudomonas* infection.

**Diagnosis** includes:

- Topical anesthetic prior to testing for visual acuity
- Fluorescent staining and examination with cobalt blue light
- Eversion of eyelid to check for foreign body
- Examine cornea and assess anterior chamber with slit lamp

**Treatments** include:

- Cycloplegic agent to relieve spasm and pain: Cyclopentolate 1%
- Erythromycin ophthalmic ointment four times daily with or without eye patch if not related to contact lens AND without eye patch if related to organic source
- Tobramycin ophthalmic ointment four times daily without eye patch if related to contact lens

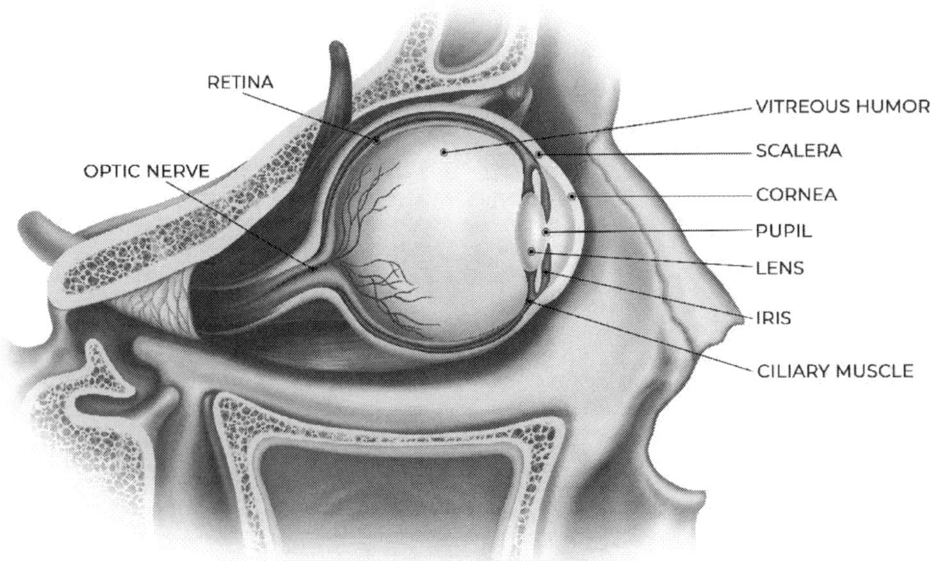


## Chemical Eye Burns

Chemical burns are caused by splashing of chemicals (solid, liquid, or fumes) into any part of the eye, often related to facial burns. Chemical burns may damage the cornea and conjunctiva, although other layers of the eye may also be damaged, depending upon the chemical and degree of saturation. Many injuries are work-related and involve alkali (greater than 7 pH), acid (less than 7 pH, such as muriatic acid or sulfuric acid), or other irritants (neutral pH) such as pepper spray. Alkali chemicals (such as ammonia, lime, and lye) usually cause the most serious injuries.

**Symptoms** include:

- Pain
- Blurring of vision
- Tearing
- Edema of eyelids

**Diagnosis** includes:

- History of event
- Eye exam showing corneal irritation

**Treatment** includes:

- Irrigation of the eye and other areas of contact with copious amounts of water or normal saline
- Litmus paper exam of eye to determine residual pH and continue irrigation until pH returns to neutral
- Cycloplegic agent to relieve spasm and pain: Cyclopentolate 1%
- Antibiotic ointment to prevent infection

## Acute Angle-Closure Glaucoma

Acute angle-closure glaucoma is a medical emergency that involves increased intraocular pressure and impairment of vision in those without history of glaucoma because of occlusion of drainage, which forces the iris forward. This condition is most common in elderly patients. **Symptoms** include eye pain (periorbital) associated with headache, nausea and vomiting, decreased visual acuity with halos, intraocular pressure greater than 21 mmHg (may be as high as 50), conjunctival injection, edema of epithelium of cornea, pupil nonreactive and mid-dilated, and shallower anterior chamber.

**Treatment** aims to reduce pressure in the eye by reducing production of aqueous humor:

- Topical beta-blocker (timolol 0.5%, one drop)
- Topical alpha-adrenergic agonist (apraclonidine 1%, one drop)
- Topical steroid (prednisolone 1%, 1 drop every 15 minutes for 1 hour and then every hour)
- Acetazolamide 500 mg IV or by mouth
- Mannitol 1-2 g/kg IV
- Pilocarpine 1-2% after pressure reduced, and before laser peripheral iridotomy, a procedure creating a hole in the iris to allow drainage of aqueous humor
- Continued monitoring of intraocular pressure every 30-60 minutes

## Infectious Conjunctivitis

Infectious conjunctivitis (pink eye) is inflammation of the conjunctiva of the eye from a bacteria or virus. Though most common in infants and children, adults are also susceptible. Infectious conjunctivitis in adults is usually caused by *Staphylococci*, *Streptococci*, *Pneumococci*, or viruses, and is extremely contagious, so diligent hand hygiene is essential.

It is difficult to differentiate between bacterial and viral infections without cultures. The patient should be kept from work for 24 hours after starting treatment or until symptoms subside:

- Red, swollen, itchy conjunctiva
- Eye pain

- Purulent discharge
- Scratchy feeling under eyelids
- Mild photophobia

Treatment is usually antibiotic drops or ointment (in the case of a bacterial source) and cool compresses, although many cases are caused by viruses and the condition often disappears without treatment in 3-5 days.

## ANTERIOR UVEITIS

Anterior uveitis (iritis) is inflammation of the iris. Iridocyclitis includes inflammation of the ciliary body in addition to the iris. Uveitis is often related to autoimmune and other disorders, such as ankylosing spondylosis, multiple sclerosis, Reiter syndrome, juvenile idiopathic arthritis, and Crohn's disease.

**Symptoms** include:

- Pain
- Photophobia with increased pain
- Reddening of eye
- Irregularly shaped pupil
- Decreased visual acuity
- Headache

The infection causes white blood cells to shed into the anterior chamber, and the numbers of these that are evident on slit lamp examination determine the degree of the disorder, graded 1 to 4 in increasing severity. Shining a bright light in the unaffected eye causes the pupil to constrict in the affected eye with an increase in pain. Applying topical anesthetic will not relieve pain.

**Treatment** includes:

- Topical steroid, such as prednisolone 1% (unless infection is also present), every 30-60 minutes during awake hours
- Cycloplegic agent to relieve spasm and pain: Cyclopentolate 1%
- Dark glasses to reduce photophobia
- Analgesia: Acetaminophen or ibuprofen

## RETINAL ARTERY OCCLUSION

Central retinal artery occlusion (CRAO) and branch retinal artery occlusion (BRAO) usually results from an embolus lodging in the central retinal artery or a branch, most commonly the temporal vessels. It is most common in elderly patients (older than 60) and is associated with hypertension and occlusion of carotid arteries.

**Symptoms** include:

- Sudden, painless vision loss on one side
- History of episodes of temporary visual deficits

**Diagnosis** includes:

- Examination with slit lamp shows whitening of retina in affected area and sometimes retinal edema. Embolus may be visible with BRAO.
- ESR to rule out temporal arteritis.
- CBC to evaluate for blood disorders and blood culture to rule out endocarditis or sepsis.
- Fluorescein angiography.

**Treatment**:

- Usually supportive without intervention.
- tPA may be used for CRAO (success limited).
- Transluminal Nd:YAG laser embolysis to clear embolus may improve vision.

## Retinal Detachment

Retinal detachment occurs when the retinal pigment epithelial (RPE) layer separates from the underlying sensory layer. There are four **types of detachment**:

- **Rhegmatogenous**: A tear occurs in the sensory retina and liquid vitreous seeps through, detaching the RPE.
- **Traction**: Bands of scar tissue provide traction that pulls on retina, usually related to diabetes, vitreous hemorrhage, or retinopathy of prematurity.
- **Exudative**: The choroid produces serous fluid under the retina, usually related to uveitis or macular degeneration.
- **Combination** of other types.

**Symptoms** include painless visual changes, such as floaters, "cobwebs," photopsia (flashes of light), shadow over vision, or loss of central vision.

**Diagnosis** includes the following:

- Assess visual acuity
- Dilated fundus exam with indirect ophthalmoscope and Goldman 3-mirror to create a detailed retinal diagram

**Treatment** generally requires a referral to retinal surgeon for surgical repair.

## Hyphema

Hyphema is the accumulation of hemorrhaging blood in the anterior chamber of the eye after an injury. It is usually caused by a projectile hitting the eye and resulting in blunt or penetrating trauma. Hyphemas are **classified** according to degree:

- **Grade 1**: Blood (layered) occupies less than one-third of chamber
- **Grade 2**: Blood (filling) occupies one-third to one-half of chamber
- **Grade 3**: Blood (layered) occupies more than one-half of chamber
- **Grade 4**: Clotted blood occupies total chamber

**Symptoms** in addition to bleeding include:

- **Increased intraocular pressure** greater than 22 mmHg initially (in about one-third of patients) followed by reduction in two to six days for those with less than three-fourths filling of chamber. Those with more than three-fourths of complete filling of chamber may have continued increase in intraocular pressure.
- **Secondary hemorrhage** may occur, especially in children and African American patients.

**Treatments** include:

- Patch and shield for injured eye
- Tylenol for analgesia (NSAIDs should be avoided)
- Topical steroids

- Systemic aminocaproic acid to prevent secondary hemorrhage
- Anti-glaucoma topical medications, such brimonidine, for increased IOP

## Penetrating or Blunt Ocular Trauma with Ruptured Globe

Penetrating or blunt ocular trauma with resultant ruptured globe (full-thickness injury to cornea or sclera) can occur from many things, such as pellets, BBs, knife wounds, gunshot wounds, and other projectiles. Sports injuries are common. Blunt trauma usually has better outcomes than penetrating. If injury is suspected, get a complete history of injury and examine the eye carefully with a slit lamp.

**Symptoms** include:

- Laceration of eyelid
- Shallow anterior chamber
- Pain varies in intensity, but may be severe
- Decreased visual acuity
- Irregularity of pupil, especially teardrop shaped
- Hyphema
- Difficulty viewing optic nerve on exam

**Diagnostic** studies include:

- Careful eye examination
- Tetanus toxoid or tetanus immune globulin as needed
- Waters view x-ray to confirm foreign body OR
- CT scan, MRI, or ultrasound to confirm rupture

**Treatment** after ruptured globe is diagnosed or suspected:

- Do NOT check IOP
- Place metal eye shield over eye for protection
- Administer cephalosporin
- Refer to ophthalmologist for surgical repair

## Laceration of the Eyelid

The eyelids are thin and provide little protection of the ocular globe from blunt or penetrating trauma, so **eyelid lacerations** should prompt complete and careful eye examination for injuries or foreign bodies prior to repair. The eyelid comprises five layers:

- Skin
- Subcutaneous tissue
- Muscle (orbicularis oculi) that controls closure of the lid and forms the medial and lateral canthus
- Tarsal plate
- Conjunctiva

Usually only **superficial horizontal lacerations** are sutured in the ED. More serious injuries should be referred to ophthalmologists or ocular plastic surgeons.

**Treatment** includes:

- Local anesthesia (supra- or infraorbital).
- Wound irrigation with NS prior to suturing.

- Suturing with 6-0 or 7-0 coated or plain nylon suture (to be removed in 3-5 days), using care to avoid suturing into globe.
- Ophthalmic topical antibiotic in place of dressing.

## Orbital Fractures

Orbital fractures most often occur with blunt force against the globe causing a rupture through the floor of the orbital bone or a direct blow to the orbital rim, often related to an assault. Injuries are most common in adolescents and young adults.

While often asymptomatic, **symptoms** may include:

- Ecchymosis and edema of eyelid
- Infraorbital anesthesia from pressure or damage to infraorbital nerve
- Decrease sensation of cheek and upper gum on injured side
- Diplopia
- Enophthalmos (sunken globe)

**Diagnosis** includes:

- Complete eye (slit lamp) and vision examination
- IOP measurement
- CT scan

**Treatment** is usually supportive and includes the following:

- Topical steroids for severe edema
- Patient advised not to blow nose for several weeks
- Surgical repair about two weeks after injury when edema has subsided for extensive fracture (at least 33% of orbital floor) or enophthalmos greater than 2 mm remaining 10-14 days post-injury

## Zygomatic Fractures

Zygomatic fracture involves the arch of bone that forms the lateral border of the eye orbit and the bony cheek prominence, most commonly associated with a blow to the lateral cheek from an altercation or accident. Fracture can result in a tilting of the eye and flattening of the cheek, which may be obscured by initial edema. Fracture may be only of the arch or may be a more extensive tripod fracture of the infraorbital rim, diastasis of the zygomaticofrontal suture, and disruption of the zygomaticotemporal arch junction. **Diagnosis** is by CT scan, which shows the extent of the fracture as well as the amount of displacement.

**Treatment** for tripod fracture is referral to surgeon for open reduction with fixation and exploration and reconstruction of orbit as needed.

## Keratitis

Keratitis is inflammation of the cornea, and it may be superficial or deep, which usually results in scarring. The multiple causes for keratitis include bacterial, fungal, viral, and parasitic infections, as well as allergic response to antigens and photokeratitis from exposure to ultraviolet rays. It can also arise from wearing contact lenses. Any corneal ulceration can allow pathogens to enter the eye and cause infection.

**Symptoms** include:

- Pain and tearing
- Photophobia
- Decreased visual acuity
- Discharge

**Diagnosis** includes:

- Careful examination with slit lamp
- Culture of discharge

**Treatment** includes the following:

- Antifungal or antibacterial drops as indicated
- Trifluridine every 2-3 hours during awake hours to maximum of 9 drops daily for herpes simplex until healing and then 4 times daily for about 1 week
- Artificial tears
- Analgesia

### *Ultraviolet Keratitis*

Ultraviolet keratitis results from injury to the corneal epithelium from exposure to ultraviolet rays from the sun (as in snow blindness where the snow reflects UV rays into the eyes) or from artificial light sources, such as tanning beds, halogen lights, or welding torches (flash burn).

**Symptoms** usually occur six to 12 hours after exposure:

- Pain
- Tearing
- Photophobia
- Decreased visual acuity
- Spasm of eyelids
- Exam shows punctate irregularities of corneal surface and corneal haze

An accurate history that details exposure to UV rays should be done.

**Diagnostic studies** include:

- Examination of eye and lids
- Slit lamp exam with fluorescein staining

**Treatment** includes:

- Cycloplegic agent to relieve spasm and pain: cyclopentolate 1%
- Antibiotic ophthalmic ointment, such as erythromycin
- Analgesia: Opiate (oxycodone) and NSAIDs (ibuprofen 600 mg 4 times daily)
- Topical NSAIDs are sometimes used

Healing should be evident within 24-48 hours.

# Environment and Toxicology Emergencies, and Communicable Diseases

## Environment

### Fluid Resuscitation for Burn Injuries

Burn victims are at risk for hypovolemia and electrolyte imbalances because of loss of body fluids through burned areas. **Fluid resuscitation** is indicated with burns of 20% or more of total body surface area (TBSA) burned. Lactated Ringers IV solution is used instead of NS, which can lead to hypernatremia and hyperchloremia. The Parkland/Baxter formula is used to calculate the volume of LR solution needed:

$$24 \text{ hour volume} = (\text{body weight [kg]}) \times (\text{TBSA burned [\%]}) \times (4 \text{ mL})$$

Example—70 kg adult with 36% TBSA burned:

$$24 \text{ hour volume} = 70 \times 36 \times 4 \text{ mL} = 10{,}080 \text{ mL}$$

Half of the volume is administered over the first 8 hours and half over the next 16 hours. Using the preceding example, this patient will receive 5,040 mL each over the first 8 hours (rate = (5040/8) = 630 mL/hr), and over the following 16 hours (rate = (5040/16) = 315 mL/hr). Fluid intake should be sufficient to produce 30-50 mL of urine per hour. In the second 24 hours, fluid volume should be 1.5-2.0 times the normal maintenance values with crystalloid with appropriate electrolyte balance.

### Burn Injuries

#### *Types and Classifications*

Burn injuries may be chemical, electrical, or thermal, and are assessed by the area, percentage of the body burned, and depth:

- **First-degree burns** are superficial and affect the epidermis, causing erythema and pain.
- **Second-degree burns** extend through the dermis (partial thickness), resulting in blistering and sloughing of epidermis.
- **Third-degree burns** affect underlying tissue, including vasculature, muscles, and nerves (full thickness).

Burns are classified according to the **American Burn Association's criteria**:

- **Minor**: Less than 10% body surface area (BSA). 2% BSA with third degree without serious risk to face, hands, feet, or perineum.
- **Moderate**: 10-20% combined second- and third-degree burns (children younger than 10 years or adults older than 40 years). 10% or less full thickness without serious risk to face, hands, feet, or perineum.
- **Major**: 20% BSA; at least 10% third-degree burns. All burns to face, hands, feet, or perineum that will result in functional/cosmetic defect. Burns with inhalation or other major trauma.

### Systemic Complications

Burn injuries begin with the skin but can affect all organs and body systems, especially with a major burn:

- **Cardiovascular**: Cardiac output may fall by 50% as capillary permeability increases with vasodilation and fluid leaks from the tissues.
- **Urinary**: Decreased blood flow causes kidneys to increase ADH, which increases oliguria. BUN and creatinine levels increase. Cell destruction may block tubules, and hematuria may result from hemolysis.
- **Pulmonary**: Injury may result from smoke inhalation or (rarely) aspiration of hot liquid. Pulmonary injury is a leading cause of death from burns and is classified according to the degree of damage:
  - *First*: Singed eyebrows and nasal hairs with possible soot in airways and slight edema
  - *Second*: (At 24 hours) Stridor, dyspnea, and tachypnea with edema and erythema of upper airway, including area of vocal cords and epiglottis
  - *Third*: (At 72 hours) Worsening symptoms if not intubated and if intubated, bronchorrhea and tachypnea with edematous, secreting tissue
- **Neurological**: Encephalopathy may develop from lack of oxygen, decreased blood volume and sepsis. Hallucinations, alterations in consciousness, seizures, and coma may result.
- **Gastrointestinal**: Ileus and ulcerations of mucosa often result from poor circulation. Ileus usually clears within 48-72 hours, but if it returns it is often indicative of sepsis.
- **Endocrine/metabolic:** The sympathetic nervous system stimulates the adrenals to release epinephrine and norepinephrine to increase cardiac output and cortisol for wound healing. The metabolic rate increases markedly. Electrolyte loss occurs with fluid loss from exposed tissue, especially phosphorus, calcium, and sodium, with an increase in potassium levels. Electrolyte imbalance can be life-threatening if burns cover >20% of BSA. Glycogen depletion occurs within 12-24 hours and protein breakdown and muscle wasting occurs without sufficient intake of protein.

### Management

Management of burn injuries must include both wound care and systemic care to avoid complications that can be life threatening. **Treatment** includes:

- Establishment of airway and treatment for inhalation injury as indicated:
  - Supplemental oxygen, incentive spirometry, nasotracheal suctioning
  - Humidification
  - Bronchoscopy as needed to evaluate bronchospasm and edema
  - β-Agonists for bronchospasm, followed by aminophylline if ineffective
  - Intubation and ventilation if there are indications of respiratory failure (This should be done prior to failure. Tracheostomy may be done if ventilation >14 days.)
- Intravenous fluids and electrolytes, based on weight and extent of burn. Parkland formula: Fluid replacement (mL) in first 24 hours = (mass in kg) × (body % burned) × 400
- Enteral feedings, usually with small lumen feeding tube into the duodenum
- NG tube for gastric decompression to prevent aspiration
- Indwelling catheter to monitor urinary output. Urinary output should be 0.5-2 mL/kg/hr
- Analgesia for reduction of pain and anxiety
- Topical and systemic antibiotics
- Wound care with removal of eschar and dressings as indicated

## Chemical Burns

Chemical burns may result from contact with acid or alkali substances. The pH scale ranges from 0 to 14 with 7 being neutral, 0 being extremely acidic, and 14 being extremely alkaline. Alkali burns tend to be more severe because acid burns denature proteins, resulting in formation of eschar that prevents deeper penetration of the acid. Alkaline burns, however, both denature proteins and hydrolyze fats, allowing for deeper penetration and tissue damage because of liquefaction necrosis. Hydrofluoric acid is similar to alkaline substances in that it also causes liquefaction necrosis. Symptoms vary depending on the substance, strength, and site of injury but often includes severe pain, tissue blistering and sloughing, and bleeding. Initial treatment includes removal of contaminated clothing and copious wound irrigation with water. If substances contain Na, K, Mg, or metallic lithium, then the burn area should be covered with mineral oil rather than irrigated. If hydrofluoric acid, copious water irrigations and soft-tissue injection or IV infusion of calcium gluconate may help reduce pain and tissue destruction. Patients may need fluid resuscitation and skin grafting. Complications include disfigurement, infection, and electrolyte imbalance.

### Electrical Burns

Electrical injuries result from electricity passing through the body from contact with live wires, lighting strikes, and short-circuiting equipment. Injuries may be high voltage (≥1000 volts) or low voltage (<1000 volts). Electrical injuries can result in extensive subdermal burns. The injury severity correlates with resistance of tissue and current amperage (AC usually causes more damage than DC). Tissue with the highest degree of resistance tends to suffer the most damage with low voltage injury, but high voltage injury can destroy all tissue. Tissue resistance (highest to lowest) include bone >fat >tendons >skin >muscles >vessels > nerves.

- **Low voltage** injuries may cause cardiac dysrhythmias (VF), external burns, tissue damage, fractures and dislocations from muscle contractions, respiratory arrest, or oral burns (children particularly). Treatment includes monitoring and cardiac care as needed, topical antimicrobials, and excision and grafting if necessary.
- **High voltage** injuries may result in additional symptoms of myonecrosis, thrombosis, compartment syndrome, nerve entrapment syndrome. Treatment may include fluid resuscitation, wound debridement, fasciotomy, and amputation, topical antibiotics, systemic antibiotics, and analgesia.

### Thermal Burns

Thermal burns are caused by heat (hot iron, stove, sun exposure) or fire. Burn injuries begin with the skin but can affect all organs and body systems, especially with a major burn. Management of burn injuries must include both wound care and systemic care to avoid complications that can be life threatening. Patients may experience open blistering wounds and severe pain. **Treatment** varies according to severity and may include:

- Establishment of airway and treatment for inhalation injury if necessary
- Cleansing of burned areas, flushing
- Debridement of open blisters (no needle aspiration)
- Tetanus immunization if needed
- Intravenous fluids and electrolytes, based on weight and extent of burn
- Enteral feedings, usually with small lumen feeding tube into the duodenum
- NG tube for gastric decompression to prevent aspiration
- Indwelling catheter to monitor urinary output. Urinary output should be 0.5-2 mL/kg/hr
- Analgesia for reduction of pain and anxiety
- Topical (usually silver sulfadiazine) and systemic antibiotics
- Wound care with removal of eschar and dressings as indicated
- Skin grafting

**Complications** include scarring, disfigurement, contractures, and infection.

### Radiation Injuries

Radiation injuries may be caused by direct radiation in which waves pass through the body (locally or to the entire body), which can result in acute radiation illness and genetic damage. **Contamination** usually occurs from radioactive dust or liquid contacting the skin. It can be absorbed into the tissues (eventually causing chronic illnesses, such as cancer) or contaminate others who contact it. Contaminated material may also be ingested. The lethal dose of 50% of those exposed within 60 days (LD50/60) is 4.5 Gy with immediate intensive treatment.

**Diagnosis** for direct radiation is symptomatic as there is no specific test; however, contamination can be measured by Geiger counter.

Syndromes of **acute radiation sickness** vary according to exposure:

- **Hematopoietic**: (at least 2 Gy exposure) affects blood cell production. 2-12 hours after exposure: anorexia, nausea, vomiting, lethargy. Symptom-free week during which blood cell production decreases causing decreased WBC and platelet count, resulting in infection and hemorrhage with weakness and dyspnea. Recovery begins in 4-5 weeks if patient survives.
- **GI**: (at least 4 Gy exposure)
  - 2-12 hours after exposure: nausea, vomiting, diarrhea, dehydration. 4-5 days, fewer symptoms but lining of GI tract sheds, leaving ulcerated tissue.
  - Severe diarrhea (bloody) and dehydration and systemic infections
- **Cerebrovascular**: (20-30 Gy exposure) always fatal
  - Alterations in mental status, nausea, vomiting, and diarrhea (bloody), progressing to shock, seizures, coma, and death

**Treatment** includes:

- Decontamination if contamination irradiation or if source of irradiation not clear
- Complete history of event, including source of radiation
- Protocol for decontamination and securing of area should be followed, including use of individual dosimeters and protective coverings
- **Localized**: burn care and analgesia
- **Internal**: gastric decontamination, collection of urine and feces for 4 days to monitor rate of radioisotopes excretion, and collection of body fluids for bioassay
- **Whole body irradiation**: supportive treatment and prophylactic measures to combat opportunistic infections, hematopoietic growth factor for bone marrow depression

## Heat-Related Illness

Children and the elderly are particularly vulnerable to heat-related illness, especially when heat is combined with humidity. Heat-related illnesses occur when heat accumulation in the body outpaces dissipation, resulting in increased temperature and dehydration, which can then lead to thermoregulatory failure and multiple organ dysfunction syndromes. Each year in the United States, about 29 children die from heat stroke after being left in automobiles. At temperatures of 72-96 °F, the temperature in a car rises 3.2 °F every 5 minutes, with 80% of rise within 30 minutes. Temperatures can reach 117 °F even on cool days. There are three **types of heat-related illness**:

- **Heat stress**: Increased temperature causes dehydration. Patient may develop swelling of hands and feet, itching of skin, sunburn, heat syncope (pale moist skin, hypotension), heat cramps, and heat tetany (respiratory alkalosis). Treatment includes removing from heat, cooling, hydrating, and replacing sodium.
- **Heat exhaustion**: Involves water or sodium depletion, with sodium depletion common in patients who are not acclimated to heat. Heat exhaustion can result in flu-like aching, nausea and vomiting, headaches, dizziness, and hypotension with cold, clammy skin and diaphoresis. Temperature may be normal or elevated to less than 106 °F. Treatment to cool the body and replace sodium and fluids must be prompt in order to prevent heat stroke. Careful monitoring is important and reactions may be delayed.

- **Heat stroke**: Involves failure of the thermoregulatory system with temperatures that may be more than 106 °F and can result in seizures, neurological damage, multiple organ failures, and death. Exertional heat stroke often occurs in young athletes who engage in strenuous activities in high heat. Young children are susceptible to nonexertional heat stroke from exposure to high heat. Treatment includes evaporative cooling, rehydration, and supportive treatment according to organ involvement.

## Hypothermia

Hypothermia occurs with exposure to low temperatures that cause the core body temperature to fall below 95 °F (35 °C). Hypothermia may be associated with immersion in cold water, exposure to cold temperature, metabolic disorders (hypothyroidism, hypoglycemia, hypoadrenalism), or CNS abnormalities (head trauma, Wernicke disease). Many patients with hypothermia are intoxicated with alcohol or drugs.

**Symptoms** of hypothermia include pallor, cold skin, drowsiness, alterations in mental status, confusion, and severe shivering. The patient can progress to shock, coma, dysrhythmias (T-wave inversion and prolongation of PR, QRS, and QT) including atrial fibrillation and AV block, and cardiac arrest.

**Diagnosis** requires low-reading thermometers to verify temperature.

**Treatment** includes:

- Passive rewarming if cardiac status stable
- Active rewarming (external) with immersion in warm water or heating blankets at 40 °C, radiant heat
- Active rewarming (internal) with warm humidified oxygen or air inhalation, heated IV fluids, and internal (bladder, peritoneal pleural, GI) lavage
- Warming with extracorporeal circuit, such as arteriovenous or venovenous shunt that warms the blood
- Supportive treatment as indicated

## Localized Cold Injuries

Frostnip is a superficial freeze injury that is reversible. Frostbite is damage to tissue caused by exposure to freezing temperatures, most often affecting the nose, ears, and distal extremities. As frostbite develops, the affected part feels numb and aches or throbs, becoming hard and insensate as the tissue freezes, resulting in circulatory impairment, necrosis of tissue, and gangrene. There are **three zones of injury:**

- **Coagulation** (usually distal): severe, irreversible cellular damage
- **Hyperemia** (usually proximal): minimal cellular damage
- **Stasis** (between other 2 zones): severe but sometimes reversible damage

**Symptoms** vary according to the degree of freezing:

- **Partial freezing** with erythema and mild edema, stinging, burning, throbbing pain
- **Full-thickness freezing** with increased edema in 3-4 hours, edema and clear blisters in 6-24 hours, desquamation with eschar formation, numbness, and then aching and throbbing pain
- Prognosis is very good for **first-degree** and good for **second-degree** frostbite
- Full-thickness and into **subdermal tissue** freezing with cyanosis, hemorrhagic blisters, skin necrosis, and "wooden" feeling, severe burning, throbbing, and shooting pains
- Freezing extends into **subcutaneous tissue**, including muscles, tendons, and bones with mottled appearance, non-blanching cyanosis, and eventual deep black eschar

Prognosis is poor for **third-degree** and **fourth-degree** freeze injuries. Determining the degree of injury can be difficult because some degree of thawing may have occurred prior to admission to the hospital.

**Treatment** includes:

- Rapid rewarming with warm water bath (40-42 °C [104-107.6 °F]) 10-30 minutes or until the frostbitten area is erythematous and pliable
- Treatment for generalized hypothermia

Treatment **after warming**:

- Debridement of clear blisters but not hemorrhagic blisters
- Aloe vera cream every 6 hours to blistered areas
- Dressings, separating digits
- Tetanus prophylaxis
- Ibuprofen 12 mg/kg daily in divided doses
- Antibiotic prophylaxis if indicated (penicillin G 500,000 units IV every 6 hours for 24 to 72 hours)

## Animal Bites

**Animal bites,** including human, are frequent causes of traumatic injury. There is not a single preferred topical therapy for traumatic wounds because they vary so widely in the type and degree of injury.

**General treatment** includes:

- **Cleanse** wound by flushing with 10 to 35 cc syringe with 18-gauge Angiocath to remove debris and bacteria using normal saline or diluted Betadine solution.
- Hand, puncture, and infected wounds or those more than 12 hours old may be closed by **secondary intention**.
- **Moisture-retentive dressings** are used as indicated by the size and extent of the wound left open. Dry dressings may be applied to injuries with closure by primary intention.
- **Topical antibiotics** may be indicated, although systemic antibiotics are commonly prescribed for animal bites.
- **Tetanus toxoid** or **immune globulin** is routinely administered.

## Spider Bites

Spider bites are frequently a misdiagnosis of a *Staphylococcus aureus* or MRSA infection, so unless the spider was observed, the wound should be cultured and antibiotics started. If the wound responds to the antibiotic, then it probably was not a spider bite. There are two main types of venomous spider bites:

- Those producing **neurological symptoms** (black widow).
- Those producing **local necrosis** (brown recluse, yellow sac, and hobo spiders).

**General treatment** includes:

- Cleanse wound, apply cool compress, and elevate body part if possible.

**Treatment for black widow bites**:

- Narcotic analgesics.
- Nitroprusside to relieve hypertension.
- Calcium gluconate 10% solution IV for abdominal cramps.
- Antivenin *Latrodectus mactans* for those with severe reaction.

**Treatment for necrotic/ulcerated bites** (e.g., brown recluse):

- There is no consensus on the best treatment, as ulceration caused by the venom may be extensive and **surgical repair** with grafts may be needed.
- Necrotic ulcers should be treated **moisture-retentive dressings** as indicated, and monitored for complications.
- **Hyperbaric oxygen therapy** (HBOT) has been used in some cases.

## SNAKE BITES

About 45,000 snake bites occur in the United States each year, with about 8,000 from poisonous snakes. In the United States, about 25 species of snakes are venomous. There are two types of snakes that can cause serious injury, classified according to the type of fangs and venom.

### *CORAL SNAKES*

Coral snakes have short fixed permanent fangs in the upper jaw and venom that is primarily neurotoxic, but may also have hemotoxic and cardiotoxic properties:

- Wounds show no fang marks but there may be scratches or semi-circular markings from the teeth.
- There may be little local reaction, but neurological symptoms may range from mild to acute respiratory and cardiovascular failure.

Treatment includes the following:

- Cleanse the wound thoroughly of dirt and debris and either leave it open to air or cover it with a dry dressing.
- Administer antivenin immediately even without symptoms, which may be delayed.
- Administer tetanus toxoid or immune globulin.
- Antibiotics are not usually indicated.

### *PIT VIPERS*

A second type of snake that can cause serious injury is the pit viper**.** Pit vipers (**rattlesnakes, copperheads, and cottonmouths)** have erectile fangs that fold until they are aroused, and venom is primarily hemotoxic and cytotoxic but may also have neurotoxic properties:

- Wounds usually show one or two fang marks.
- Edema may begin immediately or may be delayed up to six hours.
- Pain may be severe.
- There may be a wide range of symptoms, including hypotension and coagulopathy with defibrination that can lead to excessive blood loss, depending upon the type and amount of venom.
- There may be local infection and necrosis.

Treatment includes the following:

- Cleanse the wound thoroughly and apply dressings as indicated.
- Administer tetanus toxoid or immune globulin.
- Administer analgesics, such as morphine sulphate, as needed.
- Avoid NSAIDs and aspirin because of anticoagulation properties.
- Mark edema every 15 minutes.
- Administer antivenin therapy if indicated. Observe for serum sickness if horse serum used.
- Administer prophylactic antibiotics for severe tissue necrosis.
- Administer platelets, plasma, or packed RBCs for coagulopathy.

## Shark Bites

Even small shark bites can crush bones. Hit and run attacks may cause small lacerations or minimal damage, but other types of attacks can result in loss of limbs or large chunks of flesh, with loss of muscle and bone. Internal organs may be exposed and damaged. Extensive soft tissue trauma and damage to arteries and veins may occur, as well as crushing internal injuries. The wounds are often contaminated with sand, algae, fragments of shark teeth, and other materials and pathogens, such as *Mycobacterium marinum* and *Vibrio spp.* Life-threatening injuries need to be addressed first, including control of hemorrhage:

- Administer IV fluids and blood products.
- Administer tetanus toxoid or tetanus immune globulin.
- Wounds must be flushed with copious amounts of normal saline and debris removed.
- Treat for hypothermia if needed.
- X-rays are ordered to identify fractures or debris in wound.
- Fixation of fractures.
- Administer prophylactic antibiotics:
  - Ciprofloxacin
  - Trimethoprim-sulfamethoxazole
  - Doxycycline
- Surgical repair, debridement, and/or skin grafting if indicated.

## Alligator Bites

Alligators are found in ten coastal states in the southeastern United States with the largest population in Florida, where most injuries are reported. Animals between four and eight feet often bite once and release, but larger animals may bite repeatedly, engaging in typical biting and feeding activities, which result in severe injury, amputations, or death. Most wounds involve the limbs, with the hands and arms the most frequently bitten.

**Treatment** includes:

- Treat for shock and blood loss.
- Apply pressure to wound.
- Retrieve amputated limbs if possible.
- Flush wound(s) with copious amounts of normal saline to reduce contamination.
- Collect wound cultures.
- Administer prophylactic broad-spectrum antibiotics for gram-negative organisms, such as *Aeromonas hydrophila* and *Clostridium.*
- Observe for signs of infection, such as erythema, cellulitis, exudate, and necrosis.
- Administer tetanus toxoid or immune globulin.
- Repair fractures.
- Surgical repair and debridement as indicated, with wounds usually healing by secondary intention or delayed primary closure.

## Stingray Stings

Stingrays can induce injury when their tail is thrust forward, driving serrated spines into the victim, resulting in a jagged laceration. The spines of the stingray tail contain a venom that is injected upon impact, causing severe pain. The resulting wounds often become infected.

**Symptoms** include:

- Intense, excruciating pain with envenomation lasting two to three days.
- Bleeding.
- Systemic symptoms: Dizziness, GI upset, seizures, hypotension.

**Treatment** includes the following:

- **Rinse** the wound with fresh water or saline and remove visible pieces of spine with forceps or tweezers.
- **Heat immersion**: Deactivate the venom and relieve pain by immersing the wound in hot water for 30 to 90 minutes at 110-115°F (45°C). May repeat up to 2 hours.
- **Radiographs** may be necessary to locate the spine or fragment.
- Administer tetanus toxoid or tetanus immune globulin.
- Inject the wound with a **local anesthetic**, such as lidocaine or bupivacaine, to relieve severe pain.
- Administer **opiates** for pain.
- **Open wounds** are usually allowed to heal without primary closure or with loose primary closure.
- **Prophylactic antibiotics** may be given for five days to prevent infections.

## Insect Stings and Bites

### *Bee Stings*

Bees and wasps sting by puncturing the skin with a hollow stinger and injecting venom. Wasps and bumblebees can sting more than once but honeybees have barbs on their stingers, and the barbs embed the stinger into the skin. **Local reactions** to bee sting include the following:

- Raised white **wheal** with central red spot of about 10 mm appearing within a few minutes and lasting 20 minutes (honeybees).
- **Edema and erythema**, which may last several days (vespid wasps).
- Pain, swelling, and redness confined to sting site.
- Swelling may extend **beyond the sting site** and may, for example, involve swelling of an entire limb.

Some people may develop an anaphylactic reaction, including a **biphasic reaction**, in which the symptoms recede and then return two to three hours later. About 50% of deaths occur within 30 minutes of the sting, and 75% within four hours.

**Symptoms** of an allergic reaction/anaphylaxis may become increasingly severe with generalized urticaria, edema, hypotension, and respiratory distress.

**Treatment** of bee stings initially includes the following:

- Wash the site with soap and water.
- Remove stinger using 4 x 4 inch gauze wiped over the area or by scraping a sharp instrument over the area.
- NEVER squeeze the stinger or use tweezers, as this will cause more venom to go into the skin.
- Apply ice to reduce the swelling (10 to 20 minutes on, 10 to 20 minutes off, for 24 hours).
- Antihistamines may be prescribed.
- A paste of baking soda and water or meat tenderizer and water may reduce itching.
- Topical corticosteroids may relieve itching.
- Administer tetanus toxoid or tetanus immune globulin as needed.

**Allergic responses/anaphylaxis** requires immediate, aggressive medical intervention:

- Administer epinephrine.
- Administer antihistamines.
- Administer corticosteroids.
- Administer IV fluids as needed.
- Provide oxygen and other supportive treatments.

People with extensive local or anaphylactic reactions should be advised to carry an epinephrine autoinjector for emergency use if stung.

## *Scorpion Stings*

### Symptoms

- Note: Children <6 are most at risk of death from severe reactions. Symptoms vary widely depending on individual reaction and amount of venom.
- **Local (most common):** Neurotoxic effects include itching, redness, edema, and ascending hyperesthesia. Tap test: Paresthesia worsens if area tapped.
- **Cytotoxic effects** include development of macule or papule within an hour. Purpuric plaque becomes necrotic and ulcerates and venom spreads through the lymph system.
- **Nonlethal response** includes pain, induration, redness, and wheal.
- **Neurologic**: Severe wide-ranging symptoms include strokes, altered consciousness, muscle rigidity, paralysis, and seizures.
- **Multiple organ:** Can include hypertension, tachycardia, respiratory distress, generalized allergic response, dysphagia, hepatitis, priapism, acute tubular necrosis, DIC, hyperglycemia, lactic acidosis.

### Treatment

- Note: Meperidine and morphine may potentiate symptoms.
- Hospital admission for 24 hours unless symptoms very mild.
- Cool compresses, acetaminophen, topical anesthetics for pain.
- Tetanus toxoid or tetanus immune globulin as needed.
- Antivenom (available only for Centruroides).
- Complex supportive care may include intubation and ventilation.

## *Fire Ant Bites*

### Symptoms

- Note: Multiple bites, sometimes hundreds, are common. Deaths are rare but do occur if children have a severe systemic reaction or bites about the head and neck.
- **Local reaction:** A severely itching wheal develops and subsides in 30–60 minutes, followed by a blister within 4 hours. The blister fills with milky dead tissue in 8 to 24 hours with redness at base and severe itching and burning. The blister ruptures and crusts over within 72 hours but redness pain and itching may persist for days.
- **Systemic reaction**: Edema, urticaria, nausea, vomiting, bronchospasm, dyspnea, slurred speech, anaphylaxis.

### Treatment

- **Local reaction**: Cold compresses, weak bleach solution (within 15 minutes of bites), or topical anesthetic for pain. Cleanse with soap and water without breaking blisters. NSAIDS for pain. Topical corticosteroids for itching. Antihistamines. Tetanus toxoid or tetanus immune globulin as needed.
- **Systemic reaction**: As for anaphylaxis, depending on degree of symptoms, including epinephrine.

## Human Bites

Human "bites" occur when the teeth of one person injure another. This is not uncommon in contact sports. Intentional biting is common among children but usually presents mild injury. Human bites may also be the result of altercations and are referred to as "fist-bites." There are 3 common **types** of fist-bites:

- Closed fist bite resulting in small wound on the metacarpophalangeal joint of the middle finger. Bacteria enter the wound when the person extends the fingers, carrying bacteria to the extensor tendons, which can result in infection.
- Finger bite in which a finger may be partially or completely severed
- Puncture bite, usually on the face, from contact with another person's tooth

Immediate treatment of bites includes applying pressure to stop bleeding and then thoroughly flushing the wound with dilute Betadine, dilute peroxide, or normal saline solution. Protective dressings should be applied. Large wounds or those with skin flaps or signs of more serious tissue injury may require surgical repair.

# Toxicology

## Toxic Exposures

### *Carbon Monoxide Poisoning*

Carbon monoxide (CO) poisoning occurs with inhalation of fossil fuel exhausts from engines, emission of gas or coal heaters, indoor use of charcoal, and smoke and fumes. The CO binds with hemoglobin, preventing oxygen carriage and impairing oxygen delivery to tissue.

**Diagnosis** includes history, on-site oximetry reports, neurological examination, and CO neuropsychological screening battery (CONSB) done with patient breathing room air, CBC, electrolytes, ABGs, ECG, chest radiograph (for dyspnea); *pulse oximetry is not accurate in these patients.*

**Symptoms:**

- Cardiac: chest pain, palpitations, decreased capillary refill, hypotension, and cardiac arrest
- CNS: malaise, nausea, vomiting, lethargy, stroke, coma, and seizure
- Secondary injuries: Rhabdomyolysis, AKI, non-cardiogenic pulmonary edema, multiple organ failure (MOF), DIC, and encephalopathy

**Treatment** includes:

- Immediate support of airway, breathing, and circulation
- Non-barometric oxygen (100%) by non-breathing mask with reservoir or ETT if necessary
- Mild: Continue oxygen for 4 hours with reassessment
- Severe: hyperbaric oxygen therapy (usually 3 treatments) to improve oxygen delivery

### *Cyanide Poisoning*

Cyanide poisoning, from hydrogen cyanide (HCN) or cyanide salts, can result from sodium nitroprusside infusions, inhalation of burning plastics, intentional or accidental ingestion or dermal exposure, occupation exposure, ingestion of some plant products, and the manufacture of PCP. Inhalation of HCN causes immediate symptoms, and the ingestion of cyanide salts causes symptoms within minutes.

**Diagnosis** is by history, clinical examination, normal $PaO_2$ and metabolic acidosis.

**Symptoms:** Increase in severity and alter with the amount of exposure: tachycardia, hypertension, leading to bradycardia, hypotension, and cardiac arrest. Pink or cherry-colored skin because of oxygen remaining in the blood. Other symptoms include headaches, lethargy, seizures, coma, dyspnea, tachypnea, and respiratory arrest.

**Treatment** includes:

- Supportive care as indicated
- Removal of contaminated clothes
- Gastric decontamination
- Copious irrigation for topical exposure
- Antidotes:
  - Amyl nitrate ampule cracked and inhaled 30 seconds
  - Sodium nitrite (3%) 10 mL IV
  - Sodium thiosulfate (25%) 50 mL IV

### Caustic Ingestions

Caustic ingestions of acids (pH <7) such as sulfuric, acetic, hydrochloric, and hydrofluoric found in many cleaning agents and alkalis (pH >7) such as sodium hydroxide, potassium hydroxide, sodium tripolyphosphate (in detergents) and sodium hypochlorite (bleach) can result in severe injury and death. Acids cause coagulation necrosis in the esophagus and stomach and may result in metabolic acidosis, hemolysis, and renal failure if systemically absorbed. Alkali injuries cause liquefaction necrosis, resulting in deeper ulcerations, often of the esophagus, but may involve perforation and abdominal necrosis with multi-organ damage.

**Diagnosis** is by detailed history, airway examination (oral intubation if possible), arterial blood gas, electrolytes, CBC, hepatic and coagulation tests, radiograph, and CT for perforations.

**Symptoms** may vary but can include pain, dyspnea, oral burns, dysphonia, and vomiting.

**Treatment** includes:

- Supportive and symptomatic therapy
- NO ipecac, charcoal, neutralization, or dilution
- NG tube for acids only to aspirate residual
- Endoscopy in first few hours to evaluate injury/perforations
- Sodium bicarbonate for pH <7.10
- Prednisolone (alkali injuries)

### Allergic Reactions

Exposure to certain toxins, medications, illegal substances, and allergens can cause life threatening effects in some patients. The physiologic response of the patient is dependent on the agent and the degree of exposure. Tissue hypoperfusion and lactic acidosis often occur as a result of the exposure. This can lead to metabolic acidosis, shock, organ failure, and death.

**Signs and symptoms**: In allergic type reactions, urticaria, pruritus, chest, back or abdominal pain, facial flushing, shortness of breath, wheezing and stridor may occur. Beta- and alpha-adrenergic responses may occur with exposure to amphetamines, cocaine, ephedrine, and pseudoephedrine. This response is manifested by diaphoresis, hypertension, tachycardia, and mydriasis. Diarrhea, nausea, and vomiting can occur with exposure to certain toxins.

**Diagnosis**: Physical assessment and testing to discover the toxin, drug, or allergen the patient was exposed to. Labs—blood gases, BMP, complete blood count, toxicology screen, urinalysis, and allergy testing.

**Treatment**: Priority is to eliminate exposure to the drug/toxin/allergen. Antidotes (if available) may be administered in the case of toxin exposure. Activated charcoal may be administered in the case of medication/drug overdose. For allergic reactions, antihistamines and corticosteroids may be administered. Severe allergic reactions may need to be treated with epinephrine. Dialysis may be indicated in some patients. Sodium bicarbonate may be administered for the treatment of metabolic acidosis caused by many toxic reactions.

### Acetaminophen Toxicity

Acetaminophen toxicity from accidental or intentional overdose has high rates of morbidity and mortality unless promptly treated. **Diagnosis** is by history and acetaminophen level, which should be completed within 8 hours of ingestion if possible. Toxicity occurs with dosage >140 mg/kg in one dose or >7.5g in 24 hours.

**Symptoms** occur in stages:

1. (Initial) Minor gastrointestinal upset
2. (Days 2-3) Hepatotoxicity with RUQ pain and increased AST, ALT, and bilirubin

3. (Days 3-4) Hepatic failure with metabolic acidosis, coagulopathy, renal failure, encephalopathy, nausea, vomiting, and possible death
4. (Days 5-12) Recovery period for survivors

**Treatment** includes:

- GI decontamination with activated charcoal (orally or NG) <24 hours
- Toxicity is plotted on the Rumack-Matthew nomogram with serum levels >150 requiring antidote. The antidote is most effective ≤8 hours of ingestion but decreases hepatotoxicity even >24 hours.
- Antidote: 72-hour N-acetylcysteine (NAC) protocol includes 140 mg/kg initially and 70 mg/kg every 4 hours for 17 more doses (orally or IV)
- Supportive therapy: Continuous dialysis, fluids, blood pressure medications

### *Amphetamine and Cocaine Toxicity*

Amphetamine toxicity may be caused by IV, inhalation, or insufflation of various substances that include methamphetamine (MDA or "ecstasy"), methylphenidate (Ritalin), methylenedioxymethamphetamine (MDMA), and ephedrine and phenylpropanolamine. Cocaine may be ingested orally, IV or by insufflation while crack cocaine may be smoked. Amphetamines and cocaine are CNS stimulants that can cause multi-system abnormalities.

**Symptoms** may include chest pain, dysrhythmias, myocardial ischemia, MI, seizures, intracranial infarctions, hypertension, dystonia, repetitive movements, unilateral blindness, lethargy, rhabdomyolysis with acute kidney failure, perforated nasal septum (cocaine), and paranoid psychosis (amphetamines). Crack cocaine may cause pulmonary hemorrhage, asthma, pulmonary edema, barotrauma, and pneumothorax. Swallowing packs of cocaine can cause intestinal ischemia, colitis, necrosis, and perforation. **Diagnosis** includes clinical findings, CBC, chemistry panel, toxicology screening, ECG, and radiography.

**Treatment** includes:

- Gastric emptying (<1 hour). Charcoal administration
- IV access. Supplemental oxygen
- Sedation for seizures: Lorazepam 2 mg, diazepam 5 mg IV titrated in repeated doses
- Agitation: Haloperidol
- Hypertension: Nitroprusside/nicardipine, phentolamine IV
- Cocaine quinidine-like effects: Sodium bicarbonate

### *Salicylate Toxicity*

Salicylate toxicity may be acute or chronic and is caused by ingestion of OTC drugs containing salicylates, such as ASA, Pepto-Bismol, and products used in hot inhalers.

**Diagnosis** is by ferric chloride or Ames Phenistix tests. Symptoms vary according to age and amount of ingestion. Co-ingestion of sedatives may alter symptoms.

**Symptoms** include:

- <150 mg/kg: Nausea and vomiting
- 150-300 mg/kg: Vomiting, hyperpnea, diaphoresis, tinnitus, and alterations in acid-base balance
- >300 mg/kg (usually intentional overdose): Nausea, vomiting, diaphoresis, tinnitus, hyperventilation, respiratory alkalosis, and metabolic acidosis
- Chronic toxicity results in hyperventilation, tremor, and papilledema, alterations in mental status, pulmonary edema, seizures, and coma

**Treatment** includes:

- Gastric decontamination with lavage (≤1 hour) and charcoal
- Volume replacement (D5W)
- Sodium bicarbonate 1-2 mEq/kg
- Monitoring of salicylate concentration, acid-base, and electrolytes every hour
- Whole-bowel irrigation (sustained release tablets)

### *Benzodiazepine Toxicity*

Benzodiazepine toxicity may result from accidental or intentional overdose with such drugs as Xanax, Librium, Valium, Ativan, Serax, Versed, and Restoril. Mortality is usually the result of co-ingestion of other drugs.

**Diagnosis** is based on history and clinical exam, as benzodiazepine level does not correlate well with toxicity.

**Symptoms:** Non-specific neurological changes: Lethargy, dizziness, alterations in consciousness, and ataxia. Respiratory depression and hypotension are rare complications. Coma and severe central nervous depression are usually caused by co-ingestions.

**Treatment** includes:

- Gastric emptying (<1 hour)
- Charcoal
- Concentrated dextrose, thiamine, and naloxone if co-ingestions suspected, especially with altered mental status
- Monitoring for CNS/respiratory depression
- Supportive care
- Flumazenil (antagonist) 0.2 mg each minute to total 3 mg may be used in some cases but not routinely advised because of complications related to benzodiazepine dependency or co-ingestion of cyclic antidepressants. Flumazenil is contraindicated in patients with increased ICP.

### *Ethanol Overdose*

Ethanol overdose affects the central nervous system as well as other organs in the body. Alcohol is an inhibitory neurotransmitter that depresses the central nervous system. In most states, the legal intoxication blood alcohol level is defined as 100 mg/dL. Blood alcohol levels of **500 mg/dL or greater** are associated with a high mortality rate. The central nervous system depressant effect is further enhanced when alcohol is mixed with other agents.

Ethanol is absorbed through the mucosa of the mouth, stomach, and intestines, with concentrations peaking about 30-60 minutes after ingestion. If people are easily aroused, they can usually safely sleep off the effects of ingesting too much alcohol, but if the person is semi-conscious or unconscious, emergency medical treatment should be initiated.

**Symptoms** include:

- Altered mental status with slurred speech and stupor
- Nausea and vomiting
- Hypotension
- Bradycardia with arrhythmias
- Respiratory depression and hypoxia
- Cold, clammy skin or flushed skin (from vasodilation)
- Acute pancreatitis with abdominal pain
- Lack of consciousness
- Circulatory collapse

**Treatment** includes:

- Careful monitoring of arterial blood gases and oxygen saturation
- Ensure patent airway with intubation and ventilation if necessary
- Intravenous fluids
- Dextrose to correct hypoglycemia if indicated
- Maintain body temperature (warming blanket)
- Dialysis may be necessary in severe cases

### *Gastric Emptying for Toxic Substance Ingestion*

Gastric emptying for toxic substance ingestion should be done ≤60 minutes of ingestion for large life-threatening amounts of poison. The patient requires IV access, oximetry, and cardiac monitoring. Sedation (1-2 mg IV midazolam) or rapid sequence induction and endotracheal intubation may be necessary. Patients should be positioned in left lateral decubitus position with head down at 20° to prevent passage of stomach contents into duodenum, although intubated patients may be lavaged in the supine position. With a bite block in place, an orogastric Y-tube (36-40 Fr. for adults) should be inserted after estimating length. Placement should be confirmed with injection of 50 mL of air confirmed under auscultation and aspiration of gastric contents, as well as abdominal x-ray (pH may not be reliable depending on substance ingested). Irrigation is done by gravity instillation of about 200-300 mL warmed (45 °C) tap water or NS. The instillation side is clamped and drainage side opened. This is repeated until fluid returns clear. A slurry of charcoal is then instilled, and the tube is clamped and removed when procedures completed.

## Hazardous Materials

Hazardous materials, those that are ignitable, corrosive, reactive, or toxic, are any that are harmful to humans or the environment and may be solids, liquids, solid gases, or sludges. Hazardous wastes are generally transported by hazardous waste transporters in special hazardous waste containers to Treatment Storage and Disposal Facilities (TSDFs) where they are stored, inactivated, and/or recycled. Each facility should have a plan in place for appropriate **handling of hazardous materials**:

- Staff must be trained in safe handling of hazardous materials with training repeated at least annually.
- Appropriate personal protective equipment (PPE) should be available for staff members handling hazardous materials.
- Hazardous materials should be clearly labeled for easy identification.
- All hazardous materials must be safely and securely stored in appropriate environmental temperatures and conditions.
- Safety Data Sheets (SDS) must be readily available for all hazardous materials.
- Decontamination procedures must be reviewed and appropriate decontamination facilities (such as eyewash stations and showers) must be available.
- Records must be maintained for any accidental exposures (with or without injury) and reported to the appropriate authorities.

### *Biohazard Symbol*

### Biological/Biohazardous Waste

Biological wastes are those that contain or are contaminated with pathogens (human, plant, animal); rDNA; and blood, cell, or tissue products; and cultures. Biological wastes that are, or may, be infectious or rDNA contaminated (biohazardous waste) must be inactivated before disposal in hazardous waste containers. Typically, inactivation is carried out with autoclaving or treating with hypochlorite solution (bleach). Contaminated sharps must be maintained in special sharps containers to avoid injury to handlers, and inactivated before disposal. Non-infectious biological wastes, such as uncontaminated gloves, do not require deactivation and are disposed of in biological waste containers.

### Routes Biological Hazards May Take to Enter the Body

Biological hazards may **enter the body** through the following avenues:

- Airborne (through the nasal passage into the lungs)
- Ingestion (eating/drinking)
- Subcutaneous (broken skin/open wounds)
- Percutaneous (through intact skin)
- Mucosal (through the lining of the mouth and nose)

### Cleaning up Small Blood Spills

The best way to clean a small blood spill is to absorb the blood with a paper towel or gauze pad. Then disinfect the area with a disinfectant. Soap and water are not considered a disinfectant nor is alcohol. Never scrape a dry spill; this may cause an aerosol of infectious organisms. If blood is dried, use the disinfectant to moisten the dried blood.

### Internal Radiation Therapy

Internal radiation therapy **(brachytherapy)** may be utilized to treat a variety of cancers, including prostate, breast, and cervical cancer. Radiation implants may be permanent or temporary. Temporary implants may have high-dose radiation (HDR) or low-dose radiation (LDR). Systemic brachytherapy may be administered per IV with radioactive isotopes; intraluminal and intracavity, per catheters or tubes; and interstitial, per seeds, needles, small implants, or wires. Symptoms relate to the area being irradiated, but the skin and GI tract are usually the most sensitive. Bone marrow suppression may occur if the source of radiation is near bone marrow, and patients may experience fatigue and weakness. Because patients emit radiation during therapy, safeguards include:

- Specific limitations and safeguards posted at room by x-ray department outlining requirements, such as time limits for contact time
- Visitors limited to non-pregnant adults who must be 6 feet from the patient and remain in room no longer than 30 minutes each day
- Staff, limited to those who are non-pregnant, wear dosimeters for contact with patient
- Patient placed in private room
- Staff limit time in room to only that necessary to carry out care (in accordance with posted guidelines)

# Communicable Disease

## VIRAL INFECTIONS

### *HERPES SIMPLEX VIRUS INFECTIONS*

There are 2 types of the herpes simplex virus (HSV), human herpesvirus 1 and 2. **HSV-1** usually causes a **gingivostomatitis** (often referred to as "cold sores" or "fever blisters") and is transmitted through **close contact**. **HSV-2** usually causes painful **genital lesions** through **sexual contact**. Either may be found in other areas of the body.

- **Incubation** period is around 2-12 days.
- The primary infection is usually more severe (causes systemic **symptoms**) than the reactivated infection, but it may be asymptomatic. After the primary infection, the virus remains dormant in the nerve ganglia, and can be reactivated especially during times of stress, illness, immunosuppression, or sun exposure. While patients are most contagious during times of active lesions, the disease may be spread while asymptomatic. The frequency of the outbreaks usually decreases over time.
- HSV **lesions** are grouped vesicles with an erythematous base. They are usually painful, and a prodrome of tingling, pain, or burning sensations may be felt hours to a couple days before the eruption. Lesions last for approximately 2-3 weeks in primary infection (up to 4 weeks with genital HSV), and 1-2 weeks in recurrent infections.
- HSV is **diagnosed** clinically and confirmed with a + culture, PCR test, or HSV antibody tests (HSV-1 or HSV-2: IgM= active or recent infection; IgG= previous infection).
- Symptomatic **treatment**, proper wound care, and antivirals (acyclovir, valacyclovir, or famciclovir) may be given.
- **Complications** include perinatal infection, keratitis, herpetic whitlow, herpes gladiatorum, secondary infections, and encephalitis.

### *EPSTEIN-BARR INFECTION*

Epstein-Barr virus (EBV) is a **herpesvirus** (human herpesvirus 4) and is responsible for causing **infectious mononucleosis**. After the initial infection, it remains latent in B cells and epithelial cells. It has been linked to certain epithelial and lymphatic neoplasms (e.g., nasopharyngeal carcinoma, Burkitt lymphoma, Hodgkin lymphoma).

- EBV is **transmitted** through **body fluids** like saliva, so it is sometimes referred to as the kissing disease. It is most common in teenagers and college-age young adults
- **Incubation** period is typically 30-50 days.
- **Symptoms** of EBV infection range from being asymptomatic to swollen painful lymph nodes, pharyngitis (can mimic strep pharyngitis), extreme fatigue, fever, and possibly hepatosplenomegaly. The WBC count is elevated (~10,000-20,000 cells/mL) with 10-30% atypical lymphocytes in the differential.
- Confirm **diagnosis** with a Mono Spot test or EBV antibody serology tests.
- **Treatment** is supportive, and antibiotics are not helpful in treating this viral infection. Therefore, avoid unnecessary antibiotics in those with EBV, especially since administration of ampicillin or amoxicillin is often associated with a pruritic, maculopapular rash. Analgesics, warm salt water gargles, increased fluid intake, and rest will help to relieve some of the symptoms. Symptoms may last for several weeks and fatigue may last even longer. Patients should avoid contact sports for up to 2 months.
- **Complications** include hepatitis, cytopenias (e.g., thrombocytopenia), Guillain Barré syndrome, and splenic rupture.

### MEASLES, MUMPS, AND RUBELLA

**Measles (rubeola) virus** is highly contagious, is spread through **respiratory secretions** (incubation is 7-14 days), and peaks in late winter to spring. It causes a prodrome of high fever (4-7 days), cough, congestion, conjunctivitis; then Koplik spots (pathognomonic), and finally a maculopapular rash (spreads cephalocaudally). Report suspected cases immediately to the health dept. **Diagnose** with a + IgM antibody test (collected after 3 days of rash), viral culture, or PCR. **Treatment** is supportive.

**Mumps (parotitis)** is a viral infection that is spread via **saliva** (incubation is 12-24 days), and often occurs during winter and spring. It causes painful swelling of the salivary glands (parotid). Report to health dept. Supportive **treatment**. Complications include orchitis (infertility), pancreatitis, and meningitis.

**Rubella (German measles)** is a virus that spreads via **respiratory droplets** (incubation is 2-3 weeks), and peaks in the spring. There is a mild prodrome (fever, aches, sore throat, conjunctivitis, swollen nodes [esp. suboccipital, postauricular, & posterior cervical]), then a maculopapular rash (face first, then down). Report to health dept. Confirm with rubella antibodies IgM or IgG. Symptomatic care.

### INFLUENZA

Influenza is a highly contagious viral infection that affects the entire **respiratory system** from the nose to the lungs. There are 3 types of **influenza virus**: **A** (causes epidemics), **B** (only in humans), and **C**. Types A and B are seen most often and are the strains that the annual flu vaccine is most effective against; and type C is not as common and much less severe.

- Prevention is key and annual, age-appropriate influenza **vaccines** should be given to those ≥6 months; 2 vaccines are required in first-time vaccine patients if 6 mo. through 8-year-olds (separated by 28 days).
- **Incubation** period is 1-4 days and it is spread via respiratory droplets.
- Though **symptoms** can be very similar, the flu and the common cold differ in that the flu has a very sudden onset. Symptoms of influenza include a high fever (may last up to 5 days), headache, myalgias, dry cough, rhinorrhea, and fatigue. There may also be vomiting and diarrhea, although children are more prone to this.
- Clinical judgement, community patterns, and rapid influenza tests (high specificity, but lower sensitivity) aid in **diagnosis**, but RT-PCR or viral culture definitively confirm the diagnosis; pulse oximetry and CXR as needed for pulmonary issues.
- Antibiotic **treatment** is not effective unless there is a secondary bacterial infection (e.g., pneumonia). Look for signs of secondary infections (e.g., dyspnea, cyanosis, fever that goes away and returns, confusion/lethargy). Supportive treatment with rest, fluids, and analgesics. Antivirals should be considered in those who are at high risk (<5 years old, elderly, pregnant, chronic conditions). These are most effective if initiated within 24-48 hours of symptom onset. The neuraminidase inhibitors (oseltamivir, zanamivir) treat type A, type B, and avian H5N1. There is extensive resistance to the adamantanes (amantadine, rimantadine) so they are rarely used.
- **Complications** include pneumonia, ARDS, and death.

### CORONAVIRUS

A coronavirus is a common virus that causes cold-like symptoms, including a cough, runny nose, sore throat, and congestion. Most cases of coronavirus are not dangerous and are often given little attention or go entirely unnoticed. However, specific coronavirus strains have led to two worldwide pandemics. The first, **severe acute respiratory syndrome (SARS)**, appeared in China in 2002 and quickly spread worldwide. Presenting symptoms of SARS were fever, cough, dyspnea, and general malaise. It was extremely virulent, spreading easily from person to person through close contact by way of contaminated droplets produced by coughing or sneezing. SARS was also very deadly, with a case fatality rate of nearly 10%. High rates of infection occurred in health care workers and others in contact with infected patients, so prompt diagnosis and proper isolation were essential. By 2004, there were no longer any documented active cases of SARS.

The most recent coronavirus outbreak was the **COVID-19** strain, which first appeared in December of 2019, in the Chinese city of Wuhan, and quickly became a global pandemic. Presentation of COVID-19 was similar to that of SARS, with the notable additional symptom of acute loss of taste/smell as a unique identifier. Much is still unknown about this strain, including exact transmission methods (though droplet transmission is suspected), effective treatment protocols, and long-term effects.

**Precautions** to take when treating patients with pandemic coronavirus include the following:

- Contact and droplet precautions, including eye protection and appropriate personal protection equipment.
- Airborne precautions (recommended by the CDC), especially with aerosol-producing procedures (ventilators, nebulizers, intubation).
- Immediate notification of public health authorities and institution of contact tracing.
- Activity restrictions of exposed health care workers planned in coordination with public health officials.

### *Cytomegalovirus*

Cytomegalovirus (CMV) is a herpes virus, occurring in most people by the time they are adults.

- **Transmission** can occur through secretions during personal contact and from mother to baby before, during or after birth.
- Most cases have no **symptoms**, although a few infants will have fetal damage, such as jaundice, hepatitis, brain damage, or growth retardation.
- **Treatment** for those with severe infections is with ganciclovir, an antiviral drug.

### *Respiratory Syncytial Virus*

Respiratory syncytial virus (RSV) is a virus that infects the respiratory tract, causing symptoms of nasal congestion, cough, sore throat, and headache. Severe cases can lead to high fever, breathing difficulties, severe cough, and cyanosis.

- Respiratory syncytial virus may **manifest** as a cold in adults and older children; however, there are some children who are more at risk of developing complications.
- **Transmission** is through contact with droplets from an infected person's nose or throat, generally through coughing and sneezing.
- Infants born prematurely, children with chronic lung disease, children with cystic fibrosis, and children who are in an immunocompromised state because of surgery or illness are at **high risk** of breathing difficulties, poor oxygenation, and even death from RSV.

### *Fifth Disease*

Fifth disease, or **erythema infectiosum**, is a viral illness caused by parvovirus B19. It is most prevalent in the spring, with outbreaks in preschools, daycares, and elementary schools.

- The **incubation** period is 4-20 days, and it may be communicable for several days before the rash appears.
- **Transmission** occurs through oral and nasal secretions and possibly blood.
- **Symptoms** are possible fever, headache, nasal congestion, general unwell feeling, and rash starting on the cheeks (slapped cheek appearance). The rash typically spreads to the rest of the body as a lacy red rash that may come and go for up to a month.
- Use over-the-counter fever medications as needed and provide **supportive care**.
- The virus can cause fetal death if contracted during pregnancy. There is no vaccine for fifth disease, and because it is a viral infection, it is not treated with antibiotics.

### *CHICKENPOX*

Chickenpox (Varicella) is a viral infection, most prevalent in the late winter and early spring in children under 10 years of age.

- It has an **incubation** period of 10-21 days and is communicable from 1-2 days before the rash appears to after all lesions have dried up.
- **Transmission** is through direct contact and contact with respiratory droplets.
- **Symptoms** are low fever and feeling unwell, followed by the itchy rash (raised red bumps that develop vesicles which then ooze and crust over).
- The patient should be isolated until all lesions are dry. Aveeno baths and Benadryl help with the itching. Ibuprofen or acetaminophen can be used for the fever, and acyclovir is indicated in some cases. Encourage the patient not to scratch the lesions to prevent secondary infections. Provide supportive care as indicated.

### *ROSEOLA*

Roseola is a viral illness, most prevalent in children 6-24 months of age.

- The **incubation** period is about 9 days.
- **Transmission** may be through oral and nasal.
- The illness begins with a high fever for 3-5 days; the patient appears well otherwise. The fever drops and then the rash appears. The rash is a light pink maculopapular rash which lasts 1-2 days.
- Parents should **treat the fever** as needed with anti-inflammatory medications.

### *POLIOMYELITIS*

Poliomyelitis (commonly referred to as **polio**) is caused by an enterovirus and occurs most often in babies and young children.

- The **incubation** period is 3-14 days, and transmission occurs through direct contact with respiratory secretions and the oral-fecal route.
- The **symptoms** are slight fever, sore throat, general malaise, nausea and vomiting, headache, stomach ache, and constipation, but there can be severe pain, muscular weakness, and then paralysis.
- There are no drug therapies for polio. Observe for respiratory distress, provide general support measures, and provide for physical therapy.

### *ROTAVIRUS*

Rotavirus is a viral illness that causes diarrhea, fever, and vomiting in children.

- It can be extremely **contagious** within groups where large numbers of children are present, such as in daycare centers, preschools, pediatric offices, clinics, and children's units in hospitals.
- Rotavirus can be prevented through **immunization** with a vaccine, as recommended by the American Academy of Pediatrics. Immunization can prevent up to 98% of severe cases of the illness.
- Children should wash their hands before eating and after using the bathroom to avoid spreading the disease. Caregivers should wash their hands before preparing food, after changing diapers, and after using the bathroom; they should avoid letting small children place toys or other items in their mouths and should disinfect surfaces after use.

## Bacterial Infections

### Diphtheria

Diphtheria, caused by ***Corynebacterium diphtheriae***, is most prevalent in fall and winter.

- The **incubation** period is 2-7 days, possibly longer, and transmission is through direct contact with nasal, eye, and oral secretions.
- The **symptoms** are slight fever, nasal discharge, sore throat, feeling unwell, poor appetite, and swelling of the airway.
- If the disease is severe, death can result. The patient requires isolation, bed rest, fluids, antibiotics, medication for fever, and an antitoxin. The patient may also require oxygen therapy and tracheostomy if the airway is obstructed.

### Tetanus

Tetanus, caused by ***Clostridium tetani***, occurs all over the world. The spores formed by the bacillus are present in soil, dust, and the GI tracts of animals and humans.

- The **incubation** period is 3-21 days.
- **Symptoms** start with headache, irritability, jaw muscle spasms, and inability to open the mouth. This is followed by severe back muscle spasms, seizures, incontinence, and fever.
- **Treatment** requires human tetanus immune globulin, penicillin G, Valium, and placement on a ventilator. The environment should be kept quiet because the spasms are initiated by stimuli.

### Scarlet Fever

Scarlet fever, caused by **group A beta-hemolytic streptococci**, is most prevalent in school-age children during the fall, winter, and spring.

- The **incubation** period is 1-7 days, and transmission occurs through direct or indirect contact with oral and nasal secretions.
- The illness begins with a high fever, very sore throat, headache, malaise, chills and possibly vomiting and stomach pain. A rash appears in about 12 hours as sandpapery red pinpoints in creases of the skin, flushed face and then a strawberry tongue.
- Antibiotics will be prescribed, but patients should be isolated until taking the antibiotic for 24 hours. Analgesics are needed to bring down the fever and the patient should be encouraged to drink plenty of fluids.

### Whooping Cough

Whooping cough, caused by ***Bordetella pertussis*** **bacillus**, is most prevalent in infants and children who were not immunized.

- The **incubation** period is 6-20 days, and transmission occurs through direct contact with oral and nasal secretions.
- The **symptoms** are cold symptoms for 1-2 weeks, when the cough will worsen and progress to a whoop sound, usually occurring at night. Vomiting will usually follow an episode of intense coughing. As the patient recovers, the coughing will subside. In babies, a mucus plug or apnea can result in death by respiratory arrest. Hospitalization is usually required for infants less than 6 months of age and those with a severe case of pertussis.
- The patient needs isolation and bed rest, with a calm, quiet environment to limit coughing spells. Fluid intake needs to be monitored and humidified air will help.
- Watch for signs of respiratory distress and give antibiotic and pertussis immune globulin as prescribed.

### *Impetigo*

Impetigo is a skin infection that is most commonly seen in preschool children or those in young childhood.

- Impetigo causes blister-like sores on skin areas that may already be compromised, such as under the nose, on the hands or neck, or in the diaper area. It is caused by a bacterial infection, most commonly *Staphylococcus aureus* or group A *Streptococcus*. The sores may itch or the patient may already have irritation at the site, such as a diaper rash.
- To **prevent the spread of infection**, children and caregivers should wash their hands frequently and avoid scratching the sores and then touching items. Isolation by staying home from school or daycare may be necessary until the sores have crusted over. Treating skin irritations, such as poison ivy or eczema, can also prevent infection from spreading to impetigo.

## Fungal Infections

### *Cryptococcosis*

Cryptococcosis is an infection resulting from inhaling the **fungus** *Cryptococcus neoformans,* which is found worldwide in soil (can be associated with bird droppings), or *Cryptococcus gattii,* which is associated with certain trees in the Northwest.

- Cryptococcosis is most often due to *C. neoformans.* It is often found among those with compromised immune systems and is an **AIDS-defining opportunistic infection**.
- Healthy patients may be asymptomatic and the only finding may be pulmonary lesions on CXR that resolve spontaneously. The fungus can disseminate and cause meningitis, encephalitis, cutaneous lesions, and affect long bones and other tissues. **Symptoms** are based on the area of involvement. Patients may experience cough, pleuritic chest pain, weight loss, and fever if there is pulmonary involvement; headache, double vision, light sensitivity, N/V, and confusion if CNS involvement; cutaneous lesions (papules, pustules, nodules, ulcers) if the skin is involved.
- **Diagnosis** includes microscopic analysis, culture (gold standard), or an antigen test (highly sensitive; good for detecting early infection) for *Cryptococcus* using CSF, tissue, sputum, blood, or urine. Check CSF by India ink (limited sensitivity) or culture so meningitis can be ruled out. Confirm that no mass lesion is present by CT or MRI before LP is performed.
- Mild cases may only require monitoring to ensure that the infection does not spread. In more advanced cases, the infection is treated with different antifungal medications (e.g., fluconazole for pulmonary infections, amphotericin B ± flucytosine for meningitis). The patient should also be monitored for CNS infection and medication side effects. AIDS patients may need lifelong antifungals.
- **Complications** include cryptococcal meningitis, neural deficits, optic nerve damage, and hydrocephalus.

### *Histoplasmosis*

Histoplasmosis is an infection caused by inhalation of **spores** from the fungus *Histoplasma capsulatum* that is found in soil and is associated with bird and bat droppings (e.g., chicken coops, caves).

- Healthy patients are usually asymptomatic and those with symptoms are typically immunocompromised or those who've had a heavy exposure to spores. The primary **pulmonary infection** occurs 3-17 days after exposure and can present with flu-like symptoms. It is typically self-limited but may become chronic. Histoplasmosis can also spread through the **blood** and can cause progressive disseminated disease in the immunocompromised (high mortality rate); this is an **AIDS-defining illness**.
- **Diagnose** through antigen tests (urine, serum), histopathology, or cultures; order a CXR. Mild and even moderate acute pulmonary histoplasmosis may resolve on its own.
- If needed, **treat** mild to moderate infections with itraconazole and severe illness with amphotericin B.

### *Pneumocystis*

Pneumocystis jiroveci is a **fungus** (previously known as *Pneumocystis* carinii) that causes **pneumonia** (PJP, previously PCP) in the immunocompromised. Most people have been exposed to this by the age of 3 or 4.

- **Symptoms** of PJP include a dry nonproductive cough, fever, dyspnea, and weight loss.
- CXR may show diffuse bilateral infiltrates or it may be normal; and pulse oximetry may be low, especially on exertion. **Diagnosis** is confirmed with sputum histopathology using sputum induction or bronchoalveolar lavage.
- **Treat** immediately with TMP-SMX (trimethoprim/sulfamethoxazole) for 21 days if HIV + and for 14 days in other cases. Steroids may be added for HIV patients with severe PJP. HIV/AIDS patients with CD4 counts <200/μL should receive PJP prophylaxis with TMP-SMX. Dapsone and pentamidine are alternatives.
- **Complications** include ARDS and death.

### *Candidal Infections*

*Candida* is a type of yeast that may cause a variety of infections:

- **Oral thrush** is commonly seen in diabetic patients and those who are immunosuppressed (HIV or underlying neoplasm). Patients often complain of burning on the tongue or in the mouth, associated with "curd-like" white patches that can be scraped away leaving reddish tissue underneath. Diagnosis is with KOH prep. Treatment is with oral or topical antifungals, including nystatin (swish and swallow or troches).
- **Candida esophagitis** also occurs in the immunosuppressed population, and patients may complain of dysphasia, odynophagia, and chest pain. This is diagnosed on EGD and may be treated with oral or IV antifungals (ketoconazole).
- **Candidal intertrigo**, or diaper rash, presents with beefy-red lesions at skin fold areas as well as satellite lesions. Treatment is with topical antifungals.
- **Candidemia** is diagnosed with fungal blood cultures and may lead to osteomyelitis, endocarditis, and other complications. Treatment is with IV antifungals.

### *Ringworm*

Ringworm is caused by an infection from the ***Tinea* fungus**, which produces patches on the skin that have normal centers, giving the appearance of a ring.

- The fungus can cause hair loss and patches of scaly skin that may develop blisters that ooze or crust.
- It is **transmitted** by touching the affected skin or through objects that have touched the affected skin.
- Ringworm may be **diagnosed** by viewing the skin section under a Wood's lamp. Skin cultures may also be taken for examination to identify the fungus. A potassium hydroxide (KOH) exam involves scraping the affected skin and placing the skin sample in KOH to test for the presence of the fungus.

## Vector-Borne and Parasitic Infections

### *Malaria*

Malaria is a **blood-borne disease** caused by a **parasite** from the genus *Plasmodium and* found in tropical areas. There are 4 known to cause disease in humans (*P. malariae*, *P. vivax*, *P. ovale*, and *P. falciparum*). These protozoa are transmitted by the **female *Anopheles* mosquito**. They travel to the **liver** where they multiply, are released, and then infect the RBCs, where they continue to multiply. Incubation time can be as little as 9 days or as much as multiple years depending on the species of the infecting parasite.

- **Signs and symptoms** include headache, high fever with shaking chills and sweating (rigors; occurs when merozoites, an immature form of the parasite, are released from RBCs), jaundice, anemia, and hepatosplenomegaly. Take a thorough history including recent travel.

- **Diagnose** with 3 thin and thick blood smears (gold standard) stained with Giemsa (preferred) and obtained 12-24 hours apart. Labs typically show elevated LDH, thrombocytopenia, and atypical lymphocytes. Rapid antigen tests are also available as well as PCR.
- **Treat** with chloroquine. If travelling, chemoprophylaxis depends on the area of travel due to species and resistance patterns, and may include chloroquine, primaquine, mefloquine, Malarone, or doxycycline. Report infections to your local or state health department.
- **Complications** include severe anemia and hemolysis, organ failure (liver, spleen, kidneys), cerebral malaria, ARDS, and death.

### LYME DISEASE

Lyme disease occurs from a bite from a **deer tick** (blacklegged tick) infected with the **spirochete bacterium** *Borrelia burgdorferi*. It is the most common tick-borne disease in the U.S. and is more prevalent in heavily wooded areas. Adult ticks are more active during colder times whereas the nymphs (<2 mm in size) are more active in the warm, spring or summer months. Once the tick bites, it stays attached; however, it takes about 36-48 hours for nymphs and about 48-72 hours for adult ticks before the spirochete is transmitted to the person. **Incubation** period is 3-30 days. There are 3 stages to this disease: early localized, early disseminated, and chronic disseminated.

- At **Stage 1**, 75% have the characteristic expanding red rash (erythema migrans; can be large, ~30cm) which can progress to have central clearing (bull's eye), headache, fever, chills, myalgias, and fatigue.
- **Stage 2** occurs weeks to months after initial infection and involves systemic symptoms (flu-like), neck stiffness, headaches, migrating pain in muscles and joints, rashes, paresthesias, Bell's palsy, confusion, fatigue, myocarditis, and heart palpitations.
- **Stage 3** occurs months to years after initial infection and involves neurologic (e.g., encephalitis) and rheumatologic issues, especially arthritis of large joints (e.g., knee).

#### DIAGNOSIS AND TREATMENT OF LYME DISEASE

Diagnose Lyme disease using 2-tiered testing: antibodies (IgM, IgG), then Western blot. Antibiotic treatment for localized Lyme disease involves 2-3 weeks of doxycycline, amoxicillin, or cefuroxime axetil is started immediately after diagnosis. IV antibiotics may be needed for severe disease (e.g., IV ceftriaxone). Prevention is key by wearing clothes covering the skin, using tick repellents, showering soon after being outdoors in tick-prone areas, and thoroughly checking for ticks (especially in hard to see areas by using a mirror). The Lyme vaccine is no longer available and previous vaccine recipients are still at risk of contracting the disease as protection decreases over time. Complications are prevalent with untreated Lyme disease and include chronic arthritis, fatigue, chronic musculoskeletal issues, acrodermatitis chronica atrophicans, and memory and concentration issues. Report cases to the local health dept.

### ROCKY MOUNTAIN SPOTTED FEVER

Rocky Mountain spotted fever is a tick-borne illness caused by **Rickettsia rickettsii**. It tends to occur in spring and summer throughout the United States.

- **Incubation** period is about one week.
- **Symptoms** include headache, fever, nausea, vomiting, loss of appetite, muscle pain, and rash on the ankles and wrists.
- **Treatment** requires an antibiotic, usually Vibramycin.

### *Zika Virus in Pregnant Women*

Zika virus is a **flavivirus** that is transmitted by the *Aedes* mosquito and through sexual contact. This virus can be passed on to an unborn baby causing severe congenital defects while causing mild or no disease in the mother. It is advised that all pregnant women avoid traveling to areas with the Zika virus (e.g., Central and South America, Mexico, Caribbean, Africa).

- **Incubation** period is 3-14 days and symptoms may last 4-7 days. The virus has been found to remain longer in semen than in other body fluids.
- If **symptoms** are present, they may include fever, headache, myalgias, arthralgias, a maculopapular rash, and conjunctivitis. Congenital defects include severe microcephaly, severe brain abnormalities, macular scarring, hearing loss, motor disabilities (e.g., hypertonia), and contractures. Women should be screened for Zika exposure at each prenatal visit.
- **Diagnostic** testing is recommended for all asymptomatic pregnant women who have continued exposure to Zika and for all symptomatic pregnant women who have possibly been exposed to the Zika virus. Testing includes RNA NAT testing on serum and urine, and serum IgM Zika antibody testing. Prenatal ultrasound helps determine if the effects of Zika are present. Report cases to the state health department; and the CDC can be consulted.
- There is **no treatment** or cure for the Zika virus.

### *Helminth Infestations*

Helminth infestations (worms) include **roundworms** [nematodes: *Ascaris*, hookworms (cause anemia), **filariae** (cause elephantiasis)] and **flatworms** [tapeworms (cause weight loss); **flukes** (intestinal or liver)]. **Pinworms** are a type of roundworm that cause enterobiasis and is the most common helminth infestation. Pinworms are more prevalent in warmer areas of the country and infestations occur more frequently in children. The worms lay eggs within the digestive tract and then travel to the anal area where they are usually found. Pinworms are highly contagious. As a patient itches the anal area where the eggs are located, the eggs cling to the fingers and can easily be transmitted to other people either directly or through food or surfaces. The eggs can survive for 2-3 weeks on inanimate objects.

- Patients may be asymptomatic or have intense anal itching that is usually worse at night and can cause insomnia. Abdominal pain, nausea, and vomiting can also occur.
- **Diagnose** with the "tape test" which involves pressing cellophane tape over the perianal area to pick up eggs or worms and examine under the microscope. Most other helminth infestations can be diagnosed with a stool sample for ova and parasites; filariasis requires a blood smear or antigen test.
- Anthelmintic medications are given in a single dose and repeated in 2 weeks to kill the pinworms and their larvae (mebendazole, albendazole, or pyrantel pamoate). The entire family and close contacts should be treated simultaneously since pinworms are so contagious.

### *Giardia Lamblia*

*Giardia lamblia* is a **protozoan** that infects water supplies and spreads to children through the fecal-oral route. It is the most common cause of non-bacterial diarrhea in the United States, causing about 20,000 cases of infection each year in all ages.

- Children often become infected after swallowing recreational waters (pools, lakes) while swimming or putting contaminated items into the mouth. *Giardia* live and multiply within the small intestine where cysts develop.
- **Symptoms** occur 7-14 days after ingestion of 1 or more cysts and include diarrhea with greasy floating stools (rarely bloody), stomach cramps, nausea, and flatulence, lasting 2-6 weeks. A chronic infection may develop that can last for months or years.
- **Treatment** includes Furazolidone 5-8 mg/kg/day in 4 doses for 7-10 days or Metronidazole 40 mg/kg/day in 3 doses for 7-10 days. Chronic infections are often very resistant to treatment.

### *Toxoplasmosis*

Toxoplasmosis is an infection caused by the **parasite *Toxoplasma gondii***, which is commonly found in soil. It is widespread and transmitted through cat feces; however, it also may be contracted by eating undercooked meat (especially pork, lamb, or venison) or poorly washed vegetables. Toxoplasmosis can cause serious disease and can affect various organs; and immunocompromised and pregnant women and their unborn babies are especially likely to have side effects of the disease (the "T" in congenital TORCH infections).

- Healthy patients are usually asymptomatic; however, once infected the parasite can remain latent until the patient becomes immunocompromised and the parasite is reactivated causing **symptoms**. The disease can cause a flu-like illness with fever, myalgias, and lymphadenopathy. More serious effects include retinochoroiditis, brain lesions, and encephalitis. Congenital toxoplasmosis may cause retinochoroiditis, microcephaly, hydrocephalus, intellectual disability, and possibly miscarriage or stillbirth.
- **Diagnose** with serology for *Toxoplasma* antibodies IgM and IgG. Also, PCR may be used to test amniotic fluid, CSF, or tissue.
- **Treat** with pyrimethamine (preferred) plus folinic acid or sulfadiazine plus folinic acid. Pregnant women should avoid high-risk practices like changing the cat litter and should avoid sand boxes.

## Nosocomial Infections

Nosocomial infections are those that are healthcare-associated or hospital-acquired. The following is a list of common nosocomial infections.

- *Enterococci* infections include urinary infections, bacteremia, endocarditis as well as infections in wounds and the abdominal and pelvic areas.
- *Enterobacteriaceae* cause about half of the urinary tract infections and a quarter of the postoperative infections.
- *Escherichia coli* primarily causes urinary tract infections (especially related to catheters), diarrhea, and neonatal meningitis but it can also lead to pneumonia, and bacteremia (usually secondary to urinary infection).
- Group B β-hemolytic *Streptococci* (GBS) has increasingly been a cause of infections in neonatal units, causing pneumonia, meningitis, and sepsis. GBS infections may occur as wound infections after Cesarean sections, especially in those immunocompromised.
- *Staphylococcus aureus* is a major cause of nosocomial post-operative infections, both localized and systemic, and from indwelling tubes and devices.
- Methicillin-resistant *Staphylococcus aureus (MRSA)* is a common cause of surgical infections.
- *Clostridium difficile* causes more nosocomial diarrhea cases than any other microorganism.
- *Candida*, a yeast fungal pathogen, can overgrow and lead to mucocutaneous or cutaneous lesions and sepsis.
- *Aspergillus* spp., filamentous fungi, produce spores that become airborne and can invade the respiratory tract, causing pneumonia.

## Catheter-Related Infections

Intravenous catheter-related infections are a significant cause of morbidity and mortality in the hospital setting. Usually, these infections are due to *Staphylococcus aureus*, *enterococcus*, or fungal infection such as *Candida*. These infections are important because they may progress and eventually lead to bacteremia, infective endocarditis, septic pulmonary emboli, septic shock, osteomyelitis, or superficial thrombophlebitis. Therefore, vigilance should be maintained to prevent these infections. The patient may exhibit fevers, chills, and discomfort around the catheter site. The site itself may show purulence or erythema. The subclavian vein is the preferred intravenous site and the femoral is the least-preferred site due to high infection rates. Infections are diagnosed with blood cultures and catheter tip cultures. Initial treatment includes removal of the catheter and antibiotic treatment. Antibiotics should be empiric at first, then directed toward culture results. Treatment duration should be 2 weeks at first, but 4-6 weeks if there is a complicated infection.

## Infection Control Measures

**Standard infection control** measures are designed to prevent transmission of microbial substances between patients and/or medical providers. These measures are indicated for everyone and include frequent handwashing, gloves whenever bodily fluids are involved, and face shields and gowns when splashes are anticipated. For more advanced control with tuberculosis, SARS, vesicular rash disorders (such as VZV), and most recently COVID-19, **airborne precautions** should be instituted to prevent the spread of tiny droplets that can remain suspended in the air for days and travel throughout a hospital environment. Therefore, negative pressure rooms are essential, and providers and patients should wear high-efficiency N95 masks and be fitted in advance. For disorders such as influenza or other infections spread by droplets (spread by cough or sneeze) basic surgical masks should be worn (**droplet precautions**). For **contact precautions** in the setting of fecally-transmitted infection or vesicular rash diseases, gowns/gloves should be used and contact limited. White coats are not a substitute for proper gowning. In the case of a *Clostridium difficile* infection, contact precautions should be used in addition to washing hands with soap and water (rather than alcohol-based hand sanitizer) after patient contact.

## Infection Control Plan

The purpose of an infection control/surveillance plan should be clearly outlined and may be multifaceted, including the following elements:

- **Decreasing rates of infection**: The primary purpose of a surveillance plan is to identify a means to decrease nosocomial infections, including a notification system and laboratory surveillance.
- **Evaluating infection control measures**: Surveillance can evaluate effectiveness of infection control measures. (Surgical checklists, handwashing, housekeeping, ventilation).
- **Establishing endemic threshold rates**: Establishing threshold rates can help to enact control measures to reduce rates.
- **Identifying outbreaks**: About 5-10% of infections occur in outbreaks, and comparing data with established endemic threshold rates can help to identify these outbreaks if analysis is done in a regular and timely manner.
- **Achieving staff compliance**: Objective evidence may convince staff to cooperate with infection control measures.
- **Meeting accreditation standards**: Some accreditation agencies require reports of infection rates.
- **Providing defense for malpractice suits**: Providing evidence that a facility is proactive in combating infections can decrease liability.
- **Comparing infection rates with other facilities**: Comparing data helps focus attention and resources.

## PROTOCOL FOR NEEDLESTICK INJURY AND POSTEXPOSURE PROPHYLAXIS

If the healthcare provider experiences a **needlestick injury**, the individual's initial response should be to irrigate the wound with soap and water. As soon as possible, the incident must be reported to a supervisor and steps taken according to established protocol. This may include testing and/or prophylaxis, depending on the patient's health history. In some cases, the patient may also be tested for communicable diseases, such as HIV, in order to determine the risk to the healthcare provider. PEP (post-exposure prophylaxis) is available for exposure to HIV (human immunodeficiency virus) and hepatitis B virus (hepatis B immune globulin). However, no PEP is available for HCV (hepatitis C virus) although the CDC does provide a plan for management. PEP should be initiated within 72 hours of exposure. All testing and treatments associated with the needlestick injury must be provided free of cost at a hospital or medical facility.

# Professional Issues: Nurse

## Ethics

### Ethical Principles

**Autonomy** is the ethical principle that the individual has the right to make decisions about his or her own care. In the case of children or patients with dementia who cannot make autonomous decisions, parents or family members may serve as the legal decision maker. The nurse must keep the patient and/or family fully informed so that they can exercise their autonomy in informed decision-making.

**Justice** is the ethical principle that relates to the distribution of the limited resources of healthcare benefits to the members of society. These resources must be distributed fairly. This issue may arise if there is only one bed left and two sick patients. Justice comes into play in deciding which patient should stay and which should be transported or otherwise cared for. The decision should be made according to what is best or most just for the patients and not colored by personal bias.

**Beneficence** is an ethical principle that involves performing actions that are for the purpose of benefitting another person. In the care of a patient, any procedure or treatment should be done with the ultimate goal of benefitting the patient, and any actions that are not beneficial should be reconsidered. As conditions change, procedures need to be continually reevaluated to determine if they are still of benefit.

**Nonmaleficence** is an ethical principle that means healthcare workers should provide care in a manner that does not cause direct intentional harm to the patient:

- The actual act must be good or morally neutral.
- The intent must be only for a good effect.
- A bad effect cannot serve as the means to get to a good effect.
- A good effect must have more benefit than a bad effect has harm.

### Nursing Code of Ethics

There is more interest in the **ethics** involved in healthcare due to technological advances that have made the prolongation of life, organ transplants, prenatal manipulation, and saving of premature infants possible, sometimes with poor outcomes. Couple these with healthcare's limited resources, and **ethical dilemmas** abound. Ethics is the study of **morality** as the value that controls actions. The American Nurses Association Code of Ethics contains nine statements defining **principles** the nurse can use when faced with moral and ethical problems. Nurses must be knowledgeable about the many ethical issues in healthcare and about the field of ethics in general. The nurse must help a patient to reveal their values and morals to the health care team so that the patient, family, and team can resolve moral issues pertaining to the patient's care. As part of the healthcare team, the nurse has a right to express personal values and moral concerns about medical issues.

### Bioethics

Bioethics is a branch of ethics that involves making sure that the medical treatment given is the most morally correct choice given the different options that might be available and the differences inherent in the varied levels of treatment. In the health care unit, if the patients, family members, and the staff are in agreement when it comes to values and decision-making, then no ethical dilemma exists; however, when there is a difference in value beliefs between the patients/family members and the staff, there is a bioethical dilemma that must be resolved. Sometimes, discussion and explanation can resolve differences, but at times the institution's ethics committee must be brought in to resolve the conflict. The primary goal of bioethics is to determine the most morally correct action using the set of circumstances given.

## Ethical Decision-Making Model

There are many ethical decision-making models. Some general guidelines to apply in using ethical decision-making models could be the following:

- Gather information about the identified problem
- State reasonable alternatives and solutions to the problem
- Utilize ethical resources (for example, clergy or ethics committees) to help determine the ethically important elements of each solution or alternative
- Suggest and attempt possible solutions
- Choose a solution to the problem

It is important to always consider the **ethical principles** of autonomy, beneficence, nonmaleficence, justice, and fidelity when attempting to facilitate ethical decision-making with family members, caregivers, and the healthcare team.

## Ethical Assessment

While the terms *ethics* and *morals* are sometimes used interchangeably, ethics is a study of morals and encompasses concepts of right and wrong. When making **ethical assessments,** one must consider not only what people should do but also what they actually do, as these two things are sometimes at odds. Ethical issues can be difficult to assess because of personal bias, which is one of the reasons that sharing concerns with other internal sources and reaching consensus is so valuable. Issues of concern might include options for care, refusal of care, rights to privacy, adequate relief of suffering, and the right to self-determination. Internal sources might include the ethics committee, whose role is to make decisions regarding ethical issues. Risk management can provide guidance related to personal and institutional liability. External agencies might include government agencies, such as the public health department.

## Ethical Analysis of a Situation

Assessment of the situation is done to reveal the ethical, legal, and professional **conflicts** that are present. Those who are involved are identified, including the patient, family, and healthcare personnel. The decision maker is determined if it is not the patient. Information about the situation is collected to determine medical facts about the disease and condition of the patient, options for treatment, and nursing diagnoses. Any pertinent legal information is included. The patient and family's cultural, religious, and moral values are determined. Possible courses of action are listed and compared in terms of outcomes for the patient using the utilitarian or deontological theory of ethics. Professional codes of ethics are also applied. A decision is made and evaluated as to whether it is the most morally correct action. Ethical arguments for and against the decision are given and responded to by the decision maker.

## Professional Boundaries

### *Gifts*

Over time, patients may develop a bond with nurses they trust and may feel grateful to the nurse for the care provided and want to express thanks, but the nurse must make sure to maintain professional boundaries. Patients often offer **gifts** to nurses to show their appreciation, but some adults, especially those who are weak and ill or have cognitive impairment, may be taken advantage of easily. Patients may offer valuables and may sometimes be easily manipulated into giving large sums of money. Small tokens of appreciation that can be shared with other staff, such as a box of chocolates, are usually acceptable (depending upon the policy of the institution), but almost any other gifts (jewelry, money, clothes) should be declined: "I'm sorry, that's so kind of you, but nurses are not allowed to accept gifts from patients." Declining may relieve the patient of the feeling of obligation.

### Sexual Relations

When the boundary between the role of the professional nurse and the vulnerability of the patient is breached, a boundary violation occurs. Because the nurse is in the position of authority, the responsibility to maintain the boundary rests with the nurse; however, the line separating them is a continuum and sometimes not easily defined. It is inappropriate for nurses to engage in **sexual relations** with patients, and if the sexual behavior is coerced or the patient is cognitively impaired, it is **illegal**. However, more common violations with adults, particularly elderly patients, include exposing a patient unnecessarily, using sexually demeaning gestures or language (including off-color jokes), harassment, or inappropriate touching. Touching should be used with care, such as touching a hand or shoulder. Hugging may be misconstrued.

### Attention

Nursing is a giving profession, but the nurse must temper giving with recognition of professional boundaries. Patients have many needs. As acts of kindness, nurses (especially those involved in home care) often give certain patients extra attention and may offer to do **favors**, such as cooking or shopping. They may become overly invested in the patients' lives. While this may benefit a patient in the short term, it can establish a relationship of increasing **dependency** and **obligation** that does not resolve the long-term needs of the patient. Making referrals to the appropriate agencies or collaborating with family to find ways to provide services is more effective. Becoming overly invested may be evident by the nurse showing favoritism or spending too much time with the patient while neglecting other duties. On the other end of the spectrum are nurses who are disinterested and fail to provide adequate attention to the patient's detriment. Lack of adequate attention may lead to outright neglect.

### Coercion

Power issues are inherent in matters associated with professional boundaries. Physical abuse is both unprofessional and illegal, but behavior can easily border on abusive without the patient being physically injured. Nurses can easily **intimidate** older adults and sick patients into having procedures or treatments they do not want. Regardless of age, patients have the right to choose and the right to refuse treatment. Difficulties arise with cognitive impairment, and in that case, another responsible adult (often the patient's child or spouse) is designated to make decisions, but every effort should be made to gain patient cooperation. Forcing the patient to do something against his or her will borders on abuse and can sometimes degenerate into actual abuse if physical coercion is involved.

### Personal Information

When pre-existing personal or business relationships exist, other nurses should be assigned care of the patient whenever possible, but this may be difficult in small communities. However, the nurse should strive to maintain a professional role separate from the personal role and respect professional boundaries. The nurse must respect and maintain the confidentiality of the patient and family members, but the nurse must also be very careful about **disclosing personal information** about him or herself because this establishes a social relationship that interferes with the professional role of the nurse and the boundary between the patient and the nurse. The nurse and patient should never share secrets. When the nurse divulges personal information, he or she may become vulnerable to the patient, a reversal of roles.

# Evidence Based Practice

## Classes of Evidence-Based Practice

**Evidence-based practice** is treatment based on the best possible evidence, including a study of current research. Literature is searched to find evidence of the most effective treatments for specific diseases or injuries, and those treatments are then utilized to create clinical pathways that outline specific multi-departmental treatment protocols, including medications, treatments, and timelines. Evidence-based guidelines are often produced by specialty organizations that undertake the task of searching and analyzing literature to produce policies, procedures, and guidelines that become the standard of care for the disease. These guidelines are then used when a patient fits the disease criteria for that guideline.

**Evidence-based nursing** aims to improve the quality of nursing care by examining the reasons for all nursing practices and determining those that have the most positive outcomes. Evidence-based nursing focuses on the individual nurse utilizing evidence-based observations to influence decision-making.

## Evidence-Based Practice Guidelines

The creation of evidence-based practice guidelines includes the following components:

- **Focus on the topic/methodology:** This includes outlining possible interventions and treatments for review, choosing patient populations and settings, and determining significant outcomes. Search boundaries (such as types of journals, types of studies, dates of studies) should be determined.
- **Evidence review:** This includes review of literature, critical analysis of studies, and summarizing of results, including pooled meta-analysis.
- **Expert judgment:** Recommendations based on personal experience from a number of experts may be utilized, especially if there is inadequate evidence based on review, but this subjective evidence should be explicitly acknowledged.
- **Policy considerations:** This includes cost-effectiveness, access to care, insurance coverage, availability of qualified staff, and legal implications.
- **Policy:** A written policy must be completed with recommendations. Common practice is to utilize letter guidelines, with "A" being the most highly recommended, usually based on the quality of supporting evidence.
- **Review:** The completed policy should be submitted to peers for review and comments before instituting the policy.

## Critical Pathways

Clinical/critical pathway development is done by those involved in direct patient care. The pathway should require no additional staffing and cover the entire scope of an illness. Steps include:

1. Selection of patient group and diagnosis, procedures, or conditions, based on analysis of data and observations of wide variance in approach to treatment and prioritizing organization and patient needs
2. Creation of interdisciplinary team of those involved in the process of care, including physicians to develop pathway
3. Analysis of data including literature review and study of best practices to identify opportunities for quality improvement
4. Identification of all categories of care, such as nutrition, medications, and nursing
5. Discussion and reaching consensus
6. Identifying the levels of care and number of days to be covered by the pathway
7. Pilot testing and redesigning steps as indicated
8. Educating staff about standards
9. Monitoring and tracking variances in order to improve pathways

## Levels of Evidence in Evidence-Based Practice

Levels of evidence are categorized according to the scientific evidence available to support the recommendations, as well as existing state and federal laws. While recommendations are voluntary, they are often used as a basis for state and federal regulations.

- **Category IA** is well supported by evidence from experimental, clinical, or epidemiologic studies and is strongly recommended for implementation.
- **Category IB** has supporting evidence from some studies, has a good theoretical basis, and is strongly recommended for implementation.
- **Category IC** is required by state or federal regulations or is an industry standard.
- **Category II** is supported by suggestive clinical or epidemiologic studies, has a theoretical basis, and is suggested for implementation.
- **Category III** is supported by descriptive studies, such as comparisons, correlations, and case studies, and may be useful.
- **Category IV** is obtained from expert opinion or authorities only.
- **Unresolved** means there is no recommendation because of a lack of consensus or evidence.

## Outcome Evaluation

Outcome evaluation is an important component of evidence-based practice, which involves both internal and external research. All treatments are subjected to review to determine if they produce positive outcomes, and policies and protocols for outcome evaluation should be in place. **Outcome evaluation** includes the following:

- **Monitoring** over the course of treatment involves careful observation and record-keeping that notes progress, with supporting laboratory and radiographic evidence as indicated by condition and treatment.
- **Evaluating** results includes reviewing records as well as current research to determine if outcomes are within acceptable parameters.
- **Sustaining** involves discontinuing treatment but continuing to monitor and evaluate.
- **Improving** means to continue the treatment but with additions or modifications in order to improve outcomes.
- **Replacing** the treatment with a different treatment must be done if outcome evaluation indicates that current treatment is ineffective.

## Evidence-Based Nursing Interventions

Evidence-based nursing interventions enable nurses to provide high-quality patient care that is based upon research and knowledge, as opposed to giving care that is based upon tradition or information that is out of date. An evidence-based nursing approach is based on the integration of practical clinical experience with medical and clinical research; it utilizes proven clinical guidelines and assessment practices. Evidence-based nursing interventions allow nurses to make patient care decisions based on cutting-edge research that has been scientifically validated. Studies show that evidence-based nursing practice yields improved patient outcomes, enables nurses to practice up-to-date methods, improves nurse confidence and decision-making skills, and enhances Joint Commission standards.

### *Resources*

There are numerous information resources for evidence-based nursing interventions. These resources include evidence-based textbooks; databases such as CINAHL Plus, COCHRANE library, Mosby's Nursing Index, NursingConsult, and Nursing@Ovid; evidence-based nursing metasites such as the Academic Center for EBN, Joanna Briggs Institute, McGill University, ONS-EBN section, and EBN-University of Minnesota; online evidence-based nursing journals such as Clinical Nurse Specialist, Clinical Nursing Research, Evidence-Based Nursing, Journal of Nursing Care Quality, Journal of Advanced Nursing, Journal of Nursing Scholarship, Nurse

Researcher, Nursing Research, Western Journal of Nursing Research, and Worldviews on Evidence-Based Nursing; and various online tutorials.

### Obtaining Results of Research to Use in Evidence-Based Practice

When searching for **current evidence** in print and online literature, the nurse should look for **systematic reviews, analyses, and reports**. PUBMED lists all literature and can be searched for all published articles on a particular subject. These articles can be analyzed to determine treatments that have the best evidence of efficacy. Subject and methodological terms and clinical filters can be used to find necessary information, including a specific medical subject heading (MH), subheading (SH), publication type (PT), and text word (TW). The nurse should also search the National Guideline Clearinghouse, Cochrane Databases, Agency for Healthcare Research and Quality, and US Preventive Services Task Force Recommendations for evidence and guidelines. When trials of a treatment provide evidence of effectiveness, the evidence is weighed for strength and confidence. Those that provide the strongest evidence of efficacy become recommendations and guidelines for use in the field. Research is also done on a smaller scale by specialists who publish in peer-reviewed journals their research results related to the use of a particular intervention.

# Nursing Research

## Elements of Research

The following are elements of research:

- **Variable**: An entity that can be different within a population
- **Independent variable**: The variable that the researchers change to evaluate its effect
- **Dependent variable**: The variable that may be changed by alterations in the independent variable
- **Hypothesis**: The proposed explanation to describe an expected outcome in a study
- **Sample**: The selected population to be studied
- **Experimental group**: The population within the sample that undergoes the treatment or intervention
- **Control group**: The population within the sample that is not exposed to the treatment of intervention being evaluated

The nurse must be taught and must understand the process of critical analysis and know how to conduct a survey of the literature. **Basic research concepts** include:

- **Survey of valid sources**: Information from a juried journal and an anonymous website or personal website are very different sources, and evaluating what constitutes a valid source of data is critical.
- **Evaluation of internal and external validity**: Internal validity shows a cause-and-effect relationship between two variables, with the cause occurring before the effect and no intervening variable. External validity occurs when results hold true in different environments and circumstances with different populations.
- **Sample selection and sample size**: Selection and size can have a huge impact on the results, but a sample that is too small may lack both internal and external validity. Selection may be so narrowly focused that the results can't be generalized to other groups.

## Validity, Generalizability, and Replicability

Many research studies are most concerned with **internal validity** (adequate unbiased data properly collected and analyzed within the population studied), but studies that determine the efficacy of procedures or treatments, for example, should have **external validity** as well; that is, the results should be **generalizable** (true) for similar populations. **Replication** of the study under different circumstances and with different subjects and researchers should produce similar results. For various reasons, some people may be excluded from a study so that instead of randomized subjects, the subjects may be highly selected so when data is compared with another population in which there is less or more selection, results may be different. The selection of subjects, in this case, would interfere with external validity. Part of the design of a study should include considerations of whether or not it should have external validity or whether there is value for the institution based solely on internal validation.

## Hypothesis

A hypothesis should be generated about the probable cause of the disease/infection based on the information available in laboratory and medical records, epidemiologic study, literature review, and expert opinion. For example, a hypothesis should include the infective agent, the likely source, and the mode of transmission: "Wound infections with *Staphylococcus aureus* were caused by reuse and inadequate sterilization of single-use irrigation syringes used during wound care in the ICU."

**Hypothesis testing** includes data analysis, laboratory findings, and outcomes of environmental testing. It usually includes case-control studies, with 2-4 controls picked for each case of infection. They may be matched according to age, sex, or other characteristics, but they are not infected at the time they are picked for the study. Cohort studies, whose controls are picked based on having or lacking exposure, may also be instituted. If the hypothesis cannot be supported, then a new hypothesis or different testing methods may be necessary.

## Critical Reading

There are several steps to critical reading to evaluate research:

- **Consider the source** of the material. If it is in the popular press, it may have little validity compared to something published in a peer-reviewed journal.
- **Review the author's credentials** to determine if a person is an expert in the field of study.
- **Determine the thesis**, or the central claim of the research. It should be clearly stated.
- **Examine the organization** of the article, whether it is based on a particular theory, and the type of methodology used.
- **Review the evidence** to determine how it is used to support the main points. Look for statistical evidence and sample size to determine if the findings have wide applicability.
- **Evaluate** the overall article to determine if the information seems credible and useful and should be communicated to administration and/or staff.

## Major Study Types Utilized in Statistical Analysis

When conducting research, the nurse should be aware of the **types of studies** available and when each type of study is appropriate and most reliable:

- **Case-control studies** are simple. They use pre-existing cases with and without the disorder of interest. For example, case-control studies may be done with mesothelioma and exposure to possible pleural irritants. These are good for rare diseases to determine cause and effect.
- **Cross-sectional studies** utilize a cross-section of data from the population and analyze variables at one time point. They are not good for determining cause and effect, but they are useful for correlating characteristics with disorders.
- **Cohort studies** follow a cohort of a population for a period of time and attempt to make a link with diseases. As in the previous example, researchers could follow a group exposed to asbestos and study the incidence of mesothelioma.
- **Randomized controlled trial** is the gold standard, with patients assigned to the control or experimental group. This is a difficult type of test to design and implement but very useful, as the data is often well-controlled. It is the most expensive type of study.

## Bias in Research

**Selection bias** occurs when the method of selecting subjects results in a cohort that is not representative of the target population because of inherent error in design. For example, if all patients who develop urinary infections are evaluated per urine culture and sensitivities for microbial resistance, but only those patients with clinically-evident infections are included, a number of patients with sub-clinical infections may be missed, skewing the results. Selection bias is only a concern when participants in studies are specifically chosen. Many surveillance studies do not involve the selection of subjects.

**Information bias** occurs when there are errors in classification, so an estimate of association is incorrect. Non-differential misclassification occurs when there is similar misclassification of disease or exposure among both those who are diseased/exposed and those who are not. Differential misclassification occurs when there is a differing misclassification of disease or exposure among both those who are diseased/exposed and those who are not.

## QUALITATIVE AND QUANTITATIVE DATA

Both qualitative and quantitative data are used for analysis, but the focus is quite different:

- **Qualitative data**: Data are described verbally or graphically, and the results are subjective, depending upon observers to provide information. Interviews may be used as a tool to gather information, and the researcher's interpretation of data is important. Gathering this type of data can be time-intensive, and it can usually not be generalized to a larger population. This type of information gathering is often useful at the beginning of the design process for data collection.
- **Quantitative data**: Data are described in terms of numbers within a statistical format. This type of information gathering is done after the design of data collection is outlined, usually in later stages. Tools may include surveys, questionnaires, or other methods of obtaining numerical data. The researcher's role is objective.

# Compassion Fatigue

## Characteristics

**Compassion fatigue** can occur when people overly identify with the pain and suffering of others and begin to exhibit signs of stress as a result. These people are often empathetic, tend to place the needs of others above their own, and are motivated by the need to help others. Indications include:

- **Blaming** others and **complaining** excessively
- **Isolating** oneself from others and having **trouble concentrating**
- Engaging in **compulsive activities** (gambling, drinking)
- Having **nightmares**, **sleeping poorly**, and exhibiting a **change in appetite**
- Exhibiting **sadness** or **apathy**
- **Denying** any problems and having **high expectations** of self and others
- **Questioning** spiritual beliefs or **losing faith**
- Exhibiting **stress disorders**: tachycardia, headaches, insomnia, pain

Healthcare providers who exhibit compassion fatigue may need to take a break from work in order to recover some sense of self and may benefit from stress management programs, cognitive behavioral therapy, relaxation and visualization exercises, and physical exercise.

## Stress Management Strategies

While it's not possible to eliminate all stress, nurses can learn to manage stress so it has less emotional and physical impact on their lives. **Stress management** strategies include:

- **Relaxation exercises**:
    - Meditation/breathing exercises: Slow in and out while repeating a word or phrase
    - Massage: Self-massage or by others
    - Progressive relaxation techniques
- **Visualization exercises/positive thinking**: Use the power of the mind to imagine a more positive outcome.
- **Time management**: Establish priorities, make a schedule, and delegate.
- **Exercise**: Increase activity and exercise 20-30 minutes daily.
- **Breaks**: Plan regular breaks from work or other activities, 5-15 minutes.
- **Snacks**: Prepare healthy snacks and avoid high-sugar/high-fat snack foods.
- **Hobbies or interests**: Find an outlet, such as reading, music, painting, or crafts.

# Professional Issues: Patient

## Patient Rights

### Patient Rights and Responsibilities

Empowering patients and families to act as their own advocates requires that they have a clear understanding of their **rights and responsibilities.** These should be given (in print form) and/or presented (audio/video) to patients and families on admission or as soon as possible:

- **Rights** include competent, non-discriminatory medical care that respects privacy and allows participation in decisions about care and the right to refuse care. They should have clear understandable explanations of treatments, options, and conditions, including outcomes. They should be apprised of transfers, changes in care plan, and advance directives. They should have access to medical records and billing information.
- **Responsibilities** include providing honest and thorough information about health issues and medical history. They should ask for clarification if they don't understand information that is provided to them, and they should follow the plan of care that is outlined or explain why that is not possible. They should treat staff and other patients with respect.

**Review Video: Patient Advocacy**
Visit mometrix.com/academy and enter code: 202160

### Informed Consent

The patient or their legal guardian must provide informed consent for all treatment the patient receives. This includes a thorough explanation of all procedures and treatment and associated risks. Patients/guardians should be apprised of all options and allowed to have input on the decision-making process. They should be apprised of all reasonable risks and any complications that might be life threatening or increase morbidity. The American Medical Association has established **guidelines for obtaining informed consent:**

- Explanation of the diagnosis
- Nature and reason for the treatment or procedure
- Risks and benefits of the treatment or procedure
- Alternative options (regardless of cost or insurance coverage)
- Risks and benefits of alternative options, including no treatment

Obtaining informed consent is a requirement in all states; however, a patient may waive their right to informed consent. If this is the case, the nurse should document the patient's waiving of this right and proceed with the procedure. Informed consent is not necessary for procedures performed to save life or limb in which the patient or guardian is unable to consent.

### Confidentiality

Confidentiality is the obligation that is present in a professional-patient relationship. Nurses are under an obligation to protect the information they possess concerning the patient and family. Care should be taken to safeguard that information and provide the privacy that the family deserves. This is accomplished through the use of required passwords when family call for information about the patient and through the limitation of who is allowed to visit. There may be times when confidentiality must be broken to save the life of a patient, but those circumstances are rare. The nurse must make all efforts to safeguard patient records and identification. Computerized record keeping should be done in such a way that the screen is not visible to others, and paper records must be secured.

# End-of-Life Issues

## Grief

Grief is an emotional response to a **loss** that begins at the time a loss is anticipated and continues on an individual timetable. While there are identifiable stages or tasks, it is not an orderly and predictable process. It involves overcoming anger, disbelief, guilt, and a myriad of related emotions. The grieving individual may move back and forth between stages or experience several emotions at any given time. Each person's grief response is unique to their own coping patterns, stress levels, age, gender, belief system, and previous experiences with loss.

## Kubler-Ross's Five Stages of Grief

**Kubler-Ross** taught the medical community that the dying patient and family welcomes open, honest discussion of the dying process and felt that there were certain **stages** that patients and family go through. The stages may not occur in order, but may vary or some may be skipped. Stages include:

- **Denial**: The person denies the diagnosis and tries to pretend it isn't true. During this time, the person may seek a second opinion or alternative therapies. They may use denial until they are better able to emotionally cope with the reality of the disease or changes that need to be made. Patients may also wish to save family and friends from pain and worry. Both patients and family may use denial as a coping mechanism when they feel overwhelmed by the reality of the disease and threatened losses.
- **Anger**: The person is angry about the situation and may focus that rage on anyone.
- **Bargaining**: The person attempts to make deals with a higher power to secure a better outcome to their situation.
- **Depression**: The person anticipates the loss and the changes it will bring with a sense of sadness and grief.
- **Acceptance**: The person accepts the impending death and is ready to face it as it approaches. The patient may begin to withdraw from interests and family.

**Review Video: Patient Treatment and Grief**
Visit mometrix.com/academy and enter code: 648794

## Anticipatory Grief

Anticipatory grief is the mental, social, and somatic reactions of an individual as they prepare themselves for a **perceived future loss**. The individual experiences a process of intellectual, emotional, and behavioral responses in order to modify their self-concept, based on their perception of what the potential loss will mean in their life. This process often takes place ahead of the actual loss, from the time the loss is first perceived until it is resolved as a reality for the individual. This process can also blend with past loss experiences. It is associated with the individual's perception of how life will be affected by the particular diagnosis as well as the impending death. Acknowledging this anticipatory grief allows family members to begin looking toward a changed future. Suppressing this anticipatory process may inhibit relationships with the ill individual and contribute to a more difficult grieving process at a later time. However, appropriate anticipatory grieving does not take the place of grief during the actual time of death.

## Disenfranchised Grief

Disenfranchised grief occurs when the loss being experienced cannot be openly acknowledged, publicly mourned, or socially supported. Society and culture are partly responsible for an individual's response to a loss. There is a **social context** to grief; if a person incurring the loss will be putting himself or herself at risk if grief is expressed, disenfranchised grief occurs. The risk for disenfranchised grief is greatest among those whose relationship with the individual they lost was not known or regarded as significant. This is also the situation found among bereaved persons who are not recognized by society as capable of grief, such as young children, or needing to mourn, such as an ex-spouse or secret lover.

## Grief vs. Depression

Normal grief is preoccupied with self-limiting to the loss itself. Emotional responses will vary and may include open expressions of anger. The individual may experience difficulty sleeping or vivid dreams, a lack of energy, and weight loss. Crying is evident and provides some relief of extreme emotions. The individual remains socially responsive and seeks reassurance from others.

**Depression** is marked by extensive periods of sadness and preoccupation often extending beyond 2 months. It is not limited to the single event. There is an absence of pleasure or anger and isolation from previous social support systems. The individual can experience extreme lethargy, weight loss, insomnia, or hypersomnia, and has no recollection of dreaming. Crying is absent or persistent and provides no relief of emotions. Professional intervention is required to relieve depression.

## Loss

Loss is the blanket term used to denote the absence of a valued object, position, ability, attribute, or individual. The aspect of **loss** as it is associated with the death of an animal or person is a relatively new definition. Loss is an individualized and subjective experience depending on the **perceived attachment** between the individual and the missing aspect. This can range from little or no value of attachment to significant value. Loss also can be represented by the **withdrawal of a valued relationship** one had or would have had in the future. Depending on the unique and individual responses to the perception of loss and its significance, reactions to the loss will vary. Robinson and McKenna summarize the aspects of loss in three main attributes:

- Something has been removed.
- The item removed had value to that person.
- The response is individualized.

## Mourning

Mourning is a public grief response for the death of a loved one. The various aspects of the mourning process are partially determined by **personal and cultural belief systems**. Kagawa-Singer defines mourning as "the social customs and cultural practices that follow a death." Durkheim expands this to include the following: "mourning is not a natural movement of private feelings wounded by a cruel loss; it is a duty imposed by the group." Mourning involves participation in religious and culturally appropriate customs and rituals designed to publicly acknowledge the loss. These rituals signify they are adjusting to the change in their relationships created by the loss, as well as mark the beginning of the reorganization and forward movement of their lives.

## Bereavement

Bereavement is the emotional and mental state associated with having suffered a **personal loss**. It is the reactions of grief and sadness initiated by the loss of a loved one. Bereavement is a normal process of feeling deprived of something of value. The word bereave comes from the root "reave" meaning to plunder, spoil, or rob. It is recognized that the lost individual had value and a defining role in the surviving individual's life. Bereavement encompasses all the acts and emotions surrounding the feeling of loss for the individual. During this grieving period, there is an increased mortality risk. A **positive bereavement experience** means being able to recognize the significance of the loss while still recognizing the resilience and value of life.

### *Risk Factors Complicating Bereavement*

The caregiver should assess for multiple **life crises** that take energy away from the grieving process. An important factor is the grieving individual's history with past grieving experiences. Assess for other recent, unresolved, or difficult losses that may need to be addressed before the individual can move toward resolution of the current loss. Age, mental health, substance abuse, extreme anger, anxiety, or dependence on the individual facing the end of life can add additional stressors and handicap natural coping mechanisms. Income strains, community support, outside and personal responsibilities, the absence of cultural and religious beliefs, the difficulty of the disease process, and age of the loved one lost can also present additional risk factors.

## Counseling and Providing Emotional Support Regarding Grief and Loss to Children

The approach to counseling and providing emotional support regarding grief and loss to children is dependent on the age of the child. When available, children and family should be provided information about **peer support groups** (especially adolescents) and **bereavement art therapy groups** as these may be especially helpful. Healthcare professionals should use appropriate words (death, died) instead of euphemisms (passed on) when talking about the deceased and should encourage the child to ask questions. Children are often reluctant to express feelings directly, so it may be beneficial to encourage them to keep a journal about their feelings or draw pictures to express them. Parents should be encouraged to share their feelings of grief with their children rather than trying to hide their emotions and should be aware that children express grief in different ways and may regress or complain of physical ailments (stomach ache, headache) in response to grief. Children should be prepared for changes in routines or living situations, such as a stay-at-home parent having to take a job, which may occur as a result of a death or serious illness.

### *Signs of a Child Having Issues Managing Grief*

Management of **grief** comes in stages for children as well as for adults. Grief may be complicated for a child who does not understand the significance of the situation, such as in the case of a parent's death, or for someone who does not have the necessary support systems in place, as in the case of a child who has a grieving parent who consequently becomes unavailable. **Signs that a child is not coping well with grief** include extended periods of sadness, lack of interest in regular activities, sleep disturbances, loss of appetite, statements of wishing for death or joining a person who has died, difficulties with concentration, problems taking direction at school, poor school performance, and fear of being alone.

## Interventions for Patients and Family Experiencing Loss and Grief

Loss is painful and frightening. Loss can occur through death or loss of health, self-esteem, or relationships. Loss can also occur from threats, such as fire, flood, theft, or severe weather. The severity of the loss, preparation for it, and the maturity, stability, and coping mechanisms of the person all affect the grieving process. Multiple losses and substance abuse can complicate grief and recovery. Previous life experience and cultural and religious beliefs can help in resolution of grief. Many emotions are triggered, and if the loss is not acknowledged, the person may become depressed or develop health problems. **Interventions** for those experiencing grief and loss include:

- Teach patients to recognize symptoms, such as SOB, empty feelings in the chest or abdomen, deep sighing, lethargy, and weakness as signs of grief.
- Assist the patient and family to heal themselves by accepting the loss, recognizing the pain from it, making changes to adapt to and assimilate the loss, and moving toward new relationships and activity.
- Refer to groups or counseling for more intense support if needed.

## Supporting Families and Patients as They Receive Bad News

It is often best if the patient can **receive bad news** while being **supported** by family, friends, physicians, nurses, support staff, social workers, and clergy if they so desire. However, the patient may not want family members or others to be present, and this too should be respected.

- Provide privacy and ensure that there will be no interruptions.
- Provide seating for all participants.
- Do not provide too much information at once, as the opening statement may be all that the patient can comprehend at one time.
- Allow time for reactions before providing more information.
- Wait for the patient to signal the need for more information and then provide an honest answer in layman's terms. Information may not be absorbed and may need to be repeated as the patient and family are ready for it later after the initial conference.

- Use techniques of therapeutic communication. People may need others to sit and listen and provide comforting empathy many times before having a conversation about problem solving.

## Spirituality

Spirituality provides a connection of the self to a higher power and a way of finding meaning in life experiences. It provides guidance for behavior and can help to clarify one's purpose in life. It can offer hope to those who are ill or facing loss and grief and can give comfort, support, and guidance. **Spirituality** is not always connected to a religion and is highly individualized. A person may lose faith and confidence in his/her spiritual beliefs during trying times:

- Ask patients about their spiritual beliefs.
- Listen attentively and do not offer opinions about their beliefs or share your own unless invited.
- Show respect for their views and offer to obtain spiritual support by calling a spiritual leader or setting up a spiritual ritual that has meaning for them.

This support can help them to regain their beliefs and endure illness by helping them to rise above their suffering and find meaning in this experience.

## Palliative and Hospice Care

**Palliative care** attempts to make the rest of the patient's life as comfortable as possible by treating distressing symptoms to keep them controlled. It does not attempt to cure but only to control discomfort caused by the disease. Palliative care does not require terminal illness/prognosis and can be implemented for any patient with chronic disease and suffering.

**Hospice care** uses palliative care as it supports the patient and family through the dying process. Hospice teams support the daily needs of the patient and family and provide needed equipment, medical expertise, and medications to control symptoms. They offer spiritual, psychological, and social support to the patient and family as needed and desired. Assistance with end-of-life planning is given to help the patient and family accomplish goals important to them. Bereavement support is also given. The team consists of the attending physician, hospice physician advisor, nurses, social worker, clergy, hospice aides, and volunteers. Hospice care is given in the home when the patient has family who are willing to assume care with the assistance of the hospice team. Hospice care also occurs in hospice facilities, hospitals, and extended care facilities. To qualify for Hospice care, the patient must be deemed terminal and given a 6-month or less life expectancy by two separate physicians. Should the patient survive 6 months in hospice, they can be extended for two 90-day periods, and then an unlimited number of 60-day periods per physician order.

# Forensic Evidence Collection

## ABCs of Forensic Nursing (McCracken)

The ABCs of forensic nursing, developed by McCracken, provide a simple mnemonic device to help the nurse remember the steps to carry out in order to obtain forensic evidence.

- **A-Assess** the victim.
- **B**-Serve as a **bridge** or liaison between the facility and outside agencies, such as the police and ME.
- **C**-Maintain the **chain of custody** by following established protocols in obtaining and securing evidence.
- **D-Document** observations, actions.
- **E**-Obtain **evidence**.
- **F**-Provide information to **families.**
- **G-Go** to court as necessary to provide testimony.
- **H**-Learn **hospital** policies and protocols and know how and where to access them if necessary.
- **I**-Maintain a healthy **index** of suspicion and awareness of typical injuries associated with abuse and violent actions.

## Forensic Evidence and Chain of Custody

Emergency nurses come in contact with cases involving **forensic evidence** daily, but much evidence is destroyed, washed or brushed away, contaminated, or overlooked. Each facility should have protocols in place for obtaining and securing forensic evidence, and staff members should be trained. Typical items related to forensic evidence include, hairs, fibers, bullets, and clothing (blood stains, semen stains) as well as fragments of different materials, such as wood, paint, metal, or glass. Nurses should always maintain a level of suspicion when the clinical picture suggests criminal or civil liability. Evidence should be obtained properly and secured in a locked drop box or space with dispensation documented and not disturbed until retrieved by proper authorities in order to maintain the chain of custody. **Chain of custody** refers to the documented record of acquiring, securing, and transferring evidence. This record must contain a chronological paper trail that clearly outlines where and in whose custody evidence is at all times.

## Forensic Evidence Collection

| | |
|---|---|
| **Clothing** | If necessary, to cut clothing, try to do so at seams and avoid cutting through any tears, holes, or stains. Remove all clothing carefully without shaking, fold, and immediately secure each piece in a separate paper bag (not sealed in plastic). Wet clothes should be left open to dry or authorities notified immediately. |
| **Bullets** | Retrieve bullets with rubber tipped instrument and avoid contact with any metal surface, wrap in cotton, and place in secure container. If sent to pathology department, advise pathology of need to maintain chain of custody and avoid altering the surface. |
| **Weapons** | Retrieve knives or other penetrating weapons, using care not to disturb potential fingerprints. Do not wash away blood or other evidence. |
| **Gunpowder particles** | If necessary, retrieve particles on skin (such as hands) by swabbing with cotton swab or adhesive applicators and secure. |
| **Statements** | Record relevant exact statements the victim or others make. |
| **Wounds** | If protocol permits, photograph wounds and bruises. Thoroughly document all wounds and types of bruises, including size, condition, color, shape, and location. |

# Pain Assessment

## Pathophysiology of Pain

### *Nociceptors*

Nociceptors are the primary neurons, or **sensory receptors**, responding to stimuli in the skin, muscle, and joints, as well as the stomach, bladder, and uterus. These neurons have specialized responses for mechanical, thermal, or chemical stimuli. The **neuron stimulation** is a direct result of tissue injury and follows four stages: **transduction** where a change occurs, **transmission** where the impulse is transferred along the neural path, **modulation** or translation of the signal, and **perception** by the patient. When injury occurs, the nociceptors initiate the process that begins **depolarization of the peripheral nerve**. Nociceptors may consist of either A-fiber axons or C-fiber axons. The message travels along the neural pathway and creates a perception of pain. A-fiber axons carry these pain messages at a much faster rate than C-fiber axons.

### *Nociceptive Pain*

Nociceptive pain is an umbrella term for pain caused by **stimulation of the neuroreceptor**. This stimulation is a direct result of tissue injury. The severity of pain is proportionate to the extent of the injury. Nociceptive pain can be subdivided into two classifications: somatic and visceral pain. **Somatic pain** is located in the cutaneous tissues, bone joints, and muscle tissues. **Visceral pain** is specific to internal organs protected by a layer of viscera, such as the cardiovascular, respiratory, gastrointestinal, or genitourinary systems. Both types are treatable with opioids.

#### Visceral Pain

Visceral pain is associated with the internal organs. It can be very different depending on the affected organ. Not all internal organs are sensitive to pain (some lack **nociceptors**, such as the spleen, kidney, and pancreas), and may withstand a great deal of damage without causing pain. Other internal organs, such as the stomach, bladder, and ureters, can create significant pain from even the slightest damage. Visceral pain generally has a **poorly defined area**. It is also capable of referring pain to other remote locations away from the area of injury. It is described as a squeezing or cramping: a deep ache within the internal organs. The patient may complain of a generalized sick feeling or have nausea and vomiting. Visceral pain generally responds well to treatment with **opioids**.

#### Somatic Pain

Somatic pain refers to messages from pain receptors located in the **cutaneous or musculoskeletal tissues**. When the pain occurs within the musculoskeletal tissue, it is referred to as **deep somatic pain**. Metastasizing cancers commonly cause deep somatic pain. **Surface pain** refers to pain concentrated in the **dermis and cutaneous layers** such as that caused by a surgical incision. Deep somatic pain is generally described as a dull, throbbing ache that is well focused on the area of trauma. It responds well to **opioids**. Surface somatic pain is also directly focused on the injury. It is frequently described as sharper than deep somatic pain. It may also present as a burning or pricking sensation.

### *Neuropathic Pain*

Neuropathic pain results from injury to the **nervous system**. This can result from cancer cells compressing the nerves or spinal cord, from actual cancerous invasion into the nerves or spinal cord, or from chemical damage to the nerves caused by chemotherapy and radiation. Other causes include diabetes- and alcohol-related damage, trauma, neuralgias, or other illnesses affecting the neural path either centrally or peripherally. When the nerves become damaged, they are unable to carry accurate information. This results in more severe, distinct **pain messages**. The nerves may also relay pain messages long after the original cause of the pain is resolved. It can be described as sharp, burning, shooting, shocking, tingling, or electrical in nature. It may travel the length of the nerve path from the spine to a distal body part such as a hand, or down the buttocks to a foot. NSAIDs and opioids are generally ineffective against neuropathic pain, though adjuvants may enhance the therapeutic effect of opioids. Nerve blocks may also be used.

## Adverse Systemic Effects of Pain

Acute pain causes adverse systemic effects that can negatively affect many body systems.

- **Cardiovascular**: Tachycardia and increased blood pressure is a common response to pain, causing increased cardiac output and systemic vascular resistance. In those with pre-existing cardiovascular disease, such as compromised ventricular function, cardiac output may decrease. The increased myocardial need for oxygen may cause or worsen myocardial ischemia.
- **Respiratory**: Increased need for oxygen causes an increase in minute ventilation and splinting due to pain, which may compromise pulmonary function. If the chest wall movement is constrained, tidal volume falls, impairing the ability to cough and clear secretions. Bed rest further compromises ventilation.
- **Gastrointestinal**: Sphincter tone increases and motility decreases, sometimes resulting in ileus. There may be an increased secretion of gastric acids, which irritates the gastric lining and can cause ulcerations. Nausea, vomiting, and constipation may occur. Reflux may result in aspiration pneumonia. Abdominal distension may occur.
- **Urinary**: Increased sphincter tone and decreased motility result in urinary retention.
- **Endocrine**: Hormone levels are affected by pain. Catabolic hormones such as catecholamine, cortisol, and glucagon increase, and anabolic hormones such as insulin and testosterone decrease. Lipolysis increases along with carbohydrate intolerance. Sodium retention can occur because of increased ADH, aldosterone, angiotensin, and cortisol. This in turn causes fluid retention and a shift to extracellular space.
- **Hematologic**: There may be reduced fibrinolysis, increased adhesiveness of platelets, and increased coagulation.
- **Immune**: Leukocytosis and lymphopenia may occur, increasing risk of infection.
- **Emotional**: Patients may experience depression, anxiety, anger, decreased appetite, and sleep deprivation. This type of response is most common in those with chronic pain, who usually have different systemic responses from those with acute pain.

## Core Principles of Pain Assessment and Management

According to the Joint Commission, assessing pain should be a priority in patient care, and organizations must establish **policies** for assessment and treatment of pain and must educate staff members about these policies. The Joint Commission considers a **plan of care** regarding pain control an essential patient right. Hospitals should be consistent in the use of the same assessment tools throughout the organization, specific to different patient populations (for example, pediatrics and geriatrics). The latest standards (2018) of evidence-based practice include the following:

- Organizations must establish a clinical leadership team to oversee pain management and safe prescription of opioids.
- Patients must be involved in planning and setting goals and should receive education regarding safe use of opioid and non-opioid medications.
- Patients should be screened for pain in all assessments, including visits to the emergency department.
- Patients at high risk for opioid misuse or adverse effects must be identified and monitored.
- Healthcare providers should have access to prescription drug monitoring safety databases, such as the prescription databases provided by most states.
- Organizations must provide performance improvement educational programs regarding pain assessment and management and must collect and analyze data on its pain assessment and management.

## Areas Addressed When Assessing Pain

Information concerning a patient's pain can be gathered from a variety of sources, including observations, interviews with the patient and family, medical records, and observations of other health care providers. However, it is important to remember that each patient's pain is **subjective** and **personal**. Pain is defined as whatever the patient says it is. Having the patient give parameters of quality, location, duration, speed of onset, and intensity can all be beneficial in forming a treatment plan based on the patient's needs. Pain is also influenced by psychological, social, and spiritual factors. Behavioral, psychological, and subjective assessment information such as physical demeanor and vital signs can be helpful in further defining a patient's pain parameters.

## Physical Signs of Pain

The best assessment of the patient's pain is **the patient's own report**. All other information is assessed as supporting this report. However, when this method is restricted or unavailable, **physical signs and symptoms** can help the nurse's assessment capabilities. It is important to be familiar with the patient's **baseline** or resting information to give a clear picture of the changes the body may go through when experiencing significant pain. Systolic blood pressure, heart rate, and respirations may all increase above the patient's normal parameters. Tightness or tension may be felt in major muscle groups. Posturing can also occur: the patient may guard areas of the body, curl themselves up into a fetal position, or hold only certain body portions rigid. Calling out, increased volume in speech, and moaning can also be indicators. Facial expressions, such as flat affect or grimacing, and distraction from their surroundings also indicate a significant increase in stressful stimuli.

## Importance of Pain Assessments in Advanced Disease

As many as 90% of all **advanced disease patients** will experience some level of pain. The hospice and palliative care philosophy focuses on the relief of pain and provision for comfort measures for all patients who desire it to improve quality of life. Each patient has the right to accept or refuse treatment for their pain. This becomes difficult when the patient is unable to **communicate** their desires and pain level. It can be assumed that if a patient was experiencing pain when able to communicate, they will continue to experience pain when the ability to communicate has been compromised—pain will be present even in an unconscious state. Changes from previous behavioral, psychological, and subjective and objective assessment data provide the supporting information for continued pain assessments in a nonverbal patient.

## Pain Assessment Tools

### *ABCDE Mnemonic Approach to Pain Assessment*

The Agency for Healthcare Policy and Research recommends use of the **ABCDE method** for assessing and managing pain:

- **Asking** the patient about the extent of pain and assessing systematically.
- **Believing** that the degree of pain the patient reports is accurate.
- **Choosing** the appropriate method of pain control for the patient and circumstances.
- **Delivering** pain interventions appropriately and in a timely, logical manner.
- **Empowering** patients and family by helping them to have control of the course of treatment.

The **5 key elements of pain assessment** include:

- **Quality**: Words are used to describe pain, such as *burning*, *stabbing*, *deep*, *shooting*, and *sharp*. Some may complain of pressure, squeezing, and discomfort rather than pain.
- **Intensity**: Use of a 0-10 scale or other appropriate scale to quantify the degree of pain.
- **Location**: Where does the patient indicate pain?
- **Duration**: Is it constant; does it come and go; is there breakthrough pain?
- **Aggravating/alleviating factors**: What increases the intensity of pain and what relieves the pain?

### *Unidimensional Tools for Pain Assessment*

Unidimensional tools for pain assessment focus on one aspect only: the patient's level of pain. Tools include:

- **Visual analog/numeric rating scale**: A 1-10 rating scale presented visually or verbally from which the patient chooses a number to describe the degree of pain the patient is experiencing. Zero represents no pain, 1 very mild pain, and 10 the most severe pain the patient can imagine.
- **Descriptive**: Pain is described in simple terms that a patient can choose from: mild, moderate, or severe. This may be especially helpful for patients from other countries or cultures where the 1-10 scale is not generally used.
- **FACES**: A chart shows a facial expression scale of simple drawings showing faces with different emotions, such as happiness, fear, and pain. Used primarily for children over age 3 and for nonverbal adults, although both a child's and an adult's version are available. A revised version applies numeric values to expressions so that pain can be assessed according to a numeric rating scale as well.

**Review Video: How to Accurately Assess Pain**
Visit mometrix.com/academy and enter code: 693250

**Review Video: Assessment Tools for Pain**
Visit mometrix.com/academy and enter code: 634001

### *Multidimensional Tools for Pain Assessment*

**Multidimensional tools used for pain assessment** include:

- **Multidimensional pain inventory**: The patient begins by identifying a significant other and then answering 20 questions (rating scale 0-6) about the current rate of pain, the degree of interference in daily life, the ability to work, satisfaction from social/recreational activities, support level of the significant other, mood, pain during the previous week, changes brought about by pain, concerns of the significant other, ability to deal with pain, irritability, and anxiety.
- **Brief pain inventory**: Patients are assessed on the severity of pain (on a 1-10 scale), location of pain, impact of pain on daily function, pain medication, and amount of pain relief in the past 24 hours or the past week. They are asked if the pain interferes with general activity, walking, normal work, mood, interpersonal relations, sleep, or enjoyment of life.
- **McGill pain questionnaire**: The patient marks areas of internal and external pain on body diagrams and selects appropriate adjectives for 20 different sections regarding sensory, affective, and evaluative perceptions. For example, the questionnaire allows the patient to indicate if the pain is "flickering, quivering, pulsing, throbbing, beating, or pounding." The patient also rates present pain intensity (PPI) from 0 (none) to 5 (excruciating).

### *Assessment Tools for Cognitively Impaired or Nonverbal Patients*

The following are types of assessment tools available for use with cognitively impaired or nonverbal patients:

- **Discomfort Scale for Dementia of the Alzheimer Type (DS-DAT)**: For use with elderly persons experiencing dementia, decreased cognition, and decreased verbalization
- **Assessment of Discomfort in Dementia Protocol (ADD)**: Particularly designed for use with patients exhibiting difficult behaviors
- **Checklist of Nonverbal Pain Indicators (CNPI)**: Pain measurement with cognitive impairment
- **Noncommunicative Patient's Pain Assessment Instrument (NOPPAIN)**: Specifically for use by nursing assistants
- **Pain Assessment for the Dementing Elderly (PADE)**: Assessing physical pain behaviors
- **Pain Assessment Tool in Confused Older Adults (PATCOA)**: Focuses on the observation of nonverbal cues
- **Pain Assessment in Advanced Dementia (PAINAD)**: Adapted from the DS-DAT

- **Pain Assessment Checklist for Seniors with Limited Ability to Communicate (PACSLAC)**: To assess common and subtle symptoms
- **Abbey Pain Scale**: For late-stage dementia in nursing home environments

### *Neuropathic Pain Scale*

The neuropathic pain scale (NPS) is the first tool designed specifically to assess the types of pain associated with neuropathy. The NPS comprises 10 sections with 9 assessed with a 0 to 10 (not unpleasant to intolerable) scale:

- Intensity of pain
- Sharpness of pain
- Heat of pain
- Dullness of pain
- Coldness of pain
- Skin sensitivity to touch, clothing
- Itchiness
- Overall unpleasantness of pain
- Intensity of deep and surface pain

The 10th section asks for narrative descriptions of the **time quality** of pain. The patient chooses from three options:

- Feeling background pain all of the time with occasional flare-ups
- Feeling a single type of pain all the time
- Feeling a single type of pain sometimes while having some pain-free periods. The patient then is asked to describe the pain experienced

### *Pain Assessment of Neonates/Infants*

Pain assessment of neonates and infants depends on careful observation of a number of characteristics. The Neonate/Infant Pain Scale (NIPS) assesses 6 areas with a score >3 indicating pain. Five areas are scored 0-1, depending upon the degree of stress. Crying, which is often the most indicative of pain, is scored 0-2:

| Characteristic | 0 | 1 | 2 |
|---|---|---|---|
| **Expression on face** | Rested, normal | Negative, tightened muscles, grimace | |
| **Crying** | None | Intermittent, moaning, whimper | Loud, shrill continuous crying |
| **Respiratory patterns** | Relaxed, normal | Changes include irregular breathing, tachypnea, holding breath, gagging | |
| **Upper extremities** | Relaxed, random movement | Tense, rigid, or rapid extending and flexing. | |
| **Lower extremities** | Relaxed, random movement | Tense, rigid, or rapid extending and flexing. | |
| **Arousal state** | Quiet, awake or asleep with random leg movements | Restless, fussing, thrashing about. | |

### *Assessing Pain in Pediatric Patients*

When assessing the pediatric patient, the nurse must take into consideration the **chronological and developmental age** of the child. These factors help determine which measure the child might use to express pain, as well as treatments that might prove most successful. Assessment parameters must also include the presence of and parameters surrounding chronic illness, as well as neurological impairment. The nurse must identify the underlying cause of the pain, what nonpharmacological measures have been tried for pain control, and what methods can be used to deliver pharmacological interventions. The weight of the child in kilograms determines the appropriate dosages of medications. If the child is able to speak, do the child and the parents speak the same language as the health care provider, and are there any other obvious barriers to communication or pain relief measures?

#### Preteen/Adolescent Pain Scale

**Pain** is subjective and may be influenced by the individual's pain sensation threshold (the smallest stimulus that produces the sensation of pain) and tolerance threshold (the maximum degree of pain that a person can tolerate). The most common current pain assessment tool for preteens and adolescents is the 1-10 pain scale:

- 0 = no pain
- 1-2 = mild pain
- 3-5 = moderate pain
- 6-7 = severe pain
- 8-9 = very severe pain
- 10 = excruciating pain

However, assessment also includes information about onset, duration, and intensity. Identifying pain triggers and what relieves the pain is essential when developing a pain management plan. Children may show very different behaviors when they are in pain. Some may cry and moan with minor pain, and others may seem indifferent even when they are truly suffering. Thus, judging pain by behavior alone can lead to the wrong conclusions.

#### Non-Communicating Children's Pain Checklist

The **Non-Communicating Children's Pain Checklist** (NCCPC) is designed for children ages 3-8 who are cognitively impaired, but a modified version may be used for children recovering from anesthesia. The checklist contains 7 categories with sub-listings that are each scored: 0 (not occurring), 1 (occurring occasionally), 2 (occurring fairly often), 3 (occurring frequently), and NA (not applicable).

- **Vocal**: Moaning, whining, crying, screaming, yelling, or using a specific word for pain
- **Social**: Uncooperative, unhappy, withdrawn, seeking closeness, or can't be distracted
- **Facial**: Furrowed brow, eye changes, not smiling, lips tight or quivering, or clenching or grinding teeth.
- **Activity**: Not moving and quiet or agitated and fidgety.
- **Body and limbs**: Floppy, tense, rigid, spastic, pointing to a part of body that hurts, guarding part of the body, flinching, or positioning body to show pain.
- **Physiological**: Shivering, pallor, increased perspiration, tears, gasping, or holding breath
- **Eating and sleeping**: Eating less or sleeping significantly more or less than usual

The child is usually observed for 2 hours and then scored. All scores are then added together, A score of ≥7 indicates pain.

### QUESTT Pediatric Pain Assessment Tool

QUESTT is designed to focus on assessment, action, and consequent reassessment for results.

- **Question** both the child and parent about the pain experience.
- **Use** assessment tools and rating scales that are appropriate to the developmental stage and situation and understanding of the child.
- **Evaluate** the patient for both behavioral and physiological changes.
- **Secure** the parent's participation in all stages of the pain evaluation and treatment process.
- **Take the cause of the pain into consideration** during the evaluation and choice of treatment methods.
- **Take action** to treat the pain appropriately, and then evaluate the results on a regular basis.

## Barriers to Optimal Pain Assessments

Barriers to optimal pain assessments include:

- **Professional**: Health care providers may lack knowledge about pain assessment and management of different patient populations or may carry out assessments based on personal perceptions rather than validated pain assessment instruments. Some may be concerned about managing adverse effects or the patient's development of tolerance or addiction. In other cases, healthcare providers may lack empathy for patients' suffering. Lack of cultural awareness may affect interpretation of pain. For example, patients in cultures that encourage expression of pain may be assessed as having more pain than patients from cultures that value stoicism.
- **System**: The organization may lack clear policies regarding pain assessment and management, and may not have established clear guidelines for consistent use of pain assessment instruments. Additionally, supervision and accountability may be inadequate, and the organization may be concerned about costs and reimbursement for treatment.
- **Patient**: For personal or cultural reasons, patients may minimize or overstate the degree of pain, interfering with assessment. Some patients may be concerned about addiction or the effects of drugs on cognition (confusion, disorientation, lethargy) or other side effects (constipation, nausea, itching). Some may want to protect family from knowing the extent of pain.
- **Family**: Cultural biases may influence how the family responds to a patient's pain, and this can influence the patient's response as well. Families may lack understanding of the role of pain assessment and management. Some lack understanding about the difference between addiction and pain control at the end of life.
- **Society**: Concerns about drug abuse and addiction often permeate society and influence societal attitudes toward pain control and appropriate drugs to use. Laws and regulations may make access to certain drugs, such as those derived from marijuana, difficult or impossible to obtain.

## Influential Factors in Pain Perception

Factors that can influence the perception of pain include:

- **Emotional state/Attitude**: Patients who are extremely upset or anxious may be so overwhelmed they don't feel the pain, or they may experience pain as more severe than those who are relaxed and calm. If patients expect to suffer from pain, they are also more likely to report severe pain than patients who expect that their pain will be controlled.
- **Cultural expectations**: Perception may vary according to cultural beliefs about pain. For example, if a patient believes that pain is punishment, the patient may agonize over past sins. If a patient believes that pain is fate and reflects karma, then the patient may feel that bearing pain is necessary.
- **Pain threshold**: Different patients simply perceive and experience pain to different degrees. What may be a minor pain to one individual may be severe to another.

## Effects of Gender on Pain Experience

Gender can affect pain sensitivity, tolerance, distress, and exaggeration of pain, and the patient's willingness to report pain, as well as displayed nonverbal cues concerning the pain experience. Studies indicate that women generally have **lower pain thresholds** and **less tolerance** for noxious stimuli or pain factors that hinder them from doing things they enjoy. Women seek help for pain-related problems sooner than men and respond better to therapy. Women also experience more **visceral pain** than men. Men are more prone to experience **somatic pain** and show more stoicism regarding pain experiences than women. **Neuropathic pain** seems to be experienced equally between men and women. Nurses need to be careful that biases concerning gender experiences with pain do not skew their assessments of pain. However, they need to be aware that pain experiences are always individual and may differ between the sexes.

## Cultural Considerations for Pain Management

The following are cultural considerations for pain management:

- **American Indian** and **Alaskan natives** may be unwilling to show pain or request medications. Pain is a difficulty that must be endured rather than treated.
- **Asian and Pacific Islanders** may not vocalize pain and may have an interest in pursuing nontraditional and nonpharmacological treatments to help relieve pain.
- **Black and African American** cultures may tend to openly express their pain but still believe that it is to be endured. They may avoid medication because of personal fears of addiction or cultural stigmatism.
- **Hispanic cultures** may value the ability to endure pain and suffering as a personal quality of strength. Expression of pain, especially for a male, may be considered a sign of weakness. They may feel that pain is a form of divine punishment or trial.

## Psychological Factors in Experience of Pain

**Psychological factors** that may influence a patient's experience of pain include:

- **Fear**: The fear of pain and the anticipation of having pain are factors in how much pain a person feels, because the fear stimulates areas of the brain that focus attention on the body so that the patient experiences an increased sensation of pain. Fear also causes muscles to tense, blood pressure to increase, and the heart rate to increase, and all of these can exacerbate the perception of pain. While pain medications may be necessary, practicing relaxation and mindfulness exercises may help to reduce anxiety and have a positive effect.
- **Depression**: The same neurotransmitters that transmit sensations of pain are also those that transmit moods, so many people with depression present first with complaints of pain or discomfort, and this can result in chronic pain if the depression is not resolved. In some cases, pain may lead to depression, but then the depression worsens the pain so it becomes a cycle of worsening discomfort. Patients may benefit from cognitive behavioral therapy or medication such as SSRIs.

## Pain Documentation in Medical Records

Recommendations for **pain documentation** in the medical record include:

- Describe the time of onset, the location of pain, the character of the pain, and the degree of pain, using a validated pain assessment instrument (either a self-reporting instrument, such as the visual analog scale, or one based on observation, such as PAINAD).
- Document all interventions, both pharmacological (opioids, adjuvants) and nonpharmacological (positioning, massage, relaxation exercises), including the time, the dosage, and the method of administration.
- Assess and document the initial response to the medication based on the expected response time. For example, an IV medication should take effect almost immediately, but oral medications may take up to 20 minutes to take effect.

- Assess and document the duration of response based on the expected duration of the medication. For example, if a medication response is expected to last for 6 hours, the patient's pain level should be assessed at least every 2 hours and more frequently if the rate of pain increases.
- Describe any adverse effects, such as itching or nausea.

# Pharmacologic Pain Management

## WHO Pain Ladder

The WHO pain ladder was developed as an algorithm for treating pain through medications with progressively increasing potency. The approach can be used effectively with both adult and pediatric patients. Beginning with the least potent medication option, each step adds a stronger analgesic until optimum pain relief is reached.

The **WHO pain ladder** has three steps.

- **Step 1**: The patient is given a non-opioid medication which may be used alone or in conjunction with other adjuvant therapies.
- **Step 2**: If the patient reports no change in the pain level, mild- to moderate-level pain-relieving opioids are introduced along with adjuvants if they have not been previously introduced.
- **Step 3**: Uncontrolled pain is then treated with opioids for moderate to severe pain. Adjuvants may also be continued.

## Scheduling of Pain Medications

For mild to moderate pain, patients may take **acetaminophen** alternating with an **NSAID** such as ibuprofen on a regularly scheduled basis or as needed (PRN) at the onset of pain or when pain is anticipated (such as before a dressing change). However, for severe chronic pain, long-acting **opioid pain medications**, such as time-released MS Contin, Duragesic, and OxyContin, should be given regularly around the clock, because these medications help not only control but also prevent pain. The patient should not skip a dose when free of pain, because this makes control more difficult when the pain recurs. In addition to **time-scheduled medications**, the patient may need **short-acting supplementary medications**, such as Percocet, to take on a PRN basis. When taking short-acting medications, the patient should take the medication at the onset of pain, before anticipated pain, or at the onset of increased pain, rather than waiting until the pain is severe, because the goal should always be to keep the pain under control.

## Acetaminophen

Acetaminophen remains one of the safest analgesics for **long-term use**. It can be used to treat mild pain or as an adjuvant with other analgesics for more severe pain. Nonspecific musculoskeletal pain and osteoarthritis are particularly responsive to acetaminophen therapy. Acetaminophen also has a limited **anti-inflammatory nature**.

Acetaminophen should, however, be used cautiously in persons with altered liver or kidney function, as well as those with a history of significant alcohol use, regardless of liver function compromise. It should be dosed separately from any opioid analgesic, which should be given separately as well. This allows for individual titration of each drug to assess the individual needs and side effects separately.

## NSAIDs

NSAIDs act by inhibiting the cyclooxygenase (COX) enzyme, which controls prostaglandin formation. COX-1 affects platelet clumping, gastric blood flow, and mucosal integrity. COX-2 affects pain, inflammation, and fever. COX-1 and 2 inhibitors include aspirin and ibuprofen. Ibuprofen has a lower occurrence of side effects, such as gastric bleeding, than aspirin does. A COX-2 inhibitor, such as Celebrex, must be used with caution due to increased cardiovascular risks when used for over 18 months. NSAIDs are useful for both arthritis and bone cancer pain and work well with opioids for relief of postoperative and other severe pain. NSAIDs may increase the effects of antiseizure drugs and warfarin. Smaller doses are needed if kidney function is impaired.

## Local Anesthetic Pain Relief

Local anesthetics block neural conduction of pain through the application of the anesthetic directly to the nerve endings in the area of pain. It can be injected prior to minor surgery or suturing. It can be injected intercostally for thoracic or high abdominal surgeries. The addition of a vasoconstrictor prolongs effectiveness of the anesthetic. A cream containing local anesthetics (EMLA) can be rubbed on the skin to decrease pain from IV starts or lumbar punctures. It should be applied 60-90 minutes prior to the procedure. A lidocaine 5% patch is approved to relieve pain from postherpetic neuralgia. The patient applies up to 3 patches for 12 hours at a time. Local anesthetics can be applied via the use of an epidural catheter to provide pain control for surgery, childbirth, or postoperative pain control. Opioids can be infused along with the anesthetic agent. Patients using an epidural catheter for postoperative pain tend to ambulate sooner, suffer fewer complications as a result, and go home more quickly.

## OPIOIDS

### *GUIDELINES FOR OPIOID USE*

**Opioid analgesic therapy** is a widely used method of chronic pain control. By adhering to clinical guidelines, pain control can be safely optimized. **Intramuscular administration** should be used as a last resort except in the presence of a "pain emergency" when no other treatment is readily available. Such cases are rare since subcutaneous delivery is almost always an alternative. Noninvasive routes such as **transdermal** and **transmucosal**, which bypass the enteral route, are optimal for continuous pain control and are often effective in eliminating breakthrough pain as well. Changing from one opioid to another, or altering the delivery method, may become necessary under the assumption that incomplete cross-tolerance among opioids occurs. Changing analgesics or method of delivery may result in a decreased drug requirement. When altering opioid delivery regimens, use **morphine equivalents** as the common factor for all dose conversions. This method will help reduce medication errors. Side effects such as sedation, constipation, nausea, and myoclonus should be anticipated in every care plan, and require both prevention and treatment methods.

### *SIDE EFFECTS OF OPIOID ANALGESICS*

Examples of **opioid analgesics** are numerous and include morphine, hydromorphone, oxymorphone, methadone, meperidine, fentanyl, sufentanil, alfentanil, levorphanol, codeine, oxycodone, hydrocodone, propoxyphene, pentazocine, nalbuphine, and buprenorphine. Opioid analgesics have multiple effects on most of the organ systems of the body. Central nervous system (CNS) effects include respiratory depression, analgesia, euphoria, sedation, miosis, cough suppression, truncal rigidity, nausea, and vomiting. Cardiovascular effects are usually slight and include bradycardia, hypotension, reduced blood volume, and increased cerebral blood flow. Gastrointestinal effects can include constipation, decreased gastric motility, and decreased hydrochloric acid. Genitourinary effects are urinary retention and decreased renal function. Other effects are sweating, flushing, and histamine release with itching.

### *OPIOID USE DURING LAST FEW HOURS OF LIFE*

Assessment of pain continues in the **last hours of life**, and medication is adjusted according to assessment. Pain does not necessarily increase as death approaches. It can be assumed that if pain was present prior to loss of consciousness it will continue in the patient's unconscious state. It should be assessed for and treated accordingly. Research has confirmed that administering opioids at the end of life does not hasten nor prolong the dying process. The patient's **prior medication regimen** should be continued. However, adjustments may be made in consideration of reduced renal or hepatic clearance. The **route of administration** should also be assessed for appropriateness and adjusted as needed (e.g., loss of consciousness, inability to swallow).

### *ORAL TRANSMUCOSAL FENTANYL CITRATE*

Oral transmucosal fentanyl citrate consists of **fentanyl** on an oral applicator. The patient applies the dosage (starting at 200 mcg) to the **buccal mucosa** between the cheek and gum for rapid absorption and subsequent pain relief. This makes transmucosal fentanyl particularly useful for managing **breakthrough pain**. Pain relief generally begins within 5 minutes, but the patient should be instructed to wait 15 minutes after the previous dose has been completed before taking another dose. Swallowing even part of the dose rather than having it completely absorbed through the oral mucosa can affect the timing of pain relief onset. **Peak effect** occurs in 20-40 minutes with the total pain relief duration lasting 2-3 hours. Side effects can include somnolence, nausea, and dizziness. Consuming drinks such as coffee, tea, and juices that alter the oral secretion pH can also alter the absorption rate of transmucosal fentanyl.

### Methadone

Methadone is useful for treating **severe or chronic pain** and may be particularly helpful in the presence of **neuropathic pain**. It has a long-acting pain relief factor for a lower cost than many comparable medications. However, the exact dosing ratios with morphine remain unclear within the available research. Metabolism of methadone can also be swayed (either increased or decreased) by many other medications normally taken by patients with chronic conditions. Methadone can also be used to treat opioid addiction. US law for the prescription of methadone for addiction in detoxification or maintenance programs requires a special license and patient enrollment. The words "for pain" need to be clearly stated in the prescription. Methadone can cause drowsiness, weakness, headache, nausea, vomiting, constipation, sweating, and flushing, as well as sedation, decreased respirations, or an irregular heart rate.

### Oxycodone

Oxycodone, a synthetic formulation, is a long-acting opioid for **moderate to severe pain relief**. Side effects are similar to those of morphine. It has a similar pain relief ratio, with the possibility of less nausea and vomiting. Because if its **extended-release nature**, the medication cannot be cut or crushed for administration. Oxycodone does not carry any greater addiction risk than other types of opioids; however, public sensationalism related to this formulation may create hesitation for use among patients. Pharmacies may also limit the amount of this medication they will make available to an individual. Oxycodone should be used cautiously in patients with a history of hypothyroidism, Addison's disease, urethral stricture, prostatic hypertrophy, or lung or liver disease.

### Hydromorphone

Hydromorphone is available as tablets, liquid, suppository, and parenteral formulations. It offers the advantage of being synthetic, allowing for its use in the presence of a true **morphine allergy**. It is also helpful when significant side effects have occurred in the past or pain has been inadequately controlled with other medications. It may also be useful for controlling cough. However, neurotoxicity may occur, particularly myoclonus, hyperalgesia, and seizures. It should also be used cautiously in the presence of kidney, liver, heart, and thyroid disease, seizure disorders, respiratory disease, prostatic hypertrophy, or urinary problems. Common *side effects* include dizziness, lightheadedness, drowsiness, upset stomach if taken without food, vomiting, and constipation.

### Titration of Morphine for Pain Control

Morphine titration protocols vary according to the type of morphine used, the severity of pain, and the patient's tolerance:

| Type | Peak | Duration (hours) |
|---|---|---|
| **Short-acting** | 60 minutes | 4-5 |
| **Long-acting** | 3-4 hours | 8-24 |
| **IM** | 30-60 minutes | 4-5 |
| **SQ** | 50-90 minutes | 4-5 |
| **IV** | 20 minutes | 4-5 |
| **Rectal** | 20-60 minutes | 3-7 |

For example, **optimal dosage** is usually calculated by starting with short-acting oral morphine at 30 mg every 3-4 hours with doses increased by 25-50% for moderate pain or 50-100% for severe pain each time until the patient has at least 50% reduction in pain on a scale of 1-10 or a behavior scale. The dose may need to be reduced if excessive sedation occurs. Once the patient's pain is controlled on short-acting morphine and 24-hour dosage needs are calculated, the patient could be switched to extended-release. **Breakthrough pain** is usually treated with dosages that are 10% of the 24-hour dose. Dosages may be repeated or increased if there is inadequate relief of pain at the peak time. Increasing the dose prior to peak time will result in increased drowsiness.

### *Morphine Use for Chronic Cancer Pain*

One advantage of morphine for chronic cancer pain is that it has no **ceiling dose**. As tolerance to the medication increases or the disease progresses in severity, the dose can be gradually increased to an infinite level. It is also available in many different forms for administration, including intravenous, intramuscular, immediate release, sustained release, long-acting, liquid oral preparations, and suppositories. Morphine is often used as the **equivalency standard** for other opioid analgesics. Common *side effects* of morphine include sedation, respiratory depression, itching, nausea, chronic spasms or twitching of muscle groups, and constipation. Constipation is experienced by all patients receiving opioids. This inevitability should be planned for and treated aggressively. Hallucinations are common when morphine is initiated. After the first few days, most patients will overcome the respiratory depression, nausea, itching, and extreme sedation as tolerance for the medication is developed.

### *Dosages for Morphine, Codeine, Hydromorphone, and Levorphanol*

The dosages for both the enteral and parenteral routes of morphine, codeine, hydromorphone, and levorphanol are as follows:

- **Morphine**: Enteral dosage is 30 mg (available as continuous and sustained-release formulations to last 12-24 hours); parenteral dosage is 10 mg.
- **Codeine**: Enteral dosage is 200 mg (not generally recommended); parenteral dosage is 130 mg.
- **Hydromorphone**: Enteral dosage is 7.5 mg (available as a continuous-release formula lasting 24 hours); parenteral dosage is 1.5 mg.
- **Levorphanol**: In acute pain episodes, enteral dosage is 4 mg; parenteral dosage is 2 mg. For chronic pain, dosage is equivalent for both enteral and parenteral at 1 mg. Levorphanol has a long half-life, increasing the chances of dosage accumulation over time.

Adhering to the statement "If the gut works, use it," as much as 90 percent of all patients will at least start out able to use oral medications instead of other routes.

### *Calculation for Converting Medication Regimen Between Two Opioids*

Calculate the current 24-hour drug dose, or the total amount given in a 24-hour period. Multiply the current 24-hour dose times the ratio of the 24-hour equivalent dose for the new drug over the 24-hour equivalent of the old drug. This calculation provides the **equivalent 24-hour dose** for the new drug. Divide the new dose amount by the number of doses to be provided during the day. This amount equals the new **target dosage**.

$$\text{current 24 hr dose} \times \frac{\text{new drug 24 hr equiv dose}}{\text{current drug 24 hr equiv dose}} = \text{new 24 hr dose}$$

$$\frac{\text{new 24 hr dose}}{\text{doses per day}} = \text{new target dosage}$$

## Ketamine

Ketamine is a dissociative anesthetic that can provide pain relief as an alternate or complement to an opioid. The dissociative quality is an effective way to help the patient separate from the sensation of pain. Ketamine treatment begins with an initial bolus of 0.1 mg/kg IV. If there is no improvement, a second bolus with double the dosage is provided in 5 minutes. This can be repeated as needed. Boluses should be followed by a decrease in the patient's current opioid dose by 50% and an infusion of ketamine. **Infusion dosing** for ketamine is 0.015 mg/kg/min, or about 1 mg/min for a 70 kg person. If IV access cannot be attained, subcutaneous infusion is a possibility with dosing of 0.3-0.5 mg/kg. Consider concurrent treatment with a **benzodiazepine** to prevent hallucinations or frightful dreams and observe for increased secretions, as these are all possible side effects of ketamine. The secretions may be treated with glycopyrrolate, scopolamine, or atropine as needed.

## Treating Breakthrough Pain

The three basic types of breakthrough pain, and their treatment measures are as follows:

- **Incident pain**: Pain that can be specifically tied to an activity or event, such as a dressing change or physical therapy. These events can be anticipated and treated with a rapid-onset, short-acting analgesic just prior to the painful event.
- **Spontaneous pain**: This type of pain is unpredictable and cannot be pinpointed to a relationship with any certain time or event. There is no way to anticipate spontaneous pain. In the presence of neuropathic pain, adjuvant therapy may be useful. Otherwise, a rapid-onset, short-acting analgesic is used.
- **End-of-dose failure**: Pain that specifically occurs at the end of a routine analgesic dosing cycle when medication blood levels begin to taper off. Careful evaluation of end-of-dose failure can help prevent it sooner. It may indicate an increased dose tolerance and the need for medication dose alterations.

## Treating Neuropathic Pain

Treatment options for neuropathic pain are often different from the methods used to treat other types of pain. The three drug classes most commonly used and proven effective for treating neuropathic pain are **anticonvulsants**, **anesthetics**, and **antidepressants**. Some are given on an as-needed basis, but most require consistent dosing with **24-hour symptom control**. Examples of the most common medications include amitriptyline, nortriptyline, duloxetine, gabapentin, topical lidocaine, opioids, and pregabalin. Medication choice is dependent on factors such as the type and progression of the disorder and the associated physical and emotional problems, such as nerve injury, muscle weakness or spasms, anxiety, depression, or sleep disturbances.

## Treating Bone Pain

Treatment options for bone pain may depend on the causative agent related to the pain, such as the primary cancer site, severely weakened bones, or fractures. **Systemic treatment choices** include chemotherapy, radiation, and hormone therapy. **Hormone therapy** is used in the presence of estrogen and androgen receptors within the cancer cells. **Bisphosphonates**, such as ibandronate, zoledronate, and alendronate, may help strengthen the bones, slow damage, and prevent fractures; they can also help reduce pain. However, side effects can include fatigue, fever, nausea, vomiting, and anemia. **Surgery** may also be considered to remove cancerous cells or reinforce weakened areas of bone. **Opioids** and **NSAIDs/COX-2 inhibitors** are most often used for pain relief and need to be provided on a consistent basis.

Morphine combined with ibuprofen provides the benefit of a centrally acting opioid with a peripherally acting NSAID. Ibuprofen also acts as an effective adjuvant analgesic agent to enhance the relief provided by the opioid without increasing opioid side effects.

## Measures Taken During Pain Crisis

During a pain crisis, assess for a change in the mechanism or location of the pain and attempt to differentiate between **terminal anxiety** or agitation and the **physical causes** of pain. Begin with a rapid increase in **opioid treatment**. If the pain is unresponsive to opioid titration, switching to **benzodiazepines**, such as diazepam and lorazepam, may produce a more effective response. If terminal symptoms remain unresponsive, assess for **drug absorption**. While invasive routes of medication delivery are generally avoided unless necessary, the only guaranteed route of drug delivery is the IV route. If there is any question about absorption, it is appropriate to establish parenteral access. IM delivery should be considered as a last resort. When all accessible resources have been exhausted, seek a pain management consultation as quickly as possible. Alternative methods of terminal pain control include radiotherapy, anesthetic, or neuroablative procedures.

## Concerns Surrounding Use of Pain Medications with End-of-Life Patients

Common concerns surrounding the use of pain medications with end-of-life patients include:

- **Adequacy**: Patients are often concerned that medication may not be adequate to control pain and that chronic or breakthrough pain will occur. Patients may be concerned that if they take adequate pain medication, it will be less effective later when pain may be worse.
- **Sedation/addiction**: Some patients and family members are concerned about the risks of addiction, and others may be concerned about the effects of the medication on the patient's cognition, as some patients may become confused, disoriented, or sedated, depending on the medication or dosage.
- **Adverse effects**: Nausea and vomiting may be almost as debilitating to a patient as the pain it is intended to alleviate. Constipation, a common adverse effect, may be very uncomfortable for a patient. Some medications may result in itching and others may cause myoclonus, both of which are uncomfortable for the patient.

## Prescribing Controlled Substances to Patients with Advanced Illness and Addiction Challenges

In the presence of **addiction challenges**, it becomes important to choose a **long-acting opioid** that can facilitate around-the-clock dosing and minimize the need for short-term medications used for breakthrough doses. **Short-term medication** use should be very limited or eliminated entirely if possible. Whenever possible, **nondrug adjuvants** such as relaxation techniques, distraction, biofeedback, TNS, and therapeutic communication should be used in place of short-term medications. When short-term medication therapy is needed, a **nonopioid** is best. Limit the amount of medication available to the patient at any given time and monitor for compliance with pill counts and urine toxicology screens as necessary. In some instances, a referral to an addictions specialist is recommended.

## Tolerance and Pseudotolerance

**Tolerance** is the adaptation of the body to continued exposure to a drug or chemical. The effects of the drug at the same level of exposure are minimized over time. Additional dosing is required to maintain the same outcomes.

**Pseudotolerance** is the misguided perception of the health care provider that a patient's need for increasing doses of a drug is due to the development of tolerance, when the reality is that disease progression or other factors are responsible for the increase in dosing needs.

## Addiction and Pseudoaddiction

**Addiction** is a primary and constant neurobiologic disease with genetic, psychosocial, and environmental factors that create an obsessive and irrational need or preoccupation with a substance. Addictive behaviors include unrestricted, continued cravings, as well as compulsive and persistent use of a drug despite harmful experiences and side effects.

**Pseudoaddiction** is an assumption that the patient is addicted to a substance when in actuality the patient is not experiencing relief from the medication. It is prolonged, unrelieved pain that may be the result of undertreatment. This situation may lead the patient to become more aggressive in seeking medicated relief, thus resulting in the inappropriate "drug seeker" label.

## Physical Dependence

Physical dependence occurs when the body adapts to a drug, requiring increasing dosages over time to gain the same effect, and withdrawal of that drug then will result in an **abstinence syndrome** (withdrawal). Physical dependence can be described as a form of **addiction**. While physical dependence was commonly thought of as being related to narcotic drugs (such as morphine, methadone, fentanyl), many different types of drugs may cause some degree of physical dependence. For example, abruptly stopping a beta-blocker may result in cardiac arrhythmias or cardiac arrest. Abruptly stopping SSRIs may result in severe depression and anxiety. Thus, when considering stopping a patient's drugs near the end of life, physical dependence must be considered as many drugs should be **tapered** to avoid withdrawal effects. Drugs that affect the **central nervous system**, such as ethanol, barbiturates, and benzodiazepines, pose considerable risk of dependence and may result in severe withdrawal symptoms.

# Patient Safety and Injury Prevention

## Joint Commission's Patient Safety Goals

The Joint Commission has a set of **goals that impact patient safety** for each type of healthcare facility. Within the hospital environment, there are several goals that pertain:

- Each facility must have a way to identify patients that will avoid errors of identification.
- Caregivers are to give careful, accurate communications about patients and their care so that mistakes are not made.
- A system to avoid medication errors must be in place.
- Medications must be reconciled when the patient moves from place to place within the hospital or is discharged to other caregivers.
- The risk of infection must be decreased so that patients are at less risk for hospital-related infections.
- The facility must have a fall prevention program and evaluate its effectiveness.

All patients and family must be encouraged to be active in their own care to help to avoid errors. They must also know how to make sure their concerns for safety of care are heard and acted upon.

## Aspects of Patient Safety in the Hospital

Deliberate decisions by the health care providers/facility can help create an environment conducive for patient safety. Some of those aspects include:

- **Educating the patient on signaling staff**: The patient must be educated about the use of the call light, and the call light placed within easy reach. If the patient is unable to use the call light, then an alternative means of calling for help, such as a handheld bell, should be available. If the patient is unable to manage any type of signaling system, then the nurse should check on the patient at least every hour.
- **Protecting from falls and electrical hazards**: All clutter should be removed from floors and cords secured away from walkways. All electrical appliances should be checked to ensure they are working properly and have no frayed cords. Patients should be provided assistive devices, such as walkers, if necessary, to improve stability.
- **Making appropriate room assignments**: Patients with the greatest need for supervision should be placed closest to the nursing desk and within the line of sight whenever possible. In environments such as critical care, each nurse should be able to visualize their patient assignment from their nursing station.

## Medication Errors

There are about 7,000 deaths yearly in the United States attributed to **medication errors.** Studies indicate that there are errors in 1 in 5 doses of medication given to patients in hospitals. Patient safety must be ensured with proper handling and administering of medications:

- **Avoid error-prone abbreviations or symbols**. The Joint Commission has established a list of abbreviations to avoid, but mistakes are frequent with other abbreviations as well. In many cases, abbreviations and symbols should be avoided altogether or restricted to a limited approved list.
- **Prevent errors due to illegible handwriting or unclear verbal orders**. Handwritten orders should be block printed to reduce chance of error; verbal orders should be repeated back to the physician.
- **Institute barcoding and scanners** that allow the patient's wristband and medications to be scanned for verification.
- **Provide lists of similarly-named medications** to educate staff.
- Establish an **institutional policy** for the administration of medications that includes protocols for verification of drug, dosage, and patient, as well as educating the patient about the medications.

## Assessing Patients for Allergies

When assessing patients for **allergies** it's important to determine the type of symptoms they have, when the initial reaction occurred, and what type of treatment they have used in the past to manage this complication (including antihistamines). Allergies of particular interest include:

- **Food**: Ask patients about any specific foods that cause an adverse reaction as some foods may have cross-reactivity to latex (such as kiwi, papaya, avocado, and bananas), so patients may be at risk of developing latex allergy and should avoid contact with latex. Some medications may contain substances derived from food, such as eggs, fish, gelatin, lactose, and soy.
- **Latex**: Sensitivity to latex can result in mild reactions, such as itching and rash, to severe anaphylactic reactions, and is common among those with repeated contact with healthcare environments, such as those with spina bifida or multiple surgeries, so it should be suspected with these clients. While non-latex options are more readily available in most hospitals (non-latex gloves and Foley catheters, for instance), latex continues to be used in hospital materials, therefore this allergy must be assessed immediately upon arrival so that appropriate materials can be substituted if necessary.
- **Environmental**: The most common environmental allergies include pollens, dust mites, animals, cigarette smoke, cockroaches, and mold/mildew, so the nurse should be sure to ask about these as well as any other environmental allergies. Some patients are sensitive to strong colognes and perfumes, so the use of these is often regulated by hospital dress codes on units with immunocompromised patients.

## Non-Pharmacologic Prescription Precautions

Some non-pharmacologic prescriptions may contribute to accident or injury, including the following:

- **Oxygen supplies**: Oxygen may be administered at the wrong level of liters (too much or too little), and the oxygen supply may be inadvertently obstructed or disconnected. Oxygen concentrators may not have backup batteries and may fail to function if electricity goes off. If people smoke around oxygen, this increases the risk of fires. Nasal cannulas and face masks that delivery oxygen, when used over prolonged periods of time, can cause pressure injuries, therefore appropriate assessment and skin care is also necessary.
- **Assistive devices**: If equipment, such as canes and walkers, are improperly fitted, they may increase risk of falls.
- **Dialysis equipment**: Contamination of equipment is always a concern and can result in peritonitis (peritoneal dialysis) and sepsis (hemodialysis). If the lines become separated, the client may exsanguinate.
- **Hot/cold compresses**: If cold compresses are placed directly on the skin, they may damage the tissue, especially if left in place for too long. Hot compresses may cause burns if temperature is too high and may damage wounds if placed directly over them.

## Seizure Precautions

Seizure disorders are broadly categorized as partial seizures (which begin locally) or generalized seizures (which are bilateral and symmetrical and may be convulsive or non-convulsive):

- **Partial seizures** include *simple partial* (with motor, sensory, and/or autonomic symptoms but without impaired consciousness), *complex partial* (with cognitive, affective, psychosensory, and/or psychomotor symptoms, as well as impaired consciousness), or *partial secondarily generalized.*
- **Generalized seizures** include seizures that are bilateral and symmetric without local onset and may be convulsive or non-convulsive. These seizures include *tonic-clonic, tonic, clonic, absence* (petit mal), *atonic*, and *myoclonic seizures*, as well as *unclassified seizures.*

**Seizure precautions** are a standard set of safety protocol that ensure patient safety in those patients with a high risk or history of seizures. Generally, these precautions include padding the siderails, keeping the bed at the lowest position, and maintaining suctioning at the bedside Precautions also include ensuring privacy and providing supportive care in the event of a seizure, such as easing the patient to the floor and providing padding to protect the head. Side rails should be raised and pillow removed if the patient is in bed. The patient should be placed on one side with the head flexed so the tongue does not block the airway. The patient should *not* be restrained or a padded tongue-blade inserted between the teeth.

## Patient Deficits That Impede Client Safety

Certain patient deficits can inherently impede client safety, including the following:

- **Visual impairment**: Patients are at risk of trips, slips, falls, burn injuries, poisoning (mistaken containers, ingredients), and medication errors because of taking the wrong medication or wrong dosage.
- **Hearing impairment**: Patients are at increased risk of falls and may not hear danger signals, such as fire alarms, smoke detectors, police/fire sirens, and tornado warning sirens, and may, therefore, not be aware that they are in danger. Most smoke detectors emit a high-frequency alarm that cannot always be detected by those with high-frequency hearing loss.
- **Sensory/Perceptual impairment**: Patients (such as those with stroke or brain injury) may exhibit a wide variety of impairments so safety concerns may vary. For example, those with one-sided neglect may have injuries to the neglected side, such as from running into doors or other things. Those with face blindness may easily get lost if away from familiar places or people.

## R.A.C.E. Acronym for Fire Safety

RACE is an acronym used for fire safety on the hospital unit:

- **R**escue: Remove all patients from area of danger
- **A**ctivate alarm: Pull fire alarm/call 9-1-1
- **C**onfine the fire: Close doors to unit/place
- **E**vacuate/Extinguish (NFPA/OSHA fire safety): Use **PASS** for fire extinguisher
    - **P**ull
    - **A**im at the base of the flames
    - **S**queeze the trigger
    - **S**weep: Use a sweeping motion across the flames

## Ergonomics

Ergonomics is the study of preventing workplace injury and stress. In nursing, it refers to the way in which a nurse can prevent injury to self and others due to the stressors and strains required in the nursing field. Some important **ergonomic principles** include:

- **Body Mechanics:** The body should be kept in proper alignment during tasks, with a wide base of support and center of gravity low. Use larger muscles (buttocks, thighs, shoulders) for activities rather than smaller when possible. Avoid twisting or jerking movements. Maintain 90° angle in elbows and knees when sitting, elbows at the side, with back straight and looking straight ahead.
- **Lifting:** Use appropriate transfer devices; use as many people as necessary. Manual lifting should be avoided. Bend at the knees, tighten core, and keep weights close to the body – *never* bend or twist when lifting.
- **Repetition**: Avoid repetitive movements/stressors and use proper safety equipment when needed (earplugs for loud noises, etc.).

## PATIENT BOARDING AND PATIENT SAFETY

Patient boarding is maintaining a patient in the emergency department (ED), sometimes for more than 24 hours, after the patient is admitted as an inpatient, usually because staffing is inadequate on the destination unit or no bed is available. Boarding results in over-crowding in the ED and impacts the quality of care because boarded patients often have intensive needs. Psychiatric patients are often boarded because of a lack of mental-health beds. According to the Joint Commission, patient boarding is a safety risk and indicates a problem in patient flow. Boarding should not exceed 4 hours. If a patient cannot be transferred promptly then added staff should be provided to care for the boarded patients. The hospital should have plans in place to facilitate rapid transfer. If the hospital is over capacity, then contingency plans may need to be implemented, such as diverting patients to other EDs or transferring patients to other hospitals.

# Therapeutic Relationships

## Therapeutic Communication

### *Facilitating Communication*

Therapeutic communication begins with respect for the patient/family and the assumption that all communication, verbal and nonverbal, has meaning. Listening must be done empathetically. The following are some techniques that facilitate communication.

**Introduction**:

- Make a personal introduction and use the patient's name: "Mrs. Brown, I am Susan Williams, your nurse."

**Encouragement**:

- Use an open-ended opening statement: "Is there anything you'd like to discuss?"
- Acknowledge comments: "Yes," and "I understand."
- Allow silence and observe nonverbal behavior rather than trying to force conversation. Ask for clarification if statements are unclear.
- Reflect statements back (use sparingly): Patient: "I hate this hospital." Nurse: "You hate this hospital?"

**Empathy**:

- Make observations: "You are shaking," and "You seem worried."
- Recognize feelings:
    - Patient: "I want to go home."
    - Nurse: "It must be hard to be away from your home and family."
- Provide information as honestly and completely as possible about condition, treatment, and procedures and respond to the patient's questions and concerns.

**Exploration**:

- Verbally express implied messages:
    - Patient: "This treatment is too much trouble."
    - Nurse: "You think the treatment isn't helping you?"
- Explore a topic but allow the patient to terminate the discussion without further probing: "I'd like to hear how you feel about that."

**Orientation**:

- Indicate reality:
    - Patient: "Someone is screaming."
    - Nurse: "That sound was an ambulance siren."
- Comment on distortions without directly agreeing or disagreeing:
    - Patient: "That nurse promised I didn't have to walk again."
    - Nurse: "Really? That's surprising because the doctor ordered physical therapy twice a day."

**Collaboration**:

- Work together to achieve better results: "Maybe if we talk about this, we can figure out a way to make the treatment easier for you."

**Validation**:

- Seek validation: "Do you feel better now?" or "Did the medication help you breathe better?"

### Avoiding Non-therapeutic Communication

While using therapeutic communication is important, it is equally important to avoid interjecting **non-therapeutic communication**, which can block effective communication. *Avoid the following:*

- Meaningless clichés: "Don't worry. Everything will be fine." "Isn't it a nice day?"
- Providing advice: "You should..." or "The best thing to do is...." It's better when patients ask for advice to provide facts and encourage the patient to reach a decision.
- Inappropriate approval that prevents the patient from expressing true feeling or concerns:
  - Patient: "I shouldn't cry about this."
  - Nurse: "That's right! You're an adult!"
- Asking for an explanation of behavior that is not directly related to patient care and requires analysis and explanation of feelings: "Why are you so upset?"
- Agreeing with rather than accepting and responding to patient's statements can make it difficult for the patient to change his or her statement or opinion later: "I agree with you," or "You are right."
- Making negative judgments: "You should stop arguing with the nurses."
- Devaluing the patient's feelings: "Everyone gets upset at times."
- Disagreeing directly: "That can't be true," or "I think you are wrong."
- Defending against criticism: "The doctor is not being rude; he's just very busy today."
- Changing the subject to avoid dealing with uncomfortable topics;
  - Patient: "I'm never going to get well."
  - Nurse: "Your family will be here in just a few minutes."
- Making inappropriate literal responses, even as a joke, especially if the patient is at all confused or having difficulty expressing ideas:
  - Patient: "There are bugs crawling under my skin."
  - Nurse: "I'll get some bug spray,"
- Challenging the patient to establish reality often just increases confusion and frustration:
  - "If you were dying, you wouldn't be able to yell and kick!"

## Communicating with Patients with Disabilities

Guidelines for communicating with individuals with disabilities:

- Do not assume that the person with disabilities also has impaired cognition.
- Always treat the person with respect and dignity.
- Use first names with the patient if asked to do so, but start out formally as with any patient.
- Offer to shake hands even when a prosthesis is present.
- Be patient if communication is impaired.
- Offer assistance, but allow the patient to tell you what is helpful; otherwise don't assist.
- When a wheelchair is used, sit down so the patient does not have to strain their neck to speak with you.
- If providing directions, consider the obstacles that may be in the way and assist the person to find an appropriate way around them.

## Communication with Patients with Cognitive Disabilities

The person with cognitive disabilities may be easily distracted, so verbal communication should be attempted in a quiet area:

- Address people with dignity and respect.
- Do not try to discuss abstract ideas but stick with concrete topics.
- Keep words and sentences very simple and try rephrasing when necessary. People may have difficulty in distinguishing your spoken words and deriving the meaning from them.
- Be very patient with people's attempts to speak to you since they may have difficulty in processing thoughts and changing them into spoken words.
- Use objects around you and gestures to illustrate your words since the patient may also use pointing and gesturing when unable to find the words to communicate with you. The person may prefer written communication, although some may be unable to read.
- Use touch to convey your regard during communication, as this is recognized by the patient as reassurance of your care and concern for them.
- Give a few instructions at a time as to not overwhelm them.

## Communicating with Deaf or Hearing-Impaired Patients

Communicating with a person with deafness or hearing impairment:

- Try to communicate in a quiet environment if possible.
- Wave or touch the person to let him or her know you are trying to communicate.
- Determine the method the person uses to communicate: sign language, lip reading, hearing devices, or writing.
- Fingerspell or use some signs if able to do so.
- Address the person directly when you speak even though the person may be looking at an interpreter or your lips.
- Look at the person as the interpreter tells you what was said.
- Speak slowly so the interpreter can keep up with you.
- If the person reads lips, face the person and speak clearly and normally, using normal volume.
- If writing a communication, do not speak while writing.
- Do not be afraid to check that the person understands you, and ask questions if you do not understand the person.

## Communication with People with Low Vision or Blindness

Communicating with a person with low vision or blindness:

- Greet the person with low vision or blindness, identifying yourself and others present.
- Always say goodbye when you are leaving.
- Alert the person to written communications, such as warning signs or printed notices.
- Face the person and touch briefly on the arm to let the person know you are speaking to him or her if you are in a group.
- Speak at normal loudness.
- Make any directions given specific in terms of the length of walk and obstacles, such as stairs.
- Use the position of hands on a clock face to give directions (potatoes at 3 o'clock) as well as using *right* or *left*.
- Mention sounds that the person may hear in transit or on arrival at a destination.
- Do not be afraid to use the word *see*, as the person will probably use it as well.

## Communicating with a Patient on a Ventilator

When a patient on a ventilator is conscious, he or she may still be able to communicate by blinking, nodding, shaking the head, or pointing to a picture or word board:

- If the person is able to write, try to reposition the IV line to leave the dominant hand free to communicate.
- Discuss the need for communication with the physician and ask if a valve or an electric larynx can be used to permit speech.
- Help the patient practice lip reading of single words.
- Remember the patient's glasses or hearing aids when attempting to communicate.
- Enlist the aid of a speech therapist if there is frustration on the part of the patient and family due to communication difficulty.

## Communicating with Persons with Speech Problems Due to a Stroke

Methods to communicate with stroke patients with speech problems:

- **Dysarthria**: Patients have problems forming the words to speak them aloud. Give them time to communicate, offer them a picture board or other means of communicating, and give encouragement to family members who are frustrated with the difficulty of trying to communicate.
- **Expressive aphasia**: The patients' efforts at speech come out garbled when they try to say sentences, but single words may be clear. Encourage the patients to try to write and to practice the sounds of the alphabet. Resist the urge to finish sentences for the patients.
- **Receptive aphasia**: The patients have a problem comprehending the speech they hear. Communicate in simple terms and speak slowly. Test comprehension of the written word as an alternative method of communication.
- **Global aphasia**: The patient has both receptive and expressive aphasia. Use simple, clear, slow speech augmented by pictures and gestures.

## Communication Problems of Patients with Parkinson's Disease

Parkinson's disease causes problems with speaking in the majority (75-90%) of patients. The reason for this is not clear but may relate to increasing rigidity and changes in movement. Speech is often very low-pitched or hoarse, given in a monotone and with a soft voice. Speech production may decrease because of the effort required to speak. **Speech therapy** can develop exercises for the patient that can assist them in remembering to speak slowly and carefully, as patients are not always aware that their **communication** is impaired:

- Allow time for the patient to communicate, asking for repetition if you do not understand the message.
- Help family by teaching ways to facilitate communication with the patient and encouraging them to assist the patient to do the exercises provided by the therapist.
- If speech volume is very low, suggest amplification devices that can be obtained through speech therapy.

## Communication with Patients with Psychiatric Problems

Persons with psychiatric disorders appreciate being addressed with respect, dignity, and honesty:

- Speak simply and clearly, repeating as necessary.
- Encourage patients to discuss their concerns regarding treatment and medications to improve compliance.
- Use good eye contact and be attentive to your body language messages.
- Be alert, but unless the person is known to be violent, try to relax and listen to them.
- Don't try to avoid words or phrases pertaining to psychiatric problems, but if you do say something inappropriate, apologize honestly to the patient.

- Offer patients outlets for their thoughts and feelings.
- Learn more about their disorder and ways to use therapeutic communication to help them with their problem, such as re-orienting them as needed.

## Cultural Competence

Different cultures view health and illness from very different perspectives, and patients often come from a mix of many cultures, so the nurse must be not only accepting of cultural differences but must be sensitive and aware. There are a number of characteristics that are important for a nurse to have **cultural competence**:

- **Appreciating diversity**: This must be grounded in information about other cultures and understanding of their value systems.
- **Assessing own cultural perspectives**: Self-awareness is essential to understanding potential biases.
- **Understanding intercultural dynamics**: This must include understanding ways in which cultures cooperate, differ, communicate, and reach understanding.
- **Recognizing institutional culture**: Each institutional unit (hospital, clinic, office) has an inherent set of values that may be unwritten but is accepted by the staff.
- **Adapting patient service to diversity**: This is the culmination of cultural competence as it is the point of contact between cultures.

## Cultural Characteristics

### *Hispanic Patients*

Many areas of the country have large populations of Hispanics and Hispanic Americans. As always, it's important to recognize that cultural generalizations don't always apply to individuals. Recent immigrants, especially, have cultural needs that the nurse must understand:

- Many Hispanics are Catholic and may like the nurse to make arrangements for a priest to visit.
- Large extended families may come to visit to support the patient and family, so patients should receive clear explanations about how many visitors are allowed, but some flexibility may be required.
- Language barriers may exist as some may have limited or no English skills, so translation services should be available around the clock.
- Hispanic culture encourages outward expressions of emotions, so family may react strongly to news about a patient's condition, and people who are ill may expect some degree of pampering, so extra attention to the patient/family members may alleviate some of their anxiety.

**Caring for Hispanic and Hispanic American patients** requires understanding of cultural differences:

- Some immigrant Hispanics have very little formal education, so medical information may seem very complex and confusing, and they may not understand the implications or need for follow-up care.
- Hispanic culture perceives time with more flexibility than American culture, so if parents need to be present at a particular time, the nurse should specify the exact time (1:30 PM) and explain the reason rather than saying something more vague, such as "after lunch."
- People may appear to be unassertive or unable to make decisions when they are simply showing respect to the nurse by being deferent.
- In traditional families, the males make decisions, so a woman waits for the father or other males in the family to make decisions about treatment or care.
- Families may choose to use folk medicines instead of Western medical care or may combine the two.
- Children and young women are often sheltered and are taught to be respectful to adults, so they may not express their needs openly.

### *Middle Eastern Patients*

There are considerable cultural differences among Middle Easterners, but religious beliefs about the segregation of males and females are common. It's important to remember that segregating the female is meant to protect her virtue. Female nurses have low status in many countries because they violate this segregation by touching male bodies, so parents may not trust or show respect for the nurse who is caring for their family member. Additionally, male patients may not want to be cared for by female nurses or doctors, and families may be very upset at a female being cared for by a male nurse or physician. When possible, these cultural traditions should be accommodated:

- In Middle Eastern countries, males make decisions, so issues for discussion or decision should be directed to males, such as the father or spouse, and males may be direct in stating what they want, sometimes appearing demanding.
- If a male nurse must care for a female patient, then the family should be advised that *personal care* (such as bathing) will be done by a female while the medical treatments will be done by the male nurse.

**Caring for Middle Eastern patients** requires understanding of cultural differences:

- Families may practice strict dietary restrictions, such as avoiding pork and requiring that animals be killed in a ritual manner, so vegetarian or kosher meals may be required.
- People may have language difficulties requiring a translator, and same-sex translators should be used if at all possible.
- Families may be accompanied by large extended families that want to be kept informed and whom patients consult before decisions are made.
- Most medical care is provided by female relatives, so educating the family about patient care should be directed at females (with female translators if necessary).
- Outward expressions of grief are considered as showing respect for the dead.
- Middle Eastern families often offer gifts to caregivers. Small gifts (candy) that can be shared should be accepted graciously, but for other gifts, the families should be advised graciously that accepting gifts is against hospital policy.
- Middle Easterners often require less personal space and may stand very close.

### *Asian Patients*

There are considerable differences among different Asian populations, so cultural generalizations may not apply to all, but nurses caring for Asian patients should be aware of common cultural attitudes and behaviors:

- Nurses and doctors are viewed with respect, so traditional Asian families may expect the nurse to remain authoritative and to give directions and may not question, so the nurse should ensure that they understand by having them review material or give demonstrations and should provide explanations clearly, anticipating questions that the family might have but may not articulate.
- Disagreeing is considered impolite. "Yes" may only mean that the person is heard, not that they agree with the person. When asked if they understand, they may indicate that they do even when they clearly do not so as not to offend the nurse.
- Asians may avoid eye contact as an indication of respect. This is especially true of children in relation to adults and of younger adults in relation to elders.

**Caring for Asian patients** requires understanding of cultural differences:

- Patients/families may not show outward expressions of feelings/grief, sometimes appearing passive. They also avoid public displays of affection. This does not mean that they don't feel, just that they don't show their feelings.
- Families often hide illness and disabilities from others and may feel ashamed about illness.

- Terminal illness is often hidden from the patient, so families may not want patients to know they are dying or seriously ill.
- Families may use cupping, pinching, or applying pressure to injured areas, and this can leave bruises that may appear as abuse, so when bruises are found, the family should be questioned about alternative therapy before assumptions are made.
- Patients may be treated with traditional herbs.
- Families may need translators because of poor or no English skills.
- In traditional Asian families, males are authoritative and make the decisions.

## Religious Objections to Treatment

### *Jehovah's Witnesses*

Jehovah's Witnesses have traditionally shunned transfusions and blood products as part of their religious beliefs. In 2004, the *Watchtower,* a Jehovah's Witness publication, presented a guide for members. When medical care indicates the need for blood transfusion or blood products and the patient and/or family members are practicing Jehovah's Witnesses, this may present a conflict. It's important to approach the patient/family with full information and reasons for the transfusion or blood components without being judgmental, allowing them to express their feelings. In fact, studies show that while adults often refuse transfusions for themselves, they frequently allow their children to receive blood products, so one should never assume that an individual would refuse blood products based on the religion alone. Jehovah's Witnesses can receive fractionated blood cells, thus allowing hemoglobin-based blood substitutes. The following guidelines are provided to church members:

Basic **blood standards for Jehovah's Witnesses**:

- **Not acceptable**: Whole blood: red cells, white cells, platelets, plasma.
- **Acceptable**: Fractions from red cells, white cells, platelets, and plasma.

### *Christian Scientists*

Christian Science**,** a religion developed by Mary Baker Eddy in 1879, promotes the belief that sickness is most effectively treated through prayer alone. While Christian Scientists do not avoid all medical interventions, their beliefs are conservative regarding medical treatment. Most notably, Christian Scientists, for the most part, do not believe in vaccinations and may only agree to such if required by law, as they do acknowledge the importance of community health. They have widely appreciated the use of exemptions from mandatory vaccines, but as these exemptions have become more limited, religious leaders have given their members the right to decide upon vaccinations.

## Impact of Culture and Religion on Dietary Preferences

When performing a dietary assessment, the nurse should remember that culture and religion might dictate which foods and spices are used. The manner in which food is prepared, cooked, and served may also be specified. The utensils used at the meal as well as the persons who may eat together may be important. Mealtimes and required fasts should be determined. Holidays may be accompanied by particular foods. Alcohol (including extracts made with alcohol) and caffeine may be prohibited. The culture may also consider obesity a sign of affluence and success. The nurse should evaluate the foods that are eaten in light of the patient's medical condition. The patient may not wish to eat the usual hospital fare and may need to have a special diet prepared or food brought from home. The nurse can guide the patient and family to foods that are acceptable and within the patient's requirements for health.

# Abuse and Neglect

## Indicators of Abuse That May Be Identified in the Patient History

The healthcare provider should always be aware of the presence of any **indicators** that may present a potential for or an actual situation that involves **abuse**. These indicators may present in the **patient's history**. Some examples of indicators concerning their primary complaint may include the following: vague description about the cause of the problem, inconsistencies between physical findings and explanations, minimizing injuries, long period of time between injury and treatment, and over-reactions or under-reactions of family members to injuries. Other important information may be revealed in the family genome, such as family history of violence, time spent in jail or prison, and family history of violent deaths or substance abuse. The patient's health history may include previous injuries, spontaneous abortions, or history of pervious inpatient psychiatric treatment or substance abuse.

During the collection of the patient history, the financial history, the patient's family values, and the patient's relationships with family members can also reveal actual or potential **abuse indicators**.

- The **financial history** may indicate that the patient has little or no money or that they are not given access to money by a controlling family member. They may also be unemployed or utilizing an elderly family member's income for their own personal expenses.
- **Family values** may indicate strong beliefs in physical punishment, dictatorship within the home, inability to allow different opinions within the home, or lack of trust for anyone outside the family.
- **Relationships** within the family may be dysfunctional. Problems such as lack of affection between family members, co-dependency, frequent arguments, extramarital affairs, or extremely rigid beliefs about roles within the family may be present.

During the collection of the patient history, the sexual, social, and psychological history of the patient should be evaluated for any signs of actual or potential abuse.

- The **sexual history** may reveal problems such as previous sexual abuse, forced sexual acts, sexually transmitted infections (STIs), sexual knowledge beyond normal age-appropriate knowledge, or promiscuity.
- The **social history** may reveal unplanned pregnancies, social isolation as evidenced by lack of friends available to help the patient, unreasonable jealousy of significant other, verbal aggression, belief in physical punishment, or problems in school.
- During the **psychological assessment** the patient may express feelings of helplessness and being trapped. The patient may be unable to describe their future, become tearful, perform self-mutilation, have low self-esteem, and have had previous suicide attempts.

## Observations That May Indicate Abuse

During the initial assessment, observations may also be made by the provider that can provide vital information about actual or potential abuse. **General observations** may include finding that the patient history is far different from what is objectively viewed by the provider or that there is a lack of proper clothing or lack of physical care provided. The home environment may include lack of heat, water, or food. It may also reveal inappropriate sleeping arrangements or lack of an environmentally safe housing situation. Observations concerning **family communications** may reveal that the abuser answers all the questions for the whole family or that others look to the controlling member for approval or seem fearful of others. Family members may frequently argue, interrupt each other, or act out negative nonverbal behaviors while others are speaking. They may avoid talking about certain subjects that they feel are secretive.

## Indicators of Abuse That May Be Evident During the Physical Assessment

During the **physical assessment** the provider should always be aware of any **indicators of abuse**. These indicators may include increased anxiety about being examined or in the presence of the abuser; poor hygiene;

looks to abuser to answer questions for them; flinching; over or underweight; presence of bruises, welts, scars or cigarette burns; bald patches on scalp for pulling out of hair; intracranial bleeding; subconjunctival hemorrhages; black eye(s); hearing loss from untreated infection or injury; poor dental hygiene; abdominal injuries; fractures; developmental delays; hyperactive reflexes; genital lacerations or ecchymosis; and presence of STIs, rectal bruising, bleeding, edema, or poor sphincter tone.

### Domestic Violence

Men, women, elderly, children, and the disabled may all be victims of **domestic violence**. The violent person harms physically or sexually and uses threats and fear to maintain control of the victim. The violence does not improve unless the abuser gets intensive counseling. The abuser may promise not to do it again, but the violence usually gets more frequent and worsens over time. The provider should ask all patients in private about abuse, neglect, and fear of a caretaker. If abuse is suspected or there are signs present, the state may require **reporting**:

- Give victims information about community hotlines, shelters, and resources.
- Urge them to set up a plan for escape for themselves and any children, complete with supplies in a location away from the home.
- Assure victims that they are not at fault and do not deserve the abuse.
- Try to empower them by helping them to realize that they do not have to take abuse and can find support to change the situation.

### Assessment of Domestic Violence

According to the guidelines of the Family Violence Prevention Fund, **assessment** for domestic violence should be done for all adolescent and adult patients, regardless of background or signs of abuse. While females are the most common victims, there are increasing reports of male victims of domestic violence, both in heterosexual and homosexual relationships. The person doing the assessment should be informed about domestic violence and be aware of risk factors and danger signs. The interview should be conducted in private (special accommodations may need to be made for children <3 years old). The manager's office, bathrooms, and examining rooms should have information about domestic violence posted prominently. Brochures and information should be available to give to patients. Patients may present with a variety of physical complaints, such as headache, pain, palpitations, numbness, or pelvic pain. They are often depressed and may appear suicidal and may be isolated from friends and family. Victims of domestic violence often exhibit fear of spouse/partner, and may report injury inconsistent with symptoms.

### Steps to Identifying Victims of Domestic Violence

The **Family Violence Prevention Fund** has issued guidelines for identifying and assisting victims of domestic violence. There are 7 steps:

1. **Inquiry**: Non-judgmental questioning should begin with asking if the person has ever been abused—physically, sexually, or psychologically.
2. **Interview**: The person may exhibit signs of anxiety or fear and may blame himself or report that others believe he is abused. The person should be questioned if she is afraid for her life or for her children.
3. **Question**: If the person reports abuse, it's critical to ask if the person is in immediate danger or if the abuser is on the premises. The interviewer should ask if the person has been threatened. The history and pattern of abuse should be questioned, and if children are involved, whether the children are abused. Note: State laws vary, and in some states, it is mandatory to report if a child was present during an act of domestic violence as this is considered child abuse. The provider must be aware of state laws regarding domestic and child abuse, and all healthcare providers are mandatory reporters.
4. **Validate**: The interviewer should offer support and reassurance in a non-judgmental manner, telling the patient the abuse is not his or her fault.

5. **Give information**: While discussing facts about domestic violence and the tendency to escalate, the interviewer should provide brochures and information about safety planning. If the patient wants to file a complaint with the police, the interviewer should assist the person to place the call.
6. **Make referrals**: Information about state, local, and national organizations should be provided along with telephone numbers and contact numbers for domestic violence shelters.
7. **Document**: Record keeping should be legal, legible, and lengthy with a complete report and description of any traumatic injuries resulting from domestic violence. A body map may be used to indicate sites of injury, especially if there are multiple bruises or injuries.

## Injuries Consistent with Domestic Violence

There are a number of characteristic **injuries** that may indicate domestic violence, including ruptured eardrum; rectal/genital injury (burns, bites, or trauma); scrapes and bruises about the neck, face, head, trunk, arms; and cuts, bruises, and fractures of the face. The pattern of injuries associated with domestic violence is also often distinctive. The bathing-suit pattern involves injuries on parts of body that are usually covered with clothing as the perpetrator inflicts damage but hides evidence of abuse. Head and neck injuries (50%) are also common. Abusive injuries (rarely attributable to accidents) are common and include bites, bruises, rope and cigarette burns, and welts in the outline of weapons (belt marks). Bilateral injuries of arms/legs are often seen with domestic abuse. Defensive injuries are indicative of abuse.

Defensive injuries to the back of the body are often incurred as the victim crouches on the floor face down while being attacked. The soles of the feet may be injured from kicking at perpetrator. The ulnar aspect of hand or palm may be injured from blocking blows.

## Identifying and Reporting Neglect of the Basic Needs of Adults

**Neglect of the basic needs of adults** is a common problem, especially among the elderly, adults with psychiatric or mental health problems, or those who live alone or with reluctant or incapable caregivers. In some cases, **passive neglect** may occur because an elderly or impaired spouse or partner is trying to take care of a patient and is unable to provide the care needed, but in other cases, **active neglect** reflects a lack of caring which may be considered negligence or abuse. Cases of neglect should be reported to the appropriate governmental agency, such as adult protective services. Indications of neglect include the following:

- Lack of assistive devices, such as a cane or walker, needed for mobility
- Misplaced or missing glasses or hearing aids
- Poor dental hygiene and dental care or missing dentures
- Patient left unattended for extended periods of time, sometimes confined to a bed or chair
- Patient left in soiled or urine- and feces-stained clothing
- Inadequate food, fluid, or nutrition, resulting in weight loss
- Inappropriate and unkempt clothing, such as no sweater or coat during the winter and dirty or torn clothing
- A dirty, messy environment

## Identifying and Reporting Neglect or Lack of Supervision in Children

While some children may not be physically or sexually abused, they may suffer from profound **neglect** or **lack of supervision** that places them at risk. Indicators include the following:

- Appearing dirty and unkempt, sometimes with infestations of lice, and wearing ill-fitting or torn clothes and shoes
- Being tired and sleepy during the daytime
- Having untended medical or dental problems, such as dental caries
- Missing appointments and not receiving proper immunizations
- Being underweight for stage of development

**Neglect** can be difficult to assess, especially if the nurse is serving a homeless or very poor population. Home visits may be needed to ascertain if adequate food, clothing, or supervision is being provided; this may be beyond the care provided by the nurse, so suspicions should be reported to appropriate authorities, such as child protective services, so that social workers can assess the home environment.

## ELDER ABUSE

Active abuse is intentional (such as hitting) while passive abuse occurs without intention. **Elder abuse** may be difficult to diagnose, especially if the person is cognitively impaired, but symptoms can include fearfulness, disparities in reports of injuries between patient and caregiver, evidence of old or repeated injuries, poor hygiene and dental care, decubiti, malnutrition, undue concern with costs on caregiver's part, unsupportive attitude of caregiver, and caregiver's reluctance or refusal to allow patient to communicate privately with the nurse. Diagnosis includes a careful history and physical exam, including direct questioning of the patient about abuse. Treatment includes attending to injuries or physical needs, (this can vary widely) and referral to adult protective services as indicated. Reporting laws regarding elder abuse vary somewhat from one state to another, but all states have laws regarding elder abuse and most states require mandatory reporting to adult protective services by health workers.

## ELDER NEGLECT

Neglect of basic needs is a common problem of older adults who live alone or with reluctant or incapable caregivers. In some cases, passive neglect may occur because an elderly spouse is trying to take care of a patient and is unable to provide the care needed, but in other cases, active neglect reflects a lack of caring and may border on negligence and abuse. **Indications** of neglect include the following:

- Lack of assistive devices, such as cane or walker, needed for mobility
- Misplaced or missing glasses or hearing aids
- Poor dental hygiene and dental care and/or missing dentures
- Patient left unattended for extended periods of time, sometimes confined to a bed or chair
- Patient left in soiled or urine/feces-stained clothing
- Inadequate food/fluid/nutrition resulting in weight loss
- Inappropriate and unkempt clothing, such as lack of sweater or coat during the winter and dirty or torn clothing
- Dirty, messy environment

## RISK OF ELDER ABUSE

Age and disability increase the **risks of elder abuse**. People over the age of 80 are more than twice as likely to suffer abuse as younger adults. Patients with dementia, such as Alzheimer's disease, are at risk of abuse in both the home environment, where they are often cared for by adult children, and in institutions. Caregivers often lose patience and become frustrated, especially if the patient's behavior is belligerent, combative, or disruptive. This type of abuse can be very difficult to diagnose, as the patient is usually unable to corroborate abuse. In fact, even older adults who are not cognitively impaired may be afraid to report abuse because they depend on the abusers to care for them. Older adults who are dependent on others for assistance with ADLs, such as dressing, bathing, and food preparation are also particularly at risk for outright abuse and neglect. Abusers often suffer from depression and or substance abuse and may be financially dependent on the victim.

## Physical and Emotional Abuse

There are a number of different types of elder abuse. **Physical abuse** is an active form of abuse and is almost always associated with **psychological abuse** as well. Older adults, particularly those cared for by family members (often an adult child) or other caregivers, may suffer various types of assaults related to hitting, kicking, pulling hair, shoving, and pushing. Caregivers may make frequent threats to hit the older adult, sometimes brandishing a weapon, if the person doesn't cooperate and may tell the person to commit suicide. Ongoing intimidation may make the patient terrified and anxious. Sometimes, caregivers threaten to injure pets or family members, increasing patient's fear. Patients may be forcibly confined, forced into seclusion, and/or force-fed to the point that they choke on food.

**Physical symptoms** include the following:

- Ruptured eardrum
- Rectal/genital injury—burns, bites, trauma
- Scrapes and bruises about the neck, face, head, trunk, arms
- Cuts, bruises, and fractures of the face

The **pattern of injuries** is also often distinctive:

- Bathing suit pattern—injuries on parts of body that are usually covered with clothing as the perpetrator abuses but hides evidence of abuse
- Head and neck injuries (50%)

**Abusive injuries** (rarely attributable to accidents) are common:

- Bites, bruises, rope and cigarette burns, welts in the outline of weapons (belt marks)
- Bilateral injuries of arms/legs

**Defensive injuries** are indicative of abuse:

- Back of the body injury from being attacked while crouched on the floor face down
- Soles of the feet from kicking at perpetrator
- Ulnar aspect of hand or palm from blocking blows

**Psychological symptoms** include anxiety, paranoia, insomnia, low self-esteem, avoidance of eye contact, and obvious nervousness in the presence of the caregiver, who is often reluctant to leave the patient alone.

## Sexual Abuse

Sexual abuse of older adults occurs when the person receiving sexual attention is unwilling to participate or unable (because of cognizant impairment or other illness) to consent to sexual intimacy. Types of **sexual abuse** include:

- **Physical**: Fondling, kissing, and rape
- **Emotional**: Exhibitionism
- **Verbal**: Sexual harassment, using obscene language, threatening

Sexual abuse of older adults occurs most commonly to women in their 70s or 80s confined to nursing homes. Sexual abuse may also occur in home environments, but it is harder to detect. Most abusers are fellow nursing home residents (males over the age of 60), and the most common form of abuse is sexualized kissing and fondling of genitals. Because older adults have a right to sexual intimacy, in some cases what may appear to be abuse between residents may, in fact, be consensual. Caregivers may have raped or otherwise sexually abused patients, and this exercise of power over another person is always illegal abuse.

## Financial Abuse

Elder abuse often occurs when an older adult is unable to care for or protect himself. In many situations, another person takes advantage of an older adult and uses threats or manipulation to justify the activity. As older adults become unable to manage their own financial affairs, they become increasingly vulnerable to **financial abuse**, especially if they have cognitive impairment or physical impairments that impair their mobility. This kind of abuse often occurs when an older adult trusts another person for help with finances and is taken advantage of. Financial abuse includes the following:

- Outright stealing of property or persuading patients to give away possessions
- Forcing patients to sign away property
- Emptying bank and savings accounts
- Using stolen credit cards
- Convincing the person to invest money in fraudulent schemes
- Taking money for home renovations that are not done

Indications of financial abuse may be unpaid bills, unusual activity at ATMs or with credit cards, inadequate funds to meet needs, disappearance of items in the home, change in the provision of a will, and deferring to caregivers regarding financial affairs. Family or caregivers may move permanently into the patient's home and take over without sharing costs.

Some examples of financial abuse of an elderly client include when another person steals money or other valuable items, forges the patient's signature on checks or signs over Social Security income, uses the adult's name and identifying information to gain access to other accounts or to spend money, advises an older adult to invest money into accounts or schemes that are not legitimate, or commits fraud by telling an older adult that she has won money or is contributing to fraudulent organizations.

## Socioeconomic Factors That May Contribute to Elder Abuse

Elder abuse is a problem that remains largely underreported. Elder abuse may be more prevalent when abusers see older adults as helpless victims who have no control over their environment or who have no access to reporting to authorities. Some older adults and their abusers may downplay the abuse or neglect, while others may be unsure of what their options are for help and safety. There are some **socioeconomic factors** that contribute to elder abuse and neglect, allowing these situations to continue. Some examples include a stressful environment, such as a long-term-care facility that houses many high-need residents, family or caregivers that are burdened by stress or who have emotional instability, the prevalence of ageism and the idea that the elderly are incompetent or frail, the increase in diagnosed cases of chronic disease, and advances in medicine and technology that allow older persons to live longer.

## Screening Questions to Assess for Elder Abuse

The nurse who cares for older adults is in a position to detect cases of abuse or neglect that may otherwise go unreported. The nurse serves as the patient's advocate to protect him from abuse taking place that he may be powerless to control. The nurse may need to ask questions when the potential abuser is not in the room. Some questions that the nurse may ask to assess for underlying abuse or neglect include:

- Has anyone been hurting you?
- Do you feel safe where you live?
- Is there someone in your family/neighborhood that you are afraid of?
- Have you ever been threatened?
- Has anyone ever touched you in a manner that made you uncomfortable?
- Do you feel that your caregiver/family/friend is there for you when you need him or her?

## UNDERREPORTING OF ABUSE IN LONG-TERM-CARE FACILITIES

Abusive and neglectful situations that occur in nursing homes may go **underreported** for various reasons. Many longterm-care facilities care for a large number of residents, caregivers may be stressed, and units may be understaffed. These facilities provide care for high-need patients, potentially causing difficulties with time management and fully meeting the needs of every resident, which further contributes to abuse. Some residents may be in situations where they are unable to report any abuse because of speech or hearing difficulties, physical disabilities, or cognitive changes. Abuse or neglect may also occur and remain underreported in residents who do not have regular visits from families or friends. These residents may go for long periods without an outside person visiting to evaluate or notice any changes in behavior or appearance that may occur with abuse.

# Professional Issues: System

## Collaboration and Communication

### Skills Needed for Collaboration

Nurses must learn the set of skills needed for collaboration in order to move nursing forward. Nurses must take an active role in gathering data for evidence-based practice to support nursing's role in health care, and they must share this information with other nurses and health professionals in order to plan staffing levels and to provide optimal care to patients. Increased and adequate staffing has consistently been shown to reduce adverse outcomes, but there is a well-documented shortage of nurses in the United States, and more than half currently work outside the hospital setting. Increased patient loads not only increase adverse outcomes but also increase job dissatisfaction and burnout. In order to manage the challenges facing nursing, nurses must develop the following skills needed for collaboration:

- Be willing to compromise
- Communicate clearly
- Identify specific challenges and problems
- Focus on the task
- Work with teams

### Communication Skills

Collaboration requires a number of communication skills that differ from those involved in communication between nurse and patient. These skills include:

- **Using an assertive approach**: It's important for the nurse to honestly express opinions and to state them clearly and with confidence, but the nurse must do so in a calm, non-threatening manner.
- **Making casual conversation**: It's easier to communicate with people with whom one has a personal connection. Asking open-ended questions, asking about others' work, or commenting on someone's contributions helps to establish a relationship. The time before meetings, during breaks, and after meetings presents an opportunity for this type of conversation.
- **Being competent in public speaking**: Collaboration requires that a nurse be comfortable speaking and presenting ideas to groups of people. Speaking and presenting ideas competently also helps the nurse to gain credibility. Public speaking is a skill that must be practiced.
- **Communicating in writing**: The written word remains a critical component of communication, and the nurse should be able to communicate clearly and grammatically.

#### *Communication and Hand Offs*

The nurse is usually the primary staff member responsible for **external and internal hand off transitions of care**, and should ensure that communication is thorough and covers all essential information. The best method is to use a standardized format:

- **DRAW**: Diagnosis, recent changes, anticipated changes, and what to watch for.
- **I PASS the BATON**: Introduction, patient, assessment, situation, safety concerns, background, actions, timing, ownership, and next.
- **ANTICipate**: Administrative data, new clinical information, tasks, illness severity, contingency plans.
- **5 Rs**: Record, review, round together, relay to team, and receive feedback.

A reporting **form** or checklist may be utilized to ensure that no aspect is overlooked.

For external transitions, the nurse must ensure that the type of transport team and monitoring is appropriate for patient needs, and provide insight when determining the most appropriate mode of transportation: ground transfer for short distance, helicopter for medium to long distance, and fixed-wing aircraft for long distances.

### *SBAR Technique*

The SBAR technique is used to hand-off a patient from one caregiver to another to provide a systematic method so that important information is conveyed:

- **(S) Situation**: Overview of current situation and important issues
- **(B) Background**: Important history and issues leading to current situation
- **(A) Assessment**: Summary of important facts and condition
- **(R) Recommendation**: Actions needed

### *Shift Reporting*

Shift reporting should include bedside handoff when possible with oncoming staff members. The nurse handing off the patient should follow a specific format for handoff (such as I PASS the BATON) so that handoff is done in the same manner every time, as this reduces the chance of omitting important information. The shift report should include introduction of the oncoming staff to the patient, the triage category or acuity level of the patient, diagnosis (potential or confirmed), current status, laboratory and imaging (completed or pending) and results if available, and medications or treatments administered and pending. Any monitoring equipment (pulse oximetry, telemetry) should be examined. Any invasive treatments (Foley catheter, IV) should be discussed and equipment examined. The nurse should report any plans for admission, transfer, or discharge. It is essential that all staff be trained in shift reporting and the importance of consistency.

## Collaboration Between Nurse and Patient/Family

One of the most important forms of collaboration is that between the nurse and the patient/family, but this type of collaboration is often overlooked. Nurses and others in the healthcare team must always remember that the point of collaboration is to improve patient care, and this means that the patient and patient's family must remain central to all planning. For example, including family in planning for a patient takes time initially, but sitting down and asking the patient and family, "What do you want?" and using the Synergy model to evaluate patient's (and family's) characteristics can provide valuable information that saves time in the long run and facilitates planning and expenditure of resources. Families, and even young children, often want to participate in care and planning and feel validated and more positive toward the medical system when they are included.

## Collaboration with External Agencies

The nurse must initiate and facilitate collaboration with external agencies because many have direct impacts on patient care and needs:

- **Industry** can include other facilities sharing interests in patient care or pharmaceutical companies. It's important for nursing to have a dialog with drug companies about their products and how they are used in specific populations because many medications are prescribed to women, children, or the aged without validating studies for dose or efficacy.
- **Payers** have a vested interest in containing health care costs, so providing information and representing the interests of the patient is important.
- **Community groups** may provide resources for patients and families, both in terms of information and financial or other assistance.
- **Political agencies** are increasingly important as new laws are considered about nurse-patient ratios and infection control in many states.
- **Public health agencies** are partners in health care with other facilities and must be included, especially in issues related to communicable disease.

## Interdisciplinary Teams

There are a number of skills that are needed to lead and facilitate coordination of **intra- and inter-disciplinary teams**:

- Communicating openly is essential. All members must be encouraged to participate as valued members of a cooperative team.
- Avoiding interrupting or interpreting the point another is trying to make allows free flow of ideas.
- Avoiding jumping to conclusions, which can effectively shut off communication.
- Active listening requires paying attention and asking questions for clarification rather than to challenge other's ideas.
- Respecting others' opinions and ideas, even when opposed to one's own, is absolutely essential.
- Reacting and responding to facts rather than feelings allows one to avoid angry confrontations and diffuse anger.
- Clarifying information or opinions stated can help avoid misunderstandings.
- Keeping unsolicited advice out of the conversation shows respect for others and allows them to solicit advice without feeling pressured.

## Leadership Styles

Leadership styles often influence the perception of leadership values and commitment to collaboration. There are a number of different leadership styles:

- **Charismatic**: Relies on personal charisma to influence people, and may be very persuasive, but this type leader may engage followers and relate to one group rather than the organization at large, limiting effectiveness.
- **Bureaucratic**: Follows organization rules exactly and expects everyone else to do so. This is most effective in handling cash flow or managing work in dangerous work environments. This type of leadership may engender respect but may not be conducive to change.
- **Autocratic**: Makes decisions independently and strictly enforces rules. Team members often feel left out of process and may not be supportive of the decisions that are made. This type of leadership is most effective in crisis situations, but may have difficulty gaining the commitment of staff.
- **Consultative**: Presents a decision and welcomes input and questions, although decisions rarely change. This type of leadership is most effective when gaining the support of staff is critical to the success of proposed changes.
- **Participatory**: Presents a potential decision and then makes final decision based on input from staff or teams. This type of leadership is time-consuming and may result in compromises that are not entirely satisfactory to management or staff, but this process is motivating to staff who feel their expertise is valued.
- **Democratic**: Presents a problem and asks staff or teams to arrive at a solution, although the leader usually makes the final decision. This type of leadership may delay decision-making, but staff and teams are often more committed to the solutions because of their input.
- **Laissez-faire ("free reign")**: Exerts little direct control but allows employees/teams to make decisions with little interference. This may be effective leadership if teams are highly skilled and motivated, but in many cases, this type of leadership is the product of poor management skills and little is accomplished because of this lack of leadership.

## Team Building

Leading, facilitating, and participating in performance improvement teams requires a thorough understanding of the dynamics of team building:

- **Initial interactions**: This is the time when members begin to define their roles and develop relationships, determining if they are comfortable in the group.
- **Power issues**: The members observe the leader and determine who controls the meeting and how control is exercised, beginning to form alliances.
- **Organizing**: Methods to achieve work are clarified and team members begin to work together, gaining respect for each other's contributions and working toward a common goal.
- **Team identification**: Interactions often become less formal as members develop rapport, and members are more willing to help and support each other to achieve goals.
- **Excellence**: This develops through a combination of good leadership, committed team members, clear goals, high standards, external recognition, spirit of collaboration, and a shared commitment to the process.

## Team Meetings

Leading and facilitating improvement teams requires utilizing good techniques for meetings. Considerations include:

- **Scheduling**: Both the time and the place must be convenient and conducive to working together, so the leader must review the work schedules of those involved, finding the most convenient time. Venues or meeting rooms should allow for sitting in a circle or around a table to facilitate equal exchange of ideas. Any necessary technology, such as computers or overhead projectors, or other equipment, such as whiteboards, should be available.
- **Preparation**: The leader should prepare a detailed agenda that includes a list of items for discussion.
- **Conduction**: Each item of the agenda should be discussed, soliciting input from all group members. Tasks should be assigned to individual members based on their interest and part in the process in preparation for the next meeting. The leader should summarize input and begin a tentative future agenda.
- **Observation**: The leader should observe the interactions, including verbal and nonverbal communication, and respond to them.

## Common Vision

Facilitating the creation of a common vision for care within the healthcare system begins with the organization/facility, working collaboratively to create teams and an organization focused on serving the patient/family. A common vision should be the ideal in any organization, but achieving such a goal requires a true collaborative effort:

- Inclusion of all levels of staff across the organization/facility, both those in nursing and non-nursing positions
- Consensus building through discussions, inservice, and team meetings to bring about convergence of diverse viewpoints
- Facilitation that values creativity and provides encouragement during the process
- Vision statement incorporating the common vision that is accessible to all staff
- Recognition that a common vision is an organic concept that may evolve over time and should be reevaluated regularly and changed as needed to reflect the needs of the organization, patients, families, and staff

## FACILITATING CHANGE

Performance improvement processes cannot occur without organizational change, and resistance to change is common for many people, so coordinating collaborative processes requires anticipating resistance and taking steps to achieve cooperation. Resistance often relates to concerns about job loss, increased responsibilities, and general denial or lack of understanding and frustration. Leaders can prepare others involved in the process of change by taking these steps:

- Be honest, informative, and tactful, giving people thorough information about anticipated changes and how the changes will affect them, including positives.
- Be patient in allowing people the time they need to contemplate changes and express anger or disagreement.
- Be empathetic in listening carefully to the concerns of others.
- Encourage participation, allowing staff to propose methods of implementing change, so they feel some sense of ownership.
- Establish a climate in which all staff members are encouraged to identify the need for change on an ongoing basis.
- Present further ideas for change to management.

## CONFLICT RESOLUTION

Conflict is an almost inevitable product of teamwork, and the leader must assume responsibility for conflict resolution. While conflicts can be disruptive, they can produce positive outcomes by opening dialogue and forcing team members to listen to different perspectives. The team should make a plan for dealing with conflict. The best time for conflict resolution is when differences emerge but before open conflict and hardening of positions occur. The leader must pay close attention to the people and problems involved, listen carefully, and reassure those involved that their points of view are understood. Steps to conflict resolution include:

- Allow both sides to present their side of conflict without bias, maintaining a focus on opinions rather than individuals.
- Encourage cooperation through negotiation and compromise.
- Maintain the focus, providing guidance to keep the discussions on track and avoid arguments.
- Evaluate the need for re-negotiation, formal resolution process, or third-party involvement.
- Utilize humor and empathy to diffuse escalating tensions.
- Summarize the issues, outlining key arguments.
- Avoid forcing resolution if possible.

## HEALTHCARE TEAM MEMBERS

### *ROLE OF NURSING CARE TO SUPPORT THERAPIES PROVIDED BY OTHER DISCIPLINES*

Nursing care often involves providing support to therapies provided by other disciplines. The nurse works as a team member with physicians, occupational and physical therapists, respiratory therapists, social workers, and discharge planners. Floor nurses may work with nurses in other specializations, such as critical care or psychiatric nurses. As a primary coordinator of the care plan, the nurse ensures that the necessary therapies from all disciplines are administered as ordered, and maintains clear communication with all members of the patient's healthcare team. Nurses also support nutritional services by assuring that the patient receives the proper diet for the particular medical or surgical condition, and they communicate with housekeeping to ensure that the patient's environment is appropriate.

### *OCCUPATIONAL THERAPY*

The function of occupational therapy is to enable the patient to attain functional outcomes that enhance health, prevent further injury or impairment, and sustain or improve the highest attainable level of independence. The occupational therapist's role is to **facilitate interventions** that aid the patient in improving basic motor and cognitive skills and to **introduce strategies** for meeting challenges at work or at home. In cases of permanent disability or loss of mobility, the occupational therapist works with the patient on adaptive measures to improve function and the ability to perform daily living tasks. Occupational therapists may use physical exercises to improve muscle strength, balance, and dexterity, or cognitive exercises and strategies to improve problem-solving and memory. They help patients with disabilities or cognitive impairments adapt to particular environments, such as a private home or workplace, and teach patients how to use adaptive equipment like wheelchairs, orthotic devices, or computer programs.

### *Respiratory Therapy*

The function of respiratory therapy is to provide care to patients with respiratory and cardiopulmonary disorders. The role of the respiratory therapist is to diagnose, evaluate, and treat patients with these disorders, and manage their therapeutic care. The respiratory therapist administers aerosolized medications and provides bronchopulmonary hygiene and postural drainage therapy. The role of the respiratory therapist is also to provide support for mechanically-ventilated patients and to maintain an artificial or natural airway. Many respiratory therapists perform pulmonary function testing as well as hemodynamic monitoring. Some respiratory therapists obtain arterial blood gases and other blood samples, as well as assemble and maintain respiratory equipment. They also teach patients how to self-administer aerosol medications and use life-support respiratory equipment in the home environment.

### *Case Manager*

The case manager is an RN that works for a healthcare insurer as a **manager of the provision of healthcare services** to the people the company insures. One manager or a group of managers are given a caseload of patients with the same range of diagnoses. The case manager is an expert in the range of diagnoses and coordinates services to fulfill the healthcare needs of that particular group of patients. The patient is followed throughout the continuum of care to ensure quality and cost-effectiveness of treatments and care. Complications are prevented and the incidence of repeat hospitalization is decreased. The case manager utilizes evidence-based pathways, clinical pathways, or other plans to track the care and progress of the patient. They are the ones who precertify care, negotiate for payment, and authorize treatment. Patient progress reports from the hospital utilization review or other liaison to the case manager are required at periodic intervals during the hospital stay.

## Identifying the Need for Patient Referral

Issues to consider when making patient referrals include:

- **Necessity**: The referral may be needed if the patient's needs are outside of the provider's scope or practice or field of expertise and if the provider cannot provide adequate assessment and treatment for the patient's condition.
- **Insurance requirements**: The provider should determine whether the patient's carrier requires preauthorization or other steps to make sure the patient's referral is covered.
- **Selection of specialist/therapist**: The specialist, in many cases, must be selected from a group of physicians who are participating in an insurance plan if the service is to be covered completely or at all by the insurance company. When possible, the patient should be given choice of referrals.
- **Submission**: The referral should be sent along with appropriate records and releases. The provider may need to make personal contact if specialists are selective, have waiting lists, and may not approve a referral.

# Delegation

## Five Rights of Delegation

Prior to delegating tasks, the nurse should assess the needs of the patients and determine the task that needs to be completed, assure that he/she can remain accountable and can supervise the task appropriately, and evaluate effective completion. The **5 rights of delegation** include:

- **Right task**: The nurse should determine an appropriate task to delegate for a specific patient. This would not include tasks that require assessment or planning.
- **Right circumstance**: The nurse has considered the setting, resources, time factors, safety factors, and all other relevant information to determine the appropriateness of delegation. A task that is usually in one's scope (such as feeding a patient) may require assessment that makes it inappropriate to delegate (feeding a new stroke patient).
- **Right person**: The nurse is in the right position to choose the right person (by virtue of education/skills) to perform a task for the right patient.
- **Right direction**: The nurse provides a clear description of the task, the purpose, any limits, and expected outcomes.
- **Right supervision**: The nurse is able to supervise, intervene as needed, and evaluate performance of the task.

## Delegation of Tasks in Teams

On major responsibility of leadership and management in performance improvement teams is using delegation effectively. The purpose of having a team is so that the work is shared, and leaders can cripple themselves by taking on too much of the workload. Additionally, failure to delegate shows an inherent distrust in team members. Delegation includes:

- Assessing the skills and available time of the team members, determining if a task is suitable for an individual
- Assigning tasks, with clear instructions that include explanation of objectives and expectations, including a timeline
- Ensuring that the tasks are completed properly and on time by monitoring progress but not micromanaging
- Reviewing the final results and recording outcomes

Because the leader is ultimately responsible for the delegated work, mentoring, monitoring, and providing feedback and intervention as necessary during this process is a necessary component of leadership. Even when delegated tasks are not completed successfully, they represent an opportunity for learning.

# Disaster Management

## Disaster

A disaster is an event where many people are exposed to hazards that result in injury, death, and damage to property. There are a number of hazards that have the potential to lead to a disaster situation. In general, they can be **classified** as natural, technological, or caused by human conflict. Some specific examples of each are as follows:

- **Natural**: Firestorms, flood, land shift, tornado, epidemic, earthquake, volcano, hurricane, high winds, blizzard, heat wave
- **Technological**: Hazmat spills, explosions, utility failure, building collapse, transportation accident, power outage, nuclear accident, dam failure, fire, water loss, ruptured gas main
- **Human conflict**: Riots, strikes, suicide bombings, bomb threat, employee violence, mass shootings, equipment sabotage, hostage events, transportation disruption, weapons of mass destruction, computer viruses/worms

## Disaster Management Plan

### *Development*

There are many different types of disaster management plans. Regardless of the type, there are several basic steps for its **development**. To begin with, a **planning team** must be established that includes representatives from all levels within the organization. The planning team is responsible for creating a timeline for completion of the plan as well as an estimation of the costs, fees, and resources necessary to complete the plan. Once this is done, an **analysis of potential disasters** can begin. In this step, potential hazards are identified and vulnerability of the organization to disasters is assessed. A **disaster response plan** is established that includes the reduction/removal of hazardous situations. The final steps are **plan implementation and review**. The plan can be tested for efficacy through drills and mock disaster situations. It is critical to review and update the plan yearly.

### *Types*

There are several different **types of disaster management plans**, some more specific than others. They are listed and briefly described below:

- **Emergency action plan**: OSHA required, evacuation plans and emergency drills
- **Business continuity plan**: Business operation-specific, aimed at reducing losses and resuming productivity
- **Risk management plan**: Off-site effects of chemical exposures
- **Emergency response plan**: Immediate response to disasters
- **Contingency plan**: General, designed to handle events not covered in other plans
- **Federal response plan**: Coordinates federal resources
- **Spill prevention, control, and countermeasures plan**: Deals with the prevention, control, and clean-up of oil spills
- **Mutual aid plan**: Plan for shared resources between other companies/firms
- **Recovery plan**: Deals with repair and rebuilding post-disaster
- **Emergency management plan**: Plan for healthcare facilities
- **All-hazard disaster management plan**: General plan that is not hazard-specific

## Emergency Response Plans

Emergency response plans must include plans for communication, resources and assets available, safety and security measures, responsibilities of staff, utilities, and measure to support clinical activities.

### *Bomb Threats*

The response to a **bomb threat** depends on the type of bomb threat and the information gleaned from the threat. The first response is to notify the police and designated staff via landlines (avoiding cell phones, which can trigger some devices) or overhead paging. An initial search may be carried out by staff in each area to try to locate possible bombs. Administration should make the decision about evacuation, and plans for evacuation should be in place. With terrorist bombing and improvised explosive devices (IEDs), situational awareness is critical because multiple explosive devices (some undetonated) may be at the scene. IEDs may be inside backpacks, suitcases, and packages left unattended. Additionally, people wearing suicide vests or belts may mix in with other victims or people escaping the blast area.

### *Natural Disasters*

Plans vary according to type of **natural disaster**. If anticipated, extra food, clothing, and supplies should be stockpiled for both clients and staff (who may be required to stay at the facility for extended periods). A command structure should be in place. With a hurricane or tornado, clients may need to be moved away from windows and to more secure areas, such as interior hallways, during the storm. The hospital must prepare plans to evacuate clients if necessary (such as with flooding, earthquakes, or storm damage) and transfer them to other facilities and must also be prepared for an influx of clients.

### *Community Planning*

Healthcare providers, such as hospitals, should work closely with the community to identify community resources that are available for emergency response and the needs that may arise in response to disasters, including the number of people who may depend on the hospital for care.

## ICS

The **Incident Command System** (ICS) was developed by the Department of Homeland Security as a part of the **National Incident Management System**. It is a highly organized, hierarchical disaster management system that focuses on planning and organization, communication and delegation of responsibility, as well as response evaluation so that any disaster or emergency response effort runs as smoothly as possible. An **Incident Commander (IC)** is established as the person in charge. Safety officers, operations section officers, planning officers, and logistics officers are all appointed. These different officer positions are responsible for reporting back to the IC.

### Multiple-Casualty Incidents Versus Mass-Casualty Incidents

**Multiple-casualty incidents** involve more than one person, but different jurisdictions may quantify the total number of persons differently. It usually refers to the following:

- An incident involving at least three patients
- An incident involving only one jurisdiction and only one to three agencies (ambulance, fire department, and police)
- An incident requiring triage, but generally only primary triage
- Standards of care are maintained, and all patients not coded black (deceased) are transported for care

**Mass-casualty incidents** also involve more than one person, but may involve much larger numbers—dozens, if not hundreds to thousands.

- Often involves multiple jurisdictions and agencies
- Requires triage but may also involve separate waiting areas for color-coded individuals and secondary triage
- Standards of care may be modified, and patients coded black (expectant) and not expected to live may be left in the field and/or receive delayed care if they are still living after the red- and yellow-coded individuals are transported

### Principles of Triage During Mass Casualty Events

**Primary triage** is a rapid method (30-60 seconds) of prioritizing clients based on severity of condition and carried out at the scene of multiple casualty incidents. All clients are triaged and tagged according to international color-coding priority (P) guidelines on foot or wrist (not clothing):

- **P1—Red**: Immediate care needed for urgent systemic life-threatening conditions, such as airway/breathing problems, severe bleeding, severe burns (especially with breathing problems), decreased mental status, shock, and severe medical problems, Glasgow Coma Score ≤13.
- **P2—Yellow**: Delayed care and able to wait 45-60 minutes for treatment. Conditions include burns (without breathing problems), multiple bone/joint injuries, back and/or spinal cord injuries (unless in respiratory distress).
- **P3—Green**: Hold, able to wait hours for treatment of minor injuries.
- **P4—Black**: Deceased or with injuries so extensive that they are not survivable.

Resource management involves identifying a triage officer, who remains at the scene during the event, and identifying the need for additional personnel and equipment and providing those to the clients with the highest priority.

### Identifying Clients to Discharge in Disaster Situations

In the event of a **disaster situation**, the surge capacity of a hospital may need to increase markedly with a large influx of clients in need of emergency care and hospitalization, so appropriate clients must be quickly identified for possible discharge. All elective admissions and procedures should be cancelled and non-critical clients, such as those with non-life-threatening conditions or those near discharge, should be discharged or transferred to other facilities if possible. Generally, hospitalists, charge nurses, or team leaders may be in the best position to identify clients for discharge as well as the person tasked with monitoring length of stay. If an acuity-based model of client care is utilized, then those already categorized as the least acute should be quickly assessed for discharge. Ideally, each unit should have plans in place for rapid discharge so that assessment and discharge can be carried out quickly and safely.

### Terrorism

Terrorism is defined as the use of violence (or threat of violence) to frighten and coerce governments or societies into accepting the instigator's (terrorists) **demands**. The demands and goals of terrorists are often extreme and focused on areas with high population densities. This means that large companies can become potential targets of a terrorist attack. For this reason, when developing an emergency preparedness/disaster management plan, terrorist attacks should be included as a potential disaster. There are many different possible ways that terrorists can strike. Some examples are weapons of mass destruction, biological agents (i.e., bacteria, viruses, or toxins), nuclear and radiological incidents, incendiary devices, chemicals, and explosive devices.

### Organizational Plan for Bioterrorism

The ICP and the infection control team should develop specific plans for dealing with different **bioterrorism** agents, and training should be provided to staff. An organized approach should include the following:

- Be on the alert for possible bioterrorism-related infections, based on clusters of patients or symptoms.
- Use personal protection equipment, including respirators when indicated.
- Complete thorough assessment of patient, including medical history, physical examination, immunization record, and travel history.
- Provide a probable diagnosis based on symptoms and lab findings, including cultures.
- Provide treatment, including prophylaxis, while waiting for laboratory findings.
- Use transmission precautions as well as isolation for suspected biologic agents.
- Notify local, state, and federal authorities per established protocol.
- Conduct surveillance and epidemiological studies to identify at-risk populations.

- Develop plans to accommodate large numbers of patients:
  - Restricting elective admissions
  - Transferring patients to other facilities

## B-NICE Hazardous Material Incidents Associated with Terrorist Attacks

| Category | Response |
|---|---|
| **B—Biological (bacteria, viruses, fungi, toxins)** | Inhalation type—evacuate for 80 feet, shut down air-handling systems, wear appropriate PPE and SCBA, and avoid contamination.<br>Visible agent—decontaminate with soap and water. Symptoms may vary but are usually delayed. |
| **N—Nuclear/ Radiological** | Inhalation type (most common)—Isolate/Secure the area, avoid smoke/fumes, stay upwind, and use PPE and SCBA. Isolate victims and decontaminate as appropriate. Symptoms are usually delayed. |
| **I—Incendiary** | Be on alert for multiple devices and sabotaged fire suppression equipment. Symptoms include burns, pain, and trauma. |
| **C—Chemical** | Isolate/Secure the area, decontaminate victims with soap and water, and be on alert for chemical dispersal devices. Approach toward uphill and upwind. Isolate symptomatic patients from others. Symptoms vary but may include burns, blistering, vomiting, breathing difficulty, and neurological damage. |
| **E—Explosives** | Be alert for secondary devices, undetonated devices, and secondary hazards (unstable buildings and debris). Remove victims from the area, secure the perimeter, and stage away from the incident area. Decontaminate as necessary. Symptoms include burns, amputations, cuts, and penetrating and blunt trauma. |

## All-Hazards Safety Approach to Mass-Casualty Incidents

The all-hazards safety approach to mass-casualty incidents aims to provide plans that can be used to deal with all types of hazards (natural disasters, terrorist attacks, and mass-casualty incidents) as well as encompassing the four components of emergency management: mitigation, preparedness, response, and recovery. Organizations in an area coordinate to develop joint action plans that can be activated in response to incidents, with the chain of command clearly outlined. This approach lowers costs to individual organizations and provides for faster and more effective response. However, although the basic structure may be the same for responding to all hazards, there are inevitable differences between (for example) a terrorist attack with active shooters and a natural disaster, such as a hurricane, which can be anticipated and mitigated to some degree. For this reason, modifying existing incident action plans to meet the needs of a situation is essential.

## Infections with Biological Weapons

### *Anthrax*

A number of different infections could be part of a bioterrorism attack. The type of barrier/isolation needed is dependent upon the symptoms and the mode of transmission. Knowledge of typical presenting symptoms and prompt precautions are essential to prevent spread of disease. **Anthrax (Bacillus anthracis)** usually occurs from contact with animals, but as a bioterrorism weapon, anthrax would most likely be aerosolized and inhaled. It is not transferred from person to person. There are 3 types:

- **Inhalation**: Fever, cough, shortness of breath, and general debility
- **Cutaneous**: Small non-painful sores that blister and ulcerate with necrosis at the center
- **Gastrointestinal**: Nausea, vomiting, diarrhea, and abdominal pain

The inhaled form of anthrax is the most severe with about a 50% mortality rate. The vaccine for anthrax is not yet available to the public.

Precautions are as follows:

- Prophylaxis with antibiotics after exposure
- Standard precautions
- Contact precautions for wounds if there are cutaneous lesions

### Pneumonic Plague

*Yersinia pestis* causes **pneumonic plague**, which is normally carried by fleas from infected rats but can be aerosolized to use as a biologic weapon. There are 3 forms of plague, but they sometimes occur together and bubonic and septicemic plague can develop into pneumonic, which is the primary concern related to bioterrorism:

- **Bubonic** occurs when a person is bitten by an infected flea.
- **Pneumonic** occurs with inhalation and results in pneumonia with fever, headache, cough, and progressive respiratory failure.
- **Septicemic** occurs when *Y. pestis* invades the bloodstream, often after initial bubonic or pneumonic plague.

Pneumonic plague can spread easily from person to person. There is no vaccine available. Precautions include the following:

- Immediate antibiotics within first 24 hours are necessary, so early diagnosis is critical.
- Prophylaxis with antibiotics may protect those exposed.
- Droplet precautions should be used with appropriate barriers, such as surgical mask.

### Botulism

**Clostridium botulinum** produces an extremely poisonous toxin that causes botulism. The organism can be aerosolized or used to infect food. There are 3 primary forms of botulisms:

- **Foodborne botulism** results from contamination of food. This type poses the greatest threat from bioterrorism. Symptoms usually appear 12-36 hours after ingestion but may be delayed for 2 weeks, and include nausea, vomiting, dyspnea, dysphagia, slurred speech, progressive weakness, and paralysis.
- **Infant botulism** results from *C. botulinum* ingested into the intestinal tract. Constipation, poor feeding, and progressive weakness are presenting symptoms.
- **Wound botulism** results from contamination of open skin, but symptoms are similar to foodborne botulism.

Botulism is not transmitted from person to person, but contaminated food has the potential to infect many people, especially if the contaminated food is manufactured and widely distributed.

Precautions include the following:

- Antitoxin after exposure and as early in disease as possible
- Standard precautions
- Do not feed honey to infants, as there is a risk of spore ingestion

### *Tularemia*

**Francisella tularensis** causes tularemia, which is usually transmitted from small mammals to humans through insect bites, ingestion of contaminated food or water, inhalation, or handling of infected animals. Although there is no evidence of person-to-person transmission, *F. tularensis* has the potential to be aerosolized for use in bioterrorism because it is highly infective and requires only about 10 organisms to infect. Flu-like symptoms appear in 3-5 days after exposure and progress to severe respiratory infection and pneumonia. A vaccine for laboratory workers was available until recently, but the FDA is currently reviewing it, and it is unavailable in the United States.

- Prophylaxis with antibiotics within 24 hours may prevent disease.
- Standard precautions are sufficient.
- Biologic safety measures should be used for laboratory specimens.
- Autopsy procedures that may cause tissue to be aerosolized should be avoided.

### *Smallpox*

The variola virus causes **smallpox**, which has been eradicated worldwide since 1980, but has the potential for use as a biological weapon because people are no longer vaccinated. Smallpox is extremely contagious and has a high mortality rate (about 30%). Flu-like symptoms appear about 7-17 days after exposure with fever, weakness, vomiting, and rash that begins on the face and arms and spreads. The rash becomes pustular, crusts, scabs over, and then sloughs off, leaving scars. People remain infective from the first rash until all scabs are gone. The disease can spread through contact with infective fluid from lesions or from contact with clothes or bedding. Aerosol spread is theoretically possible. Precautions are as follows:

- Vaccination must be done before symptoms appear and as soon as possible after exposure as vaccination after rash appears will not affect the severity of the disease; vaccination is done by scratching the skin with a small needle on the upper arm, leaving a characteristic pox scar.
- Contact precautions should be used, which includes the use of gowns and gloves to enter the room and keeping the patient in a private or cohorted room.

### *Viral Hemorrhagic Fevers*

Viral hemorrhagic fevers are zoonoses (spread from animals to humans) and comprise a number of different diseases: Ebola, Lassa, Marburg, yellow, Argentine and Crimean-Congo. Some hemorrhagic fevers can spread person to person, notably Ebola, Marburg, and Lassa, through close contact with body fluids or contaminated items. Hemorrhagic fevers are extremely contagious multi-system diseases, and those in contact with infected patients are at risk of infection. Symptoms vary somewhat according to the disease but present with flu-like symptoms that progress to bleeding under the skin and internally, and some people develop kidney failure and central nervous system symptoms, such as coma and seizures. Treatment is supportive and mortality rates are high. Only yellow fever and Argentine have vaccines.

Precautions are as follows:

- **Maximum precautions** must be used with full barrier precautions, with care used in any handling of blood and body fluids or wastes.
- **Screening**: ask patient if they have been out of the country in the last 3-6 months.

## Disaster Recovery Aspect of Disaster Planning and Management

Disaster recovery is the final stage of any disaster response and deals with the actions necessary to return the disaster site to normal. The recovery effort can be divided into **two different periods**:

- The **restoration period** is an immediate recovery step in which the area is made safe, utilities repaired, wreckage removed, and evacuees are allowed to return.
- The **reconstruction/replacement period** is a longer process where the disaster area is rebuilt and returned to its pre-disaster condition, both physically and economically. The reconstruction period can take many years, and is dependent on the degree of damage and availability of resources for reconstruction efforts.

As a part of the disaster recovery process, steps should be taken to prevent a recurrence of the disaster in the future.

## Security Plan

A security plan is a plan that is set in place to help guide the actions of employees in case of a breach in security at a healthcare facility. All employees must be educated and comfortable with their facilities plan, in order to facilitate the safety of staff and patients alike. The security plan usually has several components:

- **Security workers**: Most facilities have securities guards who patrol the campus and help maintain patient and visitor safety. If a patient/visitor threatens violence or becomes combative, security should be called immediately.
- **Silent alarms**: Most units have "silent alarms," which are usually buttons or switches underneath the secretary's desk or in some other discreet location. These are pushed in the case of a threat to security in which a call cannot safely be made.
- **Locked units**: Certain units in the hospital (such as mother/baby, critical care units, psychiatric floors, etc.) are locked and require an access code to enter.
- **Do not acknowledge**: Certain patients may be deemed as "do not acknowledge," meaning that the nurse cannot give out any information regarding these patients, including acknowledging the patients' presence in the facility. Examples include psychiatric patients, victims of crime, celebrities, and others. If someone calls asking about the patient, it is appropriate and ethical for the nurse to state, "I do not have any information regarding a patient with that name."
- **Overhead announcements**: Many facilities have different codes that they may call overhead to alert staff of emergences/safety threats without overt language.
- **Newborn nursery security**: Measures include matching ID bands for infant and parents/caregivers, foot-printing and photographing the infant after birth, transporting infants in bassinets rather than carrying them, utilizing a tracking and security alarm system that can trigger automatic lockdown, limiting access to obstetrics and nursery areas, having staff wear easily-identifiable ID badges, and utilizing video surveillance.
- **Violence prevention**: Measures include educating staff about de-escalation techniques, having an alarm system in place, providing adequate security, utilizing video surveillance, limiting access, identifying clients who may be at risk for behaving violently, and requiring visitors' badges.
- **Controlled access**: Measures include locked areas that require a password, biologic ID (fingerprint, eye scan), access card for entry, turnstiles at entry and/or metal detectors, security personal stationed at entry points, and video surveillance of entries, exits, stairwells, hallways, elevators, and storage areas.

### *Principles of Evacuation in a Security Plan*

Principles of evacuation in a security plan, according to OSHA, should include:

- Conditions that would trigger an evacuation
- Chain of command for decision making

- Procedures for evacuation, including methods of evacuation and preferred routes. Exits should be clearly identified
- Procedures for assisting clients who are disabled and those who do not speak English
- Procedures for determining who are responsible for terminating critical operations
- Procedures for tracking personnel and clients
- Transportation plans for transferal of clients to other facilities

The path of least resistance is an important concept to understand for evacuation, especially if they involve fire and any products of combustion (smoke, heat, gas). Fire's path of least resistance is usually vertical, although fire also spreads horizontally, especially if a vertical path is not available. Water, on the other hand, also flows vertically, but downward and then horizontally if the downward flow is blocked. Clients should be evacuated according to the path of least resistance; that is, the route that is the easiest and safest.

# Federal Regulations

## Regulation of Nursing by States' Nurse Practice Act

Each state's **nurse practice act** seeks to regulate nursing within the state. It specifies the amount and type of education required to become an RN or LPN/LVN. It defines the nurse's role and responsibilities in healthcare settings. It lists actions that the nurse may take and defines advanced practice education, experience, responsibilities, and limitations. It gives nurses the authorization to perform as required. It also regulates delegation and supervision responsibilities of the nurse. Nurse practice acts are administrated by the state board of nursing, which is responsible for issuing and renewing nurse licenses as well as discipline and censure of nurses. Most state boards of nursing now have a website that provides state-specific information about licensure and nursing rights and responsibilities.

## Nurse's Accountability for Nursing Care

Nurses are part of an interdisciplinary team responsible for patient outcomes. Nurses have the responsibility for the outcomes of nursing care as a professional group. This responsibility is outlined in each state's nurse practice act, the American Nurses Association (ANA) practice guidelines, and the nurse's job description. Tools, such as the nursing care plan that includes standardized nursing diagnoses, interventions, and expected outcomes, enable the nurse to fulfill this responsibility. Empowerment to act as the patient advocate allows the nurse to point out factors in the patient's individual situation that can be addressed to further improve outcome. Critical thinking during decision-making and detailed documentation are also important. The nurse is held accountable for delegation as well as supervising care by others and evaluation of the outcomes of that care as well. The nurse has personal **accountability** in terms of ethical and moral conduct. Since clinical knowledge is crucial to critical thinking, the nurse must strive to increase knowledge continuously through professional development throughout his or her career.

## Advance Directives

In accordance to Federal and state laws, individuals have the right to self-determination in health care, including the right to make decisions about end of life care through **advance directives** such as living wills and the right to assign a surrogate person to make decisions through a durable power of attorney. Patients should routinely be questioned about an advanced directive as they may present at a healthcare provider without the document. Patients who have indicated that they desire a do-not-resuscitate (DNR) order should not receive resuscitative treatments for terminal illness or conditions in which meaningful recovery cannot occur. Patients and families of those with terminal illnesses should be questioned as to whether the patients are Hospice patients. For those with DNR requests or those withdrawing life support, staff should provide the patient palliative rather than curative measures, such as pain control and/or oxygen, and emotional support to the patient and family. Religious traditions and beliefs about death should be treated with respect.

## HIPAA

The Health Insurance Portability and Accountability Act (HIPAA) and state laws govern **who may receive healthcare information** about a person, how permission is to be obtained, how the information may be shared, and patients' rights concerning personal information. HIPAA strives to protect the **privacy** of an individual's healthcare information. Facilities must prevent this information from being accessed by unauthorized personnel. Healthcare information is required to be protected on the **administrative**, **physical**, and **technical** levels. The patient must sign a release form to allow any sharing of patient information. There are stiff penalties for violation of these laws, ranging from $100 for an unintentional violation to $50,000 for a willful violation. Facilities that violate HIPAA may also be subject to corrective actions. Penalties are governed by the Department of Health and Human Services' Office for Civil Right and the state attorneys general.

### *Application of HIPAA to Practice*

As an integral member of the health care team, the nurse must always be aware of HIPAA regulations and apply this knowledge to practice. The nurse is responsible for the following efforts to protect and maintain patient privacy:

- The nurse must read and follow facility policies regarding the transfer of patient data.
- Communication between health care personnel about a patient should always be in a private place so that this information is not overheard by those who do not have the right to share the information.
- Access to charts must be restricted to only those health care team members involved in that patient's care.
- Patient care information for unlicensed workers cannot be posted at the bedside, but must be on a care plan or the patient chart in a protected area.
- The nurse must not give information casually to anyone (e.g., visitors or family members) unless it is confirmed that they have the right to have that information.
- Family members must not be relied upon to interpret for the patient; an interpreter must be obtained to protect patient privacy.
- Computers with patient information must have passwords and safeguards to prevent unauthorized access of patient information.
- The nurse should not leave voicemail messages containing protected healthcare information for a patient but should instead ask the patient to call back.

**Review Video: What is HIPAA?**
Visit mometrix.com/academy and enter code: 412009

## OSHA

The **Occupational Safety and Health Act (OSHA)** seeks to keep workers safe and healthy while on the job. OSHA mandates that employers maintain a safe environment, workers are made fully aware of any hazards, and that access to personal protective gear is made available to workers who come into contact with hazardous materials. By following these regulations, an employer keeps injury and illness of workers to an absolute minimum. This fosters productivity, since workers are not absent due to illness or injury, employee health costs are contained, and the turnover rate is decreased, saving money spent on hiring and training new employees. OSHA is concerned about healthcare employee exposure to radiation, as well as chemical and biological agents, when caring for patients. Information is available to help hospitals and other facilities write plans that comply with best practices to deal with this and other threats to employees. Cleaning procedures, decontamination, and hazardous waste disposal are all covered by OSHA and apply to everyday hospital operation as well as disaster situations.

**Review Video: What is OSHA (Occupational Safety and Health Administration)**
Visit mometrix.com/academy and enter code: 913559

## CMS

The **Centers for Medicare and Medicaid (CMS)**, part of the U.S. Department of Health and Human Service department, see to it that healthcare regulations are observed by healthcare facilities that receive federal reimbursement. They reimburse facilities for care given to Medicare, Medicaid, and the state Children's Health Insurance Program (CHIP) recipients. They also monitor adherence to HIPAA regulations concerning healthcare information portability and confidentiality. CMS examines documentation of patient care when deciding to reimburse for care given. CMS has regulations for all types of medical facilities, and these regulations have profoundly impacted nursing practice because nurses must ensure that they comply with regulations related to the quality of patient care and concerns regarding cost-containment. Each facility should provide guidelines to assist nursing staff in meeting the specific documentation requirements of CMS.

## OBRA 1987

The **Omnibus Budget Reconciliation Act of 1987 (OBRA 1987)**, also known as the Nursing Home Reform Act, instituted requirements for nursing homes with the purpose of strengthening and protecting patient rights. These requirements are as follows: "a facility must provide each patient with a level of care that enables him or her to attain or maintain the highest practicable physical, mental, and psychosocial wellbeing." OBRA 1987 required that all nursing home patients receive an initial evaluation with yearly follow-ups. Every patient is required to have a comprehensive care plan. Patients were ensured the right to medical care and the right to be informed about and refuse medical treatment. OBRA 1987 requires each state to establish, monitor, and enforce its own licensing requirements in addition to federal standards. Each state is also required to fund, staff, and maintain investigative and Ombudsman units.

## OBRA 1990 (PSDA)

The Omnibus Budget Reconciliation Act of 1990 included the amendment called the **Patient Self Determination Act (PSDA)**. The PSDA required healthcare facilities to provide written information about advanced healthcare directives and the right to accept or reject medical or surgical treatments to all patients. Patients who make an advanced directive are leaving instructions about what medical interventions they authorize or refuse if they are incapacitated by illness or injury. They can also nominate another person to make these decisions for them in this situation. The PSDA also protected the right of patients to accept or refuse medical treatments. Healthcare facilities and hospitals are legally required to communicate these rights to all patients, to respect these rights, and to educate staff and personnel about these rights.

## EMTALA

The **Emergency Medical Treatment and Active Labor Act (EMTALA)** is designed to prevent patient "dumping" from emergency departments (ED) and is an issue of concern for risk management that requires staff training for compliance:

- Transfers from the ED may be intrahospital or to another facility.
- Stabilization of the patient with emergency conditions or active labor must be done in the ED prior to transfer, and initial screening must be given prior to inquiring about insurance or ability to pay.
- Stabilization requires treatment for emergency conditions and reasonable belief that, although the emergency condition may not be completely resolved, the patient's condition will not deteriorate during transfer.
- Women in the ED in active labor should deliver both the child and placenta before transfer.
- The receiving department or facility should be capable of treating the patient and dealing with complications that might occur.
- Transfer to another facility is indicated if the patient requires specialized services not available intrahospital, such as to burn centers.

## AHRQ

The **Agency for Healthcare Research and Quality (AHRQ)** is part of the U.S. Department of Health and Human Services. This agency is concerned about health care and primarily promotes scientific research into the safety, effectiveness, and quality of healthcare. It encourages evidence-based healthcare that produces the best possible outcome while containing healthcare costs. It makes contracts with institutions to review any published evidence on healthcare in order to produce reports used by other organizations to write guidelines. The agency operates the National Guideline Clearinghouse, which is available online. It is a repository of evidence-based guidelines that address various health conditions and diseases. These guidelines are written by many different health-related professional organizations and are used by primary healthcare providers, nurses, and healthcare facilities to guide patient treatment and care.

# Risk Management

## Continuous Quality Improvement

Continuous quality improvement is a multidisciplinary management philosophy that can be applied to all aspects of an organization, whether related to such varied areas as the cardiac unit, purchasing, or human resources. The skills used for epidemiologic research (data collection, analysis, outcomes, action plans) are all applicable to the analysis of multiple types of events, because they are based on solid scientific methods. Multidisciplinary planning can bring valuable insights from various perspectives, and strategies used in one context can often be applied to another. All staff, from housekeeping to supervising, must be alert to not only problems but also opportunities for improvement. Increasingly, departments must be concerned with cost-effectiveness as the costs of medical care continue to rise, so the quality professional in the cardiovascular unit is not in an isolated position in an institution but is just one part of the whole, facing similar concerns as those in other disciplines. Disciplines are often interrelated in their functions.

## Juran's Quality Improvement Process

Joseph Juran's quality improvement process (QIP) is a 4-step method of change (focusing on quality control) which is based on a trilogy of concepts that includes quality planning, control, and improvement. The steps to the QIP process include the following:

1. **Defining** the project and organizing includes listing and prioritizing problems and identifying a team.
2. **Diagnosing** includes analyzing problems and then formulating theories related to cause by root cause analysis and test theories.
3. **Remediating** includes considering various alternative solutions and then designing and implementing specific solutions and controls while addressing institutional resistance to change. As causes of problems are identified and remediation instituted to remove the problems, the processes should improve.
4. **Holding** involves evaluating performance and monitoring the control system in order to maintain gains.

## FOCUS Performance Improvement Model

**Find, organize, clarify, uncover, start (FOCUS)** is a performance improvement model used to facilitate change:

1. **Find**: Identifying a problem by looking at the organization and attempting to determine what isn't working well or what is wrong.
2. **Organize**: Identifying those people who have an understanding of the problem or process and creating a team to work on improving performance.
3. **Clarify**: Determining what is involved in solving the problem by utilizing brainstorming techniques, such as the Ishikawa diagram.
4. **Uncover**: Analyzing the situation to determine the reason the problem has arisen or that a process is unsuccessful.
5. **Start**: Determining where to begin in the change process.

FOCUS, by itself, is an incomplete process and is primarily used as a means to identify a problem rather than a means to find the solution. FOCUS is usually combined with PDCA (FOCUS-PDCA), so it becomes a 9-step process; however, beginning with FOCUS helps to narrow the focus, resulting in better outcomes.

## Nurse's Involvement in Quality Improvement

The following are ways in which nurses can be involved in quality improvement in their facility:

- **Identify situations** in the nursing unit that require improvement and might benefit patient outcomes (cost containment, incident reporting, etc.) if changed.
- **Identify potential items** that can be measured to be able to test the problem or to be able to monitor patient outcomes.
- **Collect data** on those measurements and determine current patient outcomes.
- **Analyze the data** and identify procedures, methods, etc., that can be utilized to potentially make positive changes in patient outcomes, doing research if necessary.
- **Make recommendations for changes** to be implemented to determine the effect on patient outcomes.
- **Implement recommendations** after approval from administrative personnel.
- **Collect data** using the same measurements and determine if the changes improved patient outcomes or not.

## Risk Management

Risk management attempts to prevent harm and legal liability by being proactive and by identifying a patient's **risk factors**. The patient is educated about these factors and ways that they can modify their behavior to decrease their risk. Treatments and interventions must be considered in terms of risk to the patient, and the patient must always know these risks in order to make healthcare decisions. Much can be done to avoid mistakes that put patients at risk. Patients should note medications and other aspects of their care so that they can help prevent mistakes. They should feel free to question care and to have their concerns heard and addressed. When mistakes are made, the actions taken to remedy the situation are very important. The physician should be made aware of the error immediately, and the patient notified according to hospital policy. Errors must be evaluated to determine how the process failed. Honesty and caring can help mitigate many errors.

## Nursing Malpractice, Negligence, Unintentional Torts, and Intentional Torts

- **Malpractice** is unethical or improper actions or lack of proper action by the nurse that may or may not be related to a lack of skills that nurses should possess.
- **Negligence** is the failure to act as any other diligent nurse would have acted in the same situation.
- Negligence can lead to an **unintentional tort**. In this case, the patient must prove that the nurse had a duty to act, a duty proven via standards of care, and that the nurse failed in this duty and harm occurred to the patient as a result of this failure.
- **Intentional torts** differ in that the duty is assumed and the nurse breached this duty via assault and battery, invasion of privacy, slander, or false imprisonment of the patient.

**Review Video: Medical Negligence**
Visit mometrix.com/academy and enter code: 928405

# Professional Issues: Triage

## Emergency Intake Assessment

### Rapid Visual Assessment: Sick vs. Not Sick

Sick vs. not sick is a rapid visual assessment method used for initial triage and is usually completed within less than a minute based on clinical indications. The primary purpose is to classify as **sick** those who appear unstable and require immediate attention and as **not sick** those who appear stable and have no or less severe illness/injury and whose care can be delayed. Decisions are made based on knowledge about expected injuries from different types of accidents, the mechanism of injury (auto accident, gunshot wound, fall), and nature of sickness that might suggest possible diagnoses. Clinical indicators to evaluate include:

- **Vital signs**: Pulse and respiration
- **Mental status**: Alert, confused, responsive, non-responsive, disoriented
- **Circulation**: Skin signs include cyanosis, pallor, erythema, and edema
- **Body position**: Sitting, standing, prone, supine, distorted
- **Evidence of trauma, mechanism of injury (trauma)**: Bleeding, open wounds, fractures
- **Nature of medical complaints (illness)**: Pain, dizziness, and dyspnea

Patients initially classified as *not sick* may be reclassified any time their conditions change.

### Pediatric Assessment Triangle (PAT)

The Pediatric Assessment Triangle (PAT) is a method used to provide a first general impression of a child's state of health and/or illness. Each parameter is evaluated as normal or abnormal with abnormal findings requiring further assessment per the primary and secondary surveys.

| | |
|---|---|
| **Appearance** | Note the child's tone, ability to interact, response to environmental stimuli, consolability, gaze, general appearance, and speech or crying. Other descriptors include listless, responding poorly, lethargic, poor muscle tone (rigid, floppy), staring. |
| **Breathing** | Note the degree of difficulty associated with breathing, including any abnormal or adventitious breath sounds, sternal retraction, nasal flaring, bobbing of head, and positioning (such as the need to sit upright to breathe). Other descriptors include stridor, grunting, crackles, wheezing, and absent breath sounds. |
| **Circulation** | Note the color of skin and any abnormalities, such as mottling, pallor, bleeding, or cyanosis. Other descriptors include circumoral cyanosis, peripheral cyanosis. |

### Assigning Triage Acuity Levels

#### *Emergency Severity Index (ESI)*

The Emergency Severity Index (ESI) is a 5-level method of triage that evaluates the patient's condition and need for resources. The 5 levels are based on decision point questions and include:

1. Unstable and needs resuscitation/lifesaving interventions immediately. Diagnoses include: Cardiac arrest, respiratory arrest, or severe distress, $SPO_2$ <90, severe trauma, overdose, hypovolemia, anaphylaxis, hypoglycemia with mental status change, signs of MI, marked bradycardia.
2. High-risk patient needs time-sensitive treatment (usually within 10 minutes) to prevent threat to life or organ. Diagnoses include chest pain, indications of stroke, fever in immunocompromised, suicidal/homicidal ideation, staff member needle stick.

3. Patient requires ≥2 resources. Patient is stable and may wait an hour or so for treatment. Note: Resources include laboratory tests, imaging, IV fluids, parenteral medications, nebulizer treatment, referral to specialist, and simple procedures (suturing, catheter insertion), or complex procedures (conscious sedation). Complex procedures are considered equivalent to 2 resources.
4. Patient requires 1 resource.
5. Patient requires no resources.

**Emergency Severity Index (decision points)**: Includes 4 questions or decision points used to assign patients to Levels 1 through 5.

- **Is the patient dying?** If yes, the patient is classified as ESI 1, ABCs assessed, and lifesaving procedures instituted: BVM, intubation, surgical airway, C-PAP, Bi-PAP, cardioversion, pacing, defibrillation, chest needle compression, pericardiocentesis, IV/blood transfusion, reversal agents. If the patient is not dying, then the next question is posed.
- **Should the patient not wait?** Assessments include determining if the patient is at high risk, confused/disoriented, and/or in severe pain or distress. If yes, the patient is classified as ESI 2. If not, the next question is posed.
- **How many resources are needed?** This evaluation depends on knowledge of usual treatment for presenting symptoms. Patients are classified at level 3, 4, or 5 based on expected needs.
- **What are the vital signs?** This includes pulse, respiration, oxygen saturation, and temperature (for children <3). If VS are unstable, patients classified as level 3 are elevated to level 2.

#### Calculating Resource Needs

In emergency medicine, **resources** include laboratory tests, imaging, IV fluids, parenteral medications, nebulizer treatment, referral to specialist, simple procedures (suturing, catheter insertion), or complex procedures (conscious sedation). Treatments that are NOT considered resources include immunizations, oral medications, prescriptions, dressings, crutches, point-of-care testing, history, and physical examination. Information gleaned from ESI triage system can help to determine needs according to volume and triage level. Average emergency department visits per level include:

- Level 3 (needing 2 or more resources): 30–40%
- Level 4 (needing 1 resource): 20%
- Level 5 (needing 0 resources): 35%

Using these percentages and the volume of patients, one can estimate the need for resources. However, not all facilities, such as level 1 trauma center, fit this pattern of distribution, so each facility should undertake research to determine the actual utilization of resources per trauma category.

### *Simple Triage and Rapid Treatment*

S.T.A.R.T. (Simple Triage and Rapid Treatment) is a method of triage used when there are multiple casualties that must be assessed rapidly and classified for treatment. Colored tags are applied to identify status. Classification is based on sequential evaluation of respirations, perfusion, and mental status (RPM):

- **Green: Minor.** Patient may have injuries, but RPMs are intact, and patient can wait for assistance.
- **Black: Deceased.** Head is repositioned, but if respirations do not occur, CPR is not started, and the triage person moves on to the next patient.
- **Red: Immediate.** If breathing resumes after head repositioning, respirations are >30 (estimated, not counted), there is no radial pulse, capillary refill >2 seconds, or if patient is unconscious or cannot follow simple commands.
- **Delayed: Other conditions.** If patient is able to follow simple commands and needs are not immediate.

### *Three-Level and Four-Level Triage*

**Three-level triage** is still used in some emergency departments with some variations. The criteria for assignment may vary somewhat as well. Generally, the 3 levels include:

- **Critical/Immediate/Emergent:** These patients have life-threatening conditions that require immediate resuscitation or intervention to prevent death or severe morbidity and have priority for treatment.
- **Urgent:** These patients have serious injuries that require treatment, but care can be delayed for a few minutes while those with more serious injuries are treated.
- **Less urgent/Non-urgent:** These patients are assigned the lowest priority because their injuries are not life threatening.

**Four-level triage** is similar. The primary difference is the addition of a resuscitation category separate from those who otherwise require critical care. For example, a patient with cardiac arrest would be classified as *resuscitation* and a myocardial infarct as *emergent.* Various color-coding systems, sometimes specific to a facility, may be used.

# Emergency Nurse Practice Test #1

**1. A forty-year-old female presents to the emergency department (ED) complaining of chest pain. After triaging the client, obtaining vital signs including a blood pressure of 90/46, and establishing an adequate airway, what is the next most important intervention for this client?**

a. registering the patient into the system
b. ordering serum blood laboratory tests
c. placing the client on a cardiac monitor, administering oxygen, and obtaining an electrocardiogram (EKG)
d. giving a sublingual nitroglycerin tablet for the immediate relief of pain

**2. The purpose of the primary assessment in any emergency is to**

a. perform a quick look-see to determine the illness or injury
b. assess for life-threatening problems that require an immediate intervention
c. make the client comfortable and remove wet clothing for the assessment
d. gain a medical and surgical history, including allergies and medication

**3. The emergency medical services (EMS) team transports an adult male with chest pain to the ED. They have initiated a large-bore intravenous (IV) line, administered oxygen, and placed the client on the cardiac monitor. Upon arrival to the ED, the initial EKG shows ST deviation in two leads, and the client is pale, clammy, and restless. What is the next intervention the ED nurse should anticipate?**

a. the nurse will give a report to the intensive care unit (ICU)
b. the nurse will give a large dose of heparin
c. the nurse will prepare the client for the cardiac catheterization laboratory (cath lab)
d. the nurse will order a repeat EKG for 8 hours in the future

**4. Which factors about troponin levels are important to consider when caring for a client being evaluated for an acute myocardial infarction (MI)?**

a. troponin level is not the most important factor when caring for a client with an acute MI
b. troponin levels elevate 3 to 12 hours after MI onset
c. troponin levels are specific to MI clients only
d. troponin levels will elevate in unstable angina as well as in an MI

**5. Which factor is NOT a risk for heart disease but also should not be excluded when considering the diagnosis of MI when a client presents with chest pain?**

a. age greater than 65
b. nonsmoking female
c. smoking any gender
d. obesity

**6. An elderly female client presents to the ED with complaints of chest pain and a history of angina. After the initial triage, what would be the next appropriate interventions?**

a. cardiac monitor, oxygen, and sublingual nitroglycerin
b. cardiac monitor, sublingual nitroglycerin, and Foley catheter
c. cardiac monitor, IV, oxygen, and sublingual nitroglycerin
d. oxygen, sublingual nitroglycerin, and Foley catheter

**7. Which condition in the pediatric population may lead to congestive heart failure and should be considered when gaining a medical history on a pediatric patient in the ED?**

a. history of prematurity
b. low weight for age
c. history of asthma
d. congenital heart defect

**8. Which intervention is the most immediate when caring for a pediatric client who appears to be in heart failure?**

a. maintain airway and breathing
b. monitor for distress
c. limit fluid intake
d. get a complete medical history

**9. Which diagnosis may describe a client with a long history of cardiac disease and heart failure who presents to the ED with fatigue, orthopnea, edema, and hypertension but without chest pain?**

a. obesity
b. asthma
c. cardiomyopathy
d. MI

**10. What is the physical consequence of any cardiac dysrhythmia that causes the need for an intervention?**

a. there is no physical consequence unless pain is involved
b. there is a decrease in cardiac output that directly relates to the hemodynamic status of the client
c. it can increase blood pressure
d. it does not affect the airway

**11. A 64-year-old client presents to the ED complaining of shortness of breath and fatigue for two days. An initial EKG shows a non-q-wave myocardial infarction (previously called a non-transmural MI). Which of the following would NOT be true about this type of MI?**

a. ST depression is visible on the ECG
b. peak CK levels are usually reached in about 12-13 hours
c. the coronary occlusion is usually complete
d. reinfarction is common

**12. Which task would NOT be performed initially by the ED nurse when a client presents with chest pain?**

a. initiate monitoring and interpret EKG rhythm strips
b. assess defibrillator for proper functioning
c. auscultate heart sounds
d. order a low-salt diet for the client

**13. A patient presents to the ER with pain that he describes as sharp and ripping on the posterior chest. There is widening on the mediastinum on the chest x-ray, and a blood pressure differential is noted. What diagnosis does the nurse suspect?**

a. myocardial infarction
b. cardiac tamponade
c. dissecting aortic aneurysm
d. tension pneumothorax

**14. The ED nurse understands that the ongoing evaluation and monitoring of a client with chest pain includes which of the following?**

a. evaluating response to a low-sodium meal
b. managing airway patency, blood pressure, and oximetry
c. being prepared to insert an IV line as needed
d. documenting the client's insurance information

**15. Which symptom(s) would be apparent with left-sided heart failure?**

a. pulmonary edema
b. venous congestion
c. absence of pain
d. absence of any notable symptoms

**16. Inspection when triaging a client with chest pain includes which of the following?**

a. observing the patient's interactions with the assistive personnel
b. looking for family interactions
c. observing skin color, signs of edema
d. asking about medical history

**17. Which statement explains abnormal liver function tests in the client with heart failure?**

a. the client may be an alcoholic
b. the abnormal results may be the result of hepatic vascular congestion
c. the client has hepatitis
d. the results are altered from the cardiac drugs the client may have taken

**18. Which statement is NOT true about dopamine?**

a. it is a vesicant
b. it produces less instances of unwanted tachycardias than norepinephrine
c. it increases contractility of the myocardium and increases cardiac output
d. it increases myocardial workload

**19. All of the following extracardiac sounds may be heard on auscultation of the heart EXCEPT**

a. pericardial friction rub.
b. venous hum.
c. clicks of valves.
d. clucks of valves.

**20. Which nursing diagnosis would be appropriate for a client with a cardiac history and shortness of breath?**

a. ineffective tissue perfusion
b. low fluid volume
c. ineffective breathing pattern
d. none of the above

**21. Which client with a possible cardiac dysrhythmia would require an immediate intervention because of a decrease in cardiac output?**

a. a 22-year-old athlete with a heart rate of 46 at rest who is pink and in no distress
b. a 42-year-old male with a heart rate of 42 who is pale and clammy
c. an 82-year-old febrile female with a heart rate of 90
d. a 15-month-old with a heart rate of 110 who is laughing and playing

**22. Which rate may indicate possible paroxysmal supraventricular tachycardia from what is understood about normal vital signs?**

a. one hundred thirty beats per minute in a three-year-old
b. one hundred beats per minute in an adult with anxiety
c. one hundred and fifty beats per minute in a newborn
d. one hundred and thirty beats per minute in an adult

**23. Which rhythm would be identified on an ECG/EKG six-second strip by a heart rate of 76 and a PR interval of 0.24, the P:QRS ratio is 1:1, the P and the QRS are normal and regular?**

a. sinus arrhythmia
b. first-degree atrioventricular block
c. sinus rhythm
d. second-degree type I Block

**24. What constitutes the description or definition of ventricular tachycardia?**

a. one or two premature ventricular contractions (PVCs) in a one-minute span
b. any heart rate over 100
c. a run of three or more PVCs with or without symptoms
d. two PVCs together as a couplet

**25. The initial intervention when a client develops ventricular fibrillation (VF) is which of the following?**

a. perform cardiopulmonary resuscitation (CPR)
b. defibrillation
c. doses of epinephrine
d. doses of atropine

**26. The term for the abdominal emergency best described as a part of the bowel telescoping into or within itself causing a bowel obstruction is which of the following?**

a. large bowel obstruction
b. small bowel obstruction
c. intussusception
d. acute abdomen

**27. Which one of the following is NOT a cause of acute gastritis?**

a. the use of NSAIDs
b. excess alcohol consumption
c. caustic ingestion of foods with excessive seasoning
d. *H. pylori* infection

**28. Which bacteria may be a leading cause of chronic gastritis?**

a. streptococcus
b. staphylococcus
c. *Helicobacter pylori*
d. gram-negative bacteria

**29. Which fact is important to remember when dealing with pediatric abdominal trauma patients?**

a. abdominal trauma in the pediatric population is rare
b. low blood pressure is a late sign of shock in the pediatric population and doesn't appear until a child has lost greater than 25% of their circulating blood
c. low blood pressure is an early sign of shock in the pediatric population and needs to be addressed immediately upon arrival to the ED
d. children have a lower percentage of water than body weight and a lower metabolic rate making the acid-base balance difficult to maintain

**30. Which is the most common cause of intestinal obstruction requiring an intervention during infancy?**

a. intussusception
b. pyloric stenosis
c. obstructive colic
d. reflux

**31. The most important initial intervention for abdominal trauma is which of the following?**

a. assessing the airway, breathing, and circulation (ABCs)
b. initiating a large-bore IV for fluid replacement
c. preparing for a computed tomography (CT) scan of the abdomen
d. inserting a Foley catheter to assess for urinary output and bladder or kidney injury

**32. Hypocalcemia may result from which acute or chronic abdominal condition?**

a. appendicitis
b. pancreatitis
c. hepatitis
d. gastritis

**33. A patient presents to the ED with acute abdominal pain, nausea, and vomiting. Which of the following tests would cause the nurse to suspect pancreatitis?**

a. WBC count of 5.0
b. hematocrit (HCT) of 40%
c. WBC count of 28.0
d. lipase 500 U/L

**34. Which medical intervention is appropriate for a client with a possible bowel obstruction after the ABCs have been established and an IV has been initiated?**

a. place the patient on bedrest
b. insert a nasogastric (NG) tube and attach to suction
c. order a clear liquid tray
d. massage the abdomen

**35. Which pharmacologic agent would be appropriate for an adult client with pancreatitis who is in severe pain?**

a. Compazine
b. aspirin
c. narcotics, avoiding morphine if possible
d. gentamicin

**36. The pain of acute diverticulitis can be described as dull or cramping. Where is the pain most likely to be located with an acute episode?**

a. right lower quadrant (RLQ)
b. right upper quadrant (RUQ)
c. left lower quadrant (LLQ)
d. left upper quadrant (LUQ)

**37. A client with bleeding esophageal varices is at risk for severe hemorrhage and even death. What specific emergency procedure should the nurse be prepared to assist with in the case of uncontrolled esophageal bleeding?**

a. insertion of a nasogastric tube for suction
b. intubation and a Sengstaken-Blakemore tube
c. administering an IV
d. doing a type and cross match for blood

**38. An 8-year-old presents to the ED with bloody diarrhea, abdominal pain, fever, and vomiting. On history, the mother mentions the child cleaned out his pet turtle's cage yesterday before lunch time. What is the nurse beginning to suspect?**

a. *Campylobacter jejuni*
b. *Clostridium difficile*
c. *Yersinia enterocolitica*
d. Nontyphoidal *salmonella*

**39. A 45-year-old man is admitted to the emergency department after a bout of bloody vomiting. He is noted to be mildly hypotensive with slight scleral icterus, palmar erythema, and hepatomegaly. There is no history of aspirin or NSAID use but he does admit to long-term alcohol abuse. The most likely source of the bleeding is:**

a. gastric ulcer
b. esophageal varices
c. gastric cancer
d. angiodysplasia

**40. A 45-year-old woman is brought to the emergency department complaining of acute, severe midabdominal pain, radiating from the epigastrium to the mid-back. There is marked guarding of the abdomen and mild Abdominal distension is present. She denies alcohol abuse or prior abdominal surgery. There has been no recent change in her bowel habits. Bowel sounds are markedly diminished. What is the most likely diagnosis and the laboratory or imaging test to establish the diagnosis?**

a. acute pancreatitis and serum amylase
b. small bowel obstruction and plain films of the abdomen
c. acute cholecystitis and ultrasound of the gall bladder
d. acute appendicitis and CT of the abdomen

**41. A 30-year-old man comes to the emergency department with the acute onset of left flank pain radiating to the groin. Microscopic hematuria is present on urinalysis. What is the most likely diagnosis?**

a. ureteral calcium oxalate calculus
b. ureteral cystine calculus
c. testicular torsion
d. cystitis

**42. A young woman with a history of lupus and recent aminoglycoside treatment of an infection develops nausea, extreme fatigue, and poor urinary output. Her serum creatinine is 4.5 mg/dL and urine output is severely diminished. An ECG shows peaked T waves, prolonged PR interval, and a slightly widened QRS complex. Which of the following would be appropriate emergency therapy?**

a. intravenous calcium
b. intravenous glucose and insulin
c. both A and B
d. neither A nor B

**43. While assessing a trauma patient, the nurse finds the client complaining of flank pain where there is also bruising noted. What intervention should the nurse be ready to perform because of these signs of injury?**

a. a CT scan of the client's head
b. a urinalysis and a complete blood count (CBC)
c. offer oral fluids to promote hydration
d. administer oxygen

**44. An important concept when evaluating for traumatic genitourinary injuries for both children and adults would be which of the following?**

a. keep the client dressed to protect privacy and avoid direct observation
b. assess the genitourinary system last, as it is the least important
c. undress the client while protecting his or her privacy and directly observe the genitals for injury
d. never insert a Foley catheter unless absolutely needed because of the risk for infection

**45. A client presenting to the ED complaining of flank pain, diaphoresis, and nausea may be experiencing which genitourinary emergency?**

a. MI
b. kidney stones
c. testicular torsion
d. ovulation

**46. Acute renal failure developing over a short period of time is the result of which of the following?**

a. calcium buildup
b. fluid overload
c. increase in nitrogenous waste products circulating
d. decrease in potassium circulating

**47. Which prerenal sign will the ED nurse recognize as the first indication of acute renal failure needing an immediate intervention?**

a. an increase in renal blood flow
b. a prolonged period of hyperperfusion
c. a prolonged period of overhydration
d. a decrease in renal blood flow and ischemia

**48. At what age are boys at the most risk for testicular torsion?**

a. the first year of life
b. the ages of five to seven years
c. the risk for testicular torsion is minimal at any age
d. the ages of seven to nine years

**49. Children are at a higher risk for kidney injury than adults. Which statement best explains this fact?**

a. Children are more active than adults.
b. Children do not hydrate appropriately.
c. The incomplete ossification of the 10th and 11th ribs during childhood.
d. Children have kidneys that are three times the normal size of adult kidneys.

**50. What is the most common symptom of a UTI?**

a. fever
b. dysuria
c. cloudy urine
d. fruity odor of urine

**51. Pyelonephritis is a serious infection that can lead to what complications during pregnancy?**

a. cystitis
b. fever
c. bleeding
d. preterm labor and preeclampsia

**52. The immediate nursing interventions for a client presenting to the ED with urinary complaints including flank pain would include which of the following?**

a. obtain a urine specimen and initiate IV fluids
b. urinalysis, IV, and pain control
c. observe for fever
d. encourage oral fluid intake

**53. Which condition would be considered a true urologic emergency requiring surgical intervention?**

a. renal calculi
b. UTI
c. bladder tumor
d. testicular torsion

**54. An adult male presenting to the ED with complaints of pain in the scrotum, a "duck waddle" gait, and fever may have what genitourinary emergency?**

a. priapism
b. epididymitis
c. inguinal hernia
d. UTI

**55. Which condition is the most emergent for a mother and fetus during the second and third trimesters of pregnancy?**

a. multiple fetuses by ultrasound
b. placenta previa
c. UTI
d. abruptio placenta

**56. What are the classic symptoms of abruptio placenta to note when assessing a pregnant client presenting to the ED with bleeding?**

a. hyperglycemia
b. hypertension
c. vaginal bleeding and uterine tenderness
d. emesis

**57. What is the most important element of neonatal resuscitation?**

a. keeping the infant warm
b. maintaining a glucose level of greater than 45
c. maintaining cardiac compressions of greater than 90
d. establishing an adequate airway and administering oxygen

**58. Which obstetric emergency is the leading cause of maternal death due to hemorrhagic shock?**

a. multiple births with retained placenta
b. ruptured ectopic pregnancy implanted in the fallopian tube
c. pelvic inflammatory disease (PID)
d. placenta previa

**59. Which symptoms are recognized as a positive indication of preeclampsia-eclampsia?**

a. low liver enzymes, abdominal pain, edema
b. low blood pressure, proteinuria, edema
c. high blood pressure, proteinuria, edema
d. high platelet count, abdominal pain, edema

**60. What symptoms may occur in late eclampsia that can be life threatening?**

a. proteinuria
b. seizures
c. hemolysis
d. headache

**61. The seriousness of hyperemesis gravidarum is related to which side effect/s?**

a. weight loss, dehydration, low thiamine
b. obesity, low thiamine, high potassium
c. overhydration, hyponatremia, edema
d. high potassium, low magnesium, edema

**62. The initial steps for neonatal resuscitation include which of the following?**

a. drying and doing chest compressions
b. drying under a heat source and establishing an airway
c. suctioning the stomach
d. weighing and measuring the infant

**63. Discharge instructions to a female client experiencing dysfunctional uterine bleeding (DUB) who has required an emergent dilation and curettage (D&C) should include which of the following?**

a. stop taking pain medication 24 hours from procedure
b. avoid eating red meat
c. return to the ED for fever greater than 100.6 °F
d. stay on bed rest for 48 hours

**64. A female client presents to the ED with complaints of white thin vaginal discharge and a foul fishy odor. What would most likely be the cause of these symptoms?**

a. nothing; this is normal
b. vaginitis
c. trichomonas vaginitis
d. bacterial vaginitis

**65. The most common pharmacologic therapies ordered for a female in the ED diagnosed with pelvic inflammatory disease (PID) would include which of the following?**

a. antifungal
b. sedation
c. analgesics and antibiotics
d. none of the above

**66. A client presenting to the ED with an eating disorder is most likely to have what other emergent medical condition, requiring an immediate intervention?**

a. dysrhythmias due to electrolyte imbalances
b. low potassium
c. dehydration
d. depression

**67. All of the following are examples of organic psychoses EXCEPT**

a. dementia.
b. schizophrenia.
c. delirium.
d. toxic drug-induced psychosis.

**68. Suicidal behavior is best described as**

a. attempts to cause death by self-inflicted injury.
b. impulsive but not harmful.
c. never planned.
d. attempts by someone other than one's self to cause injury.

**69. During a pediatric resuscitation, family members should**

a. be allowed to watch the procedure.
b. have a nursing team member assigned to explain and comfort.
c. have a specific space and be permitted to touch their child if possible.
d. all of the above.

**70. Clinical depression**

a. results in suicide risk higher in men than women.
b. can be rapidly treated with antidepressant drugs.
c. may result from alcohol and substance abuse.
d. does not require brain imaging or blood tests.

**71. A 40-year-old man comes to the emergency department complaining of chest pain and shortness of breath for about an hour. The onset occurred rapidly while he was riding on a crowded subway. He has no history of heart or other significant medical problem. His pulse and respiratory rate are increased but blood pressure and temperature are normal. His skin is damp and cool. His electrocardiogram, cardiac enzymes, chest x-ray, and other routine laboratory tests are all normal. What is the most likely diagnosis?**

a. panic attack
b. depression
c. acute coronary syndrome
d. esophageal spasm

**72. A 1-year-old child is brought to the emergency department in a comatose state. His parents state that he fell from a swing and hit his head. There is bruising of the scalp as well as retinal hemorrhages. There are additional bruised areas of the arms and legs and what appears to be a healed rib fracture on chest x-ray. An MRI indicates a subdural hematoma in the parietal portion of the brain. A pediatric neurosurgeon is asked to consult. What is the appropriate course of action for the emergency department nurse now?**

a. report possible child abuse to the appropriate agency per state law
b. detailed questioning of the parents regarding the circumstances of the injury
c. check medical records for prior emergency department visits for trauma
d. all of the above

**73. Which of the following is NOT appropriate for screening for domestic violence by the emergency department nurse?**

a. asking if the person has been hit, kicked, or otherwise hurt by someone in the past year; if so, by whom
b. asking, "Do you feel safe in your present relationship?"
c. avoid asking about intimate person violence if the patient is in the emergency department for a medical ailment, not trauma
d. asking if there is a partner from a previous relationship that makes the individual feel unsafe

**74. An elevated ventilation/perfusion (V/Q) ratio is most likely seen in**

a. pneumonia.
b. pulmonary embolus.
c. acute respiratory distress syndrome.
d. atelectasis.

**75. A patient is intubated and on mechanical ventilation. The ventilator alarm rings and the airway pressure is found to be elevated. Possible causes include the following EXCEPT**

a. endotracheal tube obstruction with sputum.
b. pneumothorax.
c. bronchospasm.
d. cuff leak.

**76. The initial assessment of any adult, infant, or child with any emergency diagnosis should include which of the following?**

a. do a complete head-to-toe assessment
b. establish the chief complaint or injury
c. administer oxygen per mask
d. establish an adequate airway

**77. Which statement best describes acute respiratory distress syndrome (ARDS)?**

a. ARDS is caused by trauma only
b. ARDS is sudden, progressive, and severe
c. ARDS is caused by an illness only
d. ARDS never results in lung scarring

**78. An elevated blood alcohol level may lead to what respiratory complication?**

a. increase in respirations
b. no effect on the respiratory system
c. decrease in respiratory effort and aspiration
d. decrease in depression

**79. A 30-week-gestation premature infant may need pharmacological interventions to improve respiratory status of the lungs. Which drug would most likely be administered in the first few hours after birth?**

a. epinephrine
b. caffeine
c. Survanta
d. vitamin K

**80. All of the following are appropriate ways to establish an initial airway on a nonresponsive client EXCEPT**

a. nasal trumpet.
b. endotracheal tube.
c. esophageal-tracheal Combitube.
d. a Replogle tube.

**81. The nurse in the ED is caring for a patient who was brought over from dialysis with a suspected acute pulmonary embolism. Which of the following tests could provide the most definitive diagnosis?**

a. D-dimer
b. ABG
c. Chest x-ray
d. Spiral CT

**82. Which airway emergency would need to be treated first with an immediate intervention in the ED?**

a. an adult with mild wheezing who denies distress
b. a child carried in by his dad who has a fever but is alert
c. a teen in a wheelchair because of a possible long bone fracture
d. a child arriving by EMS in status asthmaticus

**83. Which respiratory illness affects children under the age of two and causes inflammatory obstruction of the airway?**

a. asthma
b. bronchitis
c. pneumonia
d. bronchiolitis

**84. Which of the following are patient care management tasks?**

a. providing community education
b. identifying clients who are potential organ donors
c. cooling a client following a cardiac arrest
d. all of the above

**85. Croup is an acute respiratory illness presenting with which of the following?**

a. fever greater than 103 °F
b. barking cough
c. rash over extremities
d. total airway obstruction

**86. Anxiety may be a precipitating factor in which respiratory syndrome?**

a. chronic obstructive pulmonary disease
b. emphysema
c. hyperventilation
d. asthma

**87. Clients seen in the ED for transporting illegal drugs by swallowing packages and subsequently overdosing are called which of the following?**

a. condoms
b. body packers
c. rockets
d. ice

**88. The street drug phencyclidine (PCP) can cause which acute complication, requiring intervention?**

a. dissociation anesthesia
b. delusions and tachycardia
c. rhabdomyolysis and renal failure
d. tachypnea and urethral calculi

**89. The nurse assessing an adolescent for complaints of headache and nausea suspects the teen has been "huffing" an inhalant. Which objective data would support that suspicion?**

a. the odor of solvent on the client's face and hands
b. a normal blood urea nitrogen (BUN) and creatinine
c. a positive pregnancy test for the female teen
d. increased reflexes

**90. All of the below are present in all three types of shock EXCEPT**

a. systolic blood pressure below 110 mm Hg.
b. decreased cardiac output.
c. urine output less than 0.5 mL/kg/hr.
d. peripheral vasoconstriction and vasodilation.

**91. Hypovolemia leads to all of the following EXCEPT**

a. decreased venous return.
b. increased cardiac output.
c. diminished stroke volume.
d. decreased central venous pressure.

**92. Professional issues regarding emergency nursing include all of the following EXCEPT**

a. participating in ethical decision making.
b. evaluating the client's capacity to make decisions.
c. protecting patient confidentiality.
d. keeping abuse ED cases confidential by not reporting them to the authorities.

**93. Which of the following is true regarding management of acute respiratory distress syndrome (ARDS)?**

a. Antibiotics have proved effective in the clinical management of ARDS.
b. Patients with ARDS are usually hypovolemic, and giving volume of IVF is a cornerstone of treatment.
c. Most of the care for ARDS is supportive and preventive of other injury.
d. Higher than normal tidal volumes must be used in patients with ARDS.

**94. You are caring for a patient that has been in the ED for 2 hours. The patient was brought in by ambulance already intubated and still sedated from drugs used for RSI on arrival. At the scene the paramedics were told the patient had been using cocaine immediately before collapsing and the ambulance being called. The patient just woke up, eyes wide, grabbing at anything she can get her hands on, biting the ETT. The patient's respiratory rate is 40 and the heart rate is 120. The patient's ABG shows pH 7.48, $PaCO_2$ 50 mm Hg, and a decreased $H_2CO_3$. The nurse attempts to calm the patient verbally and by decreasing the stimuli, with no result. What intervention should the nurse expect to perform?**

a. immediately extubate the patient
b. increase the patient's tidal volume
c. give Benzodiazepines as ordered
d. decrease the patient's tidal volume

**95. A young African American man presents with a painful, persistent erection lasting 12 hours after sexual intercourse. He denies use of sildenafil (*Viagra*) or other drugs for erectile dysfunction. Which of the following diagnostic studies would be most appropriate initially?**

a. ultrasound of the penis
b. CT of the abdomen
c. sickle cell test
d. urinary catheterization for residual urine

**96. A 24-year-old woman complains of a mucopurulent vaginal discharge and painful urination for about 5 days. Her last sexual encounter was 10 days ago. Her menstrual periods are regular. She takes birth control pills and has never been pregnant. Which of the following tests are indicated?**

a. urine for culture and sensitivity and analysis
b. quick test of vaginal discharge for Chlamydia
c. vaginal swab on modified Thayer-Martin agar
d. all of the above

**97. In differentiating the HELLP syndrome from ordinary preeclampsia, which of following is true?**

a. HELLP occurs more commonly in primigravidas
b. hemolysis and thrombocytopenia are present in HELLP
c. blood pressure is normal in HELLP
d. proteinuria is absent in HELLP

**98. A 27-year-old woman presents with left-sided pelvic pain and vaginal spotting of several days duration. She has a history of pelvic inflammatory disease in her early 20s. She is now married and trying to have a child. She has not had menses for 8 weeks and a home pregnancy test is positive. Bimanual pelvic exam reveals a normal size uterus and tenderness and fullness in the left adnexal region. Her β-hCG level is markedly elevated. Which diagnosis and treatment are most likely?**

a. ectopic pregnancy and intramuscular methotrexate
b. ovarian cyst with surgical excision
c. normal 10- to 12-week pregnancy; no treatment
d. abruptio placenta; packed cell transfusion

**99. Which of the following is NOT associated with rhabdomyolysis?**

a. use of statin drugs
b. elevated creatine kinase (CK)
c. use of beta blockers
d. hyperkalemia

**100. Which of the following is NOT true in the management of a sexual assault victim?**

a. many victims do not wish to report a rape to law enforcement
b. many victims blame themselves or their actions for inviting sexual assault
c. the hospital has discretion not to report the incident if the patient does not wish to do so
d. chain of custody must be maintained by written record and time for all transfers of evidence

**101. Which of the following is effective in the management of posterior epistaxis?**

a. pinching the nose to stop the blood flow
b. topical vasoconstrictors such as phenylephrine
c. silver nitrate or electric cautery
d. insert a Merocel nasal sponge or Nasostat epistaxis nasal balloon

**102. A 2-year-old is brought to the emergency department with mild fever, persistent restlessness, crying, and pulling his left ear. He has had a cold for about a week. Examination of the ear reveals a distorted light reflex and slight bulging of the tympanic membrane. What is the proper diagnosis and treatment?**

a. otitis externa and antibiotics
b. otitis media and antibiotics
c. otitis media and myringotomy
d. acute labyrinthitis and antivertigo drug

**103. A 45-year-old man presents with severe pain after being struck in the face during an auto accident while he was driving. He also reports some numbness of the upper lip. His face is bruised and somewhat distorted and edematous with nasal and periorbital swelling and subconjunctival hemorrhages. A CT scan of the facial structures is obtained. What is the likely diagnosis?**

a. orbital blowout fracture
b. zygomatic fracture
c. mandibular fracture
d. middle third maxillary fracture (Le Fort II)

**104. A 65-year-old Asian man comes to the emergency department complaining of headache, severe pain in his right eye, and nausea of several hours' duration. The pupil is slightly dilated and fixed to light and the globe is very hard. He also notes halos of light and a diminished peripheral vision. Left eye exam is normal. What is the likely diagnosis?**

a. open-angle glaucoma
b. acute angle-closure glaucoma
c. occlusion of the central retinal artery
d. retinal detachment

**105. A 12-year-old presents with a Grade 3 hyphema, after being hit with a baseball at a game. Which of the following are true?**

a. patch and shield will not be necessary
b. Motrin should be given for pain
c. aminocaproic acid should be given to prevent secondary hemorrhage
d. system or topical antibiotics are a cornerstone of treatment for hyphema

**106. A patient has been diagnosed with temporomandibular disorder. The nurse should include all the following in the patient's discharge instructions EXCEPT**

a. use NSAIDS to relieve pain and inflammation.
b. use ice and warm compresses several times a day.
c. use a night mouthguard when able.
d. do not stretch or use jaw until pain subsides.

**107. A patient presents with a dental avulsion. The tooth came out 1 hour ago. All of the following correctly relate to reimplanting a tooth EXCEPT**

a. soak the tooth in Hank solution for 30 minutes.
b. only permanent teeth are reimplanted.
c. after reimplantation, apply splinting material over implanted teeth and 2 adjacent teeth on both sides.
d. you cannot reimplant a tooth that has been out for more than 30 minutes.

**108. A 45-year-old man presents with an eyelid laceration that is vertical and through the orbicularis oculi muscle. The patient is stable. The nurse should be prepared to**

a. Do wound irrigation with NS prior to suturing.
b. Assist the physician with suturing with a 6-0 or 7-0 coated nylon suture.
c. Apply ophthalmic topical antibiotic in place of a dressing.
d. Transfer the patient to a facility that has an ocular plastic surgeon.

**109. Which of the following is NOT associated with a vascular migraine headache?**

a. family history of migraine
b. diffuse pain associated with muscular contraction
c. unilateral, throbbing headache
d. prodromal aura

**110. A 75-year-old man has a history of several episodes of transient right-sided arm and hand weakness lasting an hour or two but with full recovery. He is diabetic and hypertensive and is taking medication for both conditions. This time the episode does not resolve and he is taken to the emergency department some 2 hours after the onset of symptoms. He is awake and able to answer questions and give a medical history. His chest is clear and no bruits are heard over the carotids. There is drift of the right arm on examination and his speech is slightly garbled. His blood pressure is 160/95 mm Hg and his pulse is irregular at 80 beats per minute. A CT of the brain reveals a small left-sided occlusion in a branch of the middle cerebral arterial circulation without hemorrhage. What should be the next step in his management?**

a. start nitroprusside to reduce his blood pressure to normal
b. begin fibrinolytic therapy with alteplase (Activase)
c. begin warfarin
d. neurosurgical consultation for carotid endarterectomy

**111. Which of the following best describes status epilepticus?**

a. a seizure that starts in one part of the body but there is no loss of consciousness
b. a seizure that starts in one part of the body and spreads to others with loss of consciousness
c. consecutive seizures without regaining consciousness
d. seizure associated with automatism such as lip smacking or facial grimacing

**112. Which of the following cranial nerves controls facial movements, lacrimation, taste, and salivation?**

a. III (oculomotor)
b. IV (trochlear)
c. VI (abducens)
d. VII (facial)

**113. A 24-year-old woman is brought to the emergency department, after an ATV accident. The patient's neurologic status, including the Glasgow Coma Scale, is quickly evaluated. Eye response is opening eyes in response to pain. Verbal response is incomprehensible sounds. Her motor response is withdrawal in response to pain. What is her score on the Glasgow Coma Scale?**

a. 7
b. 8
c. 9
d. 10

**114. A knowledge of the circulation to the brain is important in evaluating a patient with neurologic symptoms or signs. The anterior circulation to the brain is supplied by**

a. internal carotid arteries.
b. vertebral artery.
c. basilar artery.
d. external carotid arteries.

**115. A 28-year-old HIV-positive man arrives at the emergency department with a history of intermittent fevers, headache of several weeks, and increasing confusion. Which procedure is likely to give the most accurate diagnosis?**

a. CT of the brain
b. lumbar puncture (LP)
c. blood cultures
d. magnetic resonance angiography (MRA)

**116. A 25-year-old woman presents with tingling of the extremities for several weeks and weakness in both lower extremities so that walking is difficult. These symptoms started soon after a flu-like illness and have progressed to date. On exam there is bilateral weakness in the lower extremities with decreased deep tendon reflexes. What is the most likely diagnosis?**

a. cerebrovascular accident (CVA)
b. viral meningitis
c. Guillain-Barré syndrome
d. myasthenia gravis

**117. Early signs of increased intracranial pressure (ICP) include the following EXCEPT**

a. abnormal reflexes.
b. headache.
c. slurred speech.
d. sluggish pupillary light reflex.

**118. Which of the following is the most accepted method of reducing elevated ICP?**

a. hyperventilation
b. mannitol intravenous bolus
c. mannitol continuous intravenous drip
d. hypotonic saline

**119. A young man is hit on the head with a blunt object in a street mugging. He was briefly unconscious and has now arrived at the emergency department complaining of a severe headache and a dilated pupil on the side of the injury. As he is being examined, he becomes more comatose. He is stabilized and taken for a CT exam of the head and neck. What is the most likely finding?**

a. epidural hematoma
b. subdural hematoma
c. intraventricular hemorrhage
d. cervical spine injury

**120. A 17-year-old high school football player was knocked unconscious for about a minute after a vigorous tackle during a game. On recovering consciousness, he was somewhat confused and complained of mild nausea and headache. Both of these resolved within a few minutes. He was examined by the trainer and team doctor. They did not find any neurologic deficits. He wants to go back into the game. How should this player be managed?**

a. send him back into the game after a brief rest
b. bench him for the game but allow him to practice the following week
c. hospitalize him for observation and CT scanning
d. no athletics with continued observation for neurologic signs and gradual return to school and the team

**121. All of the following are appropriate measures in stabilizing a patient with a suspected cervical spine injury EXCEPT**

a. a four-person team is optimal.
b. strap the patient to the backboard at the shoulders, hips, and proximal to the knees.
c. do not attempt to remove a helmet.
d. a rigid cervical collar is applied by one person while the leader maintains in-line head position.

**122. A Hare traction splint is appropriate for which of the following fractures?**

a. mid-shaft fracture of the femur
b. distal fracture of the tibia
c. fracture of the fibula
d. fracture of the hip

**123. A farmer's arm is severed by a threshing machine at the mid-humerus. Which of the following would best preserve the amputated arm for possible reimplantation?**

a. no action; such arm injuries cannot be reimplanted
b. irrigate the arm with normal saline and pack directly in ice water
c. pack the arm directly in warm saline
d. moisten with saline, wrap in a plastic bag, and preserve on crushed ice and water

**124. In training a patient with a foot injury to use axillary crutches, which of the following is NOT true?**

a. tips of the crutches should be 6 inches to the side and 6 inches in front
b. move crutches and injured leg forward at the same time
c. each handpiece should be situated at the fingertips with the arms in full extension
d. each crutch should be 2 inches below the axilla with no weight-bearing

**125. A basketball player landed awkwardly after a rebound attempt and twisted his ankle. He is seen in the emergency department complaining of pain and tenderness of the ankle and there is swelling and discoloration around the joint. He claims he heard a snapping noise when landing and a small avulsion fracture is seen on x-ray. What is the most likely diagnosis?**

a. first-degree strain
b. second-degree strain
c. third-degree strain
d. first-degree sprain

**126. After an auto accident, x-rays of the patient's leg show a transverse fracture of the mid-femur with several bone fragments surrounding the fracture site. The skin of the leg is intact. This type fracture is called**

a. compression fracture.
b. comminuted fracture.
c. avulsion fracture.
d. open fracture.

**127. A professional soccer player hears a loud snap in his leg while dodging an opposition player during a game. This is followed by severe pain in the heel and posterior leg. He is unable to walk or use the injured foot. Thompson sign done in the emergency department is positive in the affected foot. What is the most likely diagnosis?**

a. tibial fracture
b. fibular fracture
c. ruptured Achilles tendon
d. calcaneus fracture

**128. Which of the following is true about shoulder dislocations?**

a. most are posterior dislocations
b. most are anterior dislocations
c. they are uncommon in children
d. they rarely recur

**129. Which of the following injuries is LEAST likely to occur from the initial blast or airwave from an explosion?**

a. spinal fracture
b. ruptured tympanic membrane
c. pneumothorax
d. perforated viscus

**130. Which of the following is NOT true of the compartment syndrome?**

a. occurs most often in the arm or leg
b. deep throbbing pain out of proportion to the original injury
c. pressure of 30 to 60 mm Hg requires fasciotomy
d. irreversible tissue damage does not occur until 24 to 48 hours of the injury

**131. A 12-year-old is brought to the emergency department with a history of a dog bite the previous day. The dog was the household pet and her family treated it with 70% alcohol and bandage. Today the laceration continues to hurt and appears somewhat swollen and red with a dark exudate. Which of the following would be inappropriate in the treatment of this wound?**

a. irrigation followed by suturing
b. debridement of nonviable tissue
c. amoxicillin/clavulanate (Augmentin) orally for 5 days
d. irrigation with povidone-iodine solution (Betadine)

**132. Which of the following dressings would be most appropriate for an exudative, probably infected wound?**

a. gauze
b. transparent film
c. absorption dressing
d. hydrogel

**133. Nurse-initiated analgesia protocols (NIAP) includes all of the following EXCEPT**

a. physician-ordered sedation.
b. nonopioid.
c. opioids.
d. nonpharmacologic intervention.

**134. Which of the following is true regarding pain management in infants and children?**

a. opioids are contraindicated
b. infants are less sensitive to pain than adults
c. pretreatment with local anesthetics prior to procedures, such as lumbar puncture or suturing of a laceration, is recommended
d. sedation before a painful procedure or imaging with midazolam or propofol is not recommended

**135. The Emergency Severity Index (ESI) triage system**

a. has 4 numerical categories (1 to 5) for patient evaluation.
b. patients are triaged by arrival time and expected resource consumption.
c. both A and B.
d. neither A nor B.

**136. Which of the following is NOT true regarding application of restraints to an aggressive patient?**

a. annual physical restraint training is mandatory
b. any patient death within 24 hours of being restrained must be reported
c. once restraints are applied, the patient's condition must be assessed and recorded every 4 hours
d. reasons for restraints must be documented and duration of application specified

**137. Disaster preparation and prevention measures include**

a. disaster-related supply inventory.
b. plan for housing, food, and water for staff.
c. establish communication protocol for notifying public health and law enforcement.
d. all of the above.

**138. Organ donation after cardiac death**

a. is against federal law.
b. requires the consent of the legal next of kin or an advanced directive from the donor.
c. end-of-life care and organ harvesting should be directed by the transplant surgeon.
d. Unlike brain death donations, notification of the local organ procurement organization (OPO) is unnecessary.

**139. Which of the following is NOT true for peripherally inserted central catheters (PICC) for venous access?**

a. requires a non-coring needle such as a Huber for administering fluids or withdrawing blood
b. may be single or multilumen
c. does not require surgery for removal
d. requires frequent heparin flushing and injection cap changes

**140. A chronically anemic patient is receiving a packed red blood cell (PRBC) transfusion. He suddenly develops fever and chills, tachypnea and dyspnea, and tightness in the chest. His urine flow is diminished and dark in color. What is the probable diagnosis and appropriate measures to take?**

a. air embolus; stop infusion, administer oxygen, and turn patient on left side
b. hemolytic transfusion reaction; stop transfusion, send the untransfused blood and a patient blood sample to the blood bank, monitor UOP and collect sample for the lab
c. pyrogenic transfusion reaction; stop transfusion and switch to leukocyte-poor PRBCs
d. circulatory overload; stop transfusion, consider diuretics

**141. The best method of limiting absorption in an adult who has ingested an unknown toxic substance is**

a. induced emesis with syrup of ipecac.
b. gastric lavage.
c. administer activated charcoal.
d. administer activated charcoal plus a cathartic.

**142. A young unidentified man is brought to the emergency department comatose with poor respiratory function. He has pinpoint pupils. Needle scarring is noted on his arms and legs and he appears underweight and malnourished. What are appropriate emergency care methods to treat him?**

a. endotracheal intubation with oxygen
b. activated charcoal and cathartic by nasogastric tube
c. naloxone 0.2 mg intravenously
d. all of the above

**143. An elderly patient has recently taken a large dose of imipramine (*Tofranil*) in an apparent suicide attempt. He is confused and disoriented, hypotensive, and tachycardic with flushed skin and wide pupils. While being brought in by paramedics, he has a seizure. An ECG shows a sinus tachycardia with a prolonged QRS complex and QT-interval and T-wave abnormalities. Which of the following pharmacologic agents would NOT be appropriate?**

a. lorazepam (Ativan)
b. sodium bicarbonate
c. phenytoin (Dilantin)
d. activated charcoal and sorbitol

**144. Heat stroke differs from heat exhaustion in that**

a. heat stroke occurs suddenly; heat exhaustion does not.
b. heat exhaustion occurs mostly in infants and elderly persons.
c. heat exhaustion has up to a 70% mortality rate.
d. heat exhaustion may be treated with ice water immersion.

**145. Which of the following statements is/are accurate regarding frostbite?**

a. Frostbite may be superficial, affecting the skin and subcutaneous tissue, or deep, affecting bone and tendons.
b. Frostbite-affected areas may become mottled with blistering.
c. both A and B.
d. neither A nor B.

**146. A mountain climber is rescued by helicopter several days after an incapacitating fall near the mountain top. His core body temperature in the emergency department is 78 °F (28.8 °C). Which of the following warming techniques would be most efficient?**

a. warmed humidified oxygen
b. warmed intravenous fluids
c. Bair Hugger warming blanket
d. continuous arteriovenous rewarming (CAVR)

**147. A 40-year-old man is rescued from a house fire and brought to the emergency department by paramedics. He is quite lethargic, breathing is rapid and shallow, and heart rate is regular but increased and blood pressure is moderately low. A carboxyhemoglobin (COHb) level is 40%. An endotracheal tube is placed. Which of the following would be the best treatment?**

a. hyperbaric oxygen at 3 atm for 46 minutes; repeat in 6 hours if full CNS activity not restored
b. hyperbaric oxygen at 6 atm for 1 hour; repeat in 4 hours if full CNS activity not restored
c. 100% oxygen until the COHb falls below 10%
d. 60% oxygen until the COHb falls below 10%

**148. A 30-year-old adult has extensive full thickness burns on the upper chest (neck to nipples) and the left anterior thigh and lower leg. There are no other injuries. By the rule of nines, how much of the total body surface area (TBSA) is involved and what should be the disposition of the patient?**

a. 12%; outpatient treatment
b. 20%; admit to community hospital
c. 27%; transfer to a burn center
d. 36%; transfer to a burn center

**149. Which of the following is NOT a feature of the shock syndrome?**

a. decreased antidiuretic hormone (ADH) release
b. increased epinephrine release
c. increased angiotensin II and aldosterone
d. increased glucose production

**150. Neurogenic shock may be caused by all of the following EXCEPT**

a. spinal cord injury.
b. blood loss.
c. excessive insulin with hypoglycemia.
d. brain injury.

**151. For patients with hemorrhagic shock due to trauma**

a. blood pressure should be brought to normal with fluids and banked blood.
b. mean arterial blood pressure (MAP) should be maintained at 40 mm Hg until bleeding controlled.
c. MAP should be maintained above 65 mm Hg at all times.
d. MAP should be maintained above 95 mm Hg.

**152. Which of the following is NOT recommended for routine hemodynamic monitoring of patients in shock?**

a. pulmonary artery catheter
b. central venous pressure
c. pulse oximetry
d. superior vena cava oxygen saturation ($ScvO_2$)

**153. When placing a tourniquet to control arterial bleeding from a lower leg wound**

a. it should be placed right over the wound.
b. it should be placed as distally as possible.
c. it should be placed distally but at least 5 cm proximal to the wound.
d. it should not be used.

**154. Acid-base balance in shock patients is characterized by**

a. respiratory acidosis followed by metabolic alkalosis.
b. respiratory alkalosis.
c. metabolic acidosis.
d. transient respiratory alkalosis followed by metabolic acidosis.

**155. Which of the following has NOT been shown to improve the survival of patients with septic shock?**

a. colloid rather than crystalloid therapy
b. antibiotic therapy within 1 hour of diagnosis
c. keeping the mean arterial pressure at 65 mm Hg or higher
d. administration of recombinant human activated protein C (rhAPC)

**156. The following instructions are appropriate for which type venous access?**

*Heparin 10 to 100 units/mL: use 1 to 2.5 mL after use and/or every 12 hours. After blood withdrawal or medication administration, flush with saline before heparin flush. No saline flush required before medication administration.*

a. tunneled catheter
b. Groshong catheter
c. implanted port
d. peripherally inserted central catheter (PICC)

**157. Which bone site is least desirable for intraosseous infusion in infants and young children?**

a. sternum
b. iliac crest
c. anterior tibia
d. distal femur

**158. A 60-year-old man with type 2 diabetes is taking metformin and a diuretic for hypertension. He ran out of metformin about a week ago and is waiting for his mail order to arrive. He has become lethargic and confused over the past few days with vague abdominal pain, polyuria, and polydipsia. He appears dehydrated. His blood glucose is 900 mg/dL, arterial pH is 7.35, and serum osmolality is 430 mOsm/L; serum ketones 1+ at 1:1 dilution. Serum lactate level is 1.5 mmol/L. What is the most likely diagnosis?**

a. lactic acidosis
b. diabetic ketoacidosis (DKA)
c. hyperosmolar hyperglycemia
d. none of the above

**159. A 40-year-old woman with a history of Graves' disease is brought to the emergency department with a fever of 104 °F, and she is disoriented and semi-comatose with a Glasgow score of 10. Her ECG shows atrial fibrillation with a ventricular rate of 130. Which of the following drugs should NOT be administered?**

a. beta-blocker
b. methimazole
c. iodide
d. epinephrine

**160. Which of the following coagulation factors is NOT vitamin K dependent?**

a. prothrombin (factor II)
b. prothrombin conversion accelerator (factor VII)
c. antihemophilic factor A (factor VIII)
d. antihemophilic factor B (factor IX)

**161. Which of the following is NOT a feature of the tumor lysis syndrome?**

a. occurs in malignancies with rapid cell lysis
b. hypokalemia
c. hypocalcemia
d. hyperuricemia

**162. All of the following are acute complications of sickle cell anemia EXCEPT**

a. priapism.
b. chest pain and bilateral pulmonary infiltrates.
c. bone, joint, and spine pain.
d. gastrointestinal bleeding.

**163. A cancer patient is seen in the emergency department with high fevers and malaise for 2 days. She received chemotherapy about 10 days ago. Her physical exam is not revealing but her temperature is 103 °F. A CBC shows a hemoglobin of 10 g/dL, WBC 4000 with 10% polys, 5% bands, 70% lymphs, 10% monos, and 5% other white or unidentified cells. Platelets are 60,000/mm$^3$. Which of the following is NOT immediately appropriate?**

a. blood cultures from different sites
b. electrolytes, liver and renal function tests
c. ask if she has been receiving granulocyte colony-stimulating factor (G-CSF)
d. white blood cell transfusion

**164. Which of the following devices is most likely to give accurate intracranial pressure (ICP) readings?**

a. intraventricular
b. subdural
c. epidural
d. intraparenchymal

**165. Members of a particular government office are exposed to anthrax spores when an envelope is opened. Terrorist activity is strongly suspected. Which of the following is true?**

a. inhalation anthrax is the most common form
b. human to human transfer does not occur
c. inhalation of live bacteria causes the disease
d. antibiotics are ineffective

**166. A patient presents with a history of nausea, vomiting, and diarrhea for several days after a Caribbean cruise. In the emergency department, she is weak, moderately hypotensive, and dehydrated. An ECG shows bradycardia, mild ST depression, and a U wave with some ventricular ectopic beats. What is the most likely electrolyte abnormality?**

a. hypomagnesemia
b. hyperkalemia
c. hypokalemia
d. hypocalcemia

**167. To check orthostatic vital signs, blood pressure and pulse rate should be measured after the patient is**

a. 1 minute supine, 1 minute sitting, and 1 minute standing.
b. 3 minutes supine, 1 minute sitting and/or standing.
c. 3 minutes prone and 3 minutes standing.
d. none of the above.

**168. A 7-year-old child is brought to the emergency department after multiple bee stings about 30 minutes previously. He complains of itching, swollen lips, and difficulty breathing. Wheezing and stridor are heard. In addition to giving epinephrine, treatment will include all of the following EXCEPT**

a. IV fluids.
b. intravenous corticosteroid.
c. intravenous antihistamine.
d. broad-spectrum antibiotic.

**169. A chronic renal failure patient is sent to the emergency department because his external arteriovenous fistula is not patent. A possible solution to the problem is**

a. infuse fibrinolytics.
b. surgically remove clot.
c. repair fistula; insert dual lumen subclavian catheter.
d. all of the above.

**170. Semen samples for DNA evidence in rape cases**

a. cannot be collected from clothing.
b. may be collected up to 5 to 7 days after the crime in adults.
c. may be collected up to 2 weeks after in children and adolescents.
d. may not be stored; must be given to the police directly after collection.

**171. Which of the following is true regarding informed consent?**

a. minors must always have parental consent
b. nurses should be certain the patient understands the risks, benefits, and alternatives to treatment explained by the physician
c. parents may refuse life- or limb-saving treatment for their child based on religious grounds
d. in an emergency when the patient is unable to give consent, only the doctor can decide whether to proceed

**172. The Emergency Medical Treatment and Active Labor Act (EMTALA) includes the following provisions EXCEPT**

a. participating hospitals have emergency departments and receive funding from Health and Human Services (HHS).
b. any patient who comes to the emergency department requesting examination or treatment must receive an appropriate medical screening exam to determine if an emergency situation exists.
c. to transfer an unstable patient, the receiving hospital must accept him or her and the transferring doctor must sign a form stating that the benefits of the transfer outweigh the risks.
d. verbal patient refusal of examination or treatment absolves the hospital from possible legal penalty.

**173. Clues to child abuse include the following EXCEPT**

a. multiple emergency department visits for trauma.
b. multiple fractures in various states of healing.
c. scattered scalding of the head, torso, or upper arms.
d. retinal hemorrhages.

**174. Regarding statutory disease and specific trauma reporting to health or law enforcement authorities, it is true that**

a. it is uniform in all states.
b. it does not include suicide, nonlethal gunshot wounds, or certain communicable diseases.
c. the nurse shares reporting responsibility with the physician.
d. the nurse cannot report an event or disease without physician permission.

**175. In clinical research**

a. a P value of 0.05 means there is a 95% indication the result is not due to chance.
b. a VII level of evidence is the best possible on a scale of I to VII.
c. a confidence interval of 95% indicates that 95 out of 100 subjects reacted favorably.
d. none of the above.

# Answer Key and Explanations for Test #1

**1. C**: A family member can register the patient into the system, blood tests must be done but can be done after the EKG, and, although nitroglycerin is an appropriate intervention for pain, the low blood pressure may need evaluation before choosing to give nitroglycerin. The appropriate intervention is to place the client on a cardiac monitor, give oxygen to decrease cardiac workload, and obtain an EKG to immediately evaluate the heart. The ED is a controlled setting where a physician should be readily available to look at the client, evaluate the cardiac monitor, and interpret the EKG to determine further interventions.

**2. B**: The primary assessment is done in a systematic way. Identifying a need and performing an intervention are essential before going on to the next step. Assess the airway and then intervene, assess the breathing and then intervene, and so on until you have performed a complete head-to-toe assessment to identify the immediate illness or injury and provided an immediate emergency intervention. Answer a is incorrect because it neglects the intervention aspect of the assessment. Answers c and d are incorrect because they are not aspects of the primary assessment.

**3. C**: The goal for any suspected acute coronary syndrome is a time frame of ED door to cath lab or to balloon those arteries to be 90 minutes or less. ST segment deviation in two or more leads usually indicates an acute ischemic event, which requires an angiogram or angioplasty. The nurse may give a report and may order labs and repeat EKGs, but the immediate intervention is to get the client ready for the cardiac cath lab. This may require calling in a cardiac team, undressing the patient completely, and removing jewelry. It may also include any other orders a cardiologist requires for the patient before the procedure. An ED nurse should be prepared for the possibility of this invasive procedure.

**4. B**: Troponin levels are elevated 3 to 12 hours after an acute onset of MI. Answer A is incorrect because troponin levels have taken the place of enzymes as cardiac biomarkers. However, troponin levels can also elevate in other disease states, including renal failure, making answer C incorrect. Answer D is incorrect because troponin levels actually help to distinguish between unstable angina (UA) and MI. Troponin levels do not elevate in UA.

**5. B**: A nonsmoking female may not have any risk factors, but a female complaining of chest pain should be evaluated for an acute cardiac problem, like any client with risk factors. Females present with different symptoms when having an MI and may not have classic symptoms, and they may also have an MI without having risk factors. The other answers are all risk factors for cardiac disease and acute cardiac syndromes.

**6. C**: A cardiac monitor, oxygen, and an IV should be in place for anyone complaining of chest pain and before administering nitroglycerin, especially in an elderly client, who may develop hypotension quickly. When a client does not respond to sublingual nitroglycerin, it indicates possible unstable angina and may require other interventions to relieve the pain.

**7. D**: The cause of heart failure in the pediatric population is most often a congenital heart defect. When triaging a pediatric patient, it is important to ask about congenital heart defects because often parents do not think to mention those defects that may have been surgically corrected, especially if the ED visit seems unrelated to a heart issue. The other choices may need further evaluation but may be unrelated to symptoms of heart failure.

**8. A**: The immediate intervention for a pediatric client is to maintain the airway and facilitate breathing. The other selections can be addressed after the airway and breathing are considered. Pediatric patients will compromise for a long time, and then they just stop. It is imperative to ensure that an adequate airway is in place and effective breathing is established before proceeding to the next step of the interventions.

**9. C**: Cardiomyopathy is a term that covers the diseases that have affected the myocardium and cause the symptoms listed. Dilated cardiomyopathy is the most common type of cardiomyopathies, giving symptoms of edema and heart failure. Other causes of cardiomyopathy may be toxins, acute diseases, infections, and chronic conditions. Often, diuretics are administered to reduce edema and ease breathing. The emergency treatment of a cardiomyopathy is the same as with any cardiac condition. It requires interventions to secure the airway and facilitate breathing and circulation before going on to any other intervention.

**10. B**: Dysrhythmia of any type causes a decrease in cardiac output. The emergent treatment intervention is directly related to the stability of the client's blood pressure, heart rate, and breathing ability. The other selections are incorrect.

**11. C**: With non-q-wave MIs, ST depression is usually visible on the ECG, but there are no abnormal q waves. With this type of MI, the coronary occlusion is usually incomplete (in about 70%) and many will re-infarct. Peak CK levels will usually be reached in about 12-13 hours.

**12. D**: The client should be kept on a nothing-by-mouth (NPO) status when presenting with chest pain until it is certain that surgery is not immediate. A low-salt diet would not be ordered from the ED. The other tasks should be performed as part of the preparation for any patient with chest pain.

**13. C**: Manifestations of a dissecting aortic aneurysm include a sharp/ripping posterior chest pain with a sudden onset, mediastinal widening on chest x-ray or other radiological studies, syncope, and impaired peripheral pulses or blood pressure differential.

**14. B**: In the ED, monitoring airway, blood pressure, and oximetry are essential for a client with chest pain. A meal is not usually offered, and an IV line should already be established as the protocol for a client with chest pain. Documentation of insurance is the responsibility of the admissions clerk and not an immediate concern for the ED nurse.

**15. A**: A client presenting with left-sided heart failure is often in sudden pulmonary edema with shortness of breath. Venous congestion is a symptom of right-sided failure, and heart failure can present with or without pain. There is always shortness of breath or pulmonary congestion when presenting to the ED, which require intervention.

**16. C**: The act of inspecting is looking for objective data about the client that reinforce the client's complaints. The style of clothing, how the family interacts, and asking questions may also be part of the complete assessment, but the objective data are collected by observation of the physical signs and symptoms the patient shows.

**17. B**: Hepatic congestion is a result of acute or chronic heart failure. The other answers can contribute to an abnormal liver study, but the abnormal results would be considered a result of heart failure without alcoholism, hepatitis, or medications.

**18. D**: Dopamine increases contractility and cardiac output, which improves oxygenation delivery to the tissues. It decreases cardiac workload. Dopamine is a vesicant. It is about 1/10 as likely as norepinephrine in producing tachycardias.

**19. D**: Clucks are not recognized cardiac sounds. Possible extracardiac sounds include pericardial friction rub, a venous hum, and clicks of valves.

**20. C**: An ineffective breathing pattern would be the appropriate nursing diagnosis from the information given. Shortness of breath is the only symptom revealed. After further work-up, choices a and b may also be appropriate for a nursing care plan, but ineffective breathing pattern applies to shortness of breath.

**21. B**: The client showing signs and symptoms of a decreased cardiac output (such as being pale and clammy with bradycardia) would require an intervention that may include IV access, medications, or even pacing the heart rhythm. The other choices appear to be within normal limits for the situations described.

**22. D**: A heart rate of 130 beats in an adult could be indicative of paroxysmal supraventricular tachycardia and will need investigation, possible and ECG. If SVT is identified the patient may need an intervention, including vagal maneuvers, medications, or cardioversion. Normal heart rates: Newborn: 120-160; 1-3 years: 80-140; 3-5 years: 80-120; 6- 12 years: 70-110; 13-17 years: 55-105; Adults: 60-100.

**23. B**: First-degree atrioventricular block is diagnosed partially by an EKG showing a PR interval of greater than 0.20 seconds. In a first-degree atrioventricular block, the P and QRS rhythms are normal, but there is a delay between the P and QRS.

**24. C**: A run of three or more PVCs is considered ventricular tachycardia and may need further intervention. One or two PVCs in a minute can be common and simply require further monitoring. A heart rate over 100 may be simple sinus tachycardia, or a variety of other arrhythmias, therefore more information would be required.

**25. A**: Immediately begin CPR upon noting VF until a defibrillator is available. Once the process of resuscitation is initiated and other team members arrive with a defibrillator and medications, then clients may require intubation, IV medications including epinephrine, and defibrillation. CPR is the immediate intervention before help arrives.

**26. C**: Intussusception is a mechanical bowel obstruction most often found in infants and small children. It occurs most often near the ileocecal valve or near a colon tumor or Meckel's diverticulum. It is life threatening and causes compromise to the vascular supply to the gut. It can lead to gangrene and sepsis and requires immediate surgery to correct.

**27. C**: The National Institute of Health lists the following as common causes of acute gastritis: NSAID and alcohol consumption and bacterial infections such as *H. pylori*. The ingestion of excessively seasoned or spicy foods is not a direct cause of acute gastritis.

**28. C**: *H. pylori* may be present in 30% to 50% of the population and may be a contributing factor in chronic gastritis. Chronic gastritis can lead to ulcers, hemorrhage, perforation, and obstruction.

**29. B**: It is important to remember that a low blood pressure in a child is a late sign of shock and is often not seen until the child has lost 25% of his or her body fluids. It is imperative than that fluid replacement is part of the treatment plan for a child who has sustained any trauma, particularly to the abdomen. A child has a higher percent of water compared to body weight and a higher metabolism, which makes maintaining the acid-base balance difficult. Abdominal trauma is common in children and should not be overlooked when a child complains of stomach pain. Symptoms may appear several hours after the trauma, especially if it is low impact or wasn't reported, as in an injury during gym class or a fall on the playground.

**30. B**: Pyloric stenosis is the most common obstruction during infancy. It is also known as infantile hypertrophic pyloric stenosis and is diagnosed most often between 3 and 12 weeks of life. Delay in treatment and diagnosis can lead to dehydration, shock, and mortality. The other choices are incorrect.

**31. A**: Airway and breathing followed by circulation are the most important initial interventions regardless of the type of traumatic injury sustained. Then IV, CT, and other interventions can be initiated, but the ABCs must be addressed first.

**32. B**: Pancreatitis may cause hypocalcemia due to the release of lipase into the soft tissue. This binds with the calcium and causes a decrease in ionized calcium during this process. The other conditions do not directly relate to hypocalcemia in this way.

**33. D**: The serum Lipase level is normally 30-210 U/L. An elevation greater than two times the normal value is suspect for pancreatitis and can be used along with other diagnostic tests and clinical information to make a diagnosis. An elevated WBC count would be indicative of infection or inflammation, but not specific to pancreatitis. The WBC count of 5.0 is normal.

**34. B**: It would be most appropriate to insert an NG tube and attach it to suction. The other choices would not be appropriate for a newly diagnosed client with an acute abdomen.

**35. C**: Narcotics may be used for pain with pancreatitis. Aspirin would not be appropriate due to the gastric irritability that it may cause. Compazine is an antiemetic and is not used for pain.

**36. C**: The pain of diverticulitis begins as a general discomfort localizing to the LLQ. The other choices are not correct.

**37. B**: For uncontrolled bleeding, intubation and a Sengstaken-Blakemore tube to create a mechanical tamponade are appropriate. The IV, nasogastric tube, and type and cross match should already have been done or will be done while preparing for this emergency procedure. The ABCs take first priority in the care of the patient, so protecting the airway and stopping the bleeding will be the immediate interventions for a client with uncontrolled bleeding.

**38. D**: While all of the bacteria listed can cause diarrhea, the history listed regarding the turtle, a known vector of *salmonella*, may indicate this being the offending bacteria. Symptoms usually appear 12-72 after infection. Neither *Campylobacter jejuni* nor *Clostridium difficile* usually present with bloody diarrhea. Though *Yersinia enterocolitica* may present with bloody diarrhea, it is usually green and foul.

**39. B**: Upper gastrointestinal bleeding is a very common emergency and usually requires prompt treatment. This man almost certainly has cirrhosis of the liver and is bleeding from esophageal varices. This is a complication of the portal hypertension that develops in these patients with ultimate rupture of the esophageal veins. Bleeding is often brisk and must be controlled, usually by endoscopic band ligation or sclerotherapy. Bleeding from a gastric or duodenal ulcer is usually less dramatic and results from mucosal damage caused by anti-inflammatory drugs or *Helicobacter pylori* that render the mucosa more sensitive to gastric acid. Erosion into a blood vessel causes the bleeding but it is most often slow and detected by stool occult blood tests. Gastric cancer may also be a source of upper gastrointestinal bleeding but it is rarely associated with vehement vomiting of blood and the bleeding may be intermittent. Angiodysplasia refers to dilated and tortuous blood vessels. Bleeding is from a lower gastrointestinal venous source, usually in the cecum or ascending colon.

**40. A**: This woman's signs and symptoms are typical of acute pancreatitis but other causes of acute and severe abdominal pain must be considered. The most likely cause of pancreatitis in this woman without a history of alcoholism would be gallstones, which can result in ductal hypertension and pancreatic enzyme activation. Serum amylase is nearly always markedly elevated as is the lipase, which tends to remain elevated longer. Ultrasound of the abdomen may disclose gallstones and CT reveals pancreatic edema. Acute cholecystitis is a possibility but can usually be ruled out by ultrasonography. Bowel obstruction would be uncommon with no history of prior abdominal surgery leading to adhesions, diminished bowel sounds, and no change in her usual bowel movement pattern. The pain pattern is unusual for appendicitis but anatomic position of the appendix may cause atypical pain. This possibility may usually be ruled out by abdominal CT.

**41. A**: Ureteral calculi are a quite common cause of acute emergency evaluation, usually causing flank pain with radiation to the back and/or groin. About 75% of these are calcium oxalate or phosphate; less common are struvite, uric acid, or cystine calculi. While KUB or ultrasound may show the stone, helical CT is now the preferred diagnostic method. Additional workup includes CBC, chemistry panel, urinalysis, and straining of urine to catch a passed stone for chemical analysis. Nursing attention should be directed to intravenous hydration with input and output recording and narcotic or narcotic plus NSAID (e.g., ketorolac) administration for pain. Some patients may be discharged with analgesics and instructions for hydration and calculus capture.

Testicular torsion is most common in adolescents and usually presents with testicular and groin pain with abdominal radiation; increasing pain by lifting the scrotum to the level of the pubic symphysis causes exacerbation of the pain (Prehn's sign). Cystitis may be infectious or drug-induced, but cystitis usually causes dysuria and pyuria and shows positive urine cultures.

**42. C**: This woman with lupus may already have compromised renal function and treatment with a nephrotoxic agent such as an aminoglycoside may provoke acute renal failure (ARF). In this situation, the urine output diminishes to less than 0.3 mL/kg/h for 24 hours; sometimes the patient is anuric. The serum creatinine rises sharply to 3 times normal or greater than 4 mg/dL, indicating a diminution in glomerular filtration by 75%. The ECG findings strongly suggest hyperkalemia, a characteristic accompaniment of ARF. Hyponatremia, hypocalcemia, and hyperphosphatemia, along with volume overload, are also characteristic fluid and electrolyte abnormalities of ARF. Immediate intravenous calcium will stabilize the myocardial cell membranes for a short time, decreasing the likelihood of arrhythmia, while glucose and insulin drive the potassium from the extracellular to the intracellular fluid with an onset of action of 5 to 30 minutes and lasting up to 4 hours. An oral or rectal cation exchange resin (*Kayexalate*) and emergency dialysis are longer term methods of hyperkalemic treatment.

**43. B**: Flank pain and bruising may indicate an injury to the kidney. It would be appropriate to get a urinalysis to test for blood and a CBC to determine how much bleeding may be taking place. The other choices may or may not be necessary for the complaint of flank pain.

**44. C**: It is always the best practice to undress a client, provide privacy with a gown and sheet, and directly observe for traumatic injury. Genitourinary injuries are very important and can be a source for bleeding, so this assessment should not be saved for last.

**45. B**: The symptoms described would indicate a kidney stone; flank pain is the hallmark for renal calculi. An MI is not a genitourinary emergency. Ovulation would cause pelvic pain. Torsion would not cause flank pain. Testicular torsion causes scrotal pain.

**46. C**: Acute renal failure is the result of an increase in nitrogenous waste products due to infection, sepsis, shock, or other significant medical emergencies.

**47. D**: A decrease in renal blood flow and ischemia are indications that acute renal failure can follow. Renal calculi, trauma, or a newly diagnosed mass can all lead to renal failure as can a cardiac arrest, sepsis, or any acute medical condition that caused a decrease in blood flow to vital organs for a short time.

**48. A**: The first year of life for boys is when they are the most susceptible to torsion of the testicle.

**49. C**: The incomplete ossification of the ribs allows the kidneys to be targets when a child suffers trauma. The kidney of a child is not three times larger than that of an adult but is larger in percentage of body size than that of an adult. The other choices are incorrect.

**50. B**: Dysuria is the most common symptom of a UTI. The fever may or may not be from the urinary tract, and cloudy urine may indicate dehydration. A fruity odor to the urine may indicate the presence of sugar or diabetes.

**51. D**: Preterm labor and preeclampsia are complications of pyelonephritis that may be serious to both mother and child.

**52. B**: After the ABCs are checked, the next things to be done with a client complaining of flank pain would be a urine test to detect blood, an IV for fluids, and medications for pain. The client would be kept NPO in case the flank pain is a kidney stone requiring surgery. Observation should be accompanied by offering pain control.

**53. D**: Testicular torsion needs surgical intervention within six hours to preserve the testicle. The other choices are not so critical.

**54. B**: The classic "duck waddle" indicates the client's attempt to avoid touching the scrotum while walking. This is a common indication of epididymitis. The other conditions would not cause this type of gait.

**55. D**: Abruptio placenta is the most critical condition and is the cause of 15% of fetal deaths. Mother and infant may suffer blood loss and shock.

**56. C**: Vaginal bleeding and uterine tenderness are the hallmark signs of abruptio placenta. Dark vaginal bleeding and uterine pain warrant an ultrasound, IV fluids, and an immediate Cesarean section (C-section).

**57. D**: The other choices may be appropriate at some point, but the initial and most important step in resuscitation is to establish an adequate airway.

**58. B**: A ruptured ectopic pregnancy may cause maternal death due to blood loss, shock, and subsequent cardiac arrest of the mother.

**59. C**: High blood pressure, proteinuria, and edema are the positive symptoms for preeclampsia and eclampsia.

**60. B**: Seizures and coma may be the result of eclampsia. The best prevention of this dangerous progression is the birth of the fetus through c-section.

**61. A**: The seriousness of hyperemesis gravidarum is related to weight loss, dehydration and low thiamine. Obesity, high potassium, overhydration, hyponatremia, edema, and low magnesium are not likely.

**62. B**: It is important to dry the infant under a heat source while assessing and establishing the airway. After establishing an airway, chest compressions are initiated. The other steps will be done after the airway is established.

**63. C**: A female with DUB who has required a D&C to stop the bleeding would return for a fever because of the risk of sepsis. The other choices are not correct or necessary instructions.

**64. D**: Bacterial vaginitis symptoms are thin white secretions with a foul fishy odor. Candida vaginitis symptoms include white curdy discharge without an odor. Trichomonas vaginitis displays with a green or grayish discharge that is frothy in appearance.

**65. C**: The most common pharmacologic therapies ordered for a female in the ED diagnosed with pelvic inflammatory disease (PID) would be analgesics for pain, and antibiotics to treat the infection.

**66. A**: A client presenting to the ED with an eating disorder is most likely to have dysrhythmias due to electrolyte imbalances, requiring interventions. The electrolyte imbalances depend on the patient's specific disorder, for instance, a patient who purges with bulimia nervosa versus a patient who abuses laxatives. Therefore, a full CBC should be obtained to assess and appropriately treat the underlying imbalances that may cause dysrhythmias.

**67. B**: Examples of organic psychoses include dementia, delirium and toxic drug-induced psychosis. Schizophrenia is a functional psychosis.

**68. A**: Suicidal behavior is best described as attempts to cause death by self-inflicted injury. This may be planned, or may be an impulsive decision. Attempts by someone other than one's self to cause death would be considered homicidal behavior.

**69. D**: Several major nursing and medical organizations now support the policy of allowing family members to witness procedures on and resuscitation of their child. This is thought of as an extension of family-centered care, which is desirable for pediatric emergencies. Team members should be made aware of this policy in advance in order to facilitate procedures and avoid any unpleasant confrontations that may emerge due to parenteral concern or stress. A nursing team member should be assigned to the family to explain the medical situation and reassure them, if possible. There should be a specific space assigned to the family members to observe the procedure without getting in the way of diagnostic, surgical, or resuscitative activity. If possible, parents should be allowed to touch the child if it does not impede medical procedures.

**70. C**: Clinical depression is a very common illness with a suicide risk of 5% to 12% for men and 10% to 25% for women. Suicide is most often seen in young adults (increasingly in teenagers) and elderly patients. The emergency nurse must maintain a high index of suspicion of depression because it may be masked by other factors: drug or alcohol abuse, self-mutilation, anger, and aggression. Brain imaging, electroencephalography, and blood testing may be required to rule out underlying metabolic or neurologic disease. While antidepressant drugs have played a major role in the treatment of this condition, they may take several weeks to show an effect and some patients do not appear to be helped at all. Careful examination for suicidal ideation is mandatory in these patients and psychiatric consultation and hospitalization may be required for those whose safety is in doubt.

**71. A**: This patient's history and symptoms strongly suggest a panic attack. This ailment frequently masquerades as an acute medical illness and is responsible for many emergency department visits. Careful questioning, examination, and appropriate laboratory analysis usually detects the condition. Some patients make multiple emergency department visits without significant findings. Typically, the pulse and respiratory rate are increased but blood pressure and temperature are normal. Because chest pain and dyspnea are two of the most common symptoms of panic attack, it is necessary to eliminate underlying disease with chest (or other) x-ray, ECG, and blood tests, including arterial blood gases, serum electrolytes, thyroid tests, glucose for possible hypoglycemia, and urine toxicology for stimulatory drugs, such as cocaine or amphetamines, that the patient may deny using. Once panic attack is diagnosed, intravenous benzodiazepines, such as lorazepam (*Ativan*), may be given. Reassurance of the patient is valuable. Referral to a professional mental health expert is also useful.

**72. D**: While this child may indeed have been a victim of a fall, the combination of comatose state, retinal hemorrhages, and a subdural hematoma indicate the possibility of the "shaken baby syndrome" in which violent shaking of the child leads to acceleration-deceleration injury to the brain. Coma, retinal hemorrhages, and subdural hematoma are common injuries. Child abuse is a major cause of infant morbidity and mortality and should be considered in cases in which a child has a history of frequent emergency department visits for trauma or scattered bruises and/or healed fractures that defy other explanation. Posterior or lateral rib fractures may be caused by overzealous squeezing of the infant and fractures of several bones in various stages of healing are particularly suspicious for child abuse. Localized burns without scatter or satellite burns, often attributed to spilled hot liquids, are also suspect. Even if there is only a remote possibility of abuse, most state laws require health care professionals to report the possibility to the appropriate social agency.

**73. C**: Domestic violence, nearly always perpetrated against women, is a major problem confronted by the emergency nurse. Screening for possible cases should include answers A, B and D. Interestingly, victims of intimate partner violence often present with a medical ailment, not trauma. These include back, abdominal, or pelvic pain, headaches, urinary infections, sexually transmitted disease, or symptoms consistent with posttraumatic stress disorder (PTSD). Sometimes evidence of old trauma such as healing fractures or cosmetically concealed bruises may point toward the presence of domestic violence. Many victims will deny it but sometimes compassionate questioning in a private setting will elicit a positive response. The nurse may then offer advice, refer to a social agency or shelter, or ask for a consultation by the hospital social worker.

**74. B**: The V/Q ratio is a measure of the volume of ventilation and pulmonary blood flow. A normal value is 0.8. Elevated V/Q values indicate dead space ventilation in which alveoli are ventilated but perfusion is impaired. Examples of causes of this are pulmonary embolus, hypotension, or low cardiac output as in cardiogenic shock. In each of these there is diminution of the pulmonary blood flow. A low V/Q ratio indicates shunting of the alveolar blood supply when the alveoli are perfused but not ventilated. Examples include pneumonia, atelectasis, acute respiratory distress syndrome, pulmonary hemorrhage, or pneumothorax. Other causes of impaired oxygenation are diffusion abnormalities, which block capillary-alveolar gas exchange as in pulmonary edema or pulmonary fibrosis; and poor oxygen-carrying capacity of the red blood cells as in sepsis, or carbon monoxide or cyanide poisoning.

**75. D**: Mechanical ventilation requires diligent observation of the patient and ventilator by the emergency nurse. Modern ventilators usually come with alarms that indicate high or low airway pressure. High pressure may be caused by endotracheal tube obstruction with sputum or kinks or inadvertent endobronchial displacement. The airway should be suctioned and tube placement checked. A chest x-ray is frequently helpful in determining the cause. Lung collapse, worsening of the underlying disease, and bronchospasms are also causes of elevated pressure. Leaks around the endotracheal tube cuffs will cause low airway pressure. Auto-positive end-expiratory pressure (auto-PEEP) is caused by premature inspiratory delivery before full expiration (as in asthma or COPD patients) and may lead to increased pressure and lung damage.

**76. D**: Establishing an adequate airway should always be the top priority and initial assessment of any adult, infant, or child with an emergency diagnosis. Once that airway has been established, administering oxygen would be the next step, either through mask, cannula, or ET/OT tube. Establishing the chief complaint/injury and conducting a complete head-to-toe assessment would occur once the airway has been established and the patient is stabilized enough for this information to be obtained.

**77. B**: ARDS is sudden, progressive, and severe, even leading to death. It can be caused by trauma or disease, and may result in lung scarring.

**78. C**: Decreasing respiratory effort and aspiration may be possible under the influence of large amounts of alcohol.

**79. C**: Survanta (surfactant) would be administered to this patient to improve the respiratory status of the lungs. Epinephrine, caffeine and vitamin K may also be given, but for different reasons than respiratory issues.

**80. D**: Nasal trumpet, endotracheal (ET) tube, and esophageal-tracheal Combitube are all appropriate ways to establish an initial airway for a nonresponsive client. A Replogle is not for breathing. Rather, it is used to drain saliva in infants with esophageal atresia, and is inserted into the nostril.

**81. D**: The spiral CT provides definitive diagnosis for a PE. V/Q scans and pulmonary angiograms can also confirm a diagnosis of a PE. D-dimers will be elevated with a PE but can also be elevated for other reasons, and are often elevated in renal patients on dialysis. Therefore, an elevated D-dimer would only indicate that a spiral CT is required for confirmation of a PE.

**82. D**: The child in status asthmaticus would need to be treated first as this patient has the most life-threatening airway emergency. The other patients are not displaying symptomatic respiratory distress, therefore can be treated medically before an alternate airway is considered.

**83. D**: Bronchiolitis affects children under the age of two and causes inflammatory obstruction of the airway. Asthma, bronchitis and pneumonia can affect patients of all ages.

**84. D**: Providing community education, identifying clients who are potential organ donors, and cooling a client following cardiac arrest are all of examples of patient care management tasks. Patient care management tasks can be done in both the micro (direct patient care) and macro (community education) levels.

**85. B**: A barking cough is the hallmark symptom of croup. A patient with croup may also have respiratory difficulties (shortness of breath, wheezing, labored breathing), a fever, congestion, or when progressed, drooling.

**86. C**: Although anxiety is a part of any respiratory illness because of the fear of not catching a breath, it is most often associated with hyperventilation.

**87. B**: A "body packer" is the street term for the person assigned to smuggle drugs by placing them into body cavities.

**88. C**: PCP is a hallucinogenic drug (schedule II) that, when use is stopped suddenly, can cause withdrawal symptoms that may require hospitalization. PCP causes rhabdomyolysis and renal failure, sometimes requiring dialysis as an intervention. PCP can also cause hypertension, tachycardia, and increased labored breathing.

**89. A**: Most chemicals that are "huffed" cannot be detected in normal urine and blood drug tests, so it is important for nurses to be able to identify signs of huffing. When a client presents with paint around the nose and mouth or an odor of solvent on the clothing and hair, it is suspicious for huffing an inhalant.

**90. B**: Shock is a response to an illness or injury where there is a decrease in tissue perfusion. While in septic and cardiogenic shock, cardiac output is decreased, but in distributive shock (including anaphylactic and neurogenic) there is initially an increased cardiac output.

**91. B**: Hypovolemia leads to decreased venous return, decreased cardiac output, diminished stroke volume and decreased central venous pressure. Increased cardiac output is the opposite of what happens with hypovolemia.

**92. D**: The ED is required by law to report abuse cases and must never keep abuse quiet. It is not a breach of confidentiality when reporting a case of suspected abuse. ED nurses are also involved in ethical decision making, evaluating a client's capacity to make decisions, and protecting patient confidentiality per HIPAA policy.

**93. C**: No drug has proved effective in the clinical management or prevention of ARDS. The following are therapies that are commonly used but per ARDS network there is insufficient evidence that they decrease mortality rates: corticosteroids (may increase mortality rates in some patient populations, though this is the most common given), nitrous oxide, inhaled surfactant, and anti-inflammatory medications. Treatment of the underlying condition is the only proven treatment, especially identifying and treating with appropriate antibiotics any infection, as sepsis is most common etiology for ARDS, but prophylactic antibiotics are not indicated. Conservative fluid management is indicated to reduce days on the ventilator, but does not reduce overall mortality. Pharmacologic preventive care: enoxaparin, sucralfate, and enteral nutrition support within 24 hours of ICU admission or intubation.

**94. C**: This patient is agitated and possibly paranoid following a cocaine overdose. The first action, attempting to calm the patient has failed, probably due to the patient's psychological state. The patient may be able to be extubated, but first giving the patient the benzodiazepines and then seeing if the patient were calmer would be the safer choice, as the patient may hyperventilate even without the ventilator depending upon the patient's psychological state. Giving the benzodiazepine would also help the patient relax and the heart rate decrease which would be safer for the patient as well. Changing the tidal volume would not be appropriate at this time.

**95. C**: Priapism, a prolonged and painful erection not associated with sexual desire, is an occasional reason for emergency evaluation. It is usually caused by obstruction to the venous drainage of the corpora cavernosae with accumulation of deoxygenated blood leading to swelling and pain. Urinary obstruction occurs in 50% of cases, which requires catheterization, but this is not necessarily helpful diagnostically. Ultrasound of the penis or CT of the abdomen or spine may reveal other disease but the initial test in an African American male should be for sickle cell anemia. This is a common cause of priapism because of the relative inability of the abnormal red blood cells to traverse small blood vessels, leading to obstruction and swelling. If positive, oxygen administration and even transfusion may help. Dorsal nerve block with lidocaine 1% (without epinephrine), systemic vasodilators, and needle aspiration of the corpora, followed by phenylephrine injection, are additional treatments.

**96. D**: Vaginal discharge and/or painful urination are a common female complaint, especially after recent sexual intercourse. While many such patients are seen in the gynecologist's office, the emergency department is often the medical facility of first and last resort for much of the population. The differential diagnosis includes urinary tract infection (cystitis), and vaginal infection with *Chlamydia, Gonococcus, Trichomonas, Gardnerella*, or *Mycoplasma.* While the character of the discharge may offer a clue (e.g., the greenish-yellow discharge of *Trichomonas* or the fishy–smelling, thin discharge associated with bacterial vaginosis), definite microbiological testing is required. In this patient urine tests for cystitis, most frequently caused by *E. coli*, and vaginal swab testing for *Chlamydia* and gonorrhea are indicated. Additional tests for pregnancy, HIV, HPV, and VDRL may be warranted in a female with a sexually transmitted disease.

**97. B**: The HELLP syndrome (hemolysis, elevated liver enzymes, and low platelets) is a severe form of preeclampsia in pregnant women and may be life-threatening to both mother and fetus. HELLP usually affects multigravida mothers while the usual form of preeclampsia is more common in primigravidas. It occurs in it up to 12% of women with preeclampsia-eclampsia. Respiratory distress, hypotension, and tachycardia may develop secondary to anemia and blood loss from coagulopathies. Numerous medical conditions must be ruled out and emergency cesarean section to save the fetus is often required. Delivery usually reverses the physiologic changes but not invariably, and rarely the syndrome develops postpartum. Blood pressure greater than 160/110 mm Hg, proteinuria greater than 5 g per 24 hours, pronounced edema including face and hands, persistent headaches, increased tendon reflexes, and liver symptoms including pain and abnormal liver function tests are additional features of the HELLP syndrome. The proteinuria and edema are considerably more prominent than that seen in usual preeclampsia.

**98. A**: This woman's symptoms and clinical finding are typical of an ectopic pregnancy. There is failure of endometrial implantation of the fertilized ovum, which instead begins development in an extrauterine site. The most common sites are the ampulla and isthmus of the fallopian tube, but ectopic pregnancies may be present in many other sites in the female reproductive system or even in the abdominal cavity. It often develops in patients with a history of pelvic infections and becomes symptomatic toward the end of the first trimester. Diagnosis is usually made by an elevated β-hCG level and pelvic ultrasound. Ovarian cysts may present with pain and abdominal swelling but β-hCG levels are not elevated and pelvic examination may reveal a cystic mass. Ultrasound is the usual confirmatory diagnostic method. The normal-sized uterus and ultrasonography rule out normal pregnancy or abruptio placenta (usually occurs in the third trimester). Methotrexate with follow-up β-hCG levels is a nonsurgical treatment for ectopic pregnancy but heavy bleeding or other evidence of rupture usually requires surgical intervention.

**99. C**: Rhabdomyolysis refers to skeletal muscle destruction accompanied by release of myoglobin into the circulation. It is seen in crush injuries, toxic ingestion, and burns. With the widespread use of statin drugs for hypercholesterolemia, this type of drug may currently be the most common cause. Kidney failure may result from diminished renal blood flow or tubular obstruction. Hyperkalemia and elevated CK are characteristic. Proteinuria and hematuria may be detected on urinalysis but because this is due to myoglobin, few red blood cells will be seen. Muscle aches and tenderness, often severe, are usual presenting symptoms. Treatment includes volume replacement, increasing urine flow with an osmotic diuretic such as mannitol, and alkalinization of the urine with sodium bicarbonate to prevent myoglobin precipitation in the urine. Beta blockers have not been known to cause rhabdomyolysis.

**100. C**: Nursing procedures for a sexual assault victim are complex and usually require special training to become a sexual assault nurse examiner (SANE) or sexual assault forensic examiner (SAFE). Providing psychological support and reassuring the victim that she is not responsible play a major role. Evidence collection must be done delicately and thoroughly and specimens (e.g., semen, blood, pubic hair, oral swabs) stored in paper bags or special containers (rape kits); avoid plastic bags because they may enhance bacterial or fungal contamination. Transfer of potential evidence must be recorded as to person and time; there are usually special forms for sexual assault cases that must be submitted along with potential evidence. While hospitals are nearly always required by law to report the incident and turn over the examination report and specimens to law enforcement, the patient may refuse to speak to authorities (around 40% demur according to a recent study).

**101. D**: Nosebleeds (epistaxis) are quite commonly seen in the emergency setting and are usually divided into anterior and posterior, depending on the anatomic site of the bleeding. Infection, trauma, foreign bodies, or coagulation deficiency may be the cause; however, the most common cause is nose picking. Anterior nosebleeds usually arise in the most vascular portion of the nasal mucosa (Kiesselbach plexus) and are usually acute. Nasal pinching and nose blowing followed by nasal speculum examination is the usual diagnostic procedure. If the bleeding is anterior, topical vasoconstrictors, nasal packing with petrolatum-iodoform gauze (or newer commercial products), or local cauterization with silver nitrate or electricity are appropriate treatments. For posterior nosebleeds, more common in elderly patients and usually more serious, a posterior nasal pack with a *Merocel* nasal sponge or *Nasostat* epistaxis balloon is appropriate. Sometimes surgical ligation of the bleeding vessel is required.

**102. B**: Ear infections may cause severe and persistent pain, especially in children in the 6-month to 3-year age group and are a frequent cause of emergency department visits. Loss or distortion of the light reflex and bulging of the tympanic membrane are cardinal signs of otitis media, usually caused by bacteria such as *Streptococcus influenza* or *Haemophilus influenza*. Sinusitis and purulent rhinitis may accompany the otitis. Antibiotics to cover these organisms, topical warmed otic analgesics, and antipyretics are the usual treatment modalities. Otitis externa or swimmer's ear also causes otalgia and frequently follows swimming in contaminated water or a foreign body in the ear. Keeping the ear dry and using otic analgesics and antibiotics are indicated. Ear plugs while swimming or ear drying agents after swimming or showering are the usual preventive measures. Myringotomy is a surgical procedure to keep the middle ear draining in chronic otitis media and hopefully prevent such complications as mastoiditis, meningitis, ruptured tympanic membrane, or permanent hearing loss. Labyrinthitis is an infection of the inner ear and usually causes severe vertigo, most commonly in adults.

**103. D**: Maxillary fractures are divided into three subtypes, lower third (Le Fort I), middle third (Le Fort II), and upper (Le Fort III). Plain radiographs with a Waters view or panoramic imaging have been used for diagnosis but CT has largely supplanted these techniques. This patient's symptoms and clinical findings are typical for a Le Fort II maxillary fracture. This fracture involves the central maxillary, nasal, and ethmoid bones, and nasal rhinorrhea suggests skull fracture with CSF leak. Orbital and zygomatic fractures often are found together after facial trauma. In zygomatic fractures, there is pain in the lateral cheek and an inability to close the mouth. There is swelling and crepitus over the zygomatic arch. Orbital blowout fractures cause a rise in orbital pressure, blowing out the weak orbital floor with prolapse of the orbital contents into the maxillary sinus. Periorbital edema, subluxation of the lens, dysconjugate gaze, and enophthalmos are some of the signs of an orbital blowout, often caused by a baseball or golf ball's impact on the orbit. Mandibular fractures may cause airway obstruction by forcing the tongue posteriorly. Malocclusion is a typical finding. Paresthesias of the lower lip, broken teeth, and sublingual hematoma are also observed in this type fracture.

**104. B**: Acute angle-closure glaucoma refers to blockage of the anterior chamber angle near the root of the iris. It is more common in Asian and Inuit patients. Acute blockage of the aqueous humor results in elevated intraocular pressures, and pressures above 60 mm Hg may cause damage to the eye structures and impair circulation to the retina. It is a significant cause of blindness worldwide. Treatment includes topical miotics and beta-blockers, carbonic anhydrase inhibitors, and immediate ophthalmologic consultation. Open-angle glaucoma occurs when there is impaired drainage of the aqueous humor from the anterior chamber with a resultant rise in intraocular pressure, although the drainage angle at Schlemm canal remains open. It is the second leading cause of blindness. Central retinal artery occlusion causes sudden painless blindness; the patient may give a history of transient attacks of amaurosis in the affected eye. Retinal detachment occurs when the retina tears and allows vitreous humor to separate the retina and choroid. The patient usually complains of flashing lights, floaters, or a "curtain effect" due to a diminution in the retinal light perception.

**105. C**: Hyphemia refers to bleeding in the anterior chamber of the eye. It is usually caused by blunt trauma, which leads to rupture of the blood vessels of the iris and bleeding into the clear aqueous humor. Clotting of the blood may occur, called "eight-ball hyphema." Pain, photophobia, and blurred vision are the usual symptoms. Hyphema is more easily detected in those with light-colored eyes than in those with darker hues. Rebleeding occurs in about 30% of patients up to 14 days after the original bleed. Limitation of activity, hospitalization, and bed rest are all treatments but there is controversy about which is the best. Children and African American patients are a highest risk for secondary hemorrhage so aminocaproic acid should be given. Patch and eye shield are commonly used. NSAIDs should be avoided to reduce rebleeding. Antibiotics are not needed for hyphema especially if caused by blunt trauma as in this case.

**106. D**: TMB is jaw pain caused by dysfunction of the temporomandibular joint (TMJ) and the supporting muscles and ligaments. It may be precipitated by injury, such as whiplash, or grinding or clenching of the teeth, stress, or arthritis. Treatment includes ice pack to jaw area for 10 minutes followed by jaw stretching exercises and warm compress for 5 minutes 3 to 4 times daily, avoidance of heavy chewing by eating soft foods and avoiding hard foods, such as raw carrots and nuts, NSAIDs to relieve pain and inflammation, night mouthguard, and referral for dental treatments to improve bite as necessary.

**107. D**: Dental avulsions are complete displacement of a tooth from its socket. The tooth may be reimplanted if done within 1 to 2 hours after displacement, although only permanent teeth are reimplanted, not primary. Teeth can be transported from accident site to the ED in Hank solution, saline, or milk. Cleanse tooth with sterile NS or Hank solution, handling only the crown and avoiding any disruption of fibers. If tooth has been dry for 20 to 60 minutes, soak tooth in Hank solution for 30 minutes before reimplantation. If tooth has been dry for more than 60 minutes, soak tooth in citric acid for 5 minutes, stannous fluoride 2% for 5 minutes, and doxycycline solution for 5 minutes prior to reimplantation. Remove clot in socket and gently irrigate with NS. Place tooth into socket firmly, cover with gauze, and have patient bite firmly on gauze until splinting can be applied. Apply splinting material and mold packing over implanted tooth and 2 adjacent teeth on both sides (encompasses 5 teeth).

**108. D**: Usually only superficial horizontal lacerations are sutured in the ED. As this is a vertical laceration through the muscle in a stable patient, they should be transferred, as serious injuries should be referred to ophthalmologists or ocular plastic surgeons. Treatment includes local anesthesia (supra- or infraorbital), wound irrigation with NS prior to suturing, suturing with 6-0 or 7-0 coated or plain nylon suture (to be removed in 3 to 5 days), using care to avoid suturing into globe, and ophthalmic topical antibiotic in place of dressing.

**109. B**: Headaches, especially migraines, are a very common complaint in emergency department patients. Tension headaches tend to be diffuse with skeletal muscular contraction of the head and neck and be associated with numerous underlying conditions. Vascular migraines are often unilateral with a severe throbbing quality but may become diffuse. About 12% of the US population has experienced migraines and 70% of those have a family history. Classic migraines (about 15%) are preceded by an aura, usually visual (scintillating scotomata, tunnel vision), but almost any neurologic dysfunction may occur (e.g., transient hemiparesis or paresthesias). Nausea, vomiting, and photophobia are common. Common migraines are not preceded by an aura and may be more diffuse. Migraines may be triggered by a variety of specific and nonspecific factors, including environmental (e.g., bright light, heat, sudden changes in barometric pressure), dietary (e.g., alcohol, certain cheeses, chocolate), stress, or cyclical estrogen levels. Those without a history of migraine may require CT or MRI scanning to exclude intracranial disorders, such as bleeding, stroke, or tumor.

**110. B**: This patient had several transient ischemic attacks prior to his clear-cut signs of a stroke, shown to be nonhemorrhagic in nature. Such strokes may be caused by local thrombosis, especially in arteriosclerotic vessels, or by emboli arising in the carotid artery (usually at the bifurcation of the internal and external vessels) or the heart, most often in atrial fibrillation patients with clots in the atrial appendage. Because this patient arrived in the emergency department within 3 hours from the onset of symptoms, the current recommendation is to begin fibrinolytic therapy with recombinant tissue plasminogen activator (r-TPA). Some recent studies indicate benefit from this therapy may be achieved up to 4.5 hours after the onset of symptoms. Blood pressure management in stroke patients is tricky. Most would agree with slow reduction if the value is greater than 220 systolic or 120 diastolic or the stroke is hemorrhagic in nature. For patients treated with a fibrinolytic agent, significantly elevated blood pressure should be lowered to prevent reperfusion problems. If noninvasive carotid scanning shows marked stenosis, neurosurgical consultation for endarterectomy or angioplasty with stent placement is reasonable. Subsequent warfarin treatment may be appropriate if atrial fibrillation is present.

**111. C**: Seizures are caused by abnormal neuronal function in the brain with excessive or over-synchronized neuron discharge. They are usually caused by some underlying anatomic (e.g., brain tumor) or metabolic (e.g., hypoglycemia, hyponatremia) abnormality. Partial seizures begin in a specific body part and are limited to one hemisphere of the brain. There may be loss of consciousness (complex seizure) or not (simple partial seizure). Seizures that begin in one area and progress to others in an orderly fashion are termed Jacksonian. Temporal lobe seizures are characterized by automatism and are often preceded by olfactory or auditory aura. Status epilepticus refers to a succession of tonic-clonic seizures without regaining consciousness in between or a single seizure that lasts more than 30 minutes and does not respond to conventional therapy. It is a medical emergency, and intravenous sedation, oxygen (with or without intubation), and anticonvulsant drugs are given. If these measures fail, anesthesia is sometimes employed. Naloxone, dextrose 50%, or thiamine may be given for suspected opioid overdose, hypoglycemia, and alcohol withdrawal (delirium tremens).

**112. D**: Cranial nerves originate in the brainstem and are subject to a variety of traumatic, infectious, degenerative, and metabolic abnormalities. They may be motor, sensory, or both. There are 12 pairs, numbered by Roman numerals and/or the anatomic name. The oculomotor nerve (III) innervates most of the extraocular eye muscles and also controls lid elevation and pupillary constriction as well as eye movements. The trochlear (IV) innervates the superior oblique muscle, responsible for downward inner gaze. The abducens (VI) innervates the lateral rectus muscle, responsible for lateral gaze. The facial nerve (VII) is responsible for facial movement such as eye closure or smiling as well as lacrimation, salivation, and taste. Damage to this nerve by infection, trauma, or idiopathic (often called Bell palsy) results in unilateral facial droop, inability to smile or whistle, and diminished eye closure and tear production. Most cases recover.

**113. B**: The Glasgow Coma Scale is a useful and rapid method of determining level of consciousness in comatose patients, regardless of the cause. The scale is divided into 3 major subgroups: eye opening, best motor response, and best verbal response with point scores for individual responses. This patients GCS score would be 8, using the below scale for calculation.

| | |
|---|---|
| Eye opening | 4: Spontaneous. |
| | 3: To verbal stimuli. |
| | 2: To pain (not of face). |
| | 1: No response. |
| Verbal | 5: Oriented. |
| | 4: Conversation confused, but can answer questions. |
| | 3: Uses inappropriate words. |
| | 2: Speech incomprehensible. |
| | 1: No response. |
| Motor | 6: Moves on command. |
| | 5: Moves purposefully respond pain. |
| | 4: Withdraws in response to pain. |
| | 3: Decorticate posturing (flexion) in response to pain. |
| | 2: Decerebrate posturing (extension) in response to pain. |
| | 1: No response. |

Injuries/conditions are classified according to the total score: 3-8 Coma; ≤ 8 Severe head injury; 9-12 Moderate head injury; 13-15 Mild head injury.

**114. A**: The anterior blood supply to the brain is derived from the internal carotid arteries, which split off from the common carotids at about the level of the jawbone. The carotid arteries then supply the posterior communicating artery to the circle of Willis and the anterior and middle cerebral arteries. This anterior circulation supplies most of the cerebral hemispheres, the basal ganglia, and the diencephalon. The posterior circulation is formed by the merger of the two vertebral arteries into the basilar, which then divides into the two posterior cerebral arteries. This posterior circulation supplies the occipital lobes, cerebellum, part of the temporal lobes, the spinal cord, and the brainstem. The anterior circulation supplies about 80% of the blood to the brain while the posterior supplies about 20%. Knowledge of the circulatory pathways assists in determining the location of a lesion. For example, an obstruction of the posterior circulation is likely to cause brainstem symptoms (nausea, vertigo and balance, respiratory or cardiac abnormalities), while anterior circulation obstruction is more likely to cause hemiparesis and abnormalities of speech.

**115. B**: Fever, headache, confusion, and neck stiffness are signs and symptoms of meningitis. This possibility must be addressed quickly, especially in an HIV-positive individual who is subject to numerous opportunistic infections. A lumbar puncture with culture, chemistry, and inspection of the cerebrospinal fluid (CSF) is most likely to rule in or rule out meningitis. Many neurologists would recommend doing a CT scan of the brain first to rule out brain abscess or other mass lesion that might cause herniation of the brain due to rapid decrease in the intracranial pressure. If this is the case, a neurosurgical consultation should be obtained to get CSF because an LP is contraindicated. Blood cultures may be valuable if sepsis accompanies the meningitis, and brain angiography (MRA or intravascular) may be helpful in distinguishing a mass lesion, but the diagnostic procedure of choice is examination of the CSF.

**116. C**: This woman presents with typical history and symptoms of Guillain-Barré syndrome, an idiopathic ascending paralysis, most often in the age range of 20 to 30 years. It frequently follows a respiratory or gastrointestinal infection, and decreased myelin is found at the spinal nerve roots and peripheral nerves. The paralysis may ascend to the diaphragm and intercostal muscles, requiring intubation and ventilatory support. There were many cases in the 1970s in those receiving influenza immunizations. The disorder is thought to have an autoimmune basis, and plasmapheresis with or without immunoglobulin administration may hasten recovery. It is a leading cause of nontraumatic paraplegia but the disease is relatively rare. Recovered patients may require considerable rehabilitation. Her symptoms and age are inconsistent with a stroke, although one may occur in young people because of an aneurysm rupture or bleeding from an arteriovenous malformation. Viral meningitis does not cause bilateral paraplegia but may be excluded by LP and CSF exam. Myasthenia gravis also occurs in young adults, mostly women, and usually presents with increased fatigue and ocular symptoms such as ptosis and diplopia and weakness in the jaw or facial muscles.

**117. A**: Increased ICP often follows a traumatic brain injury but may be present in other conditions such as a mass lesion in the brain. It is usually considered a medical emergency because elevated pressure may diminish cerebral blood supply and also predispose to herniation. Cerebral perfusion pressure is calculated by subtracting the ICP from the mean arterial pressure. A value of 50 mm Hg or greater is required for adequate delivery of oxygen and nutrients. As the ICP rises, there is cerebral vasodilation and increase in systolic pressure in order to compensate. Headache, slurred speech, and a sluggish pupillary light response are characteristic of early increased ICP. In addition, confusion and restlessness, nausea and vomiting, and impaired strength and sensation may occur. As the ICP continues to rise, there is continuing decline in the level of consciousness, diminished brainstem reflexes, motor posturing (flexion or extension), fixated pupil(s), projectile vomiting, and abnormal reflexes, such as the extensor plantar reflex (Babinski sign).

**118. B**: There are several ICP monitoring devices, including the intraventricular catheter, subarachnoid screw, epi-or subdural sensor and intraparenchymal insertion. The current indication for treatment is an ICP greater than 20 mm Hg for more than 5 minutes. Sedation with midazolam or lorazepam (*Ativan*) and, increasingly, propofol (*Diprivan*) is usually indicated. Bolus mannitol is a preferred treatment because of its osmotic and neuroprotective properties but continuous infusion may be harmful and is not recommended. Hypertonic (not hypotonic) saline 3% to 10% is being used more frequently, especially in children, because it has both osmotic effects and may increase mean arterial pressure (MAP). Hyperventilation, used for many years in the treatment of increased ICP, has now been demoted in priority because it may reduce cerebral blood flow without reducing ICP.

**119. A**: Direct trauma to the head is a frequent cause of brain hemorrhage with or without skull fracture. An epidural hematoma, bleeding between the skull and the dura mater, may be due to bleeding from the middle meningeal artery with a rapid hematoma formation. This is a true medical emergency because the morbidity and mortality rate is high, more than 50%. The brief lucid period followed by a comatose state is typical but does not always occur. Immediate surgical intervention is preferred for large hematomas while some smaller ones may be managed conservatively. Bleeding into the subdural space, between the dura and arachnoid meningeal layers, may be acute, subacute, or chronic. The bleeding is from ruptured bridging veins in the subdural space. While the acute form produces immediate neurologic signs, and often loss of consciousness, the subacute form (48 hours to 2 weeks postinjury) causes a slower progression of neurologic signs. Intraventricular hemorrhage is less common with acute trauma and is more likely to result from a ruptured aneurysm or arteriovenous malformation in a young person. Cervical spine injury must be ruled out in many cases of head trauma but does not cause cerebral bleeds.

**120. D**: This young man has sustained what used to be called a concussion but now the preferred terminology is mild traumatic brain injury (MTBI). This may be caused by a direct trauma to the head or an acceleration-deceleration injury. It usually causes a brief period of unconsciousness followed by a variety of physical, cognitive, or emotional symptoms, or sleep disturbance. Most of these patients do not need hospitalization but do require observation for persistent or new neurologic signs and symptoms. No participation in athletics is permitted until all these disappear. Current thinking is that there is some neurochemical and axonal damage that leads to the postconcussive syndrome. Most authorities recommend a period of brain rest after MTBI with a gradual return to work or school and especially athletics.

**121. C**: Stabilization of a patient with suspected trauma to the cervical spine is a very common emergency requirement after falls and motor vehicle accidents. The ideal team consists of four persons. A leader maintains the head and neck in-line by use of fingers under the mandible. Gross neurologic assessment can be obtained by asking the patient, if alert, to wiggle his fingers and toes and to respond to light touch on arms and legs. One assistant then applies a rigid cervical collar of the correct size to the neck of the patient. The patient is then straightened and rolled onto a rigid backboard as a unit by two assistants on one side of the patient. The patient is then strapped to the backboard at the shoulders, hips, and proximal to the knees. His head should be stabilized further with head blocks or towel rolls. Many active sports (e.g., bicycling, in-line skating, hockey, football) require helmets that must be removed to ensure stability of the cervical spine. This should be done by two people with one maintaining in-line stability and the other removing the helmet.

**122. A**: Extremity fractures are among the most common injuries seen in emergency departments. Immobilization is mandatory for most extremity, hand, or foot fractures, but bleeding and neurovascular compromise should be assessed before applying the splint. Open fractures with bone protrusion or bleeding should be initially irrigated with normal saline and covered with a sterile dressing before immobilization. Pressure should be used for bleeding; tourniquets should only be used as a last measure. The Hare splint is one of several types of traction splints but is appropriate only for fractures of the mid-shaft of the femur or proximal tibia. It is often applied by paramedics before transport to the hospital. After immobilization, there should be another check for neurovascular integrity and the extremity should be raised. Local swelling may be treated with ice packs.

**123. D**: Traumatic amputations usually occur in workers using farm or industrial machinery or in motor vehicle accidents. Many factors influence the success of reimplantation, including the nature of the amputation (a sharp cut has a better prognosis than crush injuries), the availability of a transplant team, age, and time and method of preservation of the amputated part. The optimal method of preservation is to irrigate the amputated part with cold saline, wrap in saline moistened gauze, and seal in a plastic bag. The bag is then placed on water and crushed ice and delivered to the hospital as soon as possible. Muscle can remain viable for up to 12 hours, and bone, tendon, and skin up to 24 hours if kept cold. Under warm conditions, the viability of the part is considerably reduced. Packing the part directly in ice water or ice may cause tissue damage because of freezing of cells or osmotic depletion of intracellular contents.

**124. C**: Training patients with foot or leg injuries to use axillary crutches properly is a duty that frequently falls to the emergency nurse. In fitting the crutches to the patient, each crutch should be about 2 inches (2 to 3 fingerbreadths) below the axilla with no weight-bearing on the crutch. Each handpiece should be placed so that the patient's elbow is at a 30-degree angle, usually in line with the wrist. In walking with the crutches, the tips should be placed about 6 inches in front and 6 inches to the side. In tall persons, the crutch tips may be placed up to 12 inches to the side. Standing with the weight on the good foot, the crutches and the injured foot should move forward. Then, while bearing weight on the palms of the hands, the good foot moves forward.

**125. C**: A strain is a weakening or tear in the muscle where it attaches to the tendon. While it may occur with many different traumas to the joint, athletic injuries are perhaps the most common. A third-degree strain causes complete disruption of the muscle or tendon. A snapping noise at the time of injury and an avulsion fracture may be seen on x-ray. Acute treatment for this and lesser strains is compression bandage or splint, cold packs, analgesia, and no weight-bearing for 48 or more hours. First- and second-degree strains also present with pain and minor swelling but symptoms are less severe and no fracture is seen on x-ray. Sprains occur when a joint exceeds its normal range of motion and ligaments are damaged. A first-degree sprain causes pain and swelling around the joint, usually ankle or knee, but is less severe than the symptoms and signs this patient displays. MRI is probably the best diagnostic method for distinguishing sprains from strains.

**126. B**: A fracture is a break or disruption in a bone, generally divided into closed (no break in the skin) and open (protrusion of the bone through the skin). Fractures may take different anatomic patterns, depending on the bone location, the nature of the trauma and the bone density (may be diminished with osteoporosis). Compression fractures are most common in the spine in which a fracture of one or more vertebral bodies leads to a collapse of the spine at that location. An avulsion fracture reflects a forceful contraction of muscle mass, which pulls a bone fragment to break away at the tendon's insertion site. This type of fracture is often seen with severe joint strains. This patient has a comminuted fracture in which the trauma causes more than two separated portions of the bone. Often, several small bony fragments are seen at the site of the break.

**127. C**: Rupture of the Achilles tendon is a common athletic injury, often caused by stepping off abruptly on the forefoot with the knee in full extension. An audible snap or pop is often heard with immediate heel pain radiating to the calf. The patient is unable to walk on the leg and may have a foot-ankle deformity with swelling. Thompson sign, a diagnostic maneuver, will be positive if there is a complete rupture. The patient lies supine on an examining table with both feet extending over the edge. Squeezing the calf results normally in plantar motion; with an Achilles tendon rupture, there is little if any foot motion. Tibial or fibular fractures are not uncommon and usually occur with direct trauma or excessive rotational force. They may be open or closed and cause leg swelling, pain and point tenderness, deformity, and sometimes crepitus over the involved bone. Fractures of the calcaneus occur most often in falls with the person landing on his feet. There is pain in the heel along with swelling and point tenderness.

**128. B**: Shoulder dislocations are most common in children and athletes; 55% to 60% are recurrent. The typical athletic dislocation occurs when the extended arm is abducted and externally rotated. The head of the humerus is pushed in front of the shoulder joint by the force, called an anterior dislocation, which is most common. Less common are posterior dislocations. These may occur during a seizure when the patient falls with the arm abducted and internally rotated. In all cases in adults, there is pain in the shoulder, deformity, and inability to move the arm. Management requires checking of neurovascular elements in the arm and radiographs, followed by reduction and a postreduction radiograph to check for the correct humeral positioning. The shoulder is then immobilized with a sling and swath or a shoulder immobilizer.

**129. A**: Most explosions involve a rapid release of gas that displaces an equal volume of air that travels after the blast wave. This wave is particularly strong and does the most damage to hollow organs, such as the lungs, ears, gastrointestinal tract. Concussions are common because of the pressure wave generated by the blast.

Secondary causes of injury are related to missiles released by the explosion: fragments of shell casing or metal objects inserted into a bomb, such as nails or ball bearings. Tertiary injuries are caused by a rapid displacement of the exposed individual, which causes impact with the ground or adjacent structures. These injuries are similar to those sustained in a motor vehicle accident when the victim is thrown clear and hits the ground. In addition, burns and inhalation of noxious fumes are commonly seen in blast victims.

**130. D**: The compartment syndrome results from compression of the muscular compartment by swelling or compression-restriction of the extremity after an injury. The forearm and leg are the most common sites. Pain out of proportion to the injury is common despite strong analgesics. Prolonged external pressure, frostbite or snakebite may also cause the compartment syndrome. Impaired mobility of digits, paresthesias, coolness over the area, and pallor may be seen. Pulses may be compromised but occasionally a palpable pulse is present distal to the affected area. Rapid diagnosis is mandatory because impairment of the microcirculation in the area may lead to irreversible tissue damage within 4 to 6 hours. Compartment pressure may be determined with a syringe, catheter, or special monitoring device. Pressure above 30 to 60 mm Hg is usually an indication for a fasciotomy.

**131. A**: Dog bites are extraordinarily common, although there appears to be less risk of infection than with human or cat bites. In general, wounds that occur more than 12 hours before treatment, as in this case, should be irrigated but not sutured. Although antibiotics are not always required for simple dog bites, the delay in treatment and the appearance of the wound strongly suggest infection and places the wound at higher risk. Many different antibiotics may suffice but amoxicillin/clavulanate or clindamycin plus trimethoprim/sulfamethoxazole provides good coverage for those who are penicillin allergic. Irrigation under pressure using a syringe or a commercially available pressure device is ideal. Tetanus status should be checked but because the dog is a house pet and under observation (10 days recommended), there is no need to begin antirabies intervention unless the dog shows clear signs of the disorder. If so, the animal should be euthanized and laboratory testing for the virus done.

**132. C**: Choosing the correct dressing for wound management, especially if secondary or tertiary close is employed, is important to accelerate closure and enhance healing. Gauze can absorb exudate and support debridement if applied and kept moist. However, for wounds with considerable exudate, it is not the first choice. Transparent film permits exchange of oxygen from the environment to the wound but absorbs poorly and would not be the best choice for this type of wound. Hydrogel is useful after debridement of a wound because it maintains moisture; however, it is a poor absorber of exudate and is most useful for deep or necrotic wounds. It often requires a secondary dressing. An absorption dressing would be the best choice for this wound. It can absorb large amounts of exudate, support debridement, maintain moisture, and obliterate dead space in the wound. It is ideal for infected wounds.

**133. A**: NIAP is a relatively new phenomenon pioneered in Britain and Australia and developing widespread acceptance. It refers to the administration of various analgesic measures, both pharmacologic and nonpharmacologic, by the emergency department nurse prior to physician evaluation. Depending on the particular protocol, the nurse may give patients pain relief that includes physical methods (ice/heat, positioning, and distraction); nonopioid drugs such as aspirin, acetaminophen, or NSAIDs; or opioids, usually oral combinations such as oxycodone or hydrocodone with acetaminophen. Some research protocols have even allowed intravenous morphine to be given by the nurse under specific clinical situations. NIAP has been propelled by busy waiting rooms with many pain patients waiting lengthy periods for physician evaluation. Some potential hazards of NIAP are safety issues, nurse reluctance to use or follow the protocol, patients that leave before being seen, and drug-seeking patients.

**134. C**: Pain management in infants and children has been controversial in the past but several myths have been debunked, especially that infants are less sensitive to pain because their nervous system has not fully developed, and that opioids, both oral and parenteral, are contraindicated in very young children because they do not metabolize these drugs quickly. In fact, opioid drugs may be used efficaciously at the correct pediatric doses. Analgesia and sedation prior to painful or uncomfortable diagnostic or therapeutic procedures, such as

LP, suturing lacerations, x-ray, or CT scanning are recommended. Local vapocoolants given before venipunctures or immunization are helpful, as are sucrose drops, swaddling, maternal breastfeeding, and touching the infant. The Faces pain scale for verbal patients and the Faces, Legs, Activity, Cry, Consolability (FLACC) scale for nonverbal patients are useful adjuncts in assessing the presence and severity of pain.

**135. D**: The job of triage nurse in the emergency department requires a lot of clinical knowledge and the ability to deal with stressful situations without abandoning professional standards. Because of increasingly crowded emergency departments and longer patient waiting times, the position is crucial to the smooth operation of the facility. While triage systems vary, most require an assessment of acuity (not arrival time): emergent defined as severe and life-threatening; urgent requiring care as soon as possible; and nonurgent in which routine care is needed and physician evaluation is not required immediately. One new system, the ESI, developed by emergency physicians and nurses, takes both acuity and available resources into account to sort patients into 5 possible categories: 1) requires life-saving intervention immediately; 2) high risk, confusion or lethargy, and severe pain or distress; 3) age-specific blood pressure, respiratory rate at critical levels, and oxygen saturation less than 92% are not present; 4) one resource needed; 5) no resource needed.

**136. C**: The rules regarding use of patient restraints have evolved over the past few years. Nurses and other hospital employees with patient care responsibilities must undergo annual training in their use and under what circumstances they may be applied. In general, the confused and uncooperative or aggressive patient who does not conform to treatment or is a threat to himself or herself or the medical personnel is a possible candidate. Every effort should be made to calm the patient with other methods (conversation, intervention of family members, pharmacologic agents such as olanzapine or haloperidol) before physical restraint is applied. The indication for and duration of restraint must be documented in the patient's record. Once they are applied, the patient should be checked every 15 minutes to 2 hours (depending on hospital/unit policy) and observations recorded. Any death within 24 hours of being restrained must be reported to the Centers for Medicare and Medicaid Services (CMS).

**137. D**: Disaster planning for multiple patients with a variety of injuries is now mandated by federal law and administered by Department of Homeland Security guidelines. These include algorithms for prevention, protection, response, and recovery for both personal and professional duties. It is critical in preparation for any disaster and a large influx of injured or infected patients to ensure adequate disaster-related supplies related to specific types of calamity: fire, flood, earthquake, epidemic, and terrorist attack. Often overlooked are measures to keep the professional staff supplied with places to rest, and food and water, especially in situations where travel or time is limited. Notification protocols for health agencies, law enforcement, hazardous materials teams, EMS, and 911 responders should be in place. Regular disaster drills have become standard practice for emergency and hospital personnel.

**138. B**: Because of the acute shortage and high demand for organ transplantation, organs from cardiac death patients (declaration of death is based on cessation of cardiopulmonary activity) have become quite common. Like patients with brain death, organ donation from cardiac death patients is allowed by federal law but requires the written consent of the legal next of kin. In some states, advanced permission is recorded on driver's licenses. The local OPO must be notified and the medical examiner's approval may be required by state law. Hastening death in moribund patients is allowed after suitability of the donor and legal consent has been established; this may be done by slow termination of life support. Lethal doses of pharmacologic agents are forbidden. The transplantation team must not participate in the end-of-life care of the donor but the potential donor may be taken to a surgical suite in preparation for the organ removal.

**139. A**: Central venous access is often required for emergency patients, to replace fluid and electrolytes, for blood product transfusions and blood sample collection, and to monitor hemodynamics (central venous pressure). While arm veins may be used to thread the catheter into the superior vena cava, larger veins such as the subclavian, jugular, or femoral are often preferred for reasons of speed and stability. These catheters may be single or multilumen (e.g., to draw blood from one channel and administer drugs via another). One advantage is that surgery is unnecessary for removal but they do require frequent heparin flushing and injection cap replacement. They do not require a non-coring needle like that used for totally implanted venous access devices such as a *Port-A-Cath* or *LifePort*.

**140. B**: Transfusion reactions may be of several types and some of the symptoms may overlap. In nearly every case, the transfusion should be stopped immediately and the line kept open with normal saline or other maintenance fluid. This patient's symptoms and signs strongly suggest a hemolytic transfusion reaction due to ABO incompatibility. Type-specific blood that has been cross-matched is standard for blood and packed cell transfusions, but type O Rh negative (females and males) or type O Rh positive (males) may be given in severe emergencies. Hemolytic transfusion reactions are often severe and may be life-threatening so immediate supportive therapy is required. Pyrogenic reactions are mostly due to recipient antibodies to donor leukocytes and leukocyte-poor blood product is preferred. Air embolus is usually due to catheter manipulation (often by patient) or improper infusion technique. Circulatory overload, by overzealous or too-rapid transfusion, may produce symptoms of pulmonary edema; give diuretic and other appropriate treatment for this immediately.

**141. D**: One method of reducing absorption of an orally ingested toxic substance is by gastric decontamination. This is appropriate in cases of an unknown substance and even with known drugs or toxins that are not corrosive and for which an antidote is available. Syrup of ipecac has been used for many years to induce emesis and reduce upper gastrointestinal concentration of the toxic substance. It is rarely used now and is contraindicated by many authorities because it may cause numerous complications and no studies have shown that it actually improves clinical outcomes. Gastric lavage is also a traditional method that is used less frequently now; its use is beneficial mostly for large ingestions within the first 60 minutes. Activated charcoal is the preferred substance to administer; it absorbs most poisons (except alcohols or heavy metals) and should not be used for corrosive alkali or acid substances. Because activated charcoal is constipating, mixing a cathartic such as sorbitol or magnesium citrate with activated charcoal will enhance elimination of the poison.

**142. D**: Opioid overdoses, both oral and parenteral, are among the most common problems seen in emergency departments. This patient has typical findings of chronic opioid abuse. As with most emergency department patients, the ABC of emergency patient care is the primary concern; airway maintenance is critical because respiratory depression is the main deleterious effect of these drugs. Activated charcoal is effective in absorbing opioids and should be used with a cathartic after the airway is secure to overcome the constipating effect of the opioid. Many addicts use both oral and intravenous drugs. Naloxone is an opiate antagonist that acts on the brain to reduce respiratory depression and improve the level of consciousness. Repeat or continuous doses may be needed because the drug has a short half-life. A toxicological screen for the opiate and the frequently observed multi-drug abuse should be done but serum levels are not often helpful because of the large variety of opioid drugs with varying half-lives. Clinical response is the best indicator of effective therapy.

**143. C**: Overdose of tricyclic antidepressants, often by elderly patients with suicidal intent, is less common now since the advent of SSRI drugs for depression but is still a fairly frequent medical emergency. More common is CNS dysfunction ranging from disorientation and confusion to seizures and frank coma; anticholinergic effects including flushed skin, dry mucous membranes, and mydriasis; and cardiac effects including conduction abnormalities and ventricular tachycardia. Phenytoin is contraindicated for seizures in these patients because it has sodium channel blocking activity and may worsen arrhythmias. The drugs are very well absorbed by activated charcoal; the combination of activated charcoal with sorbitol to overcome the anticholinergics effects on the bowel is useful. Sodium bicarbonate raises the blood pH and lowers the free drug concentration, improving some of the ECG abnormalities.

**144. B**: Heat exhaustion occurs mainly in young children and elderly persons, usually because they are unable to replace fluid and electrolyte loss adequately. It often occurs suddenly and is characterized by thirst, malaise, muscle cramping, nausea, and vomiting. If untreated, it may cause hypotension, mild to severe temperature elevations, syncope, and possible progression to heat stroke. Diaphoresis may or may not be present. Treatment is based on removal to a cooler environment, replacement of fluid and electrolyte losses (oral or intravenous), and placement of moist clothing on patient to enhance perspiration. Heat stroke occurs when the physiologic cooling mechanisms become impaired and it is a medical emergency. It occurs in classic form in which the individual is exposed to prolonged elevated environmental temperatures, and in exertional form, mostly seen in athletes or military personnel. Core temperatures greater than 104 °F are found but these patients are only modestly fluid depleted. Ice packs may be used; total immersion in ice water is controversial and may cause shivering, which raises the body temperature.

**145. C**: Frostbite is a common medical emergency and its seriousness depends on exposure time and temperature, protective clothing, wind chill, wet or dry body parts, and contact with metal. Superficial frostbite affects skin and subcutaneous tissue and resembles a superficial burn. It mostly occurs on fingertips and toes, ears, nose, and cheeks. The area affected becomes extremely sensitive to further cold or heat exposure and becomes mottled with blisters, which form within a few hours. Basic treatment is application with warm soaks (104 °F to 110 °F) and extremity elevation. Deep frostbite occurs with low limb temperature and affects bone, muscle, and tendons. The patient senses a burning sensation followed by warmth and numbness. Edema, blistering, and gray-black mottling leading to necrotic gangrene may occur. Rapid rewarming of the tissue is the treatment of choice. This may be quite painful and potent analgesics may be required.

**146. D**: There are numerous techniques for rewarming body hypothermia. Treatment choice is largely dependent on core body temperature and may be active or passive. For mild hypothermia (93.2 °F to 98.6 °F), removing wet clothing, warm environment, and blankets may be satisfactory; warmed humidified oxygen and warmed glucose-containing fluids are an active option. For moderate hypothermia (86 °F to 93.2 °F), heating blankets (*Bair Hugger* therapy), radiant heating lamps, and hot water bottles may be used in addition to the active methods. Numerous other methods are available, such as peritoneal lavage, gastrointestinal rewarming by irrigation, hemodialysis, and even cardiopulmonary bypass. For severe hypothermia (below 78.8 °F), as in the case above, the CAVR method is perhaps the most efficient. A catheter in the femoral artery delivers blood to a countercurrent extracorporeal rewarming chamber and the blood is then returned to the venous cordis. The patient's own heart drives the system as there is no external pump as in a heart-lung machine. Hypotension and ventricular arrhythmias are complications of extreme hypothermia.

**147. A**: Carbon monoxide poisoning is the most frequent cause of poisoning in the United States and results predominantly from house fires, vehicle exhaust (often with suicidal intent), and defective heating equipment. Hypoxia is due to the marked affinity of CO for hemoglobin (200 times that of oxygen) and impaired delivery of oxygen to the tissues. The cytochrome oxidase system of cellular respiration is also affected by CO. Symptoms are related to the amount of CO inspired and the duration of exposure, measured as the percent attached to hemoglobin. Symptoms range from headaches, nausea, and confusion at 10% to 25% COHb to cardiopulmonary arrest at levels of 60% or greater. The main therapeutic objective is to displace the CO from hemoglobin (and myoglobin) with high-flow oxygen. The half-life of COHb at room air is 5 to 6 hours, 1 hour with 100% oxygen, and less than 20 minutes with hyperbaric oxygen. Delivery at 3 atm for 46 minutes with repeat in 6 hours if symptoms persist has been found to be most effective.

**148. C**: Burns are defined by the thickness, partial for the epidermis, full for the dermis and deeper. Often it may take 48 hours or more after the injury to determine the correct level. In addition, the extent of the burn injury is very important for management and can be estimated by a variety of tables or charts. Perhaps the most well-known and simplest is the rule of nines, in which specific body areas are assigned percentages of the TBSA: 4.5% for anterior or posterior head; 18% for anterior or posterior thorax; 4.5% for anterior or posterior abdomen or for either upper extremity; and 9% for anterior or posterior leg. Scatter burns are given 1% of TBSA if they are hand size, including fingers of the examiner. Disposition of the patient is based on criteria formulated by the American Burn Association. This patient has a 27% burn area (9% for the leg, 18% for the anterior chest). An adult younger than 40 with 25% or more TBSA involvement should be transferred to a burn center if stable.

**149. A**: Clinical shock is caused by inadequate perfusion of tissues with resulting hypoxia. Tachycardia, tachypnea, poor peripheral circulation, and diminished urine output are clinical features as blood is shunted from the periphery to the three most vital organs: brain, heart, and lungs. The release of several hormones is increased in response. Epinephrine and norepinephrine are released by the adrenal gland and cause peripheral vasoconstriction, enhancing blood shifting to the critical organs and also stimulating the heart; cortisol is released by the adrenal glands, stimulating hepatic glucose production. Although the glucose level rises, there is also an increase in insulin resistance so that tissues may still be deprived of essential fuel. The increased conversion of renin from the kidney to angiotensin II and adrenal aldosterone enhance renal sodium reabsorption and restoration of fluid to the intravascular space. Decreased renal perfusion leads to increased ADH release from the posterior pituitary gland to maintain intravascular volume; consequently, urine output is diminished.

**150. B**: Most shock syndrome differentiation is based on categories: hypovolemic (blood loss, third spacing of intravascular fluid); septic (sepsis, usually with gram-negative bacteria that release endogenous pyrogens, provoking numerous cytokines and proinflammatory mediators causing vascular insufficiency); cardiogenic (impaired cardiac output, usually due to myocardial infarction); anaphylactic (excessive allergic reaction); and neurogenic (may be caused by brain injury or spinal cord injury). Excessive insulin may also produce a neurogenic shock by sharply causing hypoglycemia. The vasomotor center of the brain is depressed, diminishing sympathetic outflow that controls the vascular response. Unopposed parasympathetic discharge leads to peripheral vasodilation and impaired cardiac performance, resulting in shock.

**151. B**: In shock resuscitation, the patient response to corrective measures is probably the best index of effective therapy. A minimum MAP of 40 mm Hg is recommended by authorities in those patients who are actively bleeding. Too vigorous administration of intravenous fluids may result in dislodgement of clots, dilution of coagulation factors, venous dilation, and hypothermia. Once bleeding is controlled by surgical or nonsurgical means, higher pressures may be sought with blood and fluid administration. A higher MAP is advised for other shock states: 90 mm Hg for traumatic brain injury without hemorrhage, and greater than 65 mm Hg for most other forms of shock. Massive blood transfusion for shock patients may lead to complications such as coagulopathies, ARDS, or multiorgan failure. Vasopressors, such as dobutamine, dopamine, epinephrine, or norepinephrine, may be required to sustain blood pressure in many forms of shock.

**152. A**: While observation of the patient's heart and respiratory rates, mental status, and adequacy of peripheral circulation are clinical indicators of shock, several invasive and noninvasive methods for following effectiveness of treatment are available. Pulse oximetry is a simple and noninvasive technique to measure peripheral oxygen saturation but is subject to limitations in estimating circulation and hypoxia, especially with use of vasoactive medications or hypothermia. Central venous pressure is a useful measure of circulating volume, cardiac performance, and vascular tone. Values under the normal range of 4 to 10 cm $H_2O$ indicate a low circulating volume while values above this range may indicate excessive fluid administration, pulmonary edema, or vascular obstruction. $ScvO_2$ is measured from a catheter in the superior vena cava and a value of 70% is used to guide therapy even if clinical signs show improvement. Pulmonary artery catheters (e.g., Swan-Ganz) are not recommended for routine hemodynamic monitoring.

**153. C**: Acute management of bleeding is an extremely common task in the emergency department and often the emergency department nurse must initially address the problem. Some of the rules of tourniquet placement are: 1) do not place directly over the wound; direct pressure to the wound is preferable; 2) the tourniquet should be placed as distally as possible but 5 cm proximal to the bleeding site; 3) apply it directly to the exposed skin, not over clothing or a dressing; 4) do not apply over a joint; 5) do not apply over a foreign object; 6) release the tourniquet as soon as possible when bleeding is controlled; it may be left in place for up to 2 hours without excessive tissue damage.

**154. D**: Poor tissue perfusion and hypoxemia in shock states lead to anaerobic metabolism and increase in lactic acid and base deficit. This tissue acidosis stimulates the respiratory centers and is initially compensated by increased respiratory action, which tends to increase oxygenation and buffer the acidosis by diminishing $CO_2$ levels. Without treatment, the acidosis prevails and is the most common finding in shock patients. If the pH is very low (less than 7.1), sodium bicarbonate should be administered because lethal cardiac arrhythmias may occur; with pH values above this, treatment of the cause of the shock along with ventilation and oxygenation and fluid replacement should improve the acidosis. Persistent or very low pH levels indicate a high risk for complications such as multiorgan failure, ARDS, or DIC.

**155. A**: Frequently intensive care measures must be initiated in the emergency department because of lack of beds and other logistical or bureaucratic problems. The early goal-directed therapy (EGDT) study for septic patients with elevated lactate levels or refractory hypotension treated in the emergency department for 6 hours prior to ICU admission showed an increased survival over standard treatment (46.5% vs 30.5%). Fluid resuscitation remains a cornerstone of treatment in these patients but the debate of the superiority of colloids vs crystalloids remains unsettled. Many patients receive both (e.g., fresh frozen plasma and normal saline). Antibiotic therapy begun within 1 hour of diagnosis has also lessened mortality. Numerous antibiotic combinations may be satisfactory but adequate gram-negative coverage is essential. Maintaining the MAP at 65 mm Hg or greater and a $ScvO_2$ of at least 70% are two of the EGTD parameters. Administration of rhAPC to septic patients in whom protein C levels are low has shown some decrease in risk and mortality.

**156. D**: There are several different types of central venous access devices for fluid and electrolyte, blood product, or drug administration and withdrawal of blood samples. The tunneled catheter is surgically threaded into the subclavian vein and then into the superior vena cava or right atrium. The distal end of the catheter emerges below the clavicle with a Dacron cuff for stability. These require withdrawal of 10 mL of blood before aspirating a sample for the lab and a 5 mL flush before medication administration. A Groshong type catheter requires 5 mL saline flushes after use or once per week; no heparin needed. An implanted port requires a 500-unit heparin flush once a month if not in use and a 10 mL saline flush followed by heparin after blood withdrawal. The instructions in the question are most appropriate for a PICC.

**157. A**: Intraosseous infusion is a rapid alternative for intravenous administration, especially for infants and children whose veins are not easily accessible or in adults until more traditional venous access is obtained. An 18-gauge needle is used for infants and a 15-gauge needle for older children and adults. The sternum is quite thin in young children and insertion of the needle here is contraindicated; however, it may be used in adults. Preferable sites are the iliac crest, anterior tibia at the tibial tuberosity (best for children), external femoral condyle or medial malleolus. Needles should not be inserted through infected or burned tissue. Manual pressure or an infusion pump is often required if large volumes must be administered quickly. Alternative vascular access should be obtained within 4 hours.

**158. C**: This patient's history, presentation, and laboratory findings are fairly typical of hyperosmolar hyperglycemia. In contrast to DKA, patients with hyperosmolar hyperglycemia tend to be older, have type 2 diabetes, and often present with neurologic signs and symptoms. Usually the glucose level is above 800 mg/dL and the serum osmolality above 350 mOsm/L, but test for ketones is negative or only slightly positive and the pH is in the normal or only slightly low range. Type 2 diabetic patients have adequate insulin levels to keep them out of ketoacidosis but not enough to overcome the marked hyperglycemia due to increased insulin resistance and increased hepatic gluconeogenesis. Often this syndrome is triggered by stopping medication and exacerbated by osmotic diuresis or diuretics causing dehydration. Mortality may be as high as 60%. Lactic acidosis may be triggered by metformin but he has been off the drug for a while and levels above 4 to 5 mmol/L are usually seen with lactic acidosis.

**159. D**: This patient has extreme thyrotoxicosis, which usually is caused by underlying Grave disease with cessation of antithyroid medications. Presentation usually involves high fever, tremors, agitation, and delirium or coma. The disorder, often called thyroid storm, is life-threatening and has a 90% mortality rate if left untreated. Often a history is difficult because of the patient's condition but the clinical picture usually is enough to make the diagnosis. Beta-blockers are given to control adrenergic effects and reduce the ventricular rate. Anti-thyroid drugs such as propylthiouracil (PTU) or methimazole are given orally or by nasogastric tube to block further synthesis of thyroid hormone. The onset of action is in about 1 hour but full effect may take 3 to 6 weeks. Iodides may also be given to inhibit hormone release from the thyroid and block the conversion of T4 to T3, but these drugs should be given for at least 1 hour after the antithyroid medications. Epinephrine would not be indicated to treat this patient.

**160. C**: Blood coagulation is complex and consists of a series of reactions, sometimes called the coagulation cascade, that involve tissue and endothelial factors, plasma coagulation factors (proteins), and platelets. In addition, there is a fibrinolytic system that lyses clots. The vitamin K–dependent factors are II, VII, IX, and X (thrombokinase factor). The drug warfarin (*Coumadin*) has been used for many years to inhibit synthesis of these factors in the treatment and prevention of thromboembolic disease (deep vein thrombosis [DVT], pulmonary embolus, emboli from the heart, especially in patients with atrial fibrillation). Factor VIII is not vitamin K dependent and is the missing or dysfunctional factor in hemophilia A, usually a sex-linked inherited disorder but occasionally caused by mutation. Interestingly, factor IX is absent or defective in hemophilia B (less common than hemophilia A) and is vitamin K dependent. Vitamin K administration may reverse deficiency of the dependent factors (usually due to excessive warfarin) but is usually given only if there is significant bleeding.

**161. B**: Tumor lysis syndrome results from a large breakdown of tumor cells, usually after chemotherapy but occasionally spontaneously. It is most often seen in highly proliferative tumors. Breakdown of cells lead to marked potassium and phosphate release, leading to hyperkalemia and hyperphosphatemia. Hypocalcemia results from the binding of calcium to the phosphate. Elevated uric acid also occurs because of the breakdown of nucleic acids released from the cells. Fatigue, anorexia, muscle and abdominal cramps, dysrhythmias, flank pain, and renal failure may result. Treatment includes vigorous hydration and sodium bicarbonate to alkalinize the urine and protect against uric acid deposits in the kidney. Diuretics may also be used. Allopurinol is given to diminish the hyperuricemia; phosphate-binding agents to diminish the elevated phosphate. Hyperkalemia is treated with intravenous calcium gluconate or chloride, glucose and insulin and sodium bicarbonate to drive potassium into cells, as well as sodium polystyrene sulfonate (*Kayexalate*) to draw potassium into the gastrointestinal tract.

**162. D**: Sickle cell anemia is an autosomal disorder, found in about 1 out 500 African-Americans, in which red blood cells contain hemoglobin S instead of the normal hemoglobin A. These abnormal red cells have a shortened lifespan (10 to 20 days vs 120 for normal red cells) and a tendency to form a sickle shape, especially when provoked by hypoxia, dehydration, infection, high altitude, or exercise. The sickle cells are less deformable than normal and tend to occlude small blood vessels, causing tissue hypoxia, infarction, and necrosis. These are referred to as sickle crises and cause diffuse, often severe, pain, especially in bones and joints. An acute chest syndrome with dyspnea, pain, fever, and pulmonary infiltrates may also occur. Priapism in males may be caused by occlusion of the venous drainage of the penis. Aplastic crisis, a condition of bone marrow failure, may also occur. Gastrointestinal bleeding may occur because of aspirin or NSAID medication or stress ulceration but is not considered part of the basic disease.

**163. D**: This patient has fever and neutropenia after chemotherapy. Neutropenia is defined as an absolute neutrophil count (ANC) under 1000/mm$^3$, and a severe neutropenia less than 500/mm$^3$ is particularly dangerous. These patients must be worked up quickly and antibiotic and possibly additional therapy started as soon as possible since the situation may be life-threatening. While myelosuppressive drugs differ in the length of time between administration and the nadir of the ANC, 10 to 14 days is typical. Multiple cultures from different possible sites of origin for sepsis must be done along with chest x-ray and other imaging as indicated by examination. Broad-spectrum antibiotics, such as ceftazidime or imipenem/cilastatin, should be started after cultures are obtained. She should be asked if she has been receiving G-CSF (*Neupogen*, *Neulasta*). WBC transfusions are rarely used today since they have a very short shelf life, do not last long in the circulation, and may cause allergic reactions.

**164. A**: Intracranial pressure monitoring is indicated for traumatic brain injury with an abnormal CT of the brain or with 2 or more high-risk factors: age older than 40, posturing motor response, or systolic blood pressure less than 90. Under normal circumstances, the ICP is between 0 and 15 mm Hg. The brain can compensate to a point for additional volume but when brain compliance is exhausted the ICP rises sharply. Critical is the central perfusion pressure (CPP), which is the difference between the mean arterial pressure (MAP) and the ICP. CPP values below 50 mm Hg indicate hypoperfusion and brain ischemia. Intraventricular placement of a pressure transducer by catheter into the lateral ventricle gives the most accurate pressure readings and allows easy sampling of CSF, but is harder to place and there is a higher risk of infection than with the other devices.

**165. B**: Anthrax is a gram-positive bacterium that forms spores that may survive for long periods in soil. The disease may occur in 3 forms: 1) inhalation of spores, the least common but most deadly form; 2) cutaneous, the most common form that produces localized disease, often contracted directly from handling infected animal hides; and 3) gastrointestinal, acquired by eating the spores, usually from infected meat. Aerosolization of spores enhances their use as a biologic weapon. A flu-like syndrome followed by a short period of improvement, then a severe deterioration and death is a typical course of the inhalation type if left untreated. Mediastinitis and meningitis are complications of the inhaled form. Human to human transfer does not occur so that mass isolation is not required. Decontamination of areas of exposure is usually carried out. Antibiotics such as ciprofloxacin (*Cipro*) or doxycycline are effective but treatment should be carried out for 60 days.

**166. C**: Hypokalemia (potassium lower than 3.5 mEq/L) may result from gastrointestinal or renal loss, or from transfer from extracellular fluid to intracellular fluid. Drugs such as aldosterone, insulin, and beta2-agonists promote the latter. Gastrointestinal loss is the most likely cause in this patient and hypokalemia may be a feature of traveler's gastroenteritis. Renal loss occurs with diuretics or kidney disease and low potassium may be a feature of diabetic ketoacidosis or excess steroids. The ECG findings described are typical of low potassium but do not necessarily correlate with the degree. Potassium administration should be through a large bore or central venous catheter (it is locally irritating) by an infusion pump at 40 mEq/L not to exceed 10 to 20 mEq per hour. For severe hypokalemia, a 5 to 10 mEq bolus may be given but serial potassium and cardiac monitoring is required to avoid hyperkalemia, ventricular dysrhythmias, and death. Low serum magnesium levels may accompany hypokalemia and should be checked.

**167. B**: Measurement of pulse and blood pressure while the patient is supine for 3 minutes and then sitting and/or standing for 1 minute is a clinical method (orthostatic vital signs) to determine hypovolemia or impaired sympathetic discharge or venoconstriction in patients with syncope. Generally, lying to standing is more sensitive to orthostatic hypotension. Positive results consist of a rise in pulse rate of 30 beats per minute or blood pressure fall of 20 mm Hg on change of position. Development of dizziness or syncope on standing is also considered a positive sign. While the value of this test in predicting hypovolemia is far from perfect, it is simple to perform, and, if positive, may direct further laboratory or clinical investigation.

**168. D**: The clinical picture of this patient is that of an anaphylactic reaction to bee stings and is potentially life-threatening. The onset of symptoms within 1 hour after exposure to the allergen is particularly worrisome as are the laryngeal and pulmonary signs. The airway must be established with intubation often necessary; high-flow oxygen, cardiac monitoring, and intravenous fluids are basics. Epinephrine given intramuscularly is the most rapidly acting agent and should be given as soon as possible after the diagnosis of anaphylaxis and every 5 to 15 minutes thereafter as needed. Steroids and antihistamines are slower acting than epinephrine but are often given to alleviate itching, angioedema, and hives. IVF will be given as needed. There is no indication for antibiotics in this clinical situation unless further signs and symptoms develop.

**169. D**: Clotted vascular access devices for chronic renal failure patients undergoing dialysis are not uncommon emergency department cases. Vascular access for these patients may be carried out with a temporary external arteriovenous shunt, or permanent internal arteriovenous fistula or graft. The cephalic vein and radial artery of the forearm are the most often used. Clotting or infection of the access may occur. If a clot impedes smooth vascular flow, it must be lysed with fibrinolytic agents or removed surgically. A temporary dual lumen subclavian catheter may be inserted for 2 to 3 days. If local signs such as swelling, erythema, or tenderness suggest infection, the device is usually removed and cultures and antibiotics prescribed.

**170. B**: At one time, collection of vaginal semen from rape victims was limited to 48 hours after the crime but, because of increasingly sensitive DNA testing, many jurisdictions have increased this collection period up to 5 to 7 days. In addition, samples for DNA analysis can be collected from clothing and bed linens; the emergency nurse should collect and preserve such items. Potential evidence must be given to the police and appropriate signatures and times from all who handle the evidence must be obtained to preserve chain of custody. Evidence may be stored in a locked closet or cabinet with limited access.

**171. B**: Issues of informed consent constantly arise in the emergency department because many patients are incompetent to understand the situation; this may be due to mental illness, altered state of consciousness, or age (minors). Generally, minors require parental consent but exceptions are made for emancipated minors, serious or life-threatening emergencies, or, in some states, if the minor is mature enough to understand the treatment and possible consequences. Parents generally cannot withhold consent for lifesaving treatment on religious grounds. Usually, the emergency physician explains the nature and risks of treatment but the nurse should make sure that this is carried out and witness the patient's signature. Handing the patient an informed consent sheet without explanation may not be enough in many legal jurisdictions. In true emergency situations where the patient is unable to give consent, another authorized person such as a close relative may be satisfactory.

**172. D**: EMTALA was passed by Congress in 1986 as part of COBRA. Its intent was to prevent "patient dumping" and "economic triage" by hospitals participating in Medicare and receiving federal funds. It applies to all patients seeking emergency treatment whether they are Medicare patients or not. Triage refers to the order in which patients are seen by the physician, not whether or not they require medical examination. The patient must receive a medical screening exam before any disposition is made and the lack of insurance or out-of-plan HMO status is not a basis for transfer or discharge of the patient without medical examination. For unstable patients being transferred to another facility, the receiving hospital must accept the transfer and the emergency physician ordering the transfer must sign an approval note outlining the benefits and risks of the transfer. While a patient may refuse examination and treatment, simple verbal refusal may not be legally sufficient and every attempt should be made to obtain a written refusal, including a statement that the benefits and risks have been explained.

**173. C**: Injuries due to child neglect and/or physical abuse are extremely common in emergency departments. Often the differentiation of a true accident or disease from intentional harm is difficult and falls to the nurse to decide. While cuts and bruises are extremely common in children, multiple bruises, especially on the head, trunk, upper arms, and buttocks, should raise the possibility of abuse. Skeletal trauma suggestive of abuse includes multiple fractures at various stages of healing, posterior or lateral rib or multiple fractures in infants, presence of "grab" marks over a long bone fracture and spiral or oblique fractures. Purposely inflicted burns tend to be discrete and are not widely scattered as in true accidental scalding from spilling of hot liquids. The shaken baby syndrome (with or without direct head trauma) is suggested by multiple retinal hemorrhages. When parental account of the "accident" does not correlate with the physical findings (e.g., multiple fractures from a fall from the couch), or multiple visits for trauma occur, child abuse should be suspected.

**174. C**: Individual states have statutes concerning conditions and diseases that must be reported by the emergency department to local law enforcement (homicides, suicides, rapes, child or elder abuse) or to the coroner/medical examiner (unexpected death within 48 hours of admission or during surgery). Communicable diseases such as tuberculosis, HIV/AIDS, or unusual or resistant organisms are reportable to local health authorities and possibly the CDC. Unexpected drug reactions may be reported to the FDA. Since state requirements vary, the list of reportable conditions is kept in the emergency department for quick reference. The nurse shares responsibility for reporting with the physician and may act independently if the situation warrants. Social services may assume responsibility in certain cases.

**175. A**: New treatments and protocols are carried out on emergency patients quite frequently. Often the medical staff participates in multi-institutional trials with an established protocol and randomization of patients to the current standard treatment or the new treatment under investigation. Sometimes these studies are "double-blind," in which neither the treating physician nor the patient know which group the latter is in until the study is terminated and the "code broken." Results are often compared statistically to evaluate whether the results of a study are due to chance rather than intervention with the new treatment. The lower the *P* value, the less likely that the result is due to chance; most clinical researchers accept values less than 0.05 (5%) to indicate that the result is not due to chance. Experimental evidence may be ranked on a scale of I to VII, with I being the most reliable (usually from randomized, controlled studies) and VII being the least (clinical opinions, anecdotal reports). A confidence interval, another statistical method, refers to the degree of precision of the results (i.e., how confident the investigator is that the results are correct).

# Emergency Nurse Practice Tests #2 and #3

To take these additional Emergency Nurse practice tests, visit our bonus page:
**mometrix.com/bonus948/cen**

# How to Overcome Test Anxiety

Just the thought of taking a test is enough to make most people a little nervous. A test is an important event that can have a long-term impact on your future, so it's important to take it seriously and it's natural to feel anxious about performing well. But just because anxiety is normal, that doesn't mean that it's helpful in test taking, or that you should simply accept it as part of your life. Anxiety can have a variety of effects. These effects can be mild, like making you feel slightly nervous, or severe, like blocking your ability to focus or remember even a simple detail.

If you experience test anxiety—whether severe or mild—it's important to know how to beat it. To discover this, first you need to understand what causes test anxiety.

## Causes of Test Anxiety

While we often think of anxiety as an uncontrollable emotional state, it can actually be caused by simple, practical things. One of the most common causes of test anxiety is that a person does not feel adequately prepared for their test. This feeling can be the result of many different issues such as poor study habits or lack of organization, but the most common culprit is time management. Starting to study too late, failing to organize your study time to cover all of the material, or being distracted while you study will mean that you're not well prepared for the test. This may lead to cramming the night before, which will cause you to be physically and mentally exhausted for the test. Poor time management also contributes to feelings of stress, fear, and hopelessness as you realize you are not well prepared but don't know what to do about it.

Other times, test anxiety is not related to your preparation for the test but comes from unresolved fear. This may be a past failure on a test, or poor performance on tests in general. It may come from comparing yourself to others who seem to be performing better or from the stress of living up to expectations. Anxiety may be driven by fears of the future—how failure on this test would affect your educational and career goals. These fears are often completely irrational, but they can still negatively impact your test performance.

**Review Video: 3 Reasons You Have Test Anxiety**
Visit mometrix.com/academy and enter code: 428468

## Elements of Test Anxiety

As mentioned earlier, test anxiety is considered to be an emotional state, but it has physical and mental components as well. Sometimes you may not even realize that you are suffering from test anxiety until you notice the physical symptoms. These can include trembling hands, rapid heartbeat, sweating, nausea, and tense muscles. Extreme anxiety may lead to fainting or vomiting. Obviously, any of these symptoms can have a negative impact on testing. It is important to recognize them as soon as they begin to occur so that you can address the problem before it damages your performance.

**Review Video:** 3 Ways to Tell You Have Test Anxiety
Visit mometrix.com/academy and enter code: 927847

The mental components of test anxiety include trouble focusing and inability to remember learned information. During a test, your mind is on high alert, which can help you recall information and stay focused for an extended period of time. However, anxiety interferes with your mind's natural processes, causing you to blank out, even on the questions you know well. The strain of testing during anxiety makes it difficult to stay focused, especially on a test that may take several hours. Extreme anxiety can take a huge mental toll, making it difficult not only to recall test information but even to understand the test questions or pull your thoughts together.

**Review Video:** How Test Anxiety Affects Memory
Visit mometrix.com/academy and enter code: 609003

## Effects of Test Anxiety

Test anxiety is like a disease—if left untreated, it will get progressively worse. Anxiety leads to poor performance, and this reinforces the feelings of fear and failure, which in turn lead to poor performances on subsequent tests. It can grow from a mild nervousness to a crippling condition. If allowed to progress, test anxiety can have a big impact on your schooling, and consequently on your future.

Test anxiety can spread to other parts of your life. Anxiety on tests can become anxiety in any stressful situation, and blanking on a test can turn into panicking in a job situation. But fortunately, you don't have to let anxiety rule your testing and determine your grades. There are a number of relatively simple steps you can take to move past anxiety and function normally on a test and in the rest of life.

**Review Video:** How Test Anxiety Impacts Your Grades
Visit mometrix.com/academy and enter code: 939819

# Physical Steps for Beating Test Anxiety

While test anxiety is a serious problem, the good news is that it can be overcome. It doesn't have to control your ability to think and remember information. While it may take time, you can begin taking steps today to beat anxiety.

Just as your first hint that you may be struggling with anxiety comes from the physical symptoms, the first step to treating it is also physical. Rest is crucial for having a clear, strong mind. If you are tired, it is much easier to give in to anxiety. But if you establish good sleep habits, your body and mind will be ready to perform optimally, without the strain of exhaustion. Additionally, sleeping well helps you to retain information better, so you're more likely to recall the answers when you see the test questions.

Getting good sleep means more than going to bed on time. It's important to allow your brain time to relax. Take study breaks from time to time so it doesn't get overworked, and don't study right before bed. Take time to rest your mind before trying to rest your body, or you may find it difficult to fall asleep.

**Review Video: The Importance of Sleep for Your Brain**
Visit mometrix.com/academy and enter code: 319338

Along with sleep, other aspects of physical health are important in preparing for a test. Good nutrition is vital for good brain function. Sugary foods and drinks may give a burst of energy but this burst is followed by a crash, both physically and emotionally. Instead, fuel your body with protein and vitamin-rich foods.

Also, drink plenty of water. Dehydration can lead to headaches and exhaustion, especially if your brain is already under stress from the rigors of the test. Particularly if your test is a long one, drink water during the breaks. And if possible, take an energy-boosting snack to eat between sections.

**Review Video: How Diet Can Affect your Mood**
Visit mometrix.com/academy and enter code: 624317

Along with sleep and diet, a third important part of physical health is exercise. Maintaining a steady workout schedule is helpful, but even taking 5-minute study breaks to walk can help get your blood pumping faster and clear your head. Exercise also releases endorphins, which contribute to a positive feeling and can help combat test anxiety.

When you nurture your physical health, you are also contributing to your mental health. If your body is healthy, your mind is much more likely to be healthy as well. So take time to rest, nourish your body with healthy food and water, and get moving as much as possible. Taking these physical steps will make you stronger and more able to take the mental steps necessary to overcome test anxiety.

## Mental Steps for Beating Test Anxiety

Working on the mental side of test anxiety can be more challenging, but as with the physical side, there are clear steps you can take to overcome it. As mentioned earlier, test anxiety often stems from lack of preparation, so the obvious solution is to prepare for the test. Effective studying may be the most important weapon you have for beating test anxiety, but you can and should employ several other mental tools to combat fear.

First, boost your confidence by reminding yourself of past success—tests or projects that you aced. If you're putting as much effort into preparing for this test as you did for those, there's no reason you should expect to fail here. Work hard to prepare; then trust your preparation.

Second, surround yourself with encouraging people. It can be helpful to find a study group, but be sure that the people you're around will encourage a positive attitude. If you spend time with others who are anxious or cynical, this will only contribute to your own anxiety. Look for others who are motivated to study hard from a desire to succeed, not from a fear of failure.

Third, reward yourself. A test is physically and mentally tiring, even without anxiety, and it can be helpful to have something to look forward to. Plan an activity following the test, regardless of the outcome, such as going to a movie or getting ice cream.

When you are taking the test, if you find yourself beginning to feel anxious, remind yourself that you know the material. Visualize successfully completing the test. Then take a few deep, relaxing breaths and return to it. Work through the questions carefully but with confidence, knowing that you are capable of succeeding.

Developing a healthy mental approach to test taking will also aid in other areas of life. Test anxiety affects more than just the actual test—it can be damaging to your mental health and even contribute to depression. It's important to beat test anxiety before it becomes a problem for more than testing.

**Review Video: Test Anxiety and Depression**
Visit mometrix.com/academy and enter code: 904704

## Study Strategy

Being prepared for the test is necessary to combat anxiety, but what does being prepared look like? You may study for hours on end and still not feel prepared. What you need is a strategy for test prep. The next few pages outline our recommended steps to help you plan out and conquer the challenge of preparation.

### Step 1: Scope Out the Test

Learn everything you can about the format (multiple choice, essay, etc.) and what will be on the test. Gather any study materials, course outlines, or sample exams that may be available. Not only will this help you to prepare, but knowing what to expect can help to alleviate test anxiety.

### Step 2: Map Out the Material

Look through the textbook or study guide and make note of how many chapters or sections it has. Then divide these over the time you have. For example, if a book has 15 chapters and you have five days to study, you need to cover three chapters each day. Even better, if you have the time, leave an extra day at the end for overall review after you have gone through the material in depth.

If time is limited, you may need to prioritize the material. Look through it and make note of which sections you think you already have a good grasp on, and which need review. While you are studying, skim quickly through the familiar sections and take more time on the challenging parts. Write out your plan so you don't get lost as you go. Having a written plan also helps you feel more in control of the study, so anxiety is less likely to arise from feeling overwhelmed at the amount to cover.

### Step 3: Gather Your Tools

Decide what study method works best for you. Do you prefer to highlight in the book as you study and then go back over the highlighted portions? Or do you type out notes of the important information? Or is it helpful to make flashcards that you can carry with you? Assemble the pens, index cards, highlighters, post-it notes, and any other materials you may need so you won't be distracted by getting up to find things while you study.

If you're having a hard time retaining the information or organizing your notes, experiment with different methods. For example, try color-coding by subject with colored pens, highlighters, or post-it notes. If you learn better by hearing, try recording yourself reading your notes so you can listen while in the car, working out, or simply sitting at your desk. Ask a friend to quiz you from your flashcards, or try teaching someone the material to solidify it in your mind.

### Step 4: Create Your Environment

It's important to avoid distractions while you study. This includes both the obvious distractions like visitors and the subtle distractions like an uncomfortable chair (or a too-comfortable couch that makes you want to fall asleep). Set up the best study environment possible: good lighting and a comfortable work area. If background music helps you focus, you may want to turn it on, but otherwise keep the room quiet. If you are using a computer to take notes, be sure you don't have any other windows open, especially applications like social media, games, or anything else that could distract you. Silence your phone and turn off notifications. Be sure to keep water close by so you stay hydrated while you study (but avoid unhealthy drinks and snacks).

Also, take into account the best time of day to study. Are you freshest first thing in the morning? Try to set aside some time then to work through the material. Is your mind clearer in the afternoon or evening? Schedule your study session then. Another method is to study at the same time of day that you will take the test, so that your brain gets used to working on the material at that time and will be ready to focus at test time.

### Step 5: Study!

Once you have done all the study preparation, it's time to settle into the actual studying. Sit down, take a few moments to settle your mind so you can focus, and begin to follow your study plan. Don't give in to distractions or let yourself procrastinate. This is your time to prepare so you'll be ready to fearlessly approach the test. Make the most of the time and stay focused.

Of course, you don't want to burn out. If you study too long you may find that you're not retaining the information very well. Take regular study breaks. For example, taking five minutes out of every hour to walk briskly, breathing deeply and swinging your arms, can help your mind stay fresh.

As you get to the end of each chapter or section, it's a good idea to do a quick review. Remind yourself of what you learned and work on any difficult parts. When you feel that you've mastered the material, move on to the next part. At the end of your study session, briefly skim through your notes again.

But while review is helpful, cramming last minute is NOT. If at all possible, work ahead so that you won't need to fit all your study into the last day. Cramming overloads your brain with more information than it can process and retain, and your tired mind may struggle to recall even previously learned information when it is overwhelmed with last-minute study. Also, the urgent nature of cramming and the stress placed on your brain contribute to anxiety. You'll be more likely to go to the test feeling unprepared and having trouble thinking clearly.

So don't cram, and don't stay up late before the test, even just to review your notes at a leisurely pace. Your brain needs rest more than it needs to go over the information again. In fact, plan to finish your studies by noon or early afternoon the day before the test. Give your brain the rest of the day to relax or focus on other things, and get a good night's sleep. Then you will be fresh for the test and better able to recall what you've studied.

### Step 6: Take a Practice Test

Many courses offer sample tests, either online or in the study materials. This is an excellent resource to check whether you have mastered the material, as well as to prepare for the test format and environment.

Check the test format ahead of time: the number of questions, the type (multiple choice, free response, etc.), and the time limit. Then create a plan for working through them. For example, if you have 30 minutes to take a 60-question test, your limit is 30 seconds per question. Spend less time on the questions you know well so that you can take more time on the difficult ones.

If you have time to take several practice tests, take the first one open book, with no time limit. Work through the questions at your own pace and make sure you fully understand them. Gradually work up to taking a test under test conditions: sit at a desk with all study materials put away and set a timer. Pace yourself to make sure you finish the test with time to spare and go back to check your answers if you have time.

After each test, check your answers. On the questions you missed, be sure you understand why you missed them. Did you misread the question (tests can use tricky wording)? Did you forget the information? Or was it something you hadn't learned? Go back and study any shaky areas that the practice tests reveal.

Taking these tests not only helps with your grade, but also aids in combating test anxiety. If you're already used to the test conditions, you're less likely to worry about it, and working through tests until you're scoring well gives you a confidence boost. Go through the practice tests until you feel comfortable, and then you can go into the test knowing that you're ready for it.

## Test Tips

On test day, you should be confident, knowing that you've prepared well and are ready to answer the questions. But aside from preparation, there are several test day strategies you can employ to maximize your performance.

First, as stated before, get a good night's sleep the night before the test (and for several nights before that, if possible). Go into the test with a fresh, alert mind rather than staying up late to study.

Try not to change too much about your normal routine on the day of the test. It's important to eat a nutritious breakfast, but if you normally don't eat breakfast at all, consider eating just a protein bar. If you're a coffee drinker, go ahead and have your normal coffee. Just make sure you time it so that the caffeine doesn't wear off right in the middle of your test. Avoid sugary beverages, and drink enough water to stay hydrated but not so much that you need a restroom break 10 minutes into the test. If your test isn't first thing in the morning, consider going for a walk or doing a light workout before the test to get your blood flowing.

Allow yourself enough time to get ready, and leave for the test with plenty of time to spare so you won't have the anxiety of scrambling to arrive in time. Another reason to be early is to select a good seat. It's helpful to sit away from doors and windows, which can be distracting. Find a good seat, get out your supplies, and settle your mind before the test begins.

When the test begins, start by going over the instructions carefully, even if you already know what to expect. Make sure you avoid any careless mistakes by following the directions.

Then begin working through the questions, pacing yourself as you've practiced. If you're not sure on an answer, don't spend too much time on it, and don't let it shake your confidence. Either skip it and come back later, or eliminate as many wrong answers as possible and guess among the remaining ones. Don't dwell on these questions as you continue—put them out of your mind and focus on what lies ahead.

Be sure to read all of the answer choices, even if you're sure the first one is the right answer. Sometimes you'll find a better one if you keep reading. But don't second-guess yourself if you do immediately know the answer. Your gut instinct is usually right. Don't let test anxiety rob you of the information you know.

If you have time at the end of the test (and if the test format allows), go back and review your answers. Be cautious about changing any, since your first instinct tends to be correct, but make sure you didn't misread any of the questions or accidentally mark the wrong answer choice. Look over any you skipped and make an educated guess.

At the end, leave the test feeling confident. You've done your best, so don't waste time worrying about your performance or wishing you could change anything. Instead, celebrate the successful completion of this test. And finally, use this test to learn how to deal with anxiety even better next time.

**Review Video: 5 Tips to Beat Test Anxiety**
Visit mometrix.com/academy and enter code: 570656

## Important Qualification

Not all anxiety is created equal. If your test anxiety is causing major issues in your life beyond the classroom or testing center, or if you are experiencing troubling physical symptoms related to your anxiety, it may be a sign of a serious physiological or psychological condition. If this sounds like your situation, we strongly encourage you to seek professional help.

# Thank You

We at Mometrix would like to extend our heartfelt thanks to you, our friend and patron, for allowing us to play a part in your journey. It is a privilege to serve people from all walks of life who are unified in their commitment to building the best future they can for themselves.

The preparation you devote to these important testing milestones may be the most valuable educational opportunity you have for making a real difference in your life. We encourage you to put your heart into it—that feeling of succeeding, overcoming, and yes, conquering will be well worth the hours you've invested.

We want to hear your story, your struggles and your successes, and if you see any opportunities for us to improve our materials so we can help others even more effectively in the future, please share that with us as well. **The team at Mometrix would be absolutely thrilled to hear from you!** So please, send us an email (support@mometrix.com) and let's stay in touch.

**If you'd like some additional help, check out these other resources we offer for your exam: http://mometrixflashcards.com/CEN**

# Additional Bonus Material

Due to our efforts to try to keep this book to a manageable length, we've created a link that will give you access to all of your additional bonus material:

**mometrix.com/bonus948/cen**

Made in United States
Troutdale, OR
11/05/2023

14319877R00259